genetic. amniorentesis

Pg

HIGH-RISK PREGNANCY
AND DELIVERY

■ ■ ■

HIGH-RISK PREGNANCY AND DELIVERY

Fernando Arias, M.D., Ph.D.

Director,
Obstetrical Services,
St. John's Mercy Medical Center,
St. Louis, Missouri

with 47 illustrations

The C. V. Mosby Company

ST. LOUIS • TORONTO • PRINCETON   1984

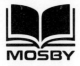

MOSBY

A TRADITION OF PUBLISHING EXCELLENCE

Editor: Carol Trumbold
Editorial assistant: Ginny Wharton
Manuscript editor: Selena V. Bussen
Book design: Jeanne E. Bush
Cover design: Suzanne Oberholtzer
Production: Teresa Breckwoldt, Carol O'Leary

Printed in the United States of America

The C.V. Mosby Company
11830 Westline Industrial Drive, St. Louis, Missouri 63146

Library of Congress Cataloging in Publication Data

Arias, Fernando, 1934-
    High-risk pregnancy and delivery.

    Bibliography: p.
    Includes index.
    1. Pregnancy, Complications of. 2. Labor, Complicated.
I. Title.
RG571.A75 1984   618.3   83-26863
ISBN 0-8016-0299-8

GW/MV/MV 9 8 7 6 5 4 3 2 1   01/D/044

CONTRIBUTORS

William L. Holcomb Jr., M.D.

Clinical Instructor,
Department of Obstetrics and Gynecology,
Washington University School of Medicine,
St. Louis, Missouri

Mark M. Jacobs, M.D.

Assistant Professor of Obstetrics and Gynecology,
Duke University,
Durham, North Carolina

Douglas C. Johnson, M.D.

Former Resident in Obstetrics and Gynecology,
Washington University School of Medicine,
Iowa City, Iowa

Alfred B. Knight, M.D.

Assistant Professor of Obstetrics and Gynecology,
Washington University School of Medicine,
St. Louis, Missouri

Denise M. Main, M.D.

Fellow in Maternal-Fetal Medicine,
Department of Obstetrics and Gynecology,
University of Pennsylvania,
School of Medicine,
Philadelphia, Pennsylvania

Elliott K. Main, M.D.

Fellow in Maternal-Fetal Medicine,
Department of Obstetrics and Gynecology,
University of Pennsylvania School of Medicine,
Philadelphia, Pennsylvania

D. Michael Nelson, M.D., Ph.D.

Assistant Professor,
Department of Obstetrics and Gynecology,
Washington University School of Medicine,
St. Louis, Missouri

Obi C. Okehi, M.D.

Former Resident in Obstetrics and Gynecology,
Washington University School of Medicine,
Macon, Georgia

William J. Ott, M.D.

Associate Professor,
Department of Obstetrics and Gynecology,
St. Louis University School of Medicine,
St. Louis, Missouri

Carlton S. Pearse, M.D.

Clinical Instructor,
Department of Obstetrics and Gynecology,
Washington University School of Medicine,
St. Louis, Missouri

Edward G. Peskin, M.D.

Clinical Instructor,
Department of Obstetrics and Gynecology,
Washington University School of Medicine,
St. Louis, Missouri

TO

my family and the memory of
my father

PREFACE

The purpose of this book is to provide residents in obstetrics and gynecology, practicing obstetricians, and interested medical students and nurses with a source of practical information about perinatal problems and their management. I wanted to emphasize therapy and give the reader protocols for the management of patients with complications of pregnancy. At the same time I wanted to provide enough information so that the rationale behind the proposed management plans could be understood. I hope that these goals have been attained.

The book is not all inclusive, and several pregnancy complications are described briefly or not at all. This is because I wanted to focus on those perinatal problems that the resident in training and the practicing obstetrician see with relatively high frequency. It is possible that other areas will be considered in future editions of this book.

Many drugs currently used in the management of pregnancy complications are not approved by the Federal Drug Administration for these indications. This should not be a limiting factor. Once a drug has been approved for marketing by the FDA and provided that it is not contraindicated during pregnancy, it may be used in the treatment of conditions that are not included in the approved labeling. This is accepted medical practice according to the Board of Trustees of the American Society of Internal Medicine, and a statement to this effect appears in the 1983 edition of the *Physicians' Desk Reference* (PDR). I have made an effort to ensure that the doses and schedules recommended in this book are in agreement with current practice. However, the reader should keep informed about changes in indications, contraindications, and doses that develop as experience accumulates.

All of the contributors to this book are my former residents or fellows when I worked at Washington University–Barnes Hospital Medical Center. I am grateful to all of them for helping me, despite the severe time constraints of their highly demanding training programs.

Since English is my second language, I needed help to correct frequent errors in grammar and composition. Helen M. Redfern filled that role and did the style editing for which I am grateful. Gratitude also goes to Pam Alvarado, Judy Kohorst, and Robyn Fischer who worked tirelessly with the word processor, trying to cope with my frequent corrections of the manuscript. I am also grateful to Carol Trumbold and Selena Bussen from the C.V. Mosby Company for making the publishing of this book so pleasurable.

This book is dedicated to my family; without their understanding and support this project most probably would be unfinished.

Fernando Arias

CONTENTS

HIGH-RISK PREGNANCY
AND DELIVERY

1

■ ■ ■

ROUTINE PRENATAL CARE AND IDENTIFICATION OF THE HIGH-RISK PATIENT

William J. Ott

One of the goals of every obstetrician is to give the best possible prenatal care. To achieve that goal the obstetrician has to know (1) how to provide routine prenatal care, (2) how to identify high-risk patients, and (3) what tests are available for fetal surveillance of these patients. This first chapter covers these three areas.

■ ROUTINE PRENATAL CARE

Ideally, prenatal care should begin long before the patient becomes pregnant. All patients of reproductive age should be encouraged to visit an obstetrician before pregnancy. Certainly those patients who are at risk because of potential obstetric or medical complications should see an obstetrician to ascertain the advisability of whether or not to attempt pregnancy. In certain situations (eg, history of genetic disease) the patient may choose not to have children at all or may decide on adoption. Despite the ideal situation, the majority of patients are seen for the first time during the concurrent pregnancy.

Good prenatal care begins with the first prenatal visit when the obstetrician looks for high-risk factors. At this time the patient's past medical records should be requested, and a careful history should be obtained.

Genetic screening

In addition to the standard obstetric and medical questions asked at the initial visit, the patient should be asked about the presence of genetic disease in herself, her husband, and both families, and if there is any indication, genetic counseling must be offered. The box on p. 2 is a questionnaire used at the Department of Obstetrics and Gynecology at Washington University in St. Louis to aid the obstetrician in genetic screening during the first prenatal visit. A more detailed treatment of this subject is found in Chapter 2.

Determining gestational age

Accurate knowledge of gestational age is the keystone in the ability of obstetricians to successfully manage the antepartum care of their patients, and it is necessary for the planning of appropriate therapy and the interpretation of tests. A number of methods can be used to determine an accurate estimated date of confinement (EDC) and an accurate gestational age.

Dating by last menstrual period. The first method of gestational dating makes use of the patient's last menstrual period (LMP). If the physician finds out that the patient's LMP was

1

2 *High-risk pregnancy and delivery*

Genetic disease screening questionnaire

1. Are you pregnant at the present time?   No _____   Yes _____
   If not, are you planning a future pregnancy?   No _____   Yes _____
2. Is your present age between 35 and 50 years   No _____   Yes _____
   old?
3. Have you ever had a child born with a birth   No _____   Yes _____
   defect or genetic disease?
      If yes, give details: _____
      _____
      _____

4. Have you had one or more miscarriages?   No _____   Yes _____
5. Have any members of you or your husband's family ever been affected with any of the following problems? (If yes, please indicate
   the affected individual's relationship to you.)

Problem	No	Yes	Relationship
Muscular dystrophy	_____	_____	_____
Hemophilia	_____	_____	_____
Spina bifida (open spine) or meningomyelocele	_____	_____	_____
Anencephaly	_____	_____	_____
Down's syndrome (mongolism)	_____	_____	_____

   Other birth defects (specify) _____
   _____
   _____

6. Please indicate below any other diseases or problems in your or your husband's family that
   you feel may be hereditary:
   _____
   _____
   _____

7. Do you wish to discuss the significance of this information with a genetic counselor?
   No _____ Yes _____ Signature: _____

---

normal, her menstrual cycles are regular, and she has not used oral contraceptives within 2 months of her LMP, Nägele's rule (first day of the LMP, plus 7 days, minus 3 months, equals EDC) can be used for the estimation of the patient's EDC and for calculating the gestational age. This information must be asked at the patient's first visit. Unfortunately, from 10% to 40% of the patients seen in prenatal clinics have either no knowledge of their LMP, or they have a history of irregular menstrual cycles, thus precluding the use of the LMP for accurate gestational dating. Even 10% to 20% of low-risk patients belonging to upper socioeconomic groups have either irregular cycles or unknown LMPs.

The accuracy of the LMP in calculating the EDC has been determined in several studies. Table 1-1 lists the distribution by number and percent of infants of singleton pregnancies delivered at each week of gestational age. In this analysis, taken from a 50% sample of live births from 36 states and the District of Columbia,[36] 58% of the patients delivered between 39 and 42 weeks. Andersen et al[1] studied 418 patients with known LMPs who delivered singleton infants with birth weights greater than 3000 grams and found that 90% delivered within 23 days of the EDC calculated from their LMP. The mean length of gestation was 284 ± 14.6 days (SD). Another study reported that 50% of 7505 patients with known LMPs delivered within 7 days of their calculated EDC.[43]

TABLE 1-1 ■ Distribution of singleton births by gestational age calculated from last menstrual period

Weeks of gestation	Number	%		
<36	57,652	6.2		
36	28,379	3.1		
37	50,335	5.4		
38	103,326	11.1		
39	183,455	19.8		
40	214,076	23.0	58.7%*	77.8%†
41	147,422	15.9		
42	74,120	8.0		
43	33,595	3.6		
44	16,493	1.8		
>44	20,216	2.2		

From Hoffman HJ, et al: Obstet Gynecol Surv 1974; 29:651.
*Delivered 39 through 41 weeks of gestation.
†Delivered 38 through 42 weeks of gestation.

Dating by physical examination. Another method for determining gestational age is by physical examination. The two most important physical findings for estimation of gestational age are (1) the correlation between uterine size and the patient's estimated gestational age and (2) the date when fetal heart tones are first audible by standard nonelectronic stethoscope.

An early pelvic examination can be an extremely important physical sign for accurate gestational dating. During the first trimester there is a good correlation between uterine size and gestational dating. At 10 weeks of gestation the top of the uterine fundus should be palpable at the level of the symphysis pubis. At 15 weeks the uterine fundal height should be midway between the symphysis pubis and the umbilicus.

Fetal heart tones are usually heard with a standard fetoscope between 18 and 20 weeks of gestation, depending on the thickness of the patient's abdominal wall. If a patient has had 20 weeks of audible fetal heart tones with a standard stethoscope, it is extremely unlikely that the gestational age is less than 38 weeks.

Dating by pregnancy test. There are several readily available commercial kits for the qualitative measurement of urinary chorionic gonadotropin (HCG) in the physician's office or clinic. Most of these rapid tests use the principle of hemagglutination, using antibodies to HCG that are mixed with the patient's urine. The sensitivity of these tests ranges from about 0.5 to 9.0 IU/ml.[26] A positive pregnancy test means that the patient is at least at 5 to 6 weeks of gestation, and if this information agrees with the duration of pregnancy as calculated from the LMP, the dates are firmly established. Also valuable is the information provided by a negative pregnancy test (less than 5 weeks of gestation) followed by a positive test (6 or more weeks of gestation).

Using sensitive radioreceptor assay techniques, some investigators[45] have been able to detect 0.12 to 0.50 IU/ml HCG as early as 5 to 7 days following conception. Newer radioimmunoassays for the beta chain of the HCG molecule can detect as little as 0.003 IU/ml. However, because of their extreme sensitivity, these new assays can actually make gestational dating more difficult. Table 1-2 lists the sensitivity and specificity of various commercially available pregnancy tests.

By using these tests together with the LMP, the patient's dates can be classified into one of three categories.

1. Poor dates: Patients with an unknown LMP or with a history of irregular menstrual cycles, those who have used oral contraceptives within 2 months of their LMP, or those who have an early pelvic examination that shows a uterine size inconsistent with the LMP.

2. Good dates: Patients with a known LMP, a history of 28- to 31-day cycles, and no recent use of oral contraceptives but without any other corroborative information (early pelvic examination, pregnancy test, ultrasound) about their dates.

3. Excellent dates: Same as good dates plus some corroborative information such as a positive HCG at 5 to 6 weeks of amenorrhea, nonelectronically auscultated fetal heart tones by the twentieth week of gestation, or an ultrasound measurement of the biparietal diameter (BPD) before 30 weeks in agreement with the dates.

A number of investigators have reviewed the accuracy of historical and clinical criteria for the evaluation of gestational age. Andersen et al.[1,2] found that the LMP when known and normal was the most accurate single method of determining gestational age. In order of accuracy the LMP was followed by uterine height, first au-

TABLE 1-2 ■ Sensitivity and predictive value of commercially available pregnancy tests

Test	Assay time (minutes)	Sensitivity (IU/ml HCG)	False positive (%)	False negative (%)
Gravindex	1.5	3.5	4.9	2.8
Pregnosis	2.5	1.5-2.5	1.0	7.5
Pregnosticon	2.0	1.0-2.0	1.0	10.3
UCG-slide	2.0	0.5	4.9	1.9
UCG-Beta slide	2.0	0.5		

From Duenhoelter JH: Contemp Obstet Gynecol 1982, 19:239.

dible heart tones, and fetal quickening (when the patient first feels fetal movement) the least accurate of all. The duration of pregnancy from the day each of these clinical signs is detected is shown below*

Clinical sign	Duration of pregnancy (days, ± SD)
First day of LMP	284.2 ± 14.6
Uterus at umbilicus	140.8 ± 14.9
Fetal heart first heard with aural fetoscope	136.2 ± 17.0
Quickening	156.3 ± 18.0

In summary, the obstetrician should carefully review the patient's LMP, check for the use of oral contraceptives within 2 months before the LMP, do an early pregnancy test, perform an early pelvic examination to evaluate uterine size, and carefully listen for fetal heart tones with an aural stethoscope at 20 weeks. When these variables are in agreement, dating of the pregnancy should be considered extremely accurate.

Dating by ultrasound. In many instances it is difficult if not impossible to obtain an accurate estimation of gestational age by clinical means. In these situations, ultrasound examination of the fetus can be extremely helpful. Ultrasound provides various fetal measurements of which BPD is the most common. The fetal BPD grows at a rate of 3.0 mm/week from 16 to 30 weeks, slows to 1.3 mm/week from 30 to 34 weeks, and is down to 1.0 mm/week after 34 weeks of gestation. Fig. 1-1 shows the growth of the fetal BPD from 15 through 40 weeks of gestation.[19] For reliable dating, an ultrasound examination should be obtained before 30 weeks of gestation.

There are two basic methods for determining

*From Anderson HF, et al: Am J Obstet Gynecol 1981; 139:173.

gestational age from the BPD measurements. One method,[58] the growth-adjusted sonographic age (GASA), uses two BPD measurements and adjusts the EDC depending on whether the fetus is small (less than the 25th percentile), average (25th to 75th percentile), or large (greater than the 75th percentile). In the second method,[42] the mean projected gestational age (MPGA), the EDC is projected after adjusting two BPD measurements to the best fit with the mean BPD value in a BPD–gestational age curve. Table 1-3 compares the accuracy in calculating the EDC using MPGA, GASA, and excellent clinical dates. The authors found no statistical difference in accuracy between the three methods and concluded that use of either GASA or MPGA gives a gestational date that is as accurate as that calculated for a patient with excellent dates. A number of investigators have found that serial ultrasound measurements of the BPD are as accurate as good clinical dating in estimating gestational age.[2,19,44] Others[42] have also found that a single BPD measurement at 16 to 24 weeks is as good in predicting the EDC as two measurements 4 weeks apart.

In addition to BPD, crown-rump (CR) length, gestational sac size, and measurements of the fetal femur length can also be used to estimate gestational age (Table 1-4). Robinson and Fleming[57] studied the use of ultrasonically measured CR length in the first trimester for calculation of the EDC and found an error of ±2 days in 95% of the patients. Other investigators in similar studies have found identical small errors between the EDC calculated from CR length and the actual delivery date.

Evaluation of the size of the gestational sac during the first trimester can also be used for gestational dating. The gestational sac can be seen at 5 to 6 weeks of gestation; it has a mean

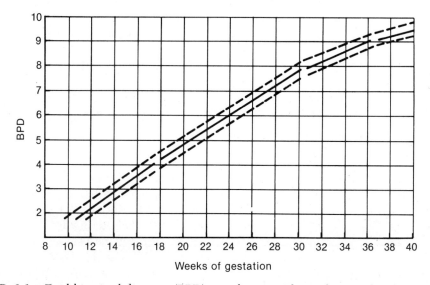

FIG. 1-1 ■ Fetal biparietal diameter (BPD) growth curve. This is the growth curve used at the ultrasound laboratory, Department of Obstetrics and Gynecology, Washington University School of Medicine. The curve was constructed using 213 successive BPD measurements in 83 women with excellent dates who delivered adequate for gestational age (AGA) babies within 1 week of their expected date of confinement. The solid line represents the mean BPD value for a given gestational age, and the upper and lower lines correspond to 2 SDs from the mean.

TABLE 1-3 ■ Interval between predicted EDC and actual delivery date by three methods

Method of predicting EDC*	Number of patients	Difference between EDC and actual delivery date			
		± 7 days	± 10 days	± 14 days	>14 days
MPGA†	60	38(63%)	48(80%)	54(90%)	6(10%)
GASA‡	60	34(56%)	41(68%)	51(85%)	9(15%)
Excellent clinical dates	60	31(51%)	38(63%)	47(78%)	13(22%)

From Kopta MM, Tomich PG, Crane JP: Obstet Gynecol 1981;57:657. Reprinted with permission from The American College of Obstetricians and Gynecologists.
*EDC, Estimated date of confinement.
†MPGA, Mean projected gestational age.
‡GASA, Growth adjusted sonographic age.

diameter of 10 mm at 6 weeks, 30 mm at 8 weeks, and 50 mm at 10 weeks of gestation.[34]

Another ultrasonic method of determining gestational age is through measurements of the femur length.[37,50] This method is especially valuable in situations in which the fetal head size is altered by a pathologic process (eg, microcephaly, hydrocephaly). Table 1-4 shows the correlation between gestational age and CR length, femur length, and BPD.

Controversy currently exists as to the efficiency and cost-effectiveness of routine ultrasound screening of all obstetric patients. Routine screening has been advocated by many investigators and is widely used in Scandinavia and the United Kingdom. British authors[3] report that of 300 patients who received routine real-time scans at a prenatal clinic in Bristol, England, almost 40% fitted into the "poor dates" category, and an additional 17% had subsequent problems during their pregnancy. Since both groups would have needed ultrasound examination anyway, they concluded that routine real-time examination was highly advantageous for good prenatal care. A report of a routine ultrasound screening program in Sweden[31] listed the

TABLE 1-4 ■ Correlation between gestational age, CR length, femur length, and BPD

Weeks of gestation	CR length (mm)	Femur length (mm)	BPD (mm)
6.5	6.1		
7.0	8.9		
7.5	11.2		
8.0	14.7		
8.5	17.6		
9.0	21.9		
9.5	25.4		
10.0	30.5		
10.5	34.6		
11.0	40.4		
11.5	45.1		
12.0	51.7		
12.5	57.0		
13.0	64.3		
13.5	70.2		
14.0	78.3	16.6	28
15.0		19.9	32
16.0		22.0	36
17.0		25.2	39
18.0		29.6	42
19.0		32.4	45
20.0		34.8	48
21.0		37.5	51
22.0		40.9	54
23.0		43.5	58
24.0		46.4	61
25.0		48.0	63
26.0		51.1	67
27.0		53.0	70
28.0		54.4	72
29.0		57.3	75
30.0		58.7	78
31.0		61.5	80
32.0		62.8	82
33.0		64.9	85
34.0		65.7	87
35.0		67.7	88
36.0		69.5	90
37.0		70.8	92
38.0		71.8	93
39.0		74.2	94
40.0		75.4	95

following advantages: (1) early identification of multiple pregnancy that resulted in a decrease of preterm delivery of twins from 33% to 10% and a concomitant tenfold decrease in perinatal mortality (from 6% to 0.6%), (2) a better estimation of gestational age, and (3) a 50% reduction in the number of x-ray examinations of pregnant women. A study from Australia found similar benefits from routine prenatal ultrasound examination.[14]

Acceptance of routine ultrasound screening in the United States has been somewhat slower than in Europe primarily because of the uncertainty of the long-term effects of ultrasound exposure to the fetus. There are few long-term follow-up studies of infants exposed to ultrasound in utero, but those that have been done have failed to show any adverse effects.[59] However, because of the theoretical possibility of intrauterine growth retardation, chromosomal damage, or other effects on the fetus, most perinatologists suggest limiting ultrasound examination to situations in which there is a reasonable indication for performing the test.

Other laboratory tests

After the initial examination and following a discussion with the patient about possible problems that may occur during pregnancy, the physician should obtain basic laboratory studies.

Hemoglobin/hematocrit tests. Hemoglobin and hematocrit are the first and in many cases the only tests necessary to evaluate the presence of anemia, a common problem encountered during pregnancy. It is important to recognize that maternal blood volume increases 30% to 60% during pregnancy,[54] and since plasma volume expands to a greater degree than red cell mass, there is a normal dilutional anemia during pregnancy. True anemia during pregnancy can be defined as a hemoglobin concentration less than 10.0 g/100 ml or a hematocrit value less than 30%. If the patient is identified as anemic, further evaluation is mandatory (see Chapter 12).

Serologic tests for infectious diseases. Since a number of infectious diseases can cause problems during gestation, it is mandatory for the obstetrician to obtain certain serologic tests. Infection may play a greater role than previously realized in perinatal mortality, as suggested by the work of Christensen[15] who found that 21% of the perinatal deaths she analyzed were directly related to infection.

Perinatal infectious agents

VIRAL

Predominantly causing malformations
  Cytomegalovirus (CMV)
  Rubella
  Varicella
  Coxsackie B virus
Predominantly causing fetal disease
  Herpes simplex
  Rubeola
  Variola (smallpox)
  Hepatitis B
  Vaccina

BACTERIAL

  Gonorrhea
  Streptococcus B
  Syphilis

PROTOZOAL

  Toxoplasmosis
  Mycoplasma
  Listeria
  Chlamydia

Screening for rubella, a significant cause of birth defects, should be routinely undertaken, since 10% to 20% of the pregnant population is at risk.[55] A serologic test for syphilis is also mandatory. Because of the increasing incidence of genital herpes infections, which can have a profound effect on the fetus, evaluation of the patient for a history of herpes should be done.[10] If either the history or the physical examination is suggestive of herpetic infection, serial cultures should be obtained.

Patients at risk for any of the viral, bacterial, or protozoal infections that adversely affect the fetus (see box above) should have appropriate cultures and serologic tests performed (see Chapter 11).

Tests for identification of blood type, Rh factor, and presence of abnormal antibodies. Routine blood testing is mandatory for investigating the possibility of Rh isoimmunization, which is the most common and usually the most severe cause of fetal erythroblastosis. Other isoantibodies can also cause significant problems, and any patient with antibodies against Kell, Duffy, or certain other antigens must have special evalu-

ation, including a consultation with a perinatologist for proper management. For more on this subject see Chapter 5.

Subsequent prenatal visits

The frequency of return visits depends on the obstetric and medical complications that may develop during pregnancy. For low-risk patients visits are usually scheduled at monthly intervals until approximately 30 weeks of gestation; the patient is then seen at biweekly intervals until 36 weeks of gestation and weekly thereafter. As previously mentioned, near 20 weeks of gestation the physician (using a standard aural stethoscope) should carefully check for audible heart tones to confirm gestational dating.

On each visit the physician should check the following:

1. Blood pressure
2. Maternal weight
3. Uterine height, measured from the symphysis pubis to the top of the fundus
4. Urine, to detect the presence of glucose and protein

The physician should question the patient about any complications that may have occurred since the previous visit, specifically the presence of vaginal bleeding, contractions, edema, headache, and leakage of fluid from the vagina.

For low-risk obstetric patients, hemoglobin and hematocrit tests should be repeated at approximately 30 to 32 weeks of gestation. There should be a slight decrease in the hemoglobin and hematocrit levels as pregnancy advances because of expanding blood volume.[54] Lack of this drop in hemoglobin and hematocrit levels may indicate development of hemoconcentration and a potential for pregnancy-induced hypertension.

Patients should also be screened for diabetes by measuring the fasting blood sugar and the blood sugar concentration 1 hour after ingesting 50 grams of glucose. This can be done in an office setting with a dextrometer, or blood samples can be sent out to a clinical laboratory. A level of greater than 90 mg/dl with fasting, greater than 140 mg/dl 1 hour after ingesting 50 grams of glucose, or other risk factors such as a glucosuria or a strong family history of diabetes indicate the need for a formal glucose tolerance test (see Chapter 7).

After 36 weeks of pregnancy the patient should have a pelvic examination on each visit to evaluate the position, consistency, and dilation of the cervix and the station of the presenting part. Pelvic examinations should also be performed earlier than 36 weeks on any patient with a suggestion of preterm labor. Following is an outline of routine antepartum care for the low-risk obstetric patient. This outline should be considered only as a guideline for patient care.

I. Initial visit
   A. Complete history and physical examination
      1. Securing of all past medical records
      2. Filling out of high-risk evaluation form (see box on p. 12)
      3. Screening for genetic disease (see box on p. 12)
   B. Initial laboratory tests
      1. Hemoglobin/hematocrit
      2. Blood type, Rh, and antibody screening
      3. Urinalysis
      4. VDRL
      5. Pap smear and gonococcus culture
      6. Ultrasound if indicated
         a. Uncertain dates
         b. Bleeding
         c. Uterine size larger or smaller than dates
         d. High-risk factors
      7. Blood sugar fasting and 1 hour after ingestion of 50 grams of glucose; glucose tolerance test if indicated
      8. Rubella HI titer
II. Schedule for repeated visits
      1. Every 4 weeks until 28 weeks
      2. Every 2 weeks until 36 weeks
      3. Weekly thereafter
III. Schedule for repeated laboratory tests
   A. Hemoglobin/hematocrit at 30 to 32 weeks
   B. Urinalysis (dip stick) at each visit
   C. Antibody screening at 24 and 28 weeks and antepartum anti-D immune globulin administration at 28 weeks if the patient is Rh negative

Many physicians have real-time ultrasound equipment in their private offices and are using it on all their pregnant patients. This seems unnecessary, but if it is done, it is important to remember that in *normal* obstetric patients two ultrasound examinations suffice—the first between 18 and 24 weeks and the second between 34 and 36 weeks. The first is to confirm the dating, to rule out multiple gestation, to screen for major congenital anomalies, and to localize the placenta; the second is to rule out intrauterine growth retardation or acceleration.

Nutrition during pregnancy

During pregnancy the nutritional needs of the fetus are met by two mechanisms. (1) In the preimplantation phase the blastocyst absorbs nutrients from the maternal fluids present in the reproductive tract. (2) From implantation until full placental development nutrition is obtained directly from maternal blood.

In the fetal lamb most of the fuel requirements are met by catabolism of glucose, lactate, and amino acids supplied by the placenta. This also appears to be true in the human fetus.[7] Under normal circumstances the physiologic changes induced by pregnancy in the maternal organism assure an adequate and steady supply of nutrients for the fetus.

Weight before pregnancy and maternal weight gain during pregnancy are the two strongest variables (excluding gestational age) related to fetal weight, which, in turn is directly related to neonatal outcome.[39,48] Two recent studies[12,27] that evaluated the pregnancy outcome of underweight mothers found a higher incidence of low birth weight infants and low Apgar scores than with patients in control groups. Both studies also showed that even if underweight women gain adequate weight during pregnancy, they are still at risk for a poor perinatal outcome. Baird[5] did an extensive review of perinatal data from Scotland and found that nutritional factors have a chronic widespread effect on large segments of the population and nutritional supplementation during a single pregnancy cannot be expected to significantly improve perinatal outcome.

Pregnancy in those patients who are greatly overweight is also frequently associated with perinatal problems.[28,32] Macrosomia, prolonged labor, postpartum hemorrhage and infection, and poor perinatal outcome are all increased in the obese pregnant patient.

With some notable exceptions most women in the United States do not suffer from protein-caloric malnutrition. However, poor eating habits are widespread. Following are some of the factors that are known to be associated with poor nutrition and call for further nutritional assessment:

Poverty
Adolescence
Low weight before pregnancy
High parity
Chronic systemic illness
Unusual nutritional habits
History of anemia or obesity
Poor reproductive history

A nutritional evaluation can be performed easily by the patient's obstetrician. A dietary history to establish the quantity and quality of the nutritional intake can be obtained using a 24-hour dietary recall.

Pregnant patients should be encouraged to eat a well-rounded diet high in protein and carbohydrates, and they should be told to avoid fasting or restricted diets. Normal weight gains range from 20 to 30 pounds depending on the mother's nutritional status before pregnancy. However, a smaller gain is enough for obese patients. The custom of weight restriction during pregnancy, popular from the 1940s to the early 1970s, should no longer be followed. Dieting during pregnancy should be avoided, and overweight

patients should be encouraged to lose weight after delivery. In the case of special diets (eg, for those patients with diabetes) a referral to a dietitian can be extremely helpful. Table 1-5 lists the standard weight for height in normal women of reproductive age.

Physical activity during pregnancy

A great deal of controversy exists concerning physical activity during normal pregnancy.[40] I recommend the following guidelines:

1. It is adequate to continue any exercise, sport, or activity that was actively practiced before pregnancy, but in the last trimester anything that requires a great deal of balance and physical coordination should be avoided.
2. It is adequate to continue within reason any customary strenuous activity.
3. It is advisable to avoid any new strenuous activity or sport during gestation.
4. It is preferable to rest as much as possible during pregnancy.

A number of medical and medicolegal problems have arisen concerning the continuation of employment during the last stages of gestation. The recommendation of the American College of Obstetrics and Gynecology is that patients may continue to work up to the onset of labor and are expected to return to work 6 weeks after delivery. Jobs that place the pregnant patient at physical risk should be avoided.

Use of drugs during pregnancy

Pregnancy presents a unique problem for the physician because a drug prescribed for the mother can affect the fetus, and occasionally these effects can be adverse. Despite this problem, physicians continue to prescribe a wide variety of drugs during pregnancy, frequently without a good understanding of their possible effects. In addition, the physician has no control over and often no knowledge of over-the-counter and "social" drugs like alcohol and tobacco, many of which are widely used by the pregnant patient although they have been proven to have an adverse effect on the fetus. There are a number of good references on the use of drugs during pregnancy,[38,65] but one reference that every obstetrician should have is *Handbook for Prescribing Medications during Pregnancy* by Berkowitz et al.[8]

TABLE 1-5 ■ Standard weight according to height in nonpregnant women of reproductive age

Height (feet)(inches)*	Weight (pounds)
4 10	104
4 11	107
5 0	110
5 1	113
5 2	116
5 3	118
5 4	123
5 5	128
5 6	132
5 7	136
5 8	140
5 9	144
5 10	148
5 11	152
6 0	156

*Without shoes.

Alcohol. Historically alcoholism has been recognized as a problem not only for the mother but also for her offspring. Today there are sufficient data to confirm the existence of the "fetal alcohol syndrome."[41,66] The abnormalities noted in the neonate include epicanthal folds, decreased length of the palpebral fissure, microcephaly, flattened maxilla, palmar crease abnormalities, immaturity of the central nervous system (hyperactivity and poor sleep patterns), and some mild mental retardation. The infants are frequently growth retarded, and this poor growth continues during childhood. Perinatal mortality can be as high as 20%.

These problems are usually associated with patients who would be classified as "chronic alcoholics." However, the exact safe level of alcohol consumption during pregnancy is unknown, and it is prudent to advise pregnant patients and those patients contemplating pregnancy to avoid its use.

Tobacco. The adverse effects of smoking on fetal growth have been well established.[16,47] Mothers who smoke have infants who are on the average 200 grams lighter than infants in control groups, and these infants are twice as likely to weigh less than 2500 grams. These are direct effects of smoking and are not related to diet or other variables[33] that may persist into childhood. In addition, there is an increased incidence of perinatal mortality, abruptio placenta, and placenta previa in mothers who smoke.

The exact cause of reduced fetal growth in women who smoke is uncertain. Hypoxia,[33] elevated carbon monoxide levels, thiocyanate, cadmium, and elevated catecholamines have all been reported to be significant causes of perinatal morbidity in women who smoke. Whatever the cause, smoking adversely affects the outcome of pregnancy. It is important to advise patients to stop or at least cut down on smoking during their pregnancy.

Over-the-counter drugs. Although most of the medications available to patients over the counter have not been reported to have systemic effects on the fetus or neonate, obstetricians should advise pregnant patients to avoid the use of these products and to consult the physician before the use of any drug. In general, the basic dictum of risk versus benefit should always be followed. U.S. women consume on the average four nonproprietary drugs during the course of their pregnancy, and this may be prevented by adequate counseling in the first prenatal visit.

■ IDENTIFICATION OF HIGH-RISK OBSTETRIC PATIENTS

Although only 10% to 30% of patients seen in the antenatal period can be classified as at risk, they account for 75% to 80% of the perinatal mortality and morbidity.[35] Early identification of these patients followed by proper management and therapy can frequently modify or prevent a poor perinatal outcome. This has been demonstrated in several studies, one of which[24,25] retrospectively analyzed the relation between infant deaths and maternal characteristics in Louisiana. A number of factors related to poor perinatal outcomes were identified, especially socioeconomic factors, and it was concluded that adequate prenatal care was the most important aspect in decreasing perinatal mortality. In another study[21] the results of intensive obstetric care on the outcome of 393 multiparous obstetric patients classified as at risk and cared for in a high-risk clinic in Syracuse, New York, were analyzed. Risk assessment was based primarily on a history of poor obstetric outcome. The conclusion was that adequate prenatal care can improve the perinatal outcome of the high-risk patient. There was a statistically significant decrease in both perinatal mortality and incidence of preterm births in pregnancies with intensified prenatal care when compared to previous pregnancies in which the care was not intense.

Goodwin et al[29] analyzed data from a number of perinatal mortality surveys, defined the "ideal" and the "high-risk" patient, and developed a relatively simple scoring system for identification of high-risk pregnancies. The main premise behind this system is that seemingly unrelated events may produce a cumulative effect during pregnancy and place the fetus at risk for a poor outcome. Also, certain factors historically known to be significantly related to poor outcome are weighed in the scoring system. The authors point out that the system was not devised to predict perinatal mortality or morbidity but to identify patients at risk for a poor outcome. The following data correspond to hypothetical low- and high-risk patients*:

---

*From Goodwin JW, Dunne JT, Thomas BW: Can Med Assoc J 1969;101:458.

Low risk	High risk
Age: 23	Age: 39
Para: 2	Para: 8
Height: 5'6"	Height: 5'0"
Weight: 120 lb	Weight: 170 lb
Lives near a hospital	Lives in isolated community
No complications in previous pregnancies	History of two premature infants and one stillbirth
More than 2 years since last pregnancy	Last baby 11 months ago
Has had several antenatal visits	One antenatal visit this pregnancy
Hemoglobin: >12 g	Hemoglobin: <9 g
No bleeding during this pregnancy	Bleeding earlier in this pregnancy
No renal disease, bacteriuria, or hypertension	Chronic pyelonephritis with decreased renal function
No abnormality of glucose tolerance	Abnormal glucose-tolerance curve

Rantakallio[56] studied 12,000 pregnant patients in North Finland using a questionnaire filled out by the patients. This simple historical questionnaire was able to identify a segment of the population (14%) that had a fourfold increase in low birth weight infants and a two-and-a-half-fold increase in perinatal morbidity.

These concepts are nothing new. The traditional role of the physician is to identify factors that place a patient at risk. Once the high-risk patient is identified, ideally the physician is able to prevent a poor outcome or at least modify it. However, in multi-physician practices in which patients may be seen by different physicians or in clinics where numerous personnel may come in contact with the patient, it is appropriate to have some type of formal screening procedure available so that the patient can be identified as at risk and not "fall through the cracks" of the system. Even in solo practice it is important to formalize the screening procedures to minimize errors. In addition, formal screening provides a record of the patient's high-risk assessment, and by frequent evaluation of patient outcome, the physician can evaluate his or her methods of practice and improve and strengthen weak areas.

In addition to Goodwin's system, a number of authors have proposed various types of screening systems for the identification of patients at risk for poor perinatal outcome. Aubry

and Pennington[4] were among the first to publish a quantitative system for identifying high-risk patients. They looked at numerous factors, including patient's age, race, marital status, parity, and past obstetric history (concentrating on reproductive loss, premature delivery, history of fetal or neonatal death, and congenital abnormalities). They also looked at obstetric and medical histories, especially infectious disease, endocrine disease (such as diabetes, thyroid, or adrenal problems), cardiovascular disease, and anemia. Socioeconomic and psychiatric factors were also included. After analyzing their first 1000 patients, they confirmed that in the population under study a relatively small proportion of patients (29%) accounted for the majority (75%) of the obstetric and neonatal problems encountered. They felt that by identifying these patients early they could focus their attention on them and perhaps improve their outcome by appropriate use of testing procedures and individualized care.

Hobel has been credited with the widespread popularization of high-risk screening. In 1973 he and others published an antepartum scoring system[35] that quantified a number of perinatal factors on a graded scale, concentrating primarily on cardiovascular, renal, and metabolic problems, poor obstetric history, anomalies of the reproductive tract, and a large number of miscellaneous problems. Hobel also developed intrapartum and neonatal scoring systems. Table 1-6 shows the results of his follow-up of patients who were divided into four categories using antepartum and intrapartum scoring. Complications in both the antepartum and intrapartum periods act together to lead to a poor perinatal outcome. The disadvantage of Hobel's scoring

TABLE 1-6 ■ Neonatal outcome of high-risk patients

	Risk		Outcome	
Group	Antepartum	Intrapartum	Morbidity (%)	Mortality (%)
I	Low	Low	5.0	0.0
II	High	Low	5.8	1.4
III	Low	High	11.6	2.3
IV	High	High	17.4	4.3

From Hobel CJ, et al: Am J Obstet Gynecol 1973;117:1.

High-risk evaluation form

Name _____ Age _____ Gravida _____ Para _____ Aborta _____

LMP _____ EDC _____ EDC by ultrasound _____

Reproductive history			Medical or surgical associated conditions			Present pregnancy		
Age:	<16	= 1	Previous gyneco-	= 1 ___		Bleeding		
	16-35	= 0	logic surgery			<20 weeks	= 1 ___	
	>35	= 2 ___	Chronic renal dis-	= 1 ___		>20 weeks	= 3 ___	
Parity:	0	= 1	ease			Anemia (<10 g %)	= 1 ___	
	1-4	= 0	Gestational diabe-	= 1 ___		Postmaturity	= 1 ___	
	>5	= 2 ___	tes (A)			Hypertension	= 2 ___	
Two or more abortions or history of infertility		= 1 ___	Class B or greater diabetes	= 3 ___		Premature rupture of membranes	= 2 ___	
			Cardiac disease	= 3 ___				
Postpartum bleeding or manual removal		= 1 ___	Other significant medical disorders (score 1 to 3 according to severity)	= ___		Polyhydramnios	= 2 ___	
						IUGR	= 3 ___	
						Multiple pregnancy	= 3 ___	
Child >9 lb		= 1 ___				Breech or malpresentation	= 3 ___	
Child <5 lb 8 oz		= 1 ___						
Toxemia or hypertension		= 2 ___				Rh isoimmunization	= 3 ___	
Previous cesarean section		= 2 ___						
Abnormal or difficult labor		= 2 ___						
COLUMN TOTAL		___			___			___

Total Scores
(Sum of the three columns)

Low risk	0-2
High risk	3-6
Severe risk	7 or more

From Coopland AT, et al: Can Med Assoc J 1977; 116:999.

system is its great detail. Though it provides a good data base for the systematic evaluation of perinatal care, the detail of the system makes it difficult to use and prone to clerical error.

Recently in the Netherlands, some investigators[67] developed a concept of "optimal scoring" in which each variable is listed as positive if its optimal condition (either presence or absence) is not identified in the patient. This is in contrast to being assigned a numerical value. The concept underlying this system is that high-risk patients tend to have a large number of nonoptimal factors in their history that result in a high "optimality score," indicating a high probability of a poor perinatal outcome. The authors' "optimality list" contains 55 items related to the antenatal condition, 11 items to the intrapartum condition, and 8 items to the infant immediately

TABLE 1-7 ■ Correlation between antepartum risk score and perinatal mortality using the Manitoba system

Antenatal risk assessment	Number of patients	Number of deaths	Perinatal mortality
High	3177	221	69/1000
Low	13,556	96	7/1000

From Morrison I, Olsen J: Obstet Gynecol 1979;53:362.

after birth. This concept involving risk assessment is relatively new and needs further evaluation before its benefits can be completely known.

I prefer the high-risk scoring system from Coopland et al,[17] first used in Manitoba, Canada, and shown in the box on p. 12. The system is similar to those of Goodwin, Aubry and Pennington, and Hobel but has the advantage of being less complicated and easier to use. Outcome statistics based on this system are similar to those of other scoring systems. Table 1-7 shows the correlation between risk scoring using the Manitoba system and perinatal mortality.[49] Neonatal morbidity also shows a twofold to tenfold increase in infants whose mothers are defined as at risk by this scoring system. The disadvantage of the Manitoba system is that it allows a large degree of subjectivity in the assessment of some of the variables. To offset this I have listed in the box on the right some common medical complications during pregnancy along with suggested numerical scores.

Patients should be screened on their initial visit and rescreened between 30 and 36 weeks of gestation. This does not diminish the need for each patient to be continuously reevaluated during the course of her pregnancy to determine if any additional complications or problems have arisen that make it necessary to transfer her from a low-risk to a high-risk classification.

Once high-risk patients are identified, the physician must select appropriate methods of management to assure an optimal maternal and neonatal outcome. Many of these patients must be referred to a perinatologist for specialized care, but some can be followed by their primary physician.

Suggested numeric value for some medical complications of pregnancy to be used with the Manitoba scoring system

PULMONARY DISEASE

Asthma	1
Tuberculosis	1
Pulmonary embolism	3

ENDOCRINE AND IMMUNOLOGIC DISEASES

Hypothyroidism	1
Hypothyroidism	1
Hyperthyroidism	
History	2
On medication	3
Collagen vascular disease	
In remission	1
Controlled (steroids)	2
Active	3

INFECTIONS

TORCH* (during this pregnancy)	3
Pyelonephritis	2
Other severe systemic infections	3

EPILEPSY

History	1
On medication	2

*Toxoplasmosis, rubella, cytomegalovirus, herpes.

■ METHODS OF FETAL SURVEILLANCE FOR HIGH-RISK PATIENTS

The different tests and procedures available for following high-risk patients can be divided into two general categories—biochemical and biophysical.

Biochemical tests

A number of biochemical tests of maternal serum, urine, and amniotic fluid have been developed to aid in following patients at risk for poor perinatal outcome. Most commonly used are the estriol and human placental lactogen (HPL) tests.

Estriol. Urinary estriol and more recently plasma-free estriol determinations are classic methods of biochemical fetal evaluation. Estriol is synthesized by the placenta primarily from fetal precursors. The vast majority of estriol precursors are derived from the fetal adrenal gland (sulfates of dehydroisoandrosterone and 16-hydroxy-dehydroisoandrosterone) and as such reflect fetal status.[62] The level of estriol measured in maternal plasma depends not only on fetal well-being but also on the integrity of the placental and maternal compartments. Abnormally low production of estriol can reflect fetal compromise, placental metabolic abnormalities (such as placental sulfatase deficiency), or abnormalities of the maternal compartment (such as maternal liver disease or derangement in the enterohepatic pathway for estriol excretion).

Historically, the measurement of maternal estriol production has been used for fetal surveillance in a number of high-risk situations, and indeed this was the first scientific test of fetal well-being available for practicing obstetricians. The test in most cases has been supplanted by biophysical tests because of the disadvantages of biochemical monitoring. However, estriol determinations are still used in some centers when postmaturity is suspected[60] and in pregnant patients who have diabetes.[23]

Human placental lactogen. HPL, or human chorionic somatomammotropin, is a protein hormone produced by the syncytiotrophoblast in increasing amounts as pregnancy advances. The production of HPL reflects placental mass and more indirectly placental function. Spellacy et al[63] have been strong proponents of the measurement of this hormone in maternal plasma as a means of antepartum fetal surveillance. A "fetal danger zone," according to Spellacy, is less than 4 μg/ml after 30 weeks of gestation and is indicative of fetal jeopardy. The best use of the HPL test has been in the screening of patients with hypertensive disease—both chronic hypertension and pregnancy-induced hypertension.[64] Recently a number of authors have looked at the use of HPL in screening for patients with intrauterine growth retardation and have reported significantly low levels of HPL in these patients.[20,30] However, other investigators have been unable to confirm the usefulness of HPL in the management of high-risk pregnancies, and the test has little use at the present time.

Other tests. A number of pregnancy-specific proteins have been examined to determine their prognostic significance in the evaluation of high-risk pregnancies. One of them is alpha fetoprotein, a glycoprotein produced in the yolk sac and the fetal liver, which is specific to the fetus.[18] Serum and amniotic fluid alpha fetoprotein concentrations have been used for the detection of fetal open neural tube defects (see Chapter 2). Normal serum concentration in the adult female is less than 10 ng/ml, but during pregnancy the level rises to 25 nanograms at 12 weeks and to 200 to 250 nanograms at 30 weeks. Recent investigations have found some prognostic significance to elevated alpha fetoprotein levels in intrauterine growth retardation and to depressed levels in preeclampsia.[11] However, other studies have reported conflicting results.

Other pregnancy-specific proteins such as alpha 1 and alpha 2 glycoproteins have also been studied as screening tools in preeclampsia and intrauterine growth retardation.[13,18] However, insufficient data exist at the present time to use these tests on a widespread clinical basis.

Biochemical testing has been replaced for the most part by biophysical tests because of the following problems associated with biochemical evaluation:

1. All biochemical tests have wide biologic ranges, and individual values may give little insight into the actual physiologic processes the fetus is undergoing. There is a need for serial evaluation, which is time consuming and expensive.
2. The delay in collecting the specimen, running the tests, and reporting the results to the physician is sometimes too long to provide the up-to-the-minute information that is necessary for the evaluation of the fetus at a high risk.

Biophysical tests

In the past decade advances in technology have provided the obstetrician with two new biophysical methods for evaluation of fetal well-being: antepartum cardiotocography and serial ultrasound screening. Biophysical testing has a distinct advantage over biochemical methods in that it provides the obstetrician with immediate information about the status of the fetus. Because of this distinct advantage and because of their high degree of specificity, biophysical tests have supplanted biochemical tests in the evaluation of most fetal high-risk situations.[51]

Antepartum cardiotocography. The use of fetal heart rate testing for antepartum evaluation of the fetus has become a standard tool in high-risk evaluation. The oxytocin challenge test (OCT) that evaluates the fetoplacental reserve by placing the fetus under the stress of an oxytocin-stimulated contraction has been partially supplanted by the nonstress test (NST) because the NST is easier to perform and has a specificity as high as the contraction stress test (CST). When normal, both tests have a 99% prognostic significance in predicting a good outcome for a fetus delivered within 1 week of the test. The predictive value of a nonreactive NST is more restricted and in most instances should be followed up by an OCT. Some differences do exist in definition and protocols for the NST. In a majority of institutions the definition of a reactive NST is two or more accelerations of 15 beats or greater lasting at least 15 seconds and associated with fetal movement during a 20-minute interval.

In a high-risk pregnancy, fetal heart rate testing may begin as soon as intervention is possible. This is usually between 28 and 30 weeks of gestation. Care must be used in evaluating an NST obtained in early gestation, since it has recently been reported[9] that there is a high percentage of false nonreactive NSTs before 30 weeks. A

suspicious NST (technical difficulty in interpretation or presence of decelerations) requires either an OCT or repeating of the NST within 24 hours, depending on the clinical situation and the degree of suspicion that the physician has regarding the severity of the high-risk situation.

It is better to use the term *contraction stress test* than oxytocin challenge test when referring to antepartum fetal stress testing. OCT has a restricted meaning because it implies that only oxytocin-induced contractions are used for the test. CST broadens this meaning and implies that the patient's spontaneous contractions may also be used as a stressful fetal stimuli. This is important because there is evidence suggesting that late decelerations after mild spontaneous contractions (Braxton-Hicks) are more significant in indicating fetal compromise than a positive OCT after oxytocin stimulation.[52]

Some authors in evaluating antepartum cardiotographs, use scoring systems that rely on baseline rate, fetal movement, baseline variability, change from the baseline, and fetal heart rate response to contractions. Quantification of the NST using scoring systems increases the specificity of the test and allows early recognition of the fetus in danger. The box below illustrates one of these scoring systems.[68]

A simplified method of performing the NST, presented by Baskett et al,[6] uses a simple office Doppler or even an aural stethoscope to record

Antepartum cardiotocography scoring system

Factor	Score* 0	Score* 1	Score* 2
Baseline rate	100 or 180	100-120 or 160-180	120-160
Fetal movement	None	1-2/20-40 min	>2/20-40 min
FHR† response to fetal movement	None	Accelerates <15 beats/min	Accelerates >15 beats/min
Baseline variability	None	<5 beats/min	>5 beats/min
FHR† response to contraction	Deceleration	No change	Acceleration

*The higher the score, the better the prognosis.
†FHR, Fetal heart rate.

From Varma TR: Int J Gynaecol Obstet 1981;19:433.

fetal heart rate accelerations. The negative predictive value of this method is similar to that of the NST using a fetal heart rate monitor.

Recently there has been some controversy about the value of the NST in certain high-risk situations such as postmaturity, intrauterine growth retardation, and diabetes. A number of fetal deaths have been reported after a reactive NST in patients with these conditions. However, the NST still remains a valid and accurate method of fetal surveillance for most high-risk situations. Even in diabetes, intrauterine growth retardation, and postmaturity, the NST coupled with the appropriate use of the OCT remains a valid method of fetal assessment. More about this subject may be found in Chapter 18.

Ultrasound. As mentioned earlier, an ultrasound examination can be invaluable in accurately determining gestational age. However, ultrasound examination can also provide important information concerning fetal weight, status, and growth. The latter subject is covered in detail in Chapter 8.

An important use of ultrasound is in the estimation of fetal weight[22] using the BPD and the fetal abdominal circumference (AC). Determination of the fetal weight can give valuable information for the management of many high-risk situations such as preterm labor and preterm rupture of the membranes. The method uses the formula of Shepard et al.[61]

$$\text{Log (birth weight)} = 1.7492 + \\ 0.166\,(\text{BPD}) + 0.046\,(\text{AC}) - \\ 2.646\,(\text{BPD} \times \text{AC})/1000$$

Ultrasonography can also be used to evaluate fetal well-being by determining the fetal biophysical profile.[46] The factors evaluated are (1) fetal breathing movement, (2) fetal movements, (3) fetal tone, (4) qualitative amniotic fluid volume, and (5) NST. The authors[46] used the biophysical profile in 216 high-risk pregnancies. The perinatal mortality ranged from 0 when all five variables were normal to 60% when all were abnormal. The biophysical profile may be the test of choice in the evaluation of some high-risk pregnancies.

In summary, with the use of clinical skills, ultrasound, and cardiotocography the obstetrician can be very accurate in the evaluation of the high-risk fetus. On the other hand, routine

use of biophysical tools for the screening of low-risk patients is controversial. I recently evaluated the effectiveness of routine serial ultrasound screening and antepartum cardiotocography in low-risk patients and found that the use of these methods did not significantly reduce the perinatal mortality in this population.[53]

■ REFERENCES

1. Andersen HF, Johnson TRB, Barclay ML, et al: Gestational age assessment: I. Analysis of individual clinical observations. Am J Obstet Gynecol 1981;139:173.
2. Andersen HF, Johnson TRB, Flora JD, et al: Gestational age assessment: II. Prediction of combined clinical observations. Am J Obstet Gynecol 1981;140:770.
3. Anderson RS, Phillips PJ: Routine real-time scanning at the first hospital visit. Br J Obstet Gynaecol 1982;89:16.
4. Aubry RH, Pennington JC: Identification and evaluation of high-risk pregnancy: the perinatal concept. Clin Obstet Gynecol 1973;16:3.
5. Baird D: Environment and reproduction. Br J Obstet Gynaecol 1980;87:1057.
6. Baskett TF, Boyce CD, Lohre MA, et al: Simplified antepartum fetal heart assessment. Br J Obstet Gynaecol 1981;88:395.
7. Battaglia F, Meschia G: Principal substrates of fetal metabolism. Physiol Rev 1978;58:499.
8. Berkowitz RL, Coustan DR, Mochezuki TK: *Handbook for prescribing medications during pregnancy*. Boston, Little Brown & Co, 1981.
9. Bishop EH: Fetal acceleration test. Am J Obstet Gynecol 1981;141:905.
10. Boehm FH, Estes W, Wright PF, et al: Management of genital herpes simplex virus infection occurring during pregnancy. Am J Obstet Gynecol 1981;141:735.
11. Brock DJ, Barron L, Raab GM: The potential of mid trimester maternal plasma α-fetoprotein measurement in predicting infants of low birth weight. Br J Obstet Gynaecol 1980;87:582.
12. Brown JE, Jacobson HN, Askue LH, et al: Influence of pregnancy weight gain on the size of infants born to underweight women. Obstet Gynecol 1981;57:13.
13. Chapman MG, O'Shea RT, Jones RW, et al: Pregnancy-specific B_1-glycoprotein as a screening tool for at-risk pregnancy. Am J Obstet Gynecol 1981;141:499.
14. Chapman MP, Sheat JH, Furness ET, et al: Routine ultrasound screening in early pregnancy. Med J Aust 1979;2:62.
15. Christensen KK: Infection as a predominant cause of perinatal mortality. Obstet Gynecol 1982;59:499.
16. Cole PV, Roberts D: Smoking during pregnancy and its effects on the fetus. Br J Obstet Gynaecol 1972;79:782.
17. Coopland AT, Peddle LJ, Baskett TF, et al: A simplified antepartum high-risk pregnancy screening form: statistical analysis of 5459 cases. Can Med Assoc J 1977;116:999.
18. Cowchacks FS: Use of maternal blood protein levels in identification and management of high-risk obstetrical patients. Clin Obstet Gynecol 1978;21:341.

19. Crane JP, Kopta MM, Welt SI, et al: Abnormal fetal growth patterns—ultrasonic diagnosis and management. Obstet Gynecol 1977;50:205.
20. Daikoku NH, Tyson JE, Graf C, et al: The relative significance of human placental lactogen in the diagnosis of retarded fetal growth. Am J Obstet Gynecol 1979;135:516.
21. DeGeorge FV, Nesbitt REL, Aubry RH: High-risk obstetrics: IV. An evaluation of the effects of intensified care on pregnancy outcome. Am J Obstet Gynecol 1971;111:650.
22. Deter RL, Hadlock FP, Harrist RB, et al: Evaluation of three methods for obtaining fetal weight estimation using dynamic image ultrasound. JCU 1981;9:421.
23. Distler W, Gabbe SG, Freeman RK, et al: Estriol in pregnancy: V. Unconjugated and total plasma estriol in the management of pregnant diabetic patients. Am J Obstet Gynecol 1978;130:424.
24. Dott AB, Fort AT: The effect of maternal demographic factors on infant mortality rates: summary of the findings of the Lousiana infant mortality study, Part I. Am J Obstet Gynecol 1975;123:847.
25. Dott AB, Fort AT: The effect of availability and utilization of prenatal care and hospital services on infant mortality rates: summary of the findings of the Lousiana infant mortality study, Part II. Am J Obstet Gynecol 1975;123:854.
26. Duenhoelter JH: Pregnancy tests—evaluating and using them. Contemp Obstet Gynecol 1982;19:239.
27. Edwards LE, Alton IR, Barrada IM, et al: Pregnancy in the underweight woman: course, outcome and growth patterns of the infant. Am J Obstet Gynecol 1979;135:297.
28. Edwards LE, Dickes WF, Alton IR, et al: Pregnancy in the massively obese: course, outcome and obesity prognosis of the infant. Am J Obstet Gynecol 1978;131:479.
29. Goodwin JW, Dunne JT, Thomas BW: Antepartum identification of the fetus at risk. Can Med Assoc J 1969;101:458.
30. Granat M, Sharf M, Diengott D, et al: Further investigation on the predictive value of human placental lactogen in high-risk pregnancy. Am J Obstet Gynecol 1977;129:647.
31. Grennert L, Persson P, Gennser G: Benefits of ultrasonic screening of a pregnant population. Acta Obstet Gynecol Scand 1978;78:5.
32. Harrison GG, Udall JN, Morrow G: Maternal obesity, weight gain in pregnancy, and infant birth weight. Am J Obstet Gynecol 1980;136:411.
33. Haworth JC, Ellestad-Sayed JJ, King J, et al: Fetal growth retardation in cigarette smoking mothers is not due to decreased food intake. Am J Obstet Gynecol 1980;137:719.
34. Hellman LM, Kobayashi M, Filliste L, et al: Growth and development of the human fetus prior to the 20th week of gestation. Am J Obstet Gynecol 1969;103:789.
35. Hobel CJ, Hyvarinen MA, Okada DM, et al: Prenatal and intrapartum high-risk screening. Am J Obstet Gynecol 1973;117:1.
36. Hoffman HJ, Stark CR, Lundin FE, et al: Analysis of birth weight, gestational age, and fetal viability, U.S. births, 1968. Obstet Gynecol Surv 1974;29:651.
37. Hohler CW, Quetel TA: Comparison of ultrasound femur length and biparietal diameter in late pregnancy. Am J Obstet Gynecol 1981;141:759.
38. Howard FM, Hill JM: Drugs during pregnancy. Obstet Gynecol Surv 1979;34:643.
39. Jacobson HN: Weight and weight gain in pregnancy. Clin Perinatol 1975;2:223.
40. Jimenez MH, Newton N: Activity and work during pregnancy and the postpartum period: a cross-cultural study of 202 societies. Am J Obstet Gynecol 1979;135:171.
41. Jones KL, Smith DW: The fetal alcohol syndrome. Teratology 1975;12:1.
42. Kopta MM, Tomich PG, Crane JP: Ultrasonic methods of predicting the estimated date of confinement. Obstet Gynecol 1981;57:657.
43. Kortenoever ME: Pregnancy of long duration and postmature infant. Obstet Gynecol Surv 1950;5:812.
44. Kurtz AB, Wapner RJ, Kurtz KJ: Analysis of biparietal diameter as an accurate indication of gestational age. JCU 1980;8:319.
45. Landesman R, Saxena BB: Results of the first 1000 radioreceptorassays for the determination of human chorionic gonadotropin: a new, rapid, reliable, and sensitive pregnancy test. Fertil Steril 1976;27:357.
46. Manning FA, Platt LD, Sipos L: Antepartum fetal evaluation: development of a fetal biophysical profile. Am J Obstet Gynecol 1980;136:787.
47. Meyer MD: How does maternal smoking affect birth weight and maternal weight gain? Evidence from the Ontario perinatal mortality study. Am J Obstet Gynecol 1978;131:888.
48. Moghissi KS: Maternal nutrition in pregnancy. Clin Obstet Gynecol 1978;21:297.
49. Morrison I, Olsen J: Perinatal mortality and antepartum risk scoring. Obstet Gynecol 1979;53:362.
50. O'Brien GD, Queenan JT: Growth of the ultrasound fetal femur length during normal pregnancy. Am J Obstet Gynecol 1981;141:833.
51. Ott WJ: Antepartum biophysical evaluation of the fetus. Perinatol/Neonatol 1978;2:11.
52. Ott WJ: Clinical experience with cardiotocometry for the evaluation of the fetus. Southern Med J 1981;47:310.
53. Ott WJ, Doyle S: Routine antepartum biophysical screening. J Reprod Med 1982;27:389.
54. Peck TM, Arias F: Hematological changes associated with pregnancy. Clin Obstet Gynecol 1979;22:785.
55. Preblud SR, Serdula MK, Frank JA, et al: Rubella vaccination in the United States: a ten-year review. Epidemiol Rev 1980;2:171.
56. Rantakallio P: Groups at risk in low-birth weight infants and perinatal mortality. Acta Paediatr Scand 1969;193(suppl):5.
57. Robinson HP, Fleming JEE: A critical evaluation of sonar "crown-rump length" measurements. Br J Obstet Gynaecol 1975;82:702.
58. Sabbagha RE, Hughey M, Deep R: Growth adjusted sonographic age: a simplified method. Obstet Gynecol 1976;51:383.

59. Scheidt PC, Stanley F, Bryla DA: One-year follow-up of infants exposed to ultrasound in utero. Am J Obstet Gynecol 1978;131:743.

60. Schneider JM, Olson RW, Curet LB: Screening for fetal and neonatal risk in the postdate pregnancy. Am J Obstet Gynecol 1978;131:473.

61. Shepard MJ, Fichards VA, Berkowitz RL, et al: An evaluation of two equations for prediction of fetal weight by ultrasound. Am J Obstet Gynecol 1982;142:47.

62. Siiteri PK, MacDonald PC: Placental estriol biosynthesis during human pregnancy. J Clin Endocrinol Metab 1966;26:751.

63. Spellacy WN, Buhi WC, Berk SA: The effectiveness of HPL measurements as an adjunct in decreasing perinatal death. Am J Obstet Gynecol 1975;121:835.

64. Spellacy WN, Teoh ES, Buhi WK, et al: Value of human chorionic somatomammotropin in management of high-risk pregnancy. Am J Obstet Gynecol 1981;109:588.

65. Sterrat GM: Prescribing problems in the second half of pregnancy and during lactation. Obstet Gynecol Surv 1976;31:1.

66. Stressguth AP, Landersman-Dwyer S, Martin JC, et al: Teratogenic effects of alcohol in human and lab animals. Science 1980;209:353.

67. Towlen BCL, Hiusjes HJ, Jurgens-v.d.Zei AD: Obstetrical conditions and neonatal neurological morbidity: an analysis with the help of optimality concept. Early Hum Dev 1980;4:207.

68. Varma, TR: Clinical experience in non-stressed antepartum cardiotocography in high-risk pregnancy. Int J Gynaecol Obstet 1981;19:433.

2

■ ■ ■

ANTENATAL DIAGNOSIS OF CONGENITAL DISEASES

Fernando Arias

According to the Consensus Development Conference on Antenatal Diagnosis, 100,000 to 150,000 infants are born every year in the United States with a significant congenital malformation, a chromosome abnormality, or a clearly defined genetic disorder. Fortunately, the number of these conditions that can be detected antenatally is growing at a rapid pace. Therefore, the obstetrician must be prepared (1) to identify specific genetic risks; (2) to discuss with the parents the implications of these risks; and (3) to refer these patients at risk to adequate facilities for expert counseling and further testing.

The obstetrician should not assume the role of a genetic counselor because this is a medical skill that requires training in human genetics. However, the obstetrician is responsible for identifying pregnant women in need of genetic counseling and for referring these patients, at an appropriate time during gestation, to the proper facilities. The obstetrician should also be ready to provide answers to a series of questions by concerned parents at the time the risk factor is identified and before consultation with the geneticist.

This chapter has been written with that view of the obstetrician's role. Rather than emphasizing genetic theory and concepts, I will briefly discuss the identification of the patient at risk

for genetic disease and then will describe genetic amniocentesis, a procedure that is a subject of profound concern to most patients referred for genetic counseling. Finally, several of the common problems seen in the obstetrician's office which require genetic counseling will be discussed, as well as some of the most common concerns of patients about drugs or substances that may cause fetal damage.

■ IDENTIFICATION OF PATIENTS AT RISK FOR CONGENITAL DISEASE IN OFFSPRING

In less than 50% of the cases, the identification of patients at risk for fetal congenital abnormalities results from the obstetrician's efforts. In the majority of cases, the possibility of genetic disease is a concern raised by the patient herself, usually because of a prior pregnancy with poor outcome, because of the existence of relatives with congenital problems, or because of the ingestion of medications or exposure to potentially harmful influences during pregnancy.

To facilitate the identification of patients at risk, we have incorporated into our antenatal record a genetic screening questionnaire (see box on p. 2). We believe this is useful for finding those patients with whom the applicability of genetic amniocentesis must be discussed according to the recommendations of the Consensus Development Conference on Antenatal Diagnosis.

The following factors identify patients who require discussion about the applicability of genetic amniocentesis:

1. Pregnancies of women 35 years of age or more
2. Previous pregnancy resulting in the birth of a child with chromosome abnormalities
3. Existence of a chromosome abnormality in either parent
4. History of Down's syndrome or other chromosome abnormality in a family member
5. History of two or more spontaneous abortions with marked alteration in fetal development in this marriage or in a previous marriage of either spouse
6. Previous birth of a child with multiple major malformations
7. Pregnancies of women who have male relatives with Duchenne muscular dystrophy or severe hemophilia or who are at increased risk of being carriers of other deleterious X-linked genes
8. Pregnancies in which couples are at risk for detectable inborn errors of metabolism (X-linked or autosomal recessive)
9. Pregnancies at increased risk for fetal neural tube defects
10. Pregnancies at increased risk for sickle cell disease in the offspring

Once the patient at risk is identified, the obstetrician must inform her and her husband about the nature of the risk factor, the need for further investigation, and the availability of referral centers to carry out these investigations. Since amniocentesis is a frequently recommended procedure in the workup of the patient at risk, the obstetrician should be ready to answer questions about the accuracy and safety of this procedure. The obstetrician also should be ready to discuss management alternatives in case further testing demonstrates the presence of fetal abnormalities.

The importance of the initial discussion between obstetrician and patient at risk cannot be overemphasized. Many patients who have negative feelings about genetic amniocentesis may change their minds after an informal conversation with the obstetrician. Many unfounded

fears can be dissipated and a very positive attitude toward the procedure can be generated in the course of this discussion. However, additional fears and a negative attitude may be developed by the patient if the obstetrician (1) cannot provide information, (2) shows a lack of security in discussing risks and benefits, or (3) defers questions with the excuse that they will be solved by the geneticist later on. It is not expected that this conversation between obstetrician and patient at risk has the content of a formal genetic counseling session; it should contain, however, enough information to allow the patient to make a decision about whether or not to accept a consultation with a professional geneticist.

■ GENETIC AMNIOCENTESIS

Genetic amniocentesis is an outpatient procedure that must be carried out at 15 to 16 weeks of gestation and after the patient has had adequate counseling by a geneticist. This counseling usually includes, in addition to a discussion about the indication for the amniocentesis, a description of the procedure, its risks, and its complications. However, if the geneticist is not an obstetrician, the responsibility for performing the genetic amniocentesis and obtaining informed consent for the procedure falls entirely on the obstetrician. In this situation, the obstetrician should be ready to answer questions concerning the procedure and reinforce the information obtained from the geneticist.

Procedure

The patient with a valid indication for genetic amniocentesis is scheduled for the procedure at 15 to 16 weeks of gestation because at this time the volume of amniotic fluid (± 200 ml) is large enough to obtain a sample without difficulties, because the cells obtained at this gestational age usually grow well in in vitro conditions, and because, if an abnormal result is found and the patient opts for abortion, it can be carried out before reaching the legal limit for a pregnancy termination.

Genetic amniocentesis should always be preceded by drawing a sample of blood for determination of maternal blood group and Rh and maternal serum alpha fetoprotein. Knowledge of the maternal Rh classification is important to determine the patient's eligibility for Rho-

GAM administration after the amniocentesis, and measurement of the maternal serum alpha fetoprotein concentration may be useful in the interpretation of the amniotic fluid results.

Amniocentesis should be preceded by a careful study of the pregnancy with real-time ultrasound. Of particular interest during the ultrasound examination are the following points:

1. Determination of the number of fetuses
2. Measurement of the fetal biparietal diameter (BPD)
3. Placental location
4. Visualization of the fetal extremities, bladder, kidneys, upper and lower spine, four heart chambers, and intracranial anatomy

If multiple gestational sacs are present, the amniocentesis procedure must involve separate puncture and analysis of the amniotic fluid of each sac. After drawing fluid from the first sac, a dye (indigo carmine) is injected into it; the fluid from the second sac should be dye free.

Measurement of the fetal BPD is important to reconfirm the gestational age. As a general rule, if the BPD is less than 3.4 cm, gestation is not at 15 to 16 weeks and amniocentesis should be rescheduled for a later date.

Placental location is an important step before genetic amniocentesis. If the placenta is located in the anterior aspect of the uterus, a search must be made for a place where the needle can be inserted while avoiding the placenta. If this is not possible, a thin placental area, away from the center of the organ and its large vessels, should be selected for the tap. The distance between the skin of the abdomen and the amniotic fluid should be measured with the electronic calipers of the ultrasound machine to avoid excessive penetration of the needle.

Finally, the ultrasound examination before amniocentesis is important in ruling out the presence of major congenital malformations such as anencephaly, meningomyelocele, open spina bifida, limb reduction defects, omphalocele, polycystic kidneys, cystic hygromas, duodenal atresia, and hydrocephaly.

Once the ultrasound examination is completed and the tap site is chosen, a sterile preparation of the lower abdomen is performed and the puncture site is anesthetized with a local infiltration of 1% mepivacaine (Carbocaine). Then a 22-gauge spinal needle is inserted with a single thrust of the operator's hand down to the distance that was determined when the thickness of the maternal tissues was measured. At this moment, particularly if the amniocentesis is transplacental, the tip of the needle must be visualized with real-time ultrasound and advanced or removed until it is clearly located in a pocket of fluid. At this time the stylet is removed and fluid should come out freely from the needle. If the fluid is bloody, it should be allowed to drain until it becomes spontaneously clear. The fluid is aspirated with a sterile glass syringe and the first 2 ml discarded because of possible contamination with maternal cells. Then three 8 ml aliquots of fluid are withdrawn, placed into separate sterile plastic tubes, and transported to the laboratory where they will be used for cytogenetic analysis and amniotic fluid alpha fetoprotein (AFP) determination. The sample for AFP determination should not be centrifuged. After the fluid is removed, the needle is withdrawn and the fetal heart motion observed with the real-time ultrasound.

Risks

In general, genetic amniocentesis is a safe procedure. However, it entails certain maternal and fetal risks and some possible technical problems.

The main maternal problems associated with genetic amniocentesis are the possibility of Rh isoimmunization in the Rh negative mother and the possibility of infection. To prevent Rh isoimmunization, maternal Rh should always be determined before the procedure and, if the patient is Rh negative, a minidose of RhoGAM (150 μg) should be administered intramuscularly after the tap. The risk of infection of the uterine cavity is very low (approximately 0.1%), especially if sterile technique is used during the procedure.

The fetal risks associated with genetic amniocentesis have been assessed in several studies, both in the United States[13,34,37] and in other countries,[30,52] involving several thousand patients. The results of these studies show that the danger to the fetus is extremely low although the procedure is not entirely risk free.

Regarding the risk of abortion following genetic amniocentesis, the National Institute of Child Health and Human Development Collaborative Study[37] and the Canadian Collaborative Study[52] show no increase in spontaneous abortion. The British Collaborative Study[30] shows a

1.5% increase in abortion rate over that of control subjects who did not have genetic amniocentesis. In the study of Golbus et al[13] the rate of spontaneous abortions was 1.5% after amniocentesis and before 28 weeks of gestation. However, the rate of spontaneous abortion was 1.2% in the week before the procedure in patients who had made appointments for counseling and amniocentesis. In conclusion, the abortion risk of genetic amniocentesis seems to be between 0.3% and 0.5%, particularly if the placenta is located in the anterior aspect of the uterus and transplacental amniocentesis is required.

Other complications associated with genetic amniocentesis are (1) amniotic fluid leakage (reported by approximately 2% to 3% of the patients), which usually disappears with bed rest; (2) unexplained fetal death during the procedure (0.7 out of 1000 cases); (3) skin puncture (1 out of 929 cases); and (4) fetal trauma with the needle, reported in only a few cases.

The technical problems associated with ge-

Consent for amniocentesis for diagnosis of fetal disorder

Amniocentesis is a test that can detect some birth defects and hereditary disorders. The test is done by withdrawing a sample of fluid from the bag of waters surrounding the fetus (baby). This fluid is obtained by introducing a needle through the abdomen and uterus (womb). Some slight discomfort is experienced when the needle is introduced.

I, _____, have been informed of the following risks and limitations of amniocentesis for the diagnosis of fetal disorders and have had the opportunity to question and discuss these with my physician and his or her assistants.

1. Although the test is being performed in a stage of pregnancy when spontaneous miscarriage sometimes occurs, amniocentesis has not been shown to increase the chance of miscarriage.
2. The possibility of injuring the fetus or umbilical cord with the needle exists; however, the chance of this happening is considered to be very small.
3. As in all surgical procedures, there is a possibility of infection. If serious enough, this could cause loss of pregnancy. This risk is very low and every precaution is taken to maintain a sterile technique.
4. Ultrasound is performed to localize the placenta (afterbirth), to determine whether twins are present and to visually guide the needle into the bag of waters. It is also used to visualize fluid pockets and to evaluate fetal heart motion before and after the test.
5. In two thirds of patients the placenta is located on the front of the uterus. In these cases it may be necessary to pass the needle through the placenta to obtain amniotic fluid. This could result in fetal bleeding. Though potentially fetal bleeding is rare, it has been known to occur.
6. It is rare that the test cannot be successfully completed because of the inability to get an adequate sample of fluid.
7. An occasional complication is leakage of either clear or blood-tinged fluid from the vagina shortly after the tap. This leakage is not considered to be a serious complication and it should cease within 24 hours. If leakage persists beyond 24 hours, it is recommended that you notify your physician.
8. In some cases the fetal cells do not grow in culture after an amniocentesis, and the procedure may have to be repeated. This occurs in not more than 1 in 50 patients.
9. Since the test screens only for selected birth defects, the results do not guarantee the birth of a normal child.
10. It is understood that there is a slight possibility that the laboratory tests could incorrectly assess the baby's health.
11. I believe the benefits of my having amniocentesis outweigh these potential risks associated with the procedure. I have had the opportunity to discuss any and all questions about these procedures and give my consent to have the procedure performed.

netic amniocentesis have to do with an occasional lack of accuracy of the test and with an occasional failure of the amniotic cells to grow adequately in vitro. The test is extremely accurate, with an overall error rate of 0.4%[13] More than half of this error rate is caused by contamination of the cultures with maternal cells. The culture failure rate for cells obtained through genetic amniocentesis is about 3.2%.[34] In these cases second amniocentesis should be performed once the lack of viability of the cultures is observed.

It is important to inform patients that the finding of a normal fetal karyotype and a normal amniotic fluid alpha fetoprotein concentration does not guarantee the birth of a normal newborn, since there are causes of birth defects and mental retardation that cannot be detected through amniocentesis. The possibilities that this may occur, however, are very low, most probably under 1%.

The box on p. 22 shows the consent form for genetic amniocentesis used in the Genetic Unit at Washington University, Department of Obstetrics and Gynecology. This form contains most of the information about risks, accuracy of the procedure, and possibilities of technical problems discussed before. Ideally, the form should be discussed with the patient and given to her several days before the scheduled amniocentesis.

■ THE PREGNANT WOMAN OF ADVANCED AGE

As shown in Table 2-1, the risk of having a child with a chromosomal abnormality increases with maternal age from 1 out of 526 at age 20, to 1 out of 18 at age 45.[50] Predominant among these chromosome defects is Down's syndrome (trisomy 21), although trisomy 18 and trisomy 13 also occur frequently.

Down's syndrome is characterized by craniofacial features evocative of an Oriental face, which include oblique palpebral fissures, small and low-set ears, protruding tongue, and broad nasal bridge. Internal anomalies are common, particularly cardiac lesions and duodenal atresia. Approximately 20% to 30% of these infants die during their first year, and 50% are dead by age 5, mainly because of respiratory infections. Those who survive infancy show mental retardation. The syndrome results from the presence

of an entire additional chromosome 21 (nondisjunctional trisomy) in about 85% of the cases, from translocation of a band from another chromosome (most commonly chromosome 14) in another 3% to 5% of the cases, and from a mosaic composition in a few cases. Most cases of nondisjunctional Down's syndrome are sporadic and show a well-defined relationship to maternal age whereas those involving translocations may be familial and show no relationship to maternal age.

In the last few years, evidence has been presented suggesting that paternal age may also be an important factor in the production of Down's syndrome; it seems that the risk of having a child with Down's syndrome increases twofold when the father's age surpasses 55 years.[29,54] Thus the father's age should be taken into consideration when talking with women at risk for Down's syndrome in the offspring; if the husband is more than 55 years old, the obstetrician should tell the couple that the risk of chromosomal abnormalities is double that which can be calculated on the basis of maternal age alone.

TABLE 2-1 ■ Risk of having a child with chromosomal abnormalities at different maternal ages

Maternal age (years)	Down's syndrome	All abnormalities except 47 XXX
20	1:1923	1:526
22	1:1538	1:500
24	1:1299	1:476
26	1:1124	1:478
28	1:990	1:435
30	1:885	1:384
32	1:725	1:322
34	1:465	1:243
35	1:365	1:178
36	1:287	1:149
38	1:177	1:105
39	1:139	1:80
40	1:109	1:63
41	1:85	1:48
42	1:67	1:39
43	1:53	1:31
44	1:41	1:24
45	1:32	1:18

From Simpson JL, Goldbus MS, Martin AO, et al: *Genetics in obstetrics and gynecology*. New York, Grune & Stratton Inc, 1982, p. 58. By permission.

Also, with the development of better cytogenetic techniques it has been possible to determine that in 24% of the cases the extra chromosome 21 in infants with Down's syndrome was received from the father.[27] This is an important fact because it allows the obstetrician to explain to patients at risk that chromosomal abnormalities, including Down's syndrome, may result from alterations in either the sperm or the egg and, in this way, the mother can avoid blaming herself for the eventual occurrence of a fetal anomaly.

It is possible that in the future, with the development of more laboratory facilities for cytogenetic studies, a trend will appear toward the antenatal search of fetuses with Down's syndrome in women under 35 years of age. The reason for this is that several studies in the United States[20,41] and in other countries[25,31] have demonstrated a substantial decrease in the average age of mothers giving birth to children with Down's syndrome. This most probably is a reflection of the relative infrequency of pregnancy after age 35. At present only about 20% of Down's infants are born to woman 35 years of age or older.[20] The problem is that there are not enough adequate laboratory facilities to perform cytogenetic studies in all women under age 35. Until this limiting factor is resolved, our policy is to recommend amniocentesis strongly to every pregnant woman 37 years old or more, to offer amniocentesis to every pregnant woman 35 to 37 years old, and to give up-to-date figures about risks of amniocentesis and risks of having an infant with chromosomal defects to every woman under 35 years of age who is pregnant. If a woman under age 35 wants to have amniocentesis, she is referred without hesitation to the geneticist for "formal" counseling and eventual performance of the procedure.

■ PATIENTS WITH HISTORY OF CHROMOSOMAL ABNORMALITY, MAJOR MALFORMATION, OR MENTAL RETARDATION IN OFFSPRING

Patients who have experienced the birth of a genetically abnormal child or who have seen the consequences of genetic disease in some member of their immediate family are usually eager to inform the obstetrician about this fact and seek genetic counseling. On a few occasions,

however, the existence of a relative with congenital malformations will only become apparent if a careful family history is obtained at the initial prenatal interview. This section examines some of the most common situations seen in an obstetric practice.

Down's syndrome

When a pregnant woman has a history of a prior child with Down's syndrome, it becomes extremely important to know what chromosomal defect was found in that particular child. As mentioned before, a child with Down's syndrome may be the product of a trisomy or may result from a chromosome translocation, and the risk of recurrence in a future pregnancy will be markedly different depending on the type of defect.

The recurrence risk for a baby with trisomy 21 Down's syndrome will depend on the age of the mother at the time of birth of the affected child and her age at the time of the present pregnancy.[32] If the pregnant woman was less than 30 years old at the time of the birth of the child with Down's syndrome and she still is under age 30, the recurrence risk is between 2% and 3%; if she becomes pregnant again after age 30, the risk will be that corresponding to her present age (Table 2-1) plus 1%.[50] If the mother was 30 years of age or older at the time of the birth of the child with Down's syndrome, her risk in a subsequent pregnancy is no higher than that of any other women of comparable age.

The recurrence risk when the Down's syndrome in a past pregnancy was caused by an unbalanced translocation will vary depending on the chromosome composition of the parents. If both parents have a normal karyotype, the translocation in the affected child occurred de novo and the risk of another affected child is less than 1%. If the mother karyotype is normal but the father has a balanced 13/21, 14/21, 15/21, or 21/22 translocation, the risk of another affected child will be 2% to 3%. If the father karyotype is normal and the mother is the carrier of a balanced 13/21, 14/21, 15/21, or 21/22 translocation, the likelihood of another affected child is 11.9%, much less than the theoretical risk of 33%. If either parent has a balanced 21/21 translocation, the risk of an affected child in a future pregnancy will be 100%. The risk of recurrence when a previous child has been born with

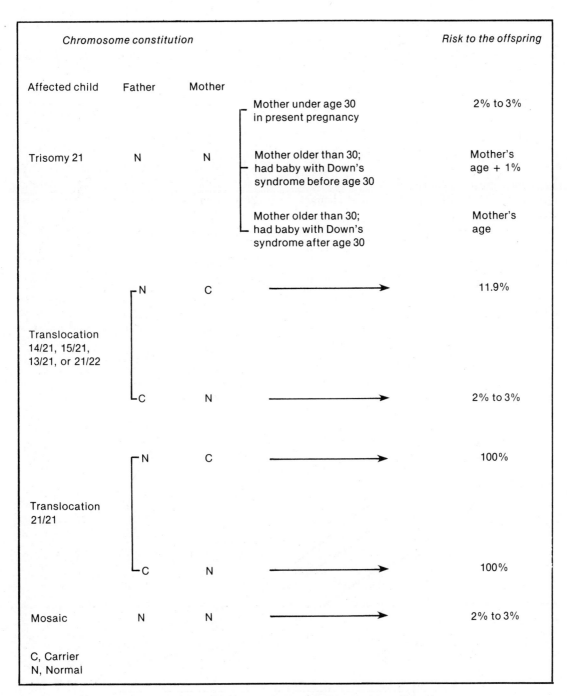

FIG. 2-1 ■ Summary of the risk of recurrence for Down's syndrome.

Down's syndrome resulting from mosaicism is unknown but probably small (2% to 3%).

Fig. 2-1 summarizes the risk of recurrence for Down's syndrome. Since in all cases the risk is greater than the risk of genetic amniocentesis, these patients must be advised to seek genetic counseling and to have genetic amniocentesis.

Neural tube defects

Neural tube defect (NTD) is a generic name to designate some malformations (anencephaly, encephalocele, and spina bifida) that result from a failure of the neural tube to close in the first 4 weeks after conception. NTDs are among the commonest major malformations of the central nervous system, and their incidence changes with race and geographic location. For example, the incidence of NTD in the United States is 2.35 out of 1000 births for the white population and 0.9 out of 1000 for the black population.[11] In Wales and Ireland, with mostly white populations, the incidence of NTD is higher, with almost 1% of the pregnant population being affected.[8]

NTD is a polygenic disorder, and the recurrence risk is lower than when a single chromosome locus is affected. The most frequently quoted recurrence risk figures come from studies carried out in England, where the prevalence of the disease is elevated. In the United States, where the frequency of NTD is much lower than in England, the recurrence risk is 1.5% to 2% when a prior child has been affected and 4% to 6% when two prior children have been affected.[51] Genetic amniocentesis must be recommended to couples who have had prior children born with NTD, since the recurrence risks are higher than risks from the procedure itself. However, in cases of encephalocele, before giving the parents the above risk figures, the obstetrician must know if the baby with encephalocele had some other anomalies such as polycystic kidneys, polydactyly, cleft palate, or congenital heart defects, because in these cases the correct diagnosis may be Meckel's syndrome, which is an autosomal recessive condition with a 25% chance of recurrence.

The main purpose of genetic amniocentesis in patients at risk of giving birth to a child with NTD is to obtain amniotic fluid to measure the concentration of alpha fetoprotein (AFP), a normal component of the amniotic fluid that is increased when the fetus has an open NTD.[6] As shown in Fig. 2-2, AFP concentration in the amniotic fluid changes with gestational age, and this makes a precise dating of the pregnancy

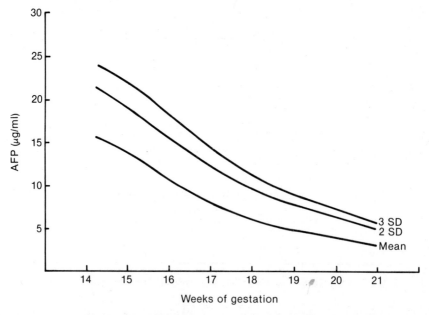

FIG. 2-2 ■ Amniotic fluid alpha fetoprotein concentration at different gestational ages. The lower line corresponds to the mean value for a given gestational age, and the middle and upper lines correspond to 2 and 3 SDs from the mean.

necessary to properly interpret the laboratory test results. The best time to measure AFP is at 16 weeks of gestation. AFP concentration will be higher than 2.5 SD from the mean value at this gestational age in 90% of the patients carrying a fetus with a NTD. The other 10% of affected infants will have closed defects, and the AFP concentration will be normal. The false positive rate for the amniotic fluid AFP test is 0.1% and in most cases is caused by contamination of the sample with fetal serum. The gradient of AFP concentration in fetal serum to amniotic fluid is 200:1. This is the reason for always drawing a maternal serum sample before genetic amniocentesis when amniotic fluid AFP is going to be measured. A normal maternal serum AFP will be reassuring if a high amniotic fluid AFP value is found as a result of fetal blood contamination.

In addition to having amniotic fluid AFP measured, patients at risk of fetal NTD must have a careful evaluation with real-time ultrasound.

This evaluation, which should precede the performance of the amniocentesis, has as its main objective the study of the intracranial anatomy and the fetal spine. The ultrasound examination allows in many cases the detection of affected infants with closed defects who give false negative AFP results.

It is very important to recognize that the meaning of an elevated amniotic fluid AFP value is not the same in patients at high risk for neural tube defects as it is in patients who have AFP measurements carried out as an additional test when the amniotic fluid is obtained for some other indication, ie, maternal age.[14] In the latter case the probability of a false positive result is high, and some corroborative evidence of the presence of a NTD must be sought before pregnancy is terminated. Therefore, when amniotic fluid AFP is abnormally high and determination of fetal hemoglobin in the fluid is negative in a patient who is *not* at high risk for NTD, a high-resolution fetal ultrasound examination must be

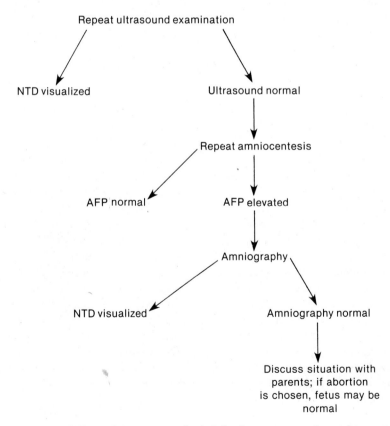

FIG. 2-3 ■ Steps to follow when amniotic fluid alpha fetoprotein is elevated in patients who are not at risk for neural tube defects.

carried out. If no lesion is found with ultrasound, a second amniocentesis must be performed to confirm the AFP elevation. If the second determination is normal, the first value most probably was a false positive. If the second determination shows again an abnormally elevated value, amniography must be performed in a last effort to corroborate the presence of a defect.[2] If the amniography is negative, the situation must be extensively discussed with the parents and the pregnancy should not be terminated unless they fully understand that it is possible that the fetus may be completely normal. A summary of the steps that should be followed in cases of unexpectedly elevated amniotic fluid AFP is shown in Fig. 2-3.

Determination of acetylcholinesterase in the amniotic fluid may also be useful in the assessment of situations with elevated AFP and no corroborative evidence of NTD. A recent paper[35] reports that the authors were capable of reclassifying adequately 89% of normal pregnancies with elevated AFP. Also, some characteristics of the amniotic fluid cells in in vitro cultures may be useful in the diagnosis of NTD.[36]

Unfortunately, 90% of all cases of NTD occur in families with no preceding affected members and under circumstances in which genetic amniocentesis is not indicated and amniotic fluid AFP is not measured. Obviously, what is required is a screening test that could be applied to the entire obstetric population. Determination of AFP in maternal *serum* offers great promise in this respect.[28,56] and, if some difficulties are overcome, this test may be broadly used in the near future.

One of the problems with maternal serum AFP screening is that 7.4% of all screened pregnancies will show elevated serum AFP levels. About one half of these individuals will be found to be normal when a second sample is analyzed. Of the remaining 4.4%, one half will be found to be normal by ultrasound and the other 2.2% will be candidates for amniocentesis and measurement of amniotic fluid AFP. About 1 out of every 10 of these patients will be found to have a fetus with NTD. These figures imply that 4.4% of all pregnancies in the United States will require specialized high-resolution ultrasonic examination of the fetal spine in search of NTD and that 30,000 to 60,000 additional amniocentesis procedures might result every year. This potential demand for services markedly exceeds the presently available ultrasound and laboratory resources.

There are also problems with the serum AFP test itself. This radioimmunoassay is a demanding test, requiring greater precision and attention than other similar procedures and requiring meticulous quality control. If these and other problems with maternal serum screening are solved, this test may become a valuable addition to prenatal management.

Hydrocephaly

Adequate counseling of parents who had a child with hydrocephaly in a prior pregnancy depends on a precise diagnosis of the abnormality. In fact, hydrocephaly may be secondary, among other causes, to aqueductal stenosis, Arnold-Chiari malformation, spina bifida, or Dandy-Walker deformity, or it may have an unknown etiology. Of particular importance is the X-linked form of hydrocephaly secondary to aqueductal stenosis, which has a recurrence risk of 12% for male infants. Other forms of hydrocephaly have a recurrence risk of about 2%.

Evaluation of the patient at risk for recurrent fetal hydrocephaly includes genetic amniocentesis and fetal sex determination in the X-linked form. However, the most important test in these cases is ultrasonic assessment of the fetal intracranial anatomy. Modern high-resolution ultrasound equipment allows measurement of the ventricular width from the beginning of the second trimester of pregnancy and detection of hydrocephalus long before the cranium becomes enlarged. The study of Johnson et al[24] demonstrated that under normal circumstances, as pregnancy advances, the ventricular size decreases significantly in relation to the size of the cerebral hemispheres.

Intrauterine treatment of fetal hydrocephalus using ventriculoamniotic shunts[10] is a spectacular advance in fetal medicine which was made possible by improved ultrasonic visualization of the fetal intracranial anatomy early in gestation. Final assessment of the advantages and risks of this form of therapy requires more extensive experience.

Cleft lip and cleft palate

Cleft lip and cleft palate occur with relatively high frequency (1 out of 1000 newborns), so most obstetricians should expect to be questioned a few times during their professional life about the recurrence risk of these abnormalities of the facial structure. The genetics and the etiology of cleft lip (with or without cleft palate) are different from those of isolated cleft palate. The recurrence risk for the former is 4% with a prior affected child, 10% with two prior affected children, and 10% if one parent and one prior child are both affected. The risk is higher in males and, if the cleft involves both the lip and the palate or is bilateral, this risk is greater than if it is unilateral or involves only the lip.[15] For cleft palate alone the recurrence risk is 2.3% if either one or two prior children are affected. If the parent and one child are affected, the risk of having a second child with cleft palate is 15%. Cleft palate is not predominant among males.[15]

Cleft lip can be detected by examination with high-resolution ultrasound as early as 16 weeks of gestation. This requires a great deal of expertise in the sonographer. However, the usefulness of antenatal diagnosis of cleft lip is in question: there are no ways to correct the problem before birth, and the decision to terminate pregnancy because of this defect is, to say the least, very difficult.

Congenital heart disease

Congenital heart disease occurs in 1 to 2 out of 1000 newborns. The most common types of congenital heart problems are ventricular septal defect, atrial septal defect, tetralogy of Fallot, patent ductus arteriosus, and pulmonary stenosis. Table 2-2 shows the risk of recurrence for several congenital heart problems.[38] In general, the risk of recurrence if one sib is affected is from 2% to 4%, depending on the type of defect. When two prior children are affected, the risk of recurrence rises to 10%.

Theoretically, ultrasound examination of the fetal heart[12] is the methodology offering the most promise for the antenatal detection of congenital heart problems. In practice, however, the advance has not been as rapid and spectacular as in other areas of fetal diagnosis.

Cystic fibrosis

Cystic fibrosis is a relatively common disorder (1 out of 2500 births) that is genetically transmitted as an autosomal recessive trait. The disease is very rare in Orientals and blacks. Cystic

TABLE 2-2 ■ Recurrent risk of some congenital heart diseases

Anomaly	Risk (%)
Ventricular septal defect	4.4
Atrial septal defect	3.2
Tetralogy of Fallot	2.7
Patent ductus arteriosus	3.4
Pulmonic stenosis	2.9
Aortic stenosis	2.2
Aortic coarctation	1.8

From Nora JJ: Pediatr Clin North Am 1971;18:1059.

TABLE 2-3 ■ Risk of having a child with cystic fibrosis (CF)

One parent	Other parent	Risk of CF in each pregnancy
No CF history	No CF history	1:1600
No CF history	First-degree relative with CF	1:240
No CF history	Sib with CF	1:120
No CF history	Has CF	1:40
Sib with CF	Sib with CF	1:9

Modified from Bowman BH, Mangos JA: N Engl J Med 1976; 294:937. Reprinted by permission.

fibrosis has eluded multiple efforts to develop an adequate test for carrier detection (among Caucasians approximately 1 in 20 individuals is heterozygous for cystic fibrosis) or for intrauterine diagnosis. Table 2-3 shows the risk of having a child with cystic fibrosis based on the prevalence of the disease and the autosomal recessive character of its inheritance.[4]

Recently, measurement of methylumbellilferylguanidobenzoate (MUGB) reactive proteases in the amniotic fluid has been described as a potentially useful method for the antenatal detection of cystic fibrosis.[35a] However, more experience with this test is necessary before it can be adopted in practice.

Sickle cell disease

Ten percent of the black population of the United States is heterozygous for the hemoglobin S gene. If two heterozygous blacks conceive a baby, the chances for such a child to have sickle cell disease are 25%. Fortunately, with recent advances in biochemical analysis and fetoscopy, it is possible to determine prenatally whether or not a baby has sickle cell disease.

Fetoscopy is a procedure consisting of the introduction of an endoscope as thin as a 16-gauge needle inside of the pregnant uterus for the purpose of visualizing the fetus and obtaining fetal blood and fetal skin biopsies. The best time to perform a fetoscopy is at 18 weeks of gestation. Once the chorionic plate of the placenta is visualized, a 26-gauge needle is threaded through a Y side arm in the cannula that contains the endoscope and is advanced under direct vision to a fetal vessel, which is pricked. Fetal blood is collected as it flows from the placental vessel into the amniotic fluid. The fetal blood is analyzed, and the diagnosis of sickle cell disease is made if the normal beta A peak is absent and only beta S is present.[5]

Fetoscopy in the hands of an experienced operator results in the collection of fetal blood successfully in 97% of cases. The procedure has a spontaneous abortion rate of 5% which is five times less than the risk of having an affected baby when both parents are carriers. The error in diagnosis with this technique is less than 1%.

A significant advance in the antenatal diagnosis of sickle cell disease has been made with the use of recombinant DNA techniques. DNA analysis allows the diagnosis of the condition using any fetal cell, since all of them, in an affected subject, must have the sickle cell gene modification. The sickle cell mutation (glutamic acid to valine in position 6 of the beta chain) reflects a change in DNA base sequence which can be accurately diagnosed using restriction endonuclease enzymes and hybridization techniques. Thus diagnosis of sickle cell disease can be made by examination of uncultured cells obtained by routine genetic amniocentesis or using chorionic villae obtained through placental biopsy.[9,58] This methodology has also been applied to the antenatal diagnosis of beta thalassemia.[42] However, the molecular diversity of the thalassemia mutations found in the United States generates considerable difficulties, making analysis of fetal blood the procedure of choice for this particular defect.

Tay-Sachs disease

Tay-Sachs disease is an inborn error of metabolism characterized by the accumulation, primarily in the neurons, of a glycolipid identified as GM_2-ganglioside. The accumulation of this substance is caused by the absence of the isoenzyme hexosaminidase A. The disease causes a cruel, invalidating, progressive deterioration of neurologic function until the infant dies, usually between 3 and 4 years of age.

Tay-Sachs disease occurs predominantly in Jews of Ashkenazi ancestry (central and eastern Europe). One of every 30 Ashkenazi Jews is a carrier for the abnormal gene, and well over 90% of all American Jews are of Ashkenazi origin. Fortunately, the heterozygous state can be recognized by a blood test, and this makes it possible to screen the population at risk. Also, the homozygous state can be recognized antenatally by amniocentesis, culture of fetal fibroblast, and analysis of hexosaminidase A.

Ideally, all Jews of Ashkenazi ancestry must be screened before marriage and pregnancy. If this has not been done and the wife is already pregnant, the husband must be screened. If he is negative (normal activity of serum hexosaminidase A), there is no risk to the fetus. If the husband is a carrier, it is necessary to determine the mother's status by measuring the enzyme activity in her leukocytes, since routine serum screening is unreliable during pregnancy. If the mother is negative, there is no risk to the fetus. If she is positive, amniocentesis must be carried out to determine if the infant is affected or not.

Mental retardation

Occasionally the obstetrician is faced with the need of giving advice to patients about the risk of recurrence of mental retardation. In the majority of cases a correct answer to this request requires careful analysis of the situation by the geneticist. However, the obstetrician may alleviate some of the couple's anxiety by giving them some general information about the subject before their visit to the geneticist.

There are several large categories of patients with mental retardation: about 20% are mentally retarded as a consequence of a chromosomal abnormality, predominantly Down's syndrome; about 20% of retarded males have X-linked mental retardation (fragile X); 10% to 15% of all cases are mentally retarded because of a single gene mutation, a category that includes the inborn errors of metabolism; 5% to 15% are patients with polygenic-multifactorial conditions affect-

TABLE 2-4 ■ Recurrence risk for mild, idiopathic mental retardation

Number of retarded subjects		Recurrence risk (%)
Parents	Children	
0	1	6
1	1	20
2	1	42

ing the development of the central nervous system; 5% to 15% are mentally retarded because of conditions such as intrauterine or neonatal infections and birth trauma. Finally, in a considerable number of cases (5% to 15%), particularly in individuals with mild or moderate mental retardation, no clearly defined etiologic agent can be found. Obviously, the chances of recurrence of mental retardation in a given family will be determined by the etiologic diagnosis. In the idiopathic group, which most probably represents individuals who belong to the lower end of the normal intelligence Gaussian distribution curve, there is a strong familial tendency for mild mental retardation (IQ of 50 to 75), as shown in Table 2-4.

■ **GENETIC ASPECTS OF REPRODUCTIVE WASTAGE**

The patient who has had several spontaneous abortions alone or in combination with stillbirths represents a relatively frequent challenge to the practicing obstetrician. The etiology of this condition is varied, and the chances of recurrence are different depending on the etiologic factors.

Patients with a history of repeated spontaneous abortions can be categorized in two groups depending on the gestational age when the abortion happened. For those in whom the abortion occurred before 12 weeks of gestation, the predominant etiology (in more than 60% of the cases) is a chromosomal defect. For those in whom the abortion occurred during the second trimester, chromosomal defects still will be an important factor (about 30% of the cases), but other causes such as incompetent cervix, anomalies of the uterine cavity, and infection will be predominant.

The chromosomal abnormalities most frequently found in first-trimester abortions are as follows:

1. *Autosomal trisomy* is a nondisjunctional defect that affects predominantly chromosome 16, although theoretically it may affect any of the autosomes; it is found in about 50% of all the abortions with chromosomal abnormalities. A large number of abortions associated with chromosomal trisomy are empty sacs (blighted ovum).
2. In *monosomy X* about 25% of all abortions with chromosomal abnormalities have a karyotype 45 X. About 1 out of every 15 fetuses with 45 X karyotype will not be aborted and will be identified after birth as individuals with Turner's syndrome. More than 60% of the abortion specimens with 45 X karyotype are sacs containing a small umbilical cord which finishes in an amorphous mass of embryonic tissue. Monosomy X may be the result of the loss of a chromosome X at the time of fertilization or may be the result of nondisjunction during either male or female meiosis.
3. *Triploidy,* a mean chromosomal count of 69, is seen in 15% to 20% of all abortions with chromosomal abnormalities. In many cases the sac is empty (blighted ovum), but if a fetus is present, it has obvious abnormalities (omphalocele, syndactyly, cleft lip and palate, etc.). In about 50% of the cases hydropic degeneration of the placenta is present. In humans the most common reason for triploidy is double fertilization of a single ovum.
4. *Tetrapolidy,* a mean chromosomal count of 92, is found in 3% to 6% of all abortions with chromosomal abnormalities. In these cases abortion occurs very early and the embryo cannot be recognized in the abortion specimen. This condition probably results from a failure of cytoplasmic division following a chromosome division in the germinal cells.
5. *Structural rearrangements of the chromosomes* and particularly unbalanced translocations and inversions account for 3% to 5% of abortions with chromosomal abnormalities.

The risk of spontaneous abortion to a woman with no history of reproductive wastage is about 12%. The study of Poland et al[43] indicates that the likelihood of a repeated abortion after a first spontaneous abortion for a woman with no living children is 19%; however, if there is a history of two consecutive spontaneous abortions, the risk increases to 35% and if the history is of three consecutive spontaneous abortions, the likelihood of a repeated abortion is 47%. These figures reveal a higher risk for recurrent abortion than those commonly quoted from the work of Warburton and Fraser,[57] which was limited to women who had at least one live-born child. In this latter situation—when there is at least one liveborn child—the risk of subsequent abortion is between 24% to 32% irrespective of the number of previous abortions. This information is summarized in Table 2-5.

In the past a woman was classified as a habitual aborter after three spontaneous abortions, and only then were efforts made to find the etiology of the problem. Today, with advances in our understanding of the problem, the diagnostic workup may be started earlier. Our approach is as follows:

1. Every patient with symptoms of threatened abortion is examined with ultrasound to determine the characteristics of the gestational sac and the presence of a fetal pole. If no fetal pole is detected at a time in gestation when it should be recognized (7 to 8 weeks), the most probable diagnosis is blighted ovum. After the abortion the products of conception are sent to the pathologist to confirm the absence of fetal parts.
2. Patients with a confirmed or strongly suggestive history of blighted ovum in a prior pregnancy are monitored with ultrasound early in the following gestation, and if a blighted ovum is present again, the patient is sent to the geneticist for determination of maternal and paternal karyotypes.

Poland et al[42] suggested initiating the evaluation of parental karyotype, hormonal status, and uterine environment after the second spontaneous abortion when both abortions have shown evidence of marked disorganization of the embryonic growth. Andrews and Roberts[1] found that one partner had a major chromosomal anomaly in 6.7% of 120 couples with at least two spontaneous abortions.

With respect to stillbirths, 5% to 10% of them have chromosomal abnormalities. Ideally, a careful gross autopsy should be performed in all

TABLE 2-5 ■ Risk of spontaneous abortion

Number of consecutive abortions	Risk of subsequent abortion (%)
No previous liveborn child	
0	12.3
1	19.0
2	35.0
3	47.0
At least one liveborn child	
0	12.3
1	23.7
2	26.2
3	32.2

cases of stillbirth, and chromosomal analysis performed if the autopsy reveals congenital anomalies. A history of recurrent stillbirths or early abortions and stillbirths is highly suspicious of chromosomal abnormalities in the parents, and genetic counseling must be offered to the couple.

■ SOME ANSWERS TO TERATOLOGIC QUESTIONS

Present-day society and individual patients are very concerned about teratogenic influences. The wide publicity given to the DES problem and the thalidomide tragedy are responsible to a large extent for this widespread concern about fetal safety from medications and other environmental influences. Thus frequently patients ask the obstetrician questions about possible embryotoxic or fetotoxic effects of drugs, nutrients, or other influences. The most frequently asked questions deal with (1) the teratogenicity of diagnostic x-ray procedures; (2) the teratogenicity of some medications prescribed during pregnancy; and (3) the teratogenicity of some other factors such as coffee, alcohol, and vaginal spermicides.

Diagnostic radiation and pregnancy

The frequency of radiation exposure in pregnancy was approximately 1% in one study carried out in the middle 1960s.[7] That frequency is probably much less at the present time because of the awareness of both patients and physicians and because of the replacement of many obstetric radiologic procedures with ultrasound.

TABLE 2-6 ■ Fetal dose* during some x-ray examinations

Type of examination	Dose (rads per examination)	
	Mean	Range
Flat plate of the abdomen	0.144	0.024-1.416
X-ray of the pelvis	0.158	0.008-1.587
Intravenous pyelogram	0.448	0.024-3.069
Barium enema	0.574	0.005-3.9218
Upper gastrointestinal series	0.091	0.001-1.228
Lumbar spine	0.608	0.002-2.901

From Hoffman D, Felten R, Cyr W: *Effects of ionizing radiation on the developing embryo and fetus: a review,* HHS publication FDA 81-8170. Rockville, Md, US Department of Health and Human Sciences, Public Health Service, Food and Drug Administration, Bureau of Radiological Health, 1981.

*Assuming that fetal dose is similar to ovarian dose.

However, once in a while the obstetrician has to counsel a patient who has had diagnostic radiologic procedures during gestation and who wants to know the fetal risks associated with those procedures.

The effects of x-ray radiation on the fetus are highly variable and depend on multiple factors, the most important being gestational age at the time of exposure and the amount of radiation received by the fetus. Gestational age is important because the chances of affecting the fetus are greater in early than in late pregnancy. Particularly important seems to be the period of organogenesis (2 to 7 weeks' postconception, 4 to 9 weeks from the last menstrual period) because of the possibility that ionizing radiation may interfere with organ development and cause malformations. The amount of radiation received by the fetus is also an important variable that changes depending on the type of x-ray examination, the number of films taken, the type of equipment used, the area of the body where the x-ray beam was directed, etc.[21] As shown in Table 2-6, the amount of radiation received by the fetus in the course of most routine diagnostic examinations rarely exceeds 5 rad and is often less than 2 rad.[19] Obviously, the possibility of adverse effects on the fetus at these radiation doses is minimal.

Patients are also concerned about the possibility that intrauterine exposure to x-ray may cause an increased risk of developing leukemia during childhood. According to Stewart et al,[55] this risk is 2 per 2000 women per rad, while the risk for a nonradiated individual is 1 per 2000 women per rad. These figures are old and should be reviewed.

The most important fact in counseling patients who have received radiation during pregnancy is to reassure them that the risk of malformation is not greater than the risk for a pregnancy that has not been exposed to x-ray unless the patient has received a dose larger than 10 rad.[16] Naturally, it is impossible to guarantee that the fetus will not have a congenital malformation.

Potential teratogenicity of some medications commonly used during pregnancy

Bendectin. Bendectin was commonly used for the treatment of nausea and vomiting in pregnancy, and since most of its use was during early pregnancy, the potential embryotoxic effect of this product was extensively studied. One of the best studies[48] found no harmful effect on the morphology or the outcome of infants whose mothers took Bendectin during pregnancy as compared with controls who did not take the medication. Other studies reached a similar conclusion. However, because of medicolegal pressures, this compound was retired from the United States market by its manufacturer.

Phenytoin. Anticonvulsant therapy is frequently used during pregnancy in patients affected by seizure disorders. It seems that when diphenylhydantoin (Dilantin) is consumed during pregnancy, it causes a twofold to fivefold increase in the frequency of congenital malformations, particularly cleft lip and cleft palate.[17,22] A "fetal hydantoin syndrome" has been described as characterized by growth retardation, mental retardation, upward slant of the eyebrows, nail or distal phalanx hypoplasia, hernias, and depressed nasal bridge. In view of the increasing evidence suggesting phenytoin embryotoxicity, the present recommendation from the American College of Obstetricians and Gynecologists is to use the less teratogenic anticonvulsant phenobarbital during pregnancy. If phenytoin is necessary for seizure control, the medication must be used in the smallest dose compatible with an adequate clinical response.

Corticosteroids. Although glucocorticoids are potent palatal teratogens in experimental animals, there is no evidence that they cause congenital malformations when administered during human pregnancy.[3] This fact should help to decrease the anxiety of some mothers in whom glucocorticoid treatment is being considered to improve fetal lung maturation. Also, when glucocorticoids are given for the purpose of accelerating the production of pulmonary surfactant, they are administered late in gestation, several weeks after organ and limb development has taken place.

Metronidazole. Metronidazole (Flagyl) is used during pregnancy for the treatment of symptomatic *Trichomonas vaginalis* infections. It is a mutagenic agent in a bacterial test system and is also a carcinogenic agent in rodents. There is no evidence that this drug increases the risk of congenital malformations in humans.[40] However, it is advisable to use symptomatic treatment for *Trichomonas* infection early in pregnancy and postpone therapy with metronidazole until the patient is at or beyond 20 weeks of gestation.

Clomiphene. There is evidence in the literature suggesting that chromosome abnormalities are increased in pregnancies that follow induced ovulation.[39] This may be caused by an increase in meiotic nondisjunctions. Further research in this area is necessary, but in the meantime it is necessary to inform women conceiving after clomiphene (Clomid) therapy that the possibility of chromosome abnormalities exists and that genetic amniocentesis is available.

Vaginal spermicides. One study found an excess of limb reduction deformities and syndromes associated with chromosomal abnormalities among the live-born infants of women who used a vaginal spermicide in the 10 months before conception when compared with control patients not using spermicides.[23] The data from the Collaborative Perinatal Project, however, give no evidence of this association.[49] It seems that, if any risk exists, it is of very low magnitude.

Coffee. The United States Food and Drug Administration, concerned about the possibility of caffeine causing birth defects, particularly limb reduction defects, in 1980 advised pregnant women to avoid caffeine-containing food and drugs during pregnancy. Two subsequent studies[26,44] have presented evidence strongly suggesting that coffee consumption during pregnancy has a minimal or no effect on the outcome of the pregnancy.

Smoking and alcohol. Although evidence incriminating smoking as a cause of congenital malformations is not solid, maternal smoking during pregnancy causes intrauterine growth retardation and an increase in the incidence of stillborn infants.[45,53] Obstetricians must advise pregnant women to discontinue smoking permanently or at least while they are pregnant. For information about the embryotoxic effects of alcohol, see Chapter 1.

Minor tranquilizers. Three studies[33,46,47] have suggested that an association exists between the ingestion of minor tranquilizers (meprobamate, chlordiazepoxide, diazepam) and increased risk of congenital anomalies. Another study[18] has failed to confirm the existence of such an association. Since the use of these drugs during pregnancy, particularly in the period of organogenesis, is not urgent or necessary, they should be avoided.

■ **REFERENCES**

1. Andrews T, Roberts DF: Chromosome analysis in couples with repeated pregnancy loss. J Biosoc Sci 1982; 14:33.
2. Balsam D, Weiss RR: Amniography in prenatal diagnosis. Radiology 1981; 141:379.
3. Bongiovanni AM, McPadden AJ: Steroids during pregnancy and possible fetal consequences. Fertil Steril 1960; 11:181.
4. Bowman BH, Mangos JA: Cystic fibrosis. N Engl J Med 1976; 294:937.
5. Alter BP, Friedman S, Hobbins JC, et al: Prenatal diagnosis of sickle-cell anemia and alpha G-Philadelphia. New Engl J Med 1976; 294:1040.
6. Brock DJH, Sutcliffe RG: Alpha-fetoprotein in the antenatal diagnosis of anencephaly and spina bifida. Lancet 1972; 2:197.
7. Brown M, Roney P, Gitlin J, et al: X-ray experience during pregnancy. JAMA 1967; 199:87.
8. Carter CO, Lawrence KM, David PA: The genetics of the major central nervous system malformations, based on the South Wales socio-genetic investigation. Dev Med Child Neurol 1967; 13(suppl):30.
9. Chang CJ, Kan YW: Antenatal diagnosis of sickle cell anemia by direct analysis of the sickle mutation. Lancet 1981; 2:1127.
10. Clewell WH, Johnson ML, Meier PR, et al: A surgical approach to the treatment of fetal hydrocephalus. N Engl J Med 1982; 306:1320.
11. *Congenital malformations surveillance report,* July 1976-June 1977. Center for Disease Control, Dec 1977, p 25.

12. Filkens KA, Brown TA, Levine OR: Real time ultrasonic evaluation of the fetal heart. Int J Obstet Gynecol 1981; 19:35.

13. Golbus MS, Loughman WD, Epstein CJ, et al: Prenatal genetic diagnosis in 3000 amniocentesis. N Engl J Med 1979; 300:157.

14. Goldberg MF, Oakley GP: Interpreting elevated amniotic fluid alpha-fetoprotein levels in clinical practice; use of the predictive value positive concept. Am J Obstet Gynecol 1979; 133:126.

15. Habib Z: Genetic counseling and genetics of cleft lip and cleft palate. Obstet Gynecol Surv 1978; 33:441.

16. Hammer-Jacobsen E: Therapeutic abortion on account of X-ray. Dan Med Bull 1959; 6:113.

17. Hanson JW, Mirianthopoulos NC, Harvey MAS, et al: Risk to the offspring of women treated with hydantoin anticonvulsants with emphasis on the fetal hydantoin syndrome. J Pediatr 1976; 89:662.

18. Hartz CS, Heinonen OP, Shapiro S, et al: Antenatal exposure to meprobamate and chlordiazepoxide in relation to malformations, mental development and childhood mortality. N Engl J Med 1975; 292:726.

19. Hoffman D, Felten R, Cyr W: *Effects of ionizing radiation on the developing embryo and fetus: a review*, HHS publication FDA 81-8170. Rockville, Md, US Dept of Health and Human Sciences, Public Health Service, Food and Drug Administration, Bureau of Radiological Health, 1981.

20. Holmes LB: Genetic counseling for the older pregnant woman: new data and questions. N Engl J Med 1978; 298:1419.

21. Jacobson A, Conley J: Estimation of fetal dose to patients undergoing diagnostic X-ray procedures. Radiology 1976; 120:683.

22. Janz D: The teratogenic risk of antiepileptic drugs. Epilepsia 1975; 16:159.

23. Jick H, Walker AM, Rothman KJ, et al: Vaginal spermicides and congenital disorders. JAMA 1981; 245:1329.

24. Johnson ML, Dunne MG, Mack LA, et al: Evaluation of fetal intracraneal anatomy by static and real-time ultrasound. J Clin Ultrasound 1980; 8:311.

25. Kuroki Y, Yamamoto Y, Matsui I, et al: Down syndrome and maternal age in Japan 1950-1973. Clin Genet 1977; 12:43.

26. Linn S, Schoenbaum SC, Monson RR, et al: No association between coffee consumption and adverse outcomes of pregnancy. N Engl J Med 1982; 306:141.

27. Magenis RE, Overton KM, Chamberlin J, et al: Parental origin of the extrachromosome in Down's syndrome. Hum Genet 1977; 37:7.

28. Masri JN, Haddow JE, Weiss RR: Screening for neural tube defects in the United States: a summary of the Scarborough Conference. Am J Obstet Gynecol 1979; 133:119.

29. Matsunaga E, Tonamura A, Oishi H, et al: Reexamination of paternal age effect in Down's syndrome. Hum Genet 1978; 40:259.

30. Medical Research Council Working Party on Amniocentesis: an assessment of the hazards of amniocentesis. Br J Obstet Gynaecol 1978; 85(suppl 2):1.

31. Mikkelsen M, Fisher G, Stene J, et al: Incidence study of Down's syndrome in Copenhagen 1960-1971: with chromosome investigation. Ann Hum Genet 1976; 40:177.

32. Mikkelsen M, Stene J: Genetic counseling in Down's syndrome. Hum Hered 1970; 20:457.

33. Milkovich L, van de Berg BJ: Effects of prenatal meprobamate and chlordiazepoxide hydrochloride on human embryonic and fetal development. N Engl J Med 1974; 291:1268.

34. Milunski A: Amniocentesis, in Milunski A (ed): *Genetic disorders and the fetus*, New York, Plenum Press, 1979, p 93.

35. Milunski A, Sapirstein VS: Prenatal diagnosis of open neural tube defects using the amniotic fluid acetylcholinesterase assay. Obstet Gynecol 1982; 59:1.

35a. Nadler HL, Walsh MJ: Intrauterine detection of cystic fibrosis. Pediatrics 1980; 66:690.

36. Narrod MJE, Friedman JM, Jimez J, et al: Rapidly adhering amniotic-fluid cells and prenatal diagnosis of neural tube defects. Lancet 1979; 2:99.

37. National Institute of Child Health and Human Development National Amniocentesis Study Group: Midtrimester amniocentesis for prenatal diagnosis—safety and accuracy. JAMA 1976; 236:1471.

38. Nora JJ: Etiologic factors in congenital heart disease. Pediatr Clin North Am 1971; 18:1059.

39. Oakley GP, Flynt JW: Increased prevalence of Down's syndrome (mongolism) among the offspring of women treated with ovulation-inducing agents. Teratology 1972; 5:264.

40. Peterson WF, Stauch JE, Ryder CD: Metronidazole in pregnancy. Am J Obstet Gynecol 1976; 126:543.

41. Piniuk AJ, Beaudet AL, Bucknall WE: Down's syndrome: changes in the incidence and contribution of advanced maternal age women. Clin Res 1975; 24:64A.

42. Pirastu M, Yuet WK, Cao A, et al: Prenatal diagnosis of B-thalasemia: detection of a single nucleotide mutation in DNA. N Engl J Med, 1983; 309:284.

43. Poland BJ, Miller JR, Jones DC, et al: Reproductive counseling in patients who have had a spontaneous abortion. Am J Obstet Gynecol 1977; 127:685.

44. Rosenberg L, Mitchel AA, Shapiro S, et al: Selected birth defects in relation to caffeine-containing beverages. JAMA 1982; 247:1429.

45. Rush D, Kaas EH: Maternal smoking: a reassessment of the association with perinatal mortality. Am J Epidemiol 1972; 96:183.

46. Saxen I: Association between oral clefts and drugs taken during pregnancy. Int J Epidemiol 1975; 4:37.

47. Safara MJ, Oakley GP: Association between cleft lip with or without cleft palate and prenatal exposure to diazepam. Lancet 1975; 2:478.

48. Shapiro S, Heinonen OP, Siskind V, et al: Antenatal exposure to doxylamine succinate and dicyclomine hydrochloride (Bendectin) in relation to congenital malformations, perinatal mortality, birth weight, and intelligence quotient score. Am J Obstet Gynecol 1977; 128:480.

49. Shapiro S, Stone D, Heinonen OP, et al: Birth defects and vaginal spermicides. JAMA 1982; 247:2381.

50. Simpson, JL, Golbus MS, Martin AO, et al (eds): *Genetics in obstetrics and gynecology*. New York, Grune & Stratton Inc., 1982, p 58.

51. Simpson JL, Golbus MS, Martin AO, et al: *Genetics in obstetrics and gynecology*. New York, Grune & Stratton Inc., 1982, p. 80.

52. Simpson NE, Dallaire L, Miller JR, et al: Prenatal diagnosis of genetic disease in Canada: report of a collaborative study. Can Med Assoc J 1976; 115:739.

53. Simpson WJA: A preliminary report on cigarette smoking and the incidence of prematurity. Am J Obstet Gynecol 1957; 73:808.

54. Stene J, Fischer G, Stene E, et al: Paternal age effect in Down's syndrome. Ann Hum Genet 1977; 40:299.

55. Stewart A, Webb J, Hewitt D: A survey of childhood malignancies. Br Med J 1958; 1:1495.

56. United Kingdom Collaborative Study on alpha-fetoprotein in relation to neural tube defects: maternal serum alpha-fetoprotein measurement in antenatal screening for anencephaly and spina bifida in early pregnancy. Lancet 1977; 1:1323.

57. Warburton D, Fraser FC: Spontaneous abortion risks in man: data from reproductive histories collected in a medical genetics unit. Am J Hum Genet 1964; 16:1.

58. Williamson R, Eskdale J, Coleman DV, et al: Direct gene analysis of chorionic villae: a possible technique for first trimester antenatal diagnosis of hemoglobinopathies. Lancet 1981; 2:1125.

3

■ ■ ■

PRETERM LABOR

Fernando Arias

Preterm labor is an important obstetric complication associated with high perinatal mortality and morbidity. Unfortunately, the literature on this subject has an abundance of unsubstantiated assumptions and a confusion in definitions that make it difficult to interpret and compare data obtained at different institutions or at different times within the same institution. A common erroneous assumption is that the majority of low birth weight infants (weighing less than 2500 grams) and preterm infants (born before 37 completed weeks of gestation) are the consequence of preterm labor of unknown origin. Preterm labor is only one of several conditions that may cause the birth of a low birth weight or preterm infant. In about 30% of the cases it is possible to find an etiologic factor for preterm labor. A further example of a common confusion is the assumption that all low birth weight infants are preterm; whereas, in reality a good number of these infants are beyond 37 weeks of gestation.

Much of the confusion in terminology has a historical origin. In 1948 the first World Health Assembly of the League of Nations defined premature as all infants with a birth weight under 2500 grams. This definition was and still is extremely useful because it identifies by means of a simple measurement a group of newborns at high risk of death and neonatal complications. Unfortunately, the definition is incorrect because the correlation between infant weight and functional maturity (the characteristic intrinsic to the term premature) is poor. In fact many infants with birth weight under 2500 grams show evidence of advanced maturity and should not be called premature. On the other hand, some babies (the typical example is the infant of the mother with diabetes) may be developmentally immature in spite of having a large birth weight.

In an attempt to correct the deficiencies of the 1948 definition, the World Health Organization recommended in 1972 that the term premature should no longer be used. Babies should be described in terms of either birth weight or gestational age. With this definition any infant weighing less than 2500 grams at birth should be called low birth weight. Any infant born before 37 completed weeks (less than 259 days) from the first day of the mother's last menstrual period (LMP) should be classified as preterm. Unfortunately, a definition of preterm based on the mother's LMP is not adequate because a large proportion of obstetric patients cite unreliable dates. This occurs mainly because of poor recollection of the incident, because they have ingested oral contraceptives shortly before pregnancy, or because of physiologic variation in the normal length of the menstrual cycle. An assessment of gestational age based on clinical and neurologic examination of the newborn[12] is much more precise. This has become standard in recent studies on preterm labor and preterm

37

infants although the World Health Organization definition remains unchanged.

When the correlation between birth weight and gestational age (as determined by clinical examination of the newborn) was analyzed, a new dimension was added to the knowledge about preterm infants. In fact it was found[32] that any newborn (term or preterm) may belong to one of the following three categories: (1) small for gestational age or SGA, (2) adequate for gestational age or AGA, and (3) large for gestational age or LGA. This finding added more complexity to the analysis of preterm infants and revealed another deficiency of the low birth weight classification. According to the new concept, a preterm infant may be large for gestational age and have a birth weight larger than 2500 grams. In this case the intant is erroneously designated as *term* on the basis of body weight.

An important source of confusion in any study of preterm labor is the definition of preterm labor and especially the definition of threatened preterm labor. Actually, the occurrence of frequent, regular, and painful uterine contractions before term (threatened premature labor) may correspond to a simple episode of false labor that resolves spontaneously and poses no threat on the continuation of the pregnancy. This outcome is possible even in cases in which cervical changes occur (preterm labor) because the contractions and the cervical changes may stop spontaneously and the pregnancy continue to term. This difficulty in separating cases of false labor from cases of true preterm labor introduces a confusing factor in the analysis of the problem and especially in the evaluation of the effectiveness of labor-inhibiting drugs.

Another source of confusion is that many studies group together patients with preterm rupture of the membranes and those with preterm labor and intact membranes. These are two different syndromes closely related to the overall problem of preterm birth and should be analyzed independently. Studies in which both conditions are considered as a single entity obscure rather than clarify the issues.

All of the previously mentioned factors and some others, such as the continuous improvement in neonatal care for small babies, make it difficult to evaluate precisely the contribution of preterm labor to perinatal mortality and morbidity. Most of the available data come from studies of low birth weight infants and reflect the contribution to the perinatal mortality and morbidity of multiple etiologic factors (preterm rupture of the membranes, fetal abnormalities, placenta previa, preterm labor, etc) rather than that of preterm labor alone.

The following are causes of low birth weight.
1. Premature rupture of the fetal membranes
2. Preterm labor
   a. Of unknown origin
   b. Secondary (urinary tract infections [UTIs], maternal febrile processes, amniotic fluid infection with intact membranes, uterine abnormalities, trauma, fetal congenital abnormalities, amniocentesis, placental pathology)
3. Preterm delivery because of fetal or maternal problems
   a. Placenta previa
   b. Hypertensive disease
   c. Abruptio placenta
   d. Fetal distress
4. Incompetent cervix
5. Multiple pregnancy
6. Infants small for gestational age

In one study carried out in South Africa,[35] preterm births accounted for 11% of all births and for 81% of the total early neonatal mortality not attributable to lethal malformations. Preterm labor was accountable for almost half of all these preterm deliveries and for 52% of all the early neonatal deaths. In a similar study from Oxford, England,[36] preterm delivery accounted for 5.1% of all births and (similar to the African study) was responsible for 85% of all early neonatal deaths. Preterm labor of unknown origin caused 38% of all preterm neonatal deaths. The difference in the prevalence of preterm delivery between Africa and England found in these studies is not surprising. As discussed later, there is a wide variation in the occurrence of preterm birth from country to country and among different ethnic and socioeconomic groups. More striking was the difference in the contribution of preterm labor to neonatal mortality—52% in South Africa and 35% in England—most probably reflecting differences in neonatal care. Unfortunately, no mention is made in any of these two papers about preterm rupture of the membranes as an etiologic agent of preterm delivery; patients with this condition were probably included in the "preterm labor of unknown etiol-

TABLE 3-1 ■ Approximate neonatal survival of preterm infants born in a tertiary care center

Gestational age (weeks)	Weight range (grams)	Survivors (%)
25 to 26	500 to 750	35
27 to 28	751 to 1000	70
29 to 30	1001 to 1250	80
31 to 32	1251 to 1500	85
33 to 34	1501 to 1750	90
35 to 36	1751 to 2000	98

TABLE 3-2 ■ Approximate incidence of major neurologic handicaps* in preterm infants who survive after being born in a tertiary care center

Gestational age at birth (weeks)	Birth weight range (grams)	With major neurologic handicap (%)
25 to 27	500 to 1000	25
28 to 32	1001 to 1500	15
32 to 34	1501 to 1750	8

*Intelligence quotient below 70, definite cerebral palsy, severe deafness, or visual loss.

ogy" group, thus introducing unreliability to the figures just mentioned.

In Washington University-Barnes Hospital Medical Center the prevalence of low birth weight infants is 12.8%. This is twice the national average (6%), reflecting that the hospital is a perinatal referral center for a large area of Missouri and Illinois. Preterm labor of unknown origin accounts for only 24.5% of all preterm deliveries.[4] The explanation for the relatively small contribution of preterm labor to the overall problem of low birth weight is that patients with rupture of the bag of waters several hours before the onset of labor were considered as a different group.

Irrespective of the cause of preterm delivery, neonatal survival for these infants is directly related to their gestational age and birth weight. Table 3-1 shows the approximate neonatal survival that should be expected in most institutions with adequate intensive neonatal facilities. Table

3-2 shows the approximate percent of survivors with major neurologic handicaps. Figures better than those shown in the tables have already been reached in certain institutions.[7,40] Despite all these advances, the most efficient system to decrease the current perinatal mortality and morbidity figures is to keep the fetus inside the uterus until it reaches a minimum of 1400 grams or 32 weeks of gestational age.[4] This implies the prevention and adequate treatment of preterm labor, preterm rupture of the membranes, and some maternal and/or fetal problems such as multiple gestation and preeclampsia, important etiologic agents of preterm delivery.

■ DEFINITIONS

prematurity Term used in the past to designate infants with a birth weight under 2500 grams. The term implies birth before maturity and should not be used.

preterm Infant born before 37 completed weeks of gestation. The weeks of gestation may be determined by calculation from the mother's LMP—a procedure that is frequently in error—or by examination of the newborn.

low birth weight Infant weighing under 2500 grams at birth. May be preterm, term (between 37 and 42 weeks) or postterm (more than 42 weeks of gestation).

adequate for gestational age (AGA) Infant with somatic development (weight, length, head circumference) adequate for his or her gestational age as determined by neonatal examination. AGA infants may be preterm, term, or postterm.

small for gestational age (SGA) Infant with somatic development below the 10th percentile of the normal variation for gestational age as determined by neonatal examination. The SGA infant may be preterm, term, or postterm.

large for gestational age (LGA) Infant with somatic development above the 90th percentile of the normal variation for gestational age as determined by neonatal examination. LGA infants may be preterm, term, or postterm.

premature labor Term designating the onset of labor before term but meaning labor before maturity; it should not be used.

preterm labor Labor (regular, painful, frequent uterine contractions causing progressive effacement and dilation of the cervix) occurring before 37 completed weeks of gestation.

threatened preterm labor Regular, painful uterine contractions occurring before 37 completed weeks of gestation and having a frequency of at least three contractions in 10 minutes.

■ MATERNAL AND FETAL CONSEQUENCES OF PRETERM LABOR

Maternal mortality and morbidity as consequences of preterm labor are rare. The most common effect on the patient is the emotional upset and feelings of inadequacy at fulfilling a reproductive role. This situation is more common in women who have suffered repeated pregnancy losses.

In contrast with the good immediate maternal prognosis, the effect of preterm labor on the fetus is devastating; neonatal mortality is high and neonatal morbidity is frequent and severe. To cover adequately the large number of problems that may occur in preterm infants as a consequence of being delivered too early is beyond the scope of this book. However, it is necessary to look closely at neonatal respiratory distress syndrome (RDS) and at intracranial bleeding because these two problems are the most important causes of neonatal mortality and morbidity in the preterm infant.

RDS

Neonatal RDS is a clinical situation characterized by grunting, retraction, nasal flaring, cyanosis in room air, and requiring oxygen to maintain an adequate partial arterial oxygen pressure. There are multiple causes for RDS such as (1) transient tachypnea of the newborn caused by wet lungs or transient intrapartum asphyxia; (2) congenital pneumonia as a result of intrauterine infection; and (3) congenital defects such as diaphragmatic hernia and Potter's syndrome. However, the most important etiologic factor is hyaline membrane disease (HMD). Chest x-ray films are essential in differentiating HMD from other causes of RDS.

The cause of HMD is inadequate production of pulmonary surfactant by the alveolar cells type II of the newborn. The surfactant is a heterogeneous mixture of lipids and proteins in which the predominant component is the phospholipid dipalmitoyl phosphatidylcholine. The surfactant spreads on the lung tissue–air interface, prevents a complete alveolar collapse during expiration, and allows the alveoli to open easily at the next inspiration. If surfactant is not present in adequate amounts, the alveoli collapse during expiration and every inspiration requires considerable effort. This situation rapidly leads to fatigue of the newborn, decreased respiratory effort, hypoxia, cyanosis, acidosis, and eventually death.

Dipalmitoyl phosphatidylcholine, also known as dipalmitoyl lecithin (DPL), is the main component of the pulmonary surfactant. After its synthesis in alveolar cells type II, DPL accumulates in osmiophilic structures called *lamellar bodies* that consist of multiple, closely packed phospholipid bilayers. The lamellar bodies are released from the cells into the alveolar fluid, and from there they eventually go into the amniotic fluid. Therefore it is possible to assess the biochemical maturation of the fetal lung by studying the amniotic fluid phospholipids. The incorporation of this fact into the day-to-day management of obstetric patients has been one of the most significant advances in reproductive medicine in this century.

The first reliable test to determine the biochemical maturation of the fetal lung was the measurement of the lecithin to sphingomyelin (L/S) ratio in the amniotic fluid.[19] This determination involves extraction of the centrifuged amniotic fluid with chloroform/methanol, precipitation of surface-acting phospholipids with cold acetone, and determination of the L/S ratio in the cold acetone precipitate by means of thin layer chromatography. The finding of a mature L/S ratio (2:1 or greater) in an amniotic fluid specimen is predictive of the absence of RDS, and that prediction is accurate in 95% of the cases. The remaining 5% of the cases in which the prediction is incorrect are infants born to mothers with diabetes or infants born after significant episodes of intrapartum asphyxia. However, the L/S ratio is not a good predictor of RDS when the value indicates lack of maturity (L/S less than 2:1). In this situation only 54% of the infants do develop RDS. This high proportion of false predictions of fetal pulmonary immaturity is a serious defect of the L/S ratio because pregnancies in which early delivery is desirable may be prolonged unnecessarily. The L/S ratio test is also noninformative if the amniotic fluid is contaminated with blood or meconium.

The 5% false positive answers with the L/S ratio (the baby develops RDS in spite of a mature ratio) can be corrected by determining the presence of phosphatidyl glycerol (PG) in the amniotic fluid sample. According to Gluck,[30,31] if

PG is present in a sample with mature L/S ratio (2:1 or greater), the infant will not develop RDS even if pregnancy was complicated by diabetes or intrapartum asphyxia. The appearance of PG in the amniotic fluid (usually occurring after 36 weeks of gestation) is the marker of the *final* or *late* biochemical maturation of the fetal lung. However, the simultaneous determination of the L/S ratio and PG does not improve the reliability of the method when the specimen is contaminated with blood or meconium. How PG works is unknown although it has been suggested that it may play a role in stabilizing the surfactant complex.

Another quantitative method of amniotic fluid phospholipid analysis has been developed in the last few years, and it may be used instead of the L/S ratio to assess fetal lung maturity in contaminated specimens and complicated pregnancies. The method involves the quantification of DPL in the amniotic fluid.[42] DPL is produced in the fetal lung and is not present in blood, meconium, or in vaginal secretions so that its concentration in the amniotic fluid cannot be changed by contamination with these biologic products. The method of determining DPL exploits the fact that this compound may be separated from other phospholipids because its unsaturated fatty acids can be selectively oxidized and the chromatographic mobility changed. A concentration of DPL greater than 500 μg/dl is predictive of fetal lung maturation. A comparison between DPL and L/S ratio determinations in amniotic fluid from complicated pregnancies or in fluid containing contaminants[42] showed significant advantages for the DPL method, which had a 97% positive predictive value (90% for the L/S ratio) and an 83% negative predictive value (55.5% for the L/S ratio). Therefore it seems that in certain situations (diabetes or fluid stained with blood or meconium) determination of PG or DPL in the amniotic fluid may be the best way of evaluating fetal lung maturity.

Some other methods may be used as substitutes for the L/S ratio. One of them is easy to perform and when positive (predicting maturity), its reliability is close to 100%. This technique is the so-called *shake test* that qualitatively estimates the stability of the bubbles formed after shaking a mixture of amniotic fluid with ethanol. A simple method for the performance of the shake test is shown in the box below. As just mentioned, the reliability of a mature shake test is almost 100%. Unfortunately, a negative test is not predictive of lung immaturity; if the shake test is negative, the fluid should be analyzed by the L/S ratio or by DPL or PG determination.

The shake test

MATERIALS

Kimax glass tubes measuring 5 cm × 1.3 cm and 95% ethanol.

PROCEDURE

Freshly obtained amniotic fluid (1 ml) is dispensed into a glass tube containing 1 ml of 95% ethanol. Recap the tube, and shake it vigorously for 30 seconds. Allow to settle for 15 seconds, and examine the air-fluid interface.

INTERPRETATION

The presence of an uninterrupted ring of bubbles around the entire meniscus of the tube is interpreted as positive. Anything less is negative.

PREDICTIVE VALUE

A positive test means that the chances of adequate fetal lung maturation are almost 100%. A negative test is unreliable because of the high number of false negative results (erroneous prediction of immaturity).

Some of the disadvantages of the shake test have been overcome with the development of the Foam Stability Index (FSI), a quantitative measure of the surfactant present in the amniotic fluid.[38] In this test the amniotic fluid is mixed with ethanol in the proportions necessary to achieve concentrations of alcohol ranging from 44% to 50%. If the test is negative (no bubbles produced after shaking the mixture) at a concentration of 44%, the risk of RDS is 73%. If the test is positive at ethanol concentrations of 44%, 45%, and 46%, the risk of RDS is 29%. If the test is positive at an ethanol concentration of 47% (the alcohol concentration used in the shake test described in the following box), the chance of developing RDS is 0.35%. This means that a positive FSI at an ethanol concentration of 47% is a better predictor of pulmonary maturity than a mature L/S ratio, but the L/S ratio is a better predictor at intermediate ranges (L/S 1.6 to 2.0) than a positive FSI at intermediate ethanol concentrations (between 44% and 46%). Both tests have a similar predictive value when the L/S is less than 1.5 and the FSI is negative at an ethanol concentration less than 44%.

Recent work[39] suggests that the FSI test may differentiate between AGA and SGA preterm infants. A positive FSI at an ethanol concentration of 47% is strongly suggestive of fetal growth retardation if the fetal weight is less than 1500 grams or the gestational age is less than or equal to 32 weeks.

It is possible to accelerate the maturation of the fetal lung in patients at high risk of being delivered before term. This capability has to a certain extent changed the end-points classically used to assess the success or failure of therapeutic plans aimed at preventing preterm delivery. Some years ago success in the management of preterm labor was the ability to prolong the pregnancy to term or near term; today success is in many cases the ability to avoid preterm delivery for the few hours necessary to obtain a fetal response to the maternal administration of glucocorticoids.

The most authoritative study on the effect of glucocorticoids on the fetal lungs is the work of Howie and Liggins in New Zealand. In their last progress report on this subject[25] they analyzed the result of their trial involving 821 mothers with unplanned preterm labor who delivered 884 infants. They had 411 mothers in a beta-methasone-treated group and 410 mothers in a control group. The perinatal mortality in infants who were delivered between 1 and 7 days after entry to the trial was significantly lower in the corticosteroid-treated group. The incidence of RDS was 8.8% in the treated versus 28.7% in the control group—a significant difference (P < 0.001). Similar studies in other parts of the world have confirmed the findings of Howie and Liggins.

There are several questions frequently asked about glucocorticoids and fetal lung maturation. One is what the minimal length of time is after the administration of the drug and the finding of a protective effect on the fetus. In Howie's and Liggins' experience there was no difference in the incidence of RDS between infants of mothers in the betamethasone-treated group and those in the control group if they were delivered less than 24 hours after the initiation of treatment. Thus 24 hours seems to be the minimal time necessary to obtain a significant effect.

Another important question is the duration of the drug effect on the fetal lungs. In the Howie and Liggins study the effectiveness of betamethasone therapy extended up to 7 days after treatment. In contrast, when infants were delivered between 7 and 21 days after treatment, there was a higher incidence of RDS in the betamethasone-treated infants (21.2%) than in the control group infants (7.1%). These data suggest that the glucocorticoid effect on the fetal lungs is transient and that if delivery is delayed more than 7 days after initiation of treatment, the dose of glucocorticoids may be repeated.

Another frequent topic of discussion among obstetricians concerns the gestational age when glucocorticoid treatment is effective. According to the data from Howie and Liggins shown in Table 3-3, the effect of therapy is more marked in infants between 30 and 32 weeks of gestation, but there are also significant reductions in RDS incidence in babies under 30 weeks and between 32 and 34 weeks. Thus glucocorticoids should be administered in any situation in which fetal lung maturation is desirable from 24 to 34 weeks of gestation. After 34 weeks, glucocorticoids have little influence on the respiratory outcome of the newborn.

The question of possible harmful effects to the fetus when the mother is given glucocortoids remains partially unanswered. However, it is re-

TABLE 3-3 ■ Incidence of RDS in live born infants delivered 24 hours to 7 days after treatment with betamethasone or placebo

Gestational age at delivery (weeks)	% with RDS		
	Betamethasone	Placebo	p
Under 30	27.8	57.7	0.04
30 to 32	8.7	56.0	0.001
32 to 34	0.0	12.9	0.04
34+	5.5	5.4	NS

From Howie RN, Liggins GF: In Anderson A, et al (eds): *Preterm Labor*, London, Royal College of Obstetricians and Gynecologists, 1977, p. 281.

assuring that in up to 9 years of follow-up Howie and Liggins have failed to demonstrate any significant problem with betamethasone-treated infants. Other related questions that are partially unsolved concern the molecular effect of the drug on the alveolar target cell, the possibility of substances different from glucocorticoids having similar effects on lung maturation, and the regulation of the movement of surfactant from the cell to the amniotic fluid.

Intraventricular hemorrhage

Many cerebral lesions are associated with and have been attributed to the complex problem of preterm delivery–RDS–perinatal asphyxia. All of them have the common denominator of hemorrhage or necrosis, and the most common seems to be the subependymal germinal matrix hemorrhage.[17] Bleeding in this area of the brain rarely contains fibrin, probably because of an abundance of plasminogen activator in the germinal tissue, and this may be the reason this type of bleeding frequently continues until the blood fills the ventricular system of the infant. However, not all subependymal hemorrhages burst into the ventricular system, and 40% are confined to their place of origin. The weight of the evidence seems to indicate that rather than birth trauma, the most important factors associated with intraventricular and subarachnoid hemorrhage in the preterm infant are intrapartum hypoxia and blood pressure fluctuations.[17,43] Hypoxia may cause damage to the vascular endothelium of the unusually thin and fragile veins of the preterm infant, and this added to the ve-

nous congestion also caused by hypoxia may result in rupture of the vessel. A contributory factor may be plasma hyperosmolarity produced by the enthusiastic use of sodium bicarbonate in the course of the infant's resuscitation.

The severity of the bleeding can be estimated by examination of the infant, by ultrasound, and by computed tomography (CT) scanning. Mild and even moderate degrees of bleeding are usually associated with good prognosis and recovery without neurologic sequelae. Severe bleeding in contrast is almost uniformly fatal; the majority of the survivors develop hydrocephalus.

The obstetrician may play a role in the prevention of intraventricular hemorrhage in the preterm infant by avoiding and aggressively treating intrapartum hypoxia. All preterm births should be carefully monitored, and a liberal policy of cesarean section should be instituted at the slightest indication of existing or threatening fetal hypoxia (see section on management of preterm labor).

■ EPIDEMIOLOGY OF PRETERM LABOR

A large number of variables are associated with preterm labor, and in some cases the association is so strong that the presence of a cause-effect relationship is suggested. In the majority of cases, however, the evidence suggesting a causative role does not exist, and the person studying preterm birth or preterm labor should be careful in recognizing and avoiding the confusion between *association* and *cause*.

There are few studies on the epidemiology and etiology of preterm labor. Most of the available information analyzes factors associated with low birth weight *deliveries* or with preterm birth[13] and not specifically those associated with preterm *labor*, which is one of the many causes of these deliveries (see p. 38). Thus when it is said that prematurity or preterm birth occurs three times more frequently in women weighing less than 112 pounds (50.8 kg) than in women who weigh more than 126 pounds (57.3 kg) at the beginning of pregnancy, it does not necessarily mean that preterm *labor* is three times more frequent in the first group than in the second. It is possible that a factor different from preterm labor is the cause of preterm delivery in this particular group of patients.

Something similar happens with the association between bleeding during pregnancy and preterm birth: in the large majority of patients who bleed during pregnancy and require early delivery, the cause of preterm birth is either placenta previa or abruptio placentae and not preterm labor. However, there are some patients with placenta previa whose placental abnormality seems to trigger the onset of uterine contractions. In these cases the association between antepartum bleeding and preterm labor may be valid. In the material that follows the variables most commonly associated with preterm *delivery* are described, but emphasis is placed on any existing relation between those variables and preterm *labor* because that is the main objective of this chapter.

Socioeconomic and ethnic factors

There is a strong association between low birth weight and low socioeconomic status. The best evidence in this respect comes from England where pregnant patients are classified according to their socioeconomic level. Classes I and II are professionals and managerial groups, class III consists of clerical workers, and classes IV and V are semiskilled and unskilled workers. The British Perinatal Mortality Survey[5] demonstrated that mothers in classes IV and V had a 10.9% incidence of preterm deliveries in contrast with a 4.3% incidence in classes I and II. What is not known is how much of this increase in low birth weight infants in the lower socioeconomic groups is the consequence of preterm labor and how much is a reflection of an increased number of SGA infants. This is pertinent if it is considered that inadequate nutrition, a predominant finding in the less privileged groups of society, is a well-known cause of fetal growth retardation. An indirect argument favoring the possibility that the majority of these low birth weight infants are SGA comes from studies in developing countries where it has been found that as many as 50% of all low birth weight infants are SGA rather than preterm.

In the United States preterm births are more common in blacks and Puerto Ricans than in whites. The question is to what extent the large incidence of low birth weight or preterm infants in the first two ethnic groups reflects a genetic or biologic predisposition or is a consequence of lower income, poor nutrition, less education, more physically demanding jobs, and other so-

cioeconomic variables. Analysis of the data collected in the Collaborative Perinatal Project, involving more than 45,000 pregnancies, indicates that economic variables cannot adequately explain the problem and suggests that babies with African ancestry have a biologic predisposition to smaller size and more advanced developmental maturity at birth than babies of Anglo-Saxon origin. This is a controversial finding, and surely there will be more about this problem in the next few years.

Maternal characteristics

An important maternal variable associated with the birth of a baby weighing less than 2500 grams is the *weight of the mother before pregnancy*. As mentioned earlier, women weighing less than 112 pounds before pregnancy have three times as many low birth weight infants as mothers who weigh more than 126 pounds before pregnancy.

Another significant association with low birth weight is maternal smoking during pregnancy. In fact, the number of births under 2500 grams is twice as frequent for smokers as for nonsmokers, and when large populations of smokers and nonsmokers are compared, the mean decrease in the weight of the baby for the smoker's group is between 150 to 250 grams with the weight reduction being proportional to the number of cigarettes smoked per day.

A less significant association between maternal characteristics and birth weight is *maternal age*. This relation follows a reverse-J curve with a high frequency of small babies (15.8%) being born to mothers under 15 years of age. The incidence of low birth weight decreases steadily with the advance in maternal age, reaches a minimum between 25 to 29 years of age (6.1%), and starts to rise reaching a new peak (9.9%) when the maternal age is between 45 and 49 years.

It is difficult to determine the existence of a cause-effect relation between any of the just described maternal characteristics and the occurrence of preterm labor. All of these maternal characteristics correlate strongly with the delivery of SGA infants and not with preterm labor. This makes sense because it is difficult to figure out a mechanism explaining how the color of the skin, the weight of the mother, or the level of her education may induce the early onset of uterine contractions.

Obstetric factors

The most important maternal variable associated with the weight of the infant at birth is *maternal weight gain during pregnancy*. Mothers who gain about 30 pounds during pregnancy have the best outcome in terms not only of baby weight but also of neonatal mortality and morbidity. In contrast, lack of weight gain or weight loss during pregnancy are important indicators of the possibility of a low birth weight (SGA) infant. Another important correlation, valid only for multiparous patients, is the *last prior birth weight*. In fact, if the last prior pregnancy ended with the birth of an infant weighing less than 2500 grams, the chances of another small baby in the present pregnancy are 24.8% if the patient is white and 33% if she is black. This is in contrast with an incidence of 5.8% if the last prior baby weight was more than 2500 grams.

Also important is the *neonatal outcome in the past prior pregnancy*. If the last pregnancy ended in neonatal death, the chances of having a low birth weight infant in the present pregnancy are 21.8%. If the prior baby is alive, the risk of a low birth weight baby in the present pregnancy is only 6.6%. Other important historical factors associated with preterm birth are *the number of previous spontaneous abortions, the number and characteristics of previous induced abortions, and the number of previous preterm deliveries*. With respect to previous spontaneous abortions, the British data[9] indicate that the incidence of preterm delivery is not increased if the maternal history reveals only first trimester abortions but increases significantly if there are as few as one mid-trimester abortion. In contrast, studies in the United States[18] have shown that there is a 2.5 times increase in the incidence of low birth weight in women with a history of at least one spontaneous abortion. However, everybody agrees that the highest risk of a preterm birth exists in the woman with a history of one or more preterm deliveries. The risk of delivering a low birth weight infant is 36.7% for women with a history of preterm delivery plus one or more abortions and is 70% for women with a history of two or more preterm births.

With respect to the relation between previous abortions and preterm birth, the information in the literature is controversial. Initial reports from Hungary indicated a low birth weight incidence of 9.3% in mothers who did not have a previous pregnancy termination. This incidence raised to 13% after one termination and to over 20% with three or more induced abortions. However, most recent reports in the United States contradict these findings and suggest that there is no difference in pregnancy outcome between patients who have a history of previous pregnancy terminations and those who do not. It is possible that the discrepancy among various studies reflects differences in the technique used for pregnancy termination, the degree of forcible dilation of the cervix, and the existence of small but perhaps significant variations in the gestational age of the subjects at the time of termination.

Some investigators have found a correlation between birth weight and *birth order* and reported a large incidence of low birth weight in the first pregnancy followed by a decrease in subsequent births and a new rise in the sixth and higher births. Other studies, however, have not found a significant relation between parity and low birth weight.

The presence of abnormal anatomic conditions of the uterus and the cervix accounts for 1% to 3% of all preterm deliveries. The most important of these conditions are the incompetent cervical os and the septate or bicornuate uterus. In spite of their low frequency, it is essential that these conditions be diagnosed because once they are identified, it is possible to establish preventive measures to avoid further occurrences of preterm births and pregnancy losses.

The diagnosis of *incompetent cervix* can be made with certainty only when the cervix is found to be dilated and the bag of waters is bulging in the vagina in the absence of labor. This condition may be responsible for some preterm deliveries occurring in patients who have had previous instrumental dilation of the cervix for pregnancy termination. The onset of the problem is insidious; usually the first sign is the appearance of a mucous plug or a mucous vaginal discharge with a few blood streaks in a patient who has reached 16 to 20 weeks of gestation in the course of a completely uncomplicated pregnancy. The mucosanguinolent discharge is quickly followed by a sensation of vaginal discomfort or pressure, and on examination the bag of waters is found coming out of the uterus through a partially or totally dilated cervix and filling the vagina. This is usually followed by rupture of the membranes and delivery.

Efforts to correct an incompetent cervix by a cervical cerclage when the bag of waters is bulging in the vagina are rarely successful, although it has been recently reported[20] that probably as many as 50% of these pregnancies can be saved if amniotic fluid is evacuated via transabdominal amniocentesis and the amniotic sac decompressed before carrying out the surgical cerclage. Although incompetent cervix is usually considered a cause of late abortion, probably as many as 50% of patients with this condition show symptoms between 20 and 26 weeks of gestation and may be classified as cases of preterm rupture of the membranes or preterm labor. The lack of a correct diagnosis allows the real condition to remain undetected in spite of several pregnancy losses.

Early pregnancy losses and preterm labor are also associated with the presence of a *septate or bicornuate uterus*. In this situation the incidence of spontaneous abortion is 27%, and the incidence of preterm labor if the pregnancy continues beyond 20 weeks varies between 16% and 20%. Different types of congenital anatomic malformations of the uterus and vagina are the result of a failure in the fusion, canalization, and absorption of the müllerian duct during embryonic development. The diagnosis of these congenital malformations is usually considered in patients with a history of repeated spontaneous abortions and preterm deliveries, although it should also be suspected in cases of fetal malpresentations, especially in breech and transverse presentations. About 50% of patients with anatomic abnormalities of the uterus may benefit from surgical correction and be able to carry a pregnancy to term. It seems that women born to mothers who ingested diethylstilbestrol (DES) during pregnancy have an unusually high incidence of anatomic abnormalities of the uterus, especially a decrease in the size of the uterine cavity that is discovered when the organ is examined by means of hysterosalpingography.[29] This may be the cause for the high incidence of early pregnancy losses and preterm deliveries reported in these patients.

Finally, an obstetric condition that is strongly associated with a high incidence of preterm labor is the presence of a *multiple gestation*. For an extensive treatment of this subject see Chapter 14.

Maternal infection

Maternal infections are associated with preterm labor and preterm delivery. Evidence shows that when acute infections with hyperpyrexia (pneumonia, appendicitis, pyelonephritis) occur during pregnancy, the uterus may start to contract before term. There is also evidence that preterm labor occurs frequently in pregnant women affected by chronic infectious processes such as tuberculosis and chronic hepatitis. It is possible that chorioamnionitis may have a greater role than so far suspected in the etiology of many cases formerly classified as preterm labor of unknown origin. In fact, amnionitis may exist without fever, leukocytosis, uterine tenderness, or any of the classic signs described for severe infections of the pregnant uterus; preterm labor (usually resistant to conventional treatment) may be the only sign indicating the presence of the infectious process. This situation termed *unrecognized amnionitis* by Ledger[6] may be the explanation behind 30% or more of all cases of preterm labor of unknown origin.

Chorioamnionitis must be suspected in patients with preterm labor that is difficult to control with high doses of beta mimetic agents. In these cases the obstetrician should overcome the fear of eliciting more contractions and withdraw some amniotic fluid, since if a Wright's or a Gram's stain of the fluid shows bacteria, the finding is diagnostic of unrecognized amnionitis. The infectious process may also be recognized postpartum by histologic examination of the placenta, which should be routine in every case of preterm labor of unknown origin. For example, Safarti[37] found histologic evidence of infection in 27% of placentas and membranes obtained after preterm deliveries as compared to an incidence of 4.7% when the placenta and membranes were obtained from normal patients delivering at term. Up to the present time a diagnosis of amnionitis in a patient in preterm labor with intact membranes has been an indication for discontinuation of tocolytic therapy and delivery. A problem of this magnitude, however, requires controlled trials of antibiotic treatment, especially since animal experiments have shown that antibiotic treatment significantly reduces neonatal death rate in animals with experimental amnionitis.

Another maternal infection strongly associated with preterm labor is *urinary tract infection* (UTI). In more than 25% of patients with preterm labor at Barnes Hospital,[2] examination of the urinary sediment was highly suggestive of urinary infection although culture-proven infection was detected in only half of the cases. Frequently trichomonas organisms are seen during microscopic examination of urine specimens obtained by catheterization in patients with preterm labor.

The data from the Collaborative Perinatal Project have clearly demonstrated the existence of an association between symptomatic and culture-proven UTI during pregnancy and preterm delivery. However, the association between asymptomatic bacteriuria and preterm delivery is a matter of controversy. In the initial research that originated this controversy, Kaas[28] suggested that asymptomatic patients with two or more successive cultures of clean voided specimens having more than 100,000 colonies per milliliter of pathogenic bacteria have two to three times the risk of preterm labor compared to patients in control groups who have negative cultures. Some investigations have supported Kaas's findings, whereas others have reached different conclusions. The overall weight of the evidence, however, seems to favor a causative role for asymptomatic UTI in preterm labor. There is evidence suggesting that UTI causes preterm labor by a mechanism involving placental and decidual lysosome breakage with liberation of enzymes capable of increasing local prostaglandin production.

Other maternal diseases

Maternal diseases peculiar to pregnancy (preeclampsia, eclampsia) or not related to pregnancy (chronic renal disease, chronic hypertension) are frequent causes of low birth weight and occasional causes of preterm labor. Most of these diseases cause a chronic alteration of the maternal oxygen-carrying capacity (heart failure, asthma, sickle cell disease) or chronically decrease the uteroplacental blood flow (chronic hypertension, preeclampsia, eclampsia) bringing as a consequence impaired fetal growth and low

birth weight. On a few occasions, however, an acute hypoxic insult or a vasoconstrictive crisis may elicit the production of spontaneous preterm labor that may or may not be superimposed on a defective fetal growth.

The most common maternal condition causing low birth weight is hypertension during pregnancy, which may be present in any of several different modalities (chronic hypertension, chronic hypertension with superimposed preeclampsia, preeclampsia, eclampsia). In a prospective study carried out in Edinburgh,[11] 69% of all children with a birth weight under 2000 grams and whose low birth weight was attributed to complications occurring in late pregnancy had mothers with a history of severe preeclampsia or severe chronic hypertension. The association between hypertension of pregnancy and low birth weight has been extensively studied by Friedman and Neff[15] using the data from the Collaborative Perinatal Project. They have found evidence indicating that this association occurs because of the effect of maternal hypertension on the fetal growth and not because hypertension causes preterm labor. Additional evidence in this respect comes from the Edinburgh[11] study in which it was found that 75% of the infants with low birth weight caused by maternal hypertension were delivered by means of deliberate induction of labor or deliberate cesarean section because of deteriorating fetal or maternal conditions and not because of the onset of spontaneous preterm labor.

Fetal problems

The possibility that the mother is carrying a fetus with major congenital abnormalities should be considered when dealing with patients in preterm labor. Birth defects are also frequently found in term SGA infants and in pregnancies complicated by rupture of the membranes early in gestation. Neural tube defects and inborn errors of metabolism such as hyperalaninemia are some of the birth defects that have been found to be associated with preterm labor. Many more congenital abnormalities have been found to be associated with low birth weight.

Anencephaly is a congenital defect that traditionally has been associated with prolonged or postterm pregnancy. However, there is a wide range of gestational age in anencephalic infants, and as many of these infants are born after pre-term labor as there are born after a prolonged pregnancy. Anencephaly should be ruled out by ultrasound examination in every patient who is admitted to the hospital with preterm labor. Potter's syndrome (renal agenesis and pulmonary hypoplasia) is another condition in which the majority of affected infants are delivered early because of preterm labor. This fact should be remembered with every patient in preterm labor with clinical or sonographic evidence of oligohydramnios.

Placental factors

Preterm delivery occurs frequently in pregnancies in which there are abnormalities in the morphology, the implantation, or the function of the placenta. Anatomic abnormalities such as battledore placenta, circumvallate placenta, and marginal insertion of the umbilical cord have been found to be associated with the occurrence of preterm labor. These are uncommon problems, and the incidence of battledore placenta, for example, is approximately 5 out of every 1000 deliveries. More common are problems associated with abnormal placental implantation, since *placenta previa* occurs in one out of every 100 deliveries.

Preterm labor is a common finding in patients with placenta previa when they are admitted to the hospital with their first episode of bleeding. In these cases cessation of the bleeding is usually concomitant with the disappearance of the contractions. This association is so common that it is tempting to speculate that the onset of uterine bleeding in patients with previa may be the result of preterm labor. In the majority of cases of previa the uterine contractions disappear with bed rest or treatment with tocolytic agents. However, in some cases contractions and bleeding persist, and early delivery is necessary for the solution of the problem.

Patients with *abruptio placentae* usually develop a tetanic contracture of the uterus that results in a significant increase of the uterine resting pressure as measured by electronic monitoring equipment. In addition to this high resting pressure, these patients also develop rhythmic uterine contractions, and most of them deliver vaginally in a relatively short time after the onset of symptoms. To consider, however,

that abruptio placentae or placenta previa is the cause of preterm labor is not correct if the problem is analyzed within a rigorous context. Even if it is accepted that placenta previa or abruptio placentae caused the onset of preterm labor, in the large majority of cases preterm delivery is the result of obstetric intervention rather than preterm labor.

There are some histologic abnormalities (accelerated maturation of the villi, excessive fibrinoid necrosis) that appear more frequently in placentas of patients delivering before term than in patients in normal control groups.[14] Frequently patients wiht preterm labor of unknown origin have small, calcified placentas with extensive areas of fibrinoid degeneration, which adhere stubbornly to the uterus and cause prolongation of the third stage of labor and retention of placental tissue.

Iatrogenic preterm delivery

A small number of preterm deliveries occur as a consequence of elective induction of labor or repeated cesarean section in patients who had an erroneous estimation of their gestational age. This problem has been steadily decreasing with the availability of ultrasound and amniotic fluid tests to evaluate the maturation of the fetal lungs. In those cases in which the dates cannot be established with certainty, the infant should not be delivered electively until evidence of adequate fetal lung maturation is obtained.

Coitus

There is a considerable amount of anecdotal evidence as well as some scientific data suggesting the existence of an association between coital activity during pregnancy and preterm delivery. For example, Goodlin et al[21] found that the incidence of orgasm after 32 weeks of gestation was significantly higher in a group of women delivering preterm infants than in a control group delivering term babies. The same investigators asked five gravids who claimed to be able to achieve orgasm at will to initiate an orgasm with the purpose of inducing labor when they were at term. Four of these women were admitted in labor within 9 hours following the orgasm, and the fifth had an episode of false labor. More recently Naeye,[34] using data from the Collaborative Perinatal Project, has shown that the frequency of amniotic fluid infection in the presence of intact membranes (unrecognized amnionitis) was significantly greater in mothers who had coitus once or more per week during the month before delivery than in those mothers who did not have coitus. Since amniotic fluid infections with intact membranes are a frequent cause of preterm labor, the implication is that coital activity during pregnancy may be a factor in the production of preterm labor.

■ DIAGNOSIS OF PRETERM LABOR

The diagnosis of preterm labor implies the ability to (1) identify patients at risk of preterm labor before the onset of signs and symptoms and (2) make the diagnosis after the onset of symptoms.

Identification of the patient at risk of preterm labor

The best predictor of preterm labor is a poor past reproductive performance, which makes it difficult to identify *nulliparous* patients at risk for preterm delivery. This is disappointing because more than 40% of all preterm labor patients are nulliparous. The impact of preventive measures is far from optimal if this large group of patients at risk remains undetected. However, when the variables associated with preterm labor are examined closely, most of them apply to both nulliparous and multiparous patients, and it is possible that a large part of our lack of ability to detect the nullipara at risk is the consequence of a failure in recognizing the presence of high-risk factors in the nulliparous patient. Factors associated with preterm labor and delivery that should be carefully investigated in every obstetric patient include the following:

1. Age less than 20 years
2. Unmarried
3. Weight less than 112 pounds (50.8 kg)
4. Smoker
5. Poor weight gain or weight loss during pregnancy
6. Previous spontaneous or induced abortion(s), especially mid-trimester abortion(s)
7. UTI during pregnancy
8. Increased spontaneous uterine activity before term

9. Multiple gestation
10. Hemoglobin less than 9 g/100 ml
11. Internal cervical os dilated one or more fingerbreadths at 30 to 32 weeks of gestation
12. History of preterm delivery in prior pregnancy
13. History of stillbirth or neonatal death in prior pregnancy

The presence of one or more of these factors automatically classifies the patient as high risk for preterm labor and demands the type of care that is described later in the section on management of preterm labor.

In the large majority of cases the onset of preterm labor is a surprise for the obstetrician. It is exceptional, however, to find a patient with preterm labor who did not show some indication of the problem several days or weeks before the onset of symptoms. Discussions of some premonitory signs of preterm labor follow.

Excessive uterine activity. The most common complaint of a patient at risk of preterm labor is excessive uterine activity, a symptom usually present several days before admission to the hospital. On many occasions the patient expresses the complaint as back pain radiating to the suprapubic region and at other times complains of "knots" over the uterus. These are unspecific symptoms, and in many cases they do not correspond to preterm labor. However, these symptoms are important and should be systematically searched for in every routine prenatal visit between 20 and 34 weeks of gestation because in many cases the patients are nulliparas who have not learned to recognize abnormally increased uterine activity and do not register it as a complaint. Unfortunately, their symptoms are frequently disregarded as a minor ailment (the famous round ligament pain). Studies[8] show that patients who have preterm deliveries have increased uterine activity for several weeks before the onset of preterm labor. Teaching the patient to recognize uterine contractions and assess the presence or absence of excessive uterine contractility is an important part of routine prenatal care. Every patient who seems to have excessive uterine contractility before 34 weeks of gestation should have a pelvic examination in search of objective signs indicating the imminence of preterm labor.

TABLE 3-4 ■ Scoring system for the evaluation of the patient at risk of preterm labor
or in preterm labor

	0	1	2
Low segment	Not developed	Starting to develop	Bulging with head engaged
Length of cervix	>1.0 cm	0.5 to 1.0 cm	<0.5 cm
Passage	External os closed	External os open; internal os closed	Both internal and external os open; admit one finger
Position of cervix	Posterior	Misposition	Anterior
Consistency of cervix	Hard	Soft	Very soft

Vaginal, rectal, or perineal pressure. Sensation of vaginal, rectal, or perineal pressure is another symptom that should be investigated in routine prenatal visits between 20 and 34 weeks. In some cases the patient spontaneously tells the obstetrician about this sensation of pressure that frequently is expressed as the feeling of "carrying the baby too low." Similar to excessive uterine activity, this symptom is in the majority of cases disregarded as a minor complaint. However, this symptom should be followed by a pelvic examination because it may correspond to early engagement of the fetal head preceding the onset of preterm labor.

Mucous vaginal discharge. Excessive mucous vaginal discharge is the least reliable of the symptoms announcing the onset of preterm labor, but it becomes valuable when any of the other symptoms (excessive uterine activity, vaginal or rectal pressure) are also present. The abundant mucous discharge is the result of the loss of the cervical mucous plug as a consequence of early effacement and dilation.

Development of the low uterine segment. If any of the previously mentioned symptoms (excessive uterine activity, sensation of vaginal or rectal pressure, onset of mucous vaginal discharge) or a combination of them is present, the obstetrician should proceed to a vaginal examination. It is possible to identify a large number of patients destined to develop preterm labor before the onset of classic symptoms by means of a pelvic examination.[1,44,45] Also, doing a pelvic examination the obstetrician is able to find concrete evidence as to whether to accept the patient's complaints or to disregard them as a minor problem. In the pelvic examination the obstetrician is looking not only for dilation and effacement of the cervix but more important for the development of the low uterine segment, the earliest sign indicative of the existence of abnormal uterine activity before the onset of preterm labor.

When examined between 20 and 34 weeks of gestation, the large majority of nulliparous patients have a cervix located posteriorly, at least 1 centimeter long, and closed. In the normal multiparous patient the cervix may have varied degrees of dilation and effacement. However, all pregnant patients regardless of their parity develop their low uterine segment a few days before parturition. When the low segment has not developed, the fingers of the examiner may be introduced up into the vaginal fornices without finding any resistance whatsoever. If the low uterine segment has developed, the fingers of the examiner will find the upper and sometimes the middle third of the vagina filled with the thinned low uterine segment that contains the presenting part and interposes between the examiner's fingers and the vaginal fornices. In a majority of cases development of the low segment occurs simultaneously with the engagement of the presenting part.

The finding of a developed low segment in a patient who complains of excessive frequency of contractions or excessive vaginal pressure means that preterm labor is imminent and demands initiation of treatment that should be similar to that received by the patient with threatened preterm labor. A useful scoring system to quantify cervical changes is shown in Table 3-4.

Diagnosis of threatened and established preterm labor

The patient with threatened preterm labor has developed an amount of uterine activity so large that she feels the need to come to the hospital for diagnosis and treatment. The difference between threatened and established preterm labor is the effect of the abnormal uterine activity on the cervix. The patient with *threatened* preterm labor has uterine contractions every 3 to 5 minutes and on pelvic examination the low uterine segment is developed, but there is no progressive effacement and dilation of the cervix, which occur only in *established* preterm labor.

A problem with threatened preterm labor is its differentiation from *false labor*. In fact, a significant number of patients coming to the hospital with preterm uterine contractions have uncoordinated uterine activity that does not cause changes in the cervix and usually disappears spontaneously and without treatment. The key to the differential diagnosis between *threatened* preterm labor and *false* labor is the pelvic examination. If the low uterine segment is developed, it should be assumed that the patient is in *threatened* preterm labor and demands aggressive treatment. If there is no development of the low uterine segment and no cervical changes occur during 2 to 4 hours of observation, the patient most probably has *false* labor.

The diagnosis of *established preterm labor* is usually simple and requires the presence of changes in cervical dilation and effacement in addition to abnormal uterine activity. The chances for achieving a substantial prolongation of pregnancy are limited when this diagnosis is made. The effort of the clinician should be directed toward recognition of the early stages of the problem (patients at risk and those with threatened preterm labor) when intervention may be more successful. Recent work from Herron et al[24] confirms that efforts at prevention are successful in significantly decreasing the rate of preterm deliveries.

■ MANAGEMENT OF PRETERM LABOR

Management of preterm labor depends on the clinical picture exhibited by the patient at the time of identification of the problem. In most cases the obstetrician is confronted with (1) patients at risk of preterm labor and (2) patients with threatened or established preterm labor.

Management of the patient at risk of preterm labor

It is possible to recognize a large number of patients destined to develop preterm labor be-

fore the onset of their symptoms. In fact, about 60% of all patients admitted to a hospital with preterm labor have risk factors that could have been recognized at the initiation of their prenatal care (see p. 49). Furthermore, the majority of women destined to develop preterm labor who have no identifiable high-risk factors may be detected before the onset of symptoms with a systematic search for excessive uterine activity and its effects on the low uterine segment. Unfortunately, the ability to define a group of patients at high risk for preterm delivery does not imply that proven, effective, and safe preventive measures are readily available. Only three modes of therapy or combinations of them are available for the prevention of preterm labor. They are bed rest, beta mimetics, and progesterone.

Bed rest. Bed rest is a method frequently recommended for the prevention of preterm labor. In theory bed rest should increase blood flow to the fetoplacental unit and by this means exert an influence on uterine contractility. In practice there is little doubt that bed rest in the lateral position usually decreases uterine contractility. However, controlled studies made on twin pregnancies concerning the role of bed rest on preterm labor have produced conflicting results with some showing prolongation of pregnancy and others not having this effect. It is possible that women carrying twins are not the ideal patients for testing the effect of bed rest on uterine contractility. It is also possible that this type of study (along with most studies on the treatment and prevention of preterm labor) is biased from the beginning because patients with preterm labor are a heterogenous group requiring different modalities of treatment in accordance with different etiologic factors. More research in this area is much needed.

Beta mimetic agents. The literature on the prevention of preterm labor by the prophylactic administration of beta mimetics is contradictory. Studies on twins have shown that these compounds are more effective in the prevention of preterm delivery than bed rest at the hospital.[41] Other studies using different populations have found no beneficial effect. As mentioned before, the etiologic heterogeneity of preterm patients in labor necessitates the adoption of strict patient selection criteria in studies designed to prove the effectiveness of any method or med-

FIG. 3-1 ■ Management protocol for patients with threatened or established preterm labor.

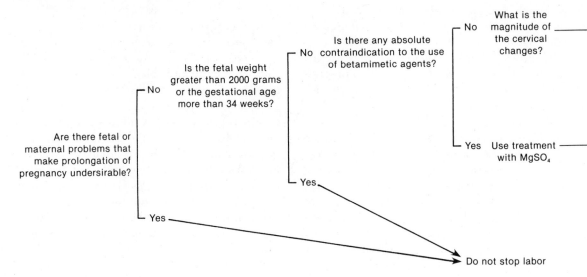

ication used for prevention or treatment of preterm labor.

Progesterone. There is a wealth of information concerning the effect of progesterone on uterine contractility. Animal research has shown that this hormone plays a key role in pregnancy maintenance and the onset of parturition. A fall in maternal plasma levels of progesterone preceding parturition has been clearly shown in sheep, goats, rabbits, and rats. In sheep the events leading to parturition begin with an increase in cortisol production by the fetal adrenal. Cortisol stimulates the activity of certain placental enzymes that transform progesterone into androstenedione and then into estrogen; this causes a decline in progesterone and an increase in estrogen levels with the latter provoking an increased production of placental prostaglandins. The prostaglandins diffuse into the myometrium and start the uterine activity characteristic of labor. Unfortunately, the mechanism of initiation of labor in the human does not follow the same pathway as in sheep. Several studies on plasma levels of progesterone before human parturition have produced contradictory results and have generated doubts about the existence of a progesterone withdrawal in the human as a prerequisite for parturition. However, it is possible that in situ withdrawal may occur in the human uterus without a significant change in peripheral levels of the hormone.

Progesterone has been used and continues to be used in the prophylaxis and treatment of preterm labor. The use of the hormone in the prevention of preterm labor received a solid base with the work of Johnson et al.[27] These investigators found significant differences in the frequency of preterm deliveries, mean duration of pregnancy, mean birth weight, and perinatal mortality in patients at high risk for preterm delivery who were randomly divided into progesterone-treated and placebo-treated groups in a double blind study protocol. They used 17 alpha hydroxyprogesterone caproate (Delalutin) 250 mg intramuscularly every week from the time of registration in the antenatal clinic until 37 weeks of gestation or delivery, whichever occurred first.

The only disadvantage of the prophylactic administration of progesterone is the potential for teratogenic effects on the fetus. This teratogenicity has not been proved, but there are data showing increases in the incidence of cardiac and great vessels abnormalities in infants born to mothers receiving progestins early in gestation.[23] There is no proof, but it seems possible that if prophylaxis with progestins is delayed until fetal organogenesis is completed, the possibility of adverse effects of the drug on the fetus will be negligible.

In conclusion, patients at risk of preterm labor should receive an explanation about the beneficial effects and the potential risks of progesterone administration during pregnancy, and if

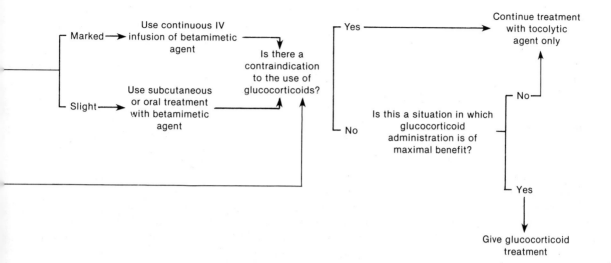

they consent, they should receive the medication according to the protocol just mentioned (250 mg Delalutin intramuscularly every week). Treatment should not start earlier than 16 weeks of gestation and be continued until 36 weeks of gestation or delivery, whichever comes first.

Management of patients with threatened or established preterm labor

The patient who comes to the hospital before 34 weeks of gestation with regular uterine contractions occurring every 3 or 4 minutes and with changes in pelvic examination indicating that those contractions have an effect on the cervix should be managed following a sequence of decision-making steps. The first question to be answered in this management protocol (Fig. 3-1) is the following:

> **Are there fetal or maternal problems that make prolongation of pregnancy undesirable?**

An appropriate answer to this question requires obtaining a complete history and carrying out a thorough physical examination of the patient with threatened preterm labor. The presence of maternal diseases such as hyperthyroidism, chronic hypertension, preeclampsia, chronic renal disease, systemic lupus erythematous, cardiac conditions causing moderate to severe functional impairment, and sickle cell

disease makes it undesirable to prolong pregnancy. One rationale behind this generalization is that in these cases the fetus has been growing within a hostile environment and has exceeded the capacity of such an environment to effectively contribute to its growth and development. Within this context the initiation of labor is nature's way to optimize the chances for fetal survival. Another reason for a policy of no prolongation of pregnancy in women affected by chronic diseases is that labor has started because the limited functional capacity of the maternal organism has been exceeded.

These explanations seem logical and are supported by a large amount of anecdotal experiences, but they were produced at a time when the ability of the obstetrician to evaluate fetal and maternal function was limited. There are many instances when in spite of the presence of maternal disease, preterm labor must be arrested and rapid surfactant induction attempted. These growing exceptions to the general rule should be managed within a tertiary care center where facilities and expertise for close maternal and fetal monitoring are available.

The possible existence of fetal problems that make it undesirable to prolong pregnancy in patients with preterm labor must also be considered. In general, the discovery of a major congenital malformation (microcephaly, anencephaly, hydrocephaly, polycystic kidney disease, meningomyelocele, omphalocele, etc) is an indication for avoiding interference with preterm labor. However this generalization does not apply to all cases of congenitally malformed infants because there are some situations (diaphragmatic hernia, omphalocele) in which the congenital defect may be treated successfully in the neonatal period, and arrest of labor and prolongation of pregnancy may help to improve the overall condition of the neonate.

If the clinical and laboratory evaluations reveal fetal or maternal problems that make the continuation of pregnancy undesirable, the patient should be allowed to continue laboring, the neonatologist should be informed of the imminent delivery of a preterm infant, and the obstetrician should be ready to treat intrapartum hypoxia if it occurs.

If no fetal or maternal problems that make the prolongation of pregnancy undesirable are detected, the next question is the following:

> **Is the fetal weight greater than 2000 grams or the gestational age greater than 34 weeks?**

This question is usually answered when the diagnosis of preterm labor is made. However, it is important to repeat the question after performing an ultrasound examination of the fetus. This test adds evidence to the assessment of gestational age based on historical factors and examination of the patient. With the help of ultrasonic measurements of the fetal biparietal diameter and abdominal circumference, the question of fetal weight and gestational age should be answered before initiation of therapy. Quite often measures to stop labor, which cause significant maternal morbidity, are undertaken following inadequate evaluation of fetal weight and gestational age. Today thanks to developments in neonatal care it is extremely unusual to lose an infant weighing more than 2000 grams or having a gestational age of 34 or more weeks. Therefore efforts to arrest preterm labor never should be of a magnitude large enough to generate maternal morbidity in situations in which the fetus weighs 2000 grams or more or the gestational age is 34 weeks or more. If the fetus is smaller than 2000 grams and the gestational age is under 34 weeks, the following is the next question to be answered:

> **Is there any absolute contraindication to the use of beta mimetic agents?**

Beta mimetics are the drugs of choice in the treatment of threatened and established preterm labor. However, they are powerful medications, and several conditions contraindicate their use in an absolute or relative form. One of these conditions is *chronic cardiac disease*. The increase in heart rate and the drop in afterload caused by beta-adrenergic agents may be enough to precipitate congestive heart failure. We[26] and others have shown that even patients without detectable cardiac abnormalities may develop pulmonary edema when preterm labor is treated with beta mimetic drugs. There is also a contraindication to the use of beta mimetic agents in patients with high cardiac output situations. Examples of this are pregnant patients with *hyperthyroidism* or with *sickle cell anemia*.

Another contraindication to the use of beta mimetics is the patient with active internal or external bleeding whose vasodilation may increase the magnitude of the blood loss. A clear example is the patient with abruptio placenta. In cases of placenta previa, however, there may be a place for beta mimetic therapy if the bleeding is minimal or moderate and if it is thought to be a consequence of increased uterine contractility (see Chapter 15). When the bleeding is severe, there is no place for beta mimetic therapy in the management of placenta previa.

Patients with insulin-dependent *diabetes* are another group at high risk for complications with the use of beta mimetic drugs. When treated with beta mimetics, especially intravenous beta mimetics, patients with diabetes develop hyperglycemia, glycosuria, and ketonuria and require considerable increases in the amount and frequency of insulin administration. Patients with *gestational diabetes* who receive beta mimetic agents for the treatment of preterm labor usually require subcutaneous insulin, whereas patients with insulin-dependent diabetes under the same circumstances usually require continuous intravenous insulin infusions. This is caused by the powerful effect of these drugs on carbohydrate metabolism (glycogenolysis, excessive formation of lactic acid) and fatty acid

---

Diazoxide for preterm labor

PREPARATION

Add 1 ampule of diazoxide (Hyperstat) containing 300 mg to 250 ml of 0.5N saline solution. This gives a solution containing approximately 1.1 mg of diazoxide per milliliter.

INITIAL DOSE

Give the diazoxide via piggyback with a Harvard or IVAC pump, at a rate of 6 to 7 ml/minute for a 60 kg patient (0.125 mg/kg and per minute).

REPEATED DOSE

Do not repeat the treatment within 6 hours after finishing the initial dose. The patient should not receive more than four doses in 24 hours.

---

metabolism (lipolysis, ketonemia, ketonuria). Beta mimetics are contraindicated in the unstable pregnant patient with diabetes, and their use in stable patients requires frequent monitoring of blood sugar and potassium levels and aggressive use of insulin therapy to avoid serious fetal and maternal side effects.

Another contraindication to the use of beta mimetic drugs in the treatment of preterm labor is a patient with *chorioamnionitis*. Clinical evidence or a strong suspicion of the presence of infection of the products of conception is at the present time an absolute contraindication to any pharmacologic effort to prolong pregnancy.

Finally, it should be remembered that pregnant patients receiving *psychiatric treatment and taking monoamine oxidase inhibitors* may have difficulties in adequately metabolizing beta mimetic drugs. Pregnant patients already taking beta mimetics for the treatment of *asthma* may develop tachyphylaxis with increased doses.

If the answer to the initial question of whether or not there is any contraindication to the use of beta mimetic drugs is yes, a medication different from beta mimetic agents should be selected as the main mode of treatment. The alternatives to beta mimetic agents are diazoxide, prostaglandin synthesis inhibitors, magnesium sulfate, ethanol, and progesterone.

Diazoxide. A medication widely used for the treatment of malignant and severe hypertension, diazoxide, is a powerful inhibitor of uterine contractility both in vivo and in vitro. The dose

used to stop uterine contractions (box above) is 5 mg/kg body weight, and it should be given by continuous IV infusion at a rate of 0.125 mg/kg/minute (1 ampule of diazoxide [300 mg] dissolved in 250 ml of 0.5N saline solution administered at 6 ml/minute for a 60 kg patient). Given slowly by IV, the drug has a negligible effect on maternal blood pressure and uteroplacental circulation. However, the medication has not been extensively used for the treatment of preterm labor and may have undesirable side effects. One of these side effects is maternal hyperglycemia that may stimulate fetal insulin production with subsequent neonatal hypoglycemia. Another potentially harmful effect is the expansion of intravascular volume caused by the medication. Also the possibility of hypotension is present when using diazoxide. Therefore the use of this drug should be restricted to research protocols.

Prostaglandin synthesis inhibitors. Prostaglandin synthesis inhibitors are compounds shown to be effective in the arrest of preterm labor. The drug most widely used for this purpose is indomethacin.[46] The most common treatment consists of a loading dose of 100 mg of indomethacin via rectal suppository followed by 25 mg orally every 6 hours for a total of 3 days. The main disadvantage of prostaglandin synthesis inhibitors in the treatment of preterm labor is the possibility of adverse effects on the fetal circulation, specifically constriction of the ductus arteriosus and development of pulmonary

---

Magnesium sulfate for preterm labor

LOADING DOSE

Give 4 grams (40 ml of a 10% solution) IV slowly over 10 to 20 minutes.

MAINTENANCE DOSE

Add 200 ml of 10% magnesium sulfate to 800 ml of 5% dextrose in water, and give 100 ml/ hour (2 g/hour).

MONITOR EVERY HOUR

a. Urine output (should be at least 30 ml/hour).
b. Deep tendon reflexes (should be present and 1+ to 2+).
c. Respiration rate (should exceed 15/minute).

MAGNESIUM TOXICITY

To reverse magnesium toxicity administer 1 to 2 grams of calcium gluconate by slow (5 minutes) IV push.

MAGNESIUM BLOOD LEVELS

Therapeutic: 6 to 8 mEq/L.
Loss of deep tendon reflexes: 10 mEq/L.
Respiratory failure: 12 mEq/L.

---

hypertension. The literature on this subject is contradictory, but until fetal toxicity is carefully evaluated by controlled studies, the use of indomethacin or its analogues in the treatment of preterm labor should be restricted to experimental protocols.

Magnesium sulfate. The use of magnesium sulfate for the treatment of preterm labor originated in the observation that preeclamptic patients in labor have a decrease in intensity and frequency of uterine contractions after receiving magnesium sulfate. Furthermore, the medication has a quiescent effect on isolated myometrial strips. Information from limited clinical trials suggests that magnesium sulfate may be useful in the treatment of preterm labor. However, larger and better designed research protocols are necessary for truly assessing effectiveness. Magnesium sulfate is toxic for both mother and fetus (see Chapter 6), and it should be administered under close monitoring. In our opinion, magnesium sulfate is a poor labor inhibitor, and its use should be limited to patients for whom beta mimetics are contraindicated or as a complement to beta mimetic agents when the patient response to them is not adequate. The box above is a guide to magnesium sulfate treatment of preterm labor.

Ethanol. Most of the experimental evidence suggesting a role for ethanol in the treatment of preterm labor is the product of the work of Fuchs.[16] A careful analysis of his data and that of other investigators fails, however, to clearly show that ethanol is better than placebo for the arrest of preterm labor. Furthermore, the use of ethanol causes important side effects. In fact, nausea, vomiting, aspiration of gastric content, and severe lactic acidosis occur frequently in mothers treated with IV alcohol. Also, alcohol intoxication with respiratory depression of the neonate is often observed in preterm infants born to mothers treated with IV alcohol. In our opinion, the risk-benefit ratio is against the routine use of alcohol in the treatment of preterm labor, and it is recommended only as an alternate mode of therapy for those patients for whom beta mimetics are contraindicated. For this purpose 100 ml of 100% ethanol are mixed with 900 ml of dextrose in water. The initial dose is 7.5 ml/kg/hour for 2 hours, followed by 1.5 ml/kg/hour. The length of a treatment should not exceed 12 hours (see box on p. 57).

Ethanol for preterm labor

PREPARATION

Add 100 ml of 100% ethyl alcohol to 900 ml of D_5W, or add 50 ml of 100% ethyl alcohol to 900 ml of 5% alcohol in D_5W.

LOADING DOSE

Administer 15 ml/kg over the first 2 hours. For a 60 kg mother this means 450 ml/hour for 2 hours.

MAINTENANCE DOSE

Give 1.5 ml/kg and per hour. For a 60 kg mother this represents 90 ml/hour. This infusion should be maintained for 6 hours after the contractions have stopped, and then the patient should be gradually weaned off. The total length of the treatment should not exceed 12 hours.

RELOADING DOSE

If contractions recur within 10 hours of discontinuation of the alcohol infusion, the repeat initial dose should be 10% of the original dose times the number of hours from discontinuation:

$$\frac{\text{loading dose}}{10} \times \text{hours off alcohol}$$

The maintenance dose and the length of treatment are not changed in repeat courses.

Progesterone. Although there is evidence that progesterone administration may be useful in the *prevention* of preterm labor, there is no proof that the medication is effective in the *treatment* of this condition. However, progesterone continues to be widely used for the treatment of preterm labor in spite of the lack of data supporting its benefits. It is possible that lack of ability to saturate myometrial receptor sites rather than a real drug failure is the reason for the lack of effectiveness of this treatment.

In summary, the only available alternatives to beta mimetics are ethanol, magnesium sulfate, and diazoxide. These are powerful drugs with capacity for serious side effects and probably lacking the effectiveness of beta mimetics. In the future anticalcium drugs may become another acceptable alternative to beta mimetics.

If the answer to the original question of whether or not there is contraindication to the use of beta mimetic agents is no, the following question should be answered:

What is the magnitude of the cervical changes (effacement and dilation)?

A useful system to assess cervical changes is shown in Table 3-4. More than six points in the scoring system indicate advanced cervical changes, and the patient becomes a candidate for continuous IV infusion of beta mimetic drugs. If preterm labor is not accompanied by marked cervical changes, beta mimetics should be given orally or subcutaneously.

In patients with little cervical changes terbutaline should be used 250 μg subcutaneously every 4 hours, or ritodrine can be given 20 mg orally every 2 to 4 hours for a minimum of 24 hours. At the end of this period, if the uterine contractions have disappeared, the patient is given terbutaline tablets 2.5 to 5.0 mg every 6 hours or 10 to 20 mg of ritodrine every 4 hours. With subcutaneous and oral terbutaline and with oral ritodrine the incidence and severity of side effects are not unusually large. The most common complaints are a sensation of nervousness and tremor. Occasionally mild hyperglycemia, glycosuria, and ketonuria are seen, but they do not require insulin treatment unless the patient has diabetes. In most cases oral administration of a beta mimetic agent should continue until the patient reaches 34 weeks of gestation. If a

Use of terbutaline in the treatment of preterm labor

PREPARATION OF SOLUTION

Dissolve 5 ampules of terbutaline (5 mg) in 500 ml of Ringer's lactate solution. This preparation contains 10 μg of terbutaline per milliliter.

CONTINUOUS INTRAVENOUS INFUSION

Using a Harvard pump, start IV infusion at a rate of 5 μg/minute (0.5 ml/minute; 30 ml/hour). Increase every 10 minutes by 5 μg/minute (0.17 ml/min; 10.2 ml/hour) until a rate of 15 μg/minute (1.5 ml/minute; 90 ml/hour) is reached. If contractions have not disappeared with this dose, a double strength solution (5 mg in 250 ml of Ringer's lactate solution) should be prepared to avoid excessive intravenous fluid administration. Further increases should continue until contractions disappear, toxicity appears, maternal pulse rate exceeds 120 beats/minute, or a dose of 30 μg/minute is reached. Once an adequate dose is reached, it should be maintained for 12 hours after the contractions stop. Do not taper down before switching to oral or subcutaneous treatment.

SUBCUTANEOUS TREATMENT

Discontinue the infusion of terbutaline IV, and 15 minutes later give 250 μg subcutaneously. Continue giving the same amount every 3 to 4 hours as necessary to keep the pulse rate between 100 and 120 beats/minute.

ORAL TREATMENT

Give a 5 mg tablet of terbutaline, and 30 minutes later discontinue the intravenous or subcutaneous administration. Give the same dosage every 4 hours for the first 24 hours as long as the pulse rate does not exceed 120 beats/minute. Then adjust the dosage to 2.5 to 5.0 mg every 3 to 6 hours depending on the patient's response to therapy.

Use of ritodrine in the treatment of preterm labor

PREPARATION OF SOLUTION

Dissolve 3 ampules of ritodrine (150 mg) in 500 ml of Ringer's lactate solution. The preparation contains 300 μg of ritodrine per milliliter.

CONTINUOUS INTRAVENOUS INFUSION

Using a Harvard pump, start intravenous infusion at a rate of 100 μg/minute (0.33 ml/minute; 20 ml/hour). Increase every 10 minutes by 50 μg/minute (0.17 ml/minute; 10.2 ml/hour) until the contractions stop, the pulse rate exceeds 120 beats/minute, toxicity appears, or a maximal rate of 350 μg/minute (1.17 ml/minute; 102 ml/hour) is reached. Once an adequate dose is reached, it should be maintained for 12 hours after the contractions stop. Do not taper down before switching to the oral treatment.

ORAL TREATMENT

Give two tablets of ritodrine (20 mg), and 30 minutes later discontinue the intravenous infusion. Continue the administration of two tablets every 2 hours for the first 24 hours after intravenous treatment as long as the pulse rate does not exceed 120 beats/minute. Then adjust the dosage, and use 10 to 20 mg every 2 to 4 hours as necessary.

treatable cause of preterm labor (ie, UTI) is found and successfully treated, it may be possible to discontinue the medication before the patient reaches 34 weeks.

There is experimental evidence showing that prolonged use of beta mimetic agents may lead to destruction of beta receptor sites and production of drug resistance. Other research has suggested that progesterone may increase the rate of formation of myometrial beta receptors. For these reasons it is possible that progesterone (Delalutin 250 mg intramuscularly every week) should be given to all patients receiving beta mimetic agents for the treatment of preterm labor.

If the low uterine segment is prominent the cervix is effaced 80% or more, and it is dilated 2 or more centimeters, the patient should be given a beta mimetic agent by continuous IV infusion. It is better to start with a low dose (5 to 10 µg/minute terbutaline, 50 to 100 µg/minute ritodrine) and increase gradually the amount of medication until a dose adequate to stop the uterine contractions is found. A summary of the details concerning terbutaline and ritodrine administration is shown in the boxes on p. 58.

The best monitor of the beta mimetic's blood level is the maternal pulse rate. It should remain between 100 and 120 beats per minute. Doses that do not raise the pulse rate to 100 beats per minute or more are usually ineffective. Doses causing marked tachycardia (more than 120 beats per minute) are dangerous because the cardiovascular tolerance of the patient is being exceeded.

A *baseline serum potassium level* should be obtained before initiation of beta mimetic therapy, and repeated determinations should be carried out every 6 hours during the duration of intravenous therapy. Serum potassium usually drops 0.5 to 1.0 mEq/L in the first few hours of treatment and remains at this level or decreases further but usually no more than another 0.5 mEq/L during the following 24 hours of therapy. It seems that the fall in potassium levels does not correspond to a real ion loss although the literature is not in agreement in this respect. Patients who develop pulmonary edema under beta mimetic therapy have low potassium levels. It is preferable to maintain the potassium concentration close to normal and administer 40 to 80 mEq of potassium in one of the IV fluid bottles if the potassium concentration falls under 3.0 mEq/L.

The hemoglobin/hematocrit values of patients in preterm labor should be determined before initiation of beta mimetic treatment and continued every 6 hours thereafter. If anemia (hemoglobin value under 10 grams, hematocrit value under 30%) exists, it should be corrected with a blood transfusion because anemia decreases blood viscosity and becomes an important contributory factor to high output heart failure during beta mimetic therapy. Also, during preterm labor therapy, water and electrolytes are retained, and this tendency may be aggravated if a large amount of IV fluids is given to the patient. A significant drop in hemoglobin/hematocrit values during beta mimetic therapy should be taken seriously because it usually indicates the presence of significant intravascular fluid retention that may precede the development of pulmonary edema and require diuretic therapy.

A *measure of blood or plasma sugar concentration* should be obtained before initiation of beta mimetic therapy and every 4 hours thereafter. The lipolytic and glycogenolytic properties of beta mimetic agents have a marked and immediate effect on the patient's blood sugar level and generate a tendency toward ketoacidosis and insulin resistance. A mild elevation (less than 200 mg/dl) in blood sugar levels is almost the universal response of patients receiving intravenous beta mimetics for the treatment of preterm labor. This elevation is more marked in patients with gestational and insulin-dependent diabetes.

Once the main mode of therapy has been selected, the next step in the management of threatened or established preterm labor is to evaluate if the patient is a suitable candidate for glucocorticoid treatment for the purpose of accelerating the maturation of the fetal lungs. Therefore the next question is the following:

> **Is there contraindication to the use of glucocorticoids?**

The most common and important contraindication to the use of glucocorticoids in the pregnant patient is the presence of bacterial or viral infections. Glucocorticoids modify the inflammatory response and alter the ability of the or-

---

Glucocorticoids for fetal lung surfactant induction in preterm labor

INITIAL DOSE

Dexamethasone 12 mg intramuscularly in two consecutive dosages 24 hours apart, or Celestone (commercial product containing 6 mg betamethasone phosphate and 6 mg betamethasone acetate per milliliter), 12 mg intramuscularly in two consecutive dosages 24 hours apart.

REPEATED DOSE

Dexamethasone 12 mg intramuscularly every week after initial treatment, or Celestone 12 mg intramuscularly every week after the initial treatment.

---

ganism to respond adequately to an infectious challenge. It is especially important to remember this contraindication in patients with tuberculosis or herpes zoster because these are situations in which the morbidity caused by steroid administration may be considerable.

Another contraindication to the use of glucocorticoids is the presence of a peptic ulcer. Guaiac testing of the stool and antiacid administration should be routine in the patient receiving steroids for the purpose of fetal lung maturation.

If the answer to the question of whether or not there is a contraindication to the use of glucocorticoids is no, the following question must be answered:

Is this a situation in which glucocorticoid administration is of maximal benefit?

Depp et al[10] have categorized patients who are candidates for glucocorticoid administration for the purpose of fetal lung maturation in three groups: (1) patients deriving no benefit, (2) patients receiving minimal benefit, and (3) patients having maximal benefit. In our opinion, this is an important analysis that must be carried out in every patient being treated for preterm labor. Glucocorticoid administration must be limited to patients who are going to obtain maximal benefit from their use.

Patients who receive no benefit from glucocorticoid treatment include those in whom the drug is contraindicated, those with adequate fetal pulmonary maturity, and those who deliver their babies in less than 24 hours or in more

than 7 days after receiving the steroid. Patients who have minimal benefit from therapy are those with more than 34 weeks of gestation and an unknown state of fetal lung maturity. Finally, patients who have maximal benefit are those under 34 weeks of gestation with immature fetal lungs who deliver their babies more than 24 hours and less than 7 days after steroid treatment.

In the study of Depp et al, 84.7% of patients at risk of preterm delivery and between 28 and 33 weeks of gestation and 94.3% of those between 34 and 37 weeks were excluded from steroid treatment. The most common reason for exclusion was a predicted time of delivery less than 24 hours or more than 7 days from the time of treatment. This prediction was correct in a large majority of cases. Only 10.9% of all patients were considered to be ideal candidates for glucocorticoid treatment.

If it is decided that the patient will have maximal benefit from glucocorticoids, a mixture of betamethasone phosphate (6 mg) and betamethasone acetate (6 mg) must be given intramuscularly in two consecutive dosages 24 hours apart (box above). Others prefer to use dexamethasone that exerts the same effect as betamethasone on the fetal lung and has less prolonged maternal effects.

Since it seems that the effect of glucocorticoids on the fetal lung is transient, it may be useful to use a "booster" every week in those patients who remain undelivered 7 days after steroid treatment. Betamethasone (12 mg intramuscularly) or dexamethasone (12 mg intramuscularly) may be used for this purpose.

The need for amniocentesis to evaluate fetal

lung maturity in patients with preterm labor requires careful individual analysis. A majority of patients under 32 weeks of gestation have immature lungs, and L/S ratio determination in these patients is probably unnecessary. However, the closer the gestational age to 34 weeks, the greater the possibility of fetal lung maturity and the justification for amniocentesis. The indication for amniocentesis following glucocorticoid treatment is questionable. We[3] and others have shown that glucocorticoids have little effect on the L/S ratio and that the test is not useful for assessing the fetal response to therapy.

Blood sugar levels should be monitored carefully during preterm labor treatment with beta mimetics and glucocorticoids. This combination causes profound alterations in carbohydrate and lipid metabolism, especially in patients with diabetes. Also, all glucocorticoids used to accelerate fetal lung maturation cause water retention. The most notorious in this respect is hydrocortisone succinate. Fluid retention may be severe and become an important factor in the development of pulmonary edema.[26] Therefore patients receiving glucocorticoids and beta mimetics for preterm labor should have daily measurements of their body weight and fluid intake and output carefully monitored. Any evidence of a large intravascular volume expansion should be treated with limitation of the fluid intake and if necessary administration of furosemide. The box above summarizes the details of the procedure of fetal lung surfactant induction with glucocorticoids.

■ DELIVERY OF THE PRETERM INFANT

Labor and delivery may be a severe traumatic insult to the preterm infant. This is clearly demonstrated for preterm infants in *breech* presentation as discussed in Chapter 17. There are some suggestions that cesarean section may be the best way to deliver infants under 1500 grams who are in *vertex* presentations. This is a controversial area, and further studies are required.

Preterm infants tolerate intrapartum hypoxia more poorly than infants at term.[22,33] This important fact should be remembered because abnormal monitoring patterns that in a term infant are not a sign for intervention may indicate deep trouble in the preterm infant.[22] Unfortunately, in many instances preterm infants are not monitored carefully, and the electronic instruments

are used mostly for low risk term infants who need them least. This is regrettable because the preterm infant is the perinatal patient with the largest need for adequate monitoring, and it is possible that neurologic damage may be prevented in some cases by timely intervention at the slightest sign of intrapartum distress.

If cesarean section is necessary for the delivery of a preterm infant, serious consideration should be given to the type of surgery to be carried out. In fact, if the low uterine segment has not developed, the best incision on the uterus is a *low vertical* approach.[22] This name is actually a misnomer because the large majority of low vertical incisions become classic incisions by the time the procedure is finished. As a consequence, there is little difference in the incidence of uterine rupture in a subsequent pregnancy between patients with classic and low vertical cesarean section incisions. In spite of its complications, the low vertical approach should be used for the abdominal delivery of preterm infants when the low segment is thick. Delivery of these babies through a low transverse incision is traumatic and frequently requires a vertical extension.

■ REFERENCES

1. Anderson ABM, Turnbull AC: Relationship between length of gestation and cervical dilation, uterine contractions and other factors during pregnancy. Am J Obstet Gynecol 1969;105:1207.
2. Arias F, Knight A: The use of terbutaline in the management of premature labor, In Zuspan FP, Christian CD (eds): *Reid's Controversy in Obstetrics and Gynecology*. Philadelphia, WB Saunders Co., 1983, pp. 31-43.
3. Arias F, Pineda J, Johnson LW: Changes in amniotic fluid lecithin/sphyngomyelin ratio and dipalmitoyl lecithin associated with maternal betamethasone therapy. Am J Obstet Gynecol 1979;133:894.
4. Arias F, Tomich P: Etiology and outcome of low birth weight and pre-term infants. Obstet Gynecol 1982; 60:277.
5. Baird D: Environmental and obstetrical factors in prematurity with special reference to the experience in Aberdeen. Bull WHO 1962;26:291.
6. Bobitt JR, Ledger W.S.: Amniotic fluid analysis: its role in maternal and neonatal infection. Obstet Gynecol 1978;51:56.
7. Bowes WA, Halgrison M, Simmons MA: Results of the intensive perinatal management of very-low-weight infants (500 to 1500 grams). J Reprod Med 1979;23:245.
8. Bruns PD, Taylor ES, Anker RM, et al: Uterine contractility, circulation, and urinary steroids in premature delivery. Am J Obstet Gynecol 1957;73:579.

9. Butler N, Bonham D: *Perinatal Mortality*. Edinburgh, E & S Livingstone, 1963, p. 288.

10. Depp R, Boehm JJ, Nosek JA, et al: Antenatal corticosteroids to prevent neonatal respiratory distress syndrome: risk versus benefit considerations. Am J Obstet Gynecol 1980;137:338.

11. Drillien MD: Prenatal and perinatal factors in etiology and outcome of low birth weight. Clin Perinatol 1974;1:197.

12. Dubowitz LMS, Dubowitz V, Goldberg CG: Clinical assessment of gestational age in the newborn infant. J Pediatr 1970;77:1.

13. Fedrick J, Anderson ABM: Factors associated with spontaneous pre-term birth. Br J Obstet Gynaecol 1976;83:342.

14. Fox H: The placenta in premature onset of labor. Br J Obstet Gynaecol 1969;76:240.

15. Friedman EA, Neff RK: *Pregnancy Hypertension*, Littleton, Mass., PSG Publishing Co, Inc, 1977, pp. 62, 200.

16. Fuchs F: Prevention of prematurity. Am J Obstet Gynecol 1976;126:809.

17. Fujimura M, Salisbury DM, Robinson RO, et al: Clinical events relating to intraventricular hemorrhage in the newborn. Arch Dis Child 1979;54:409.

18. Funderburk SJ, Guthrie D, Maldrum D: Suboptimal pregnancy outcome among women with prior abortions and premature births. Am J Obstet Gynecol 1976;126:55.

19. Gluck L, Kulovich MV, Borer RC, et al: Diagnosis of the respiratory distress syndrome by amniocentesis. Am J Obstet Gynecol 1971;109:440.

20. Goodlin RC: Cervical incompetence, hourglass membranes, and amniocentesis. Obstet Gynecol 1979;54:748.

21. Goodlin RC, Keller DW, Raffin M: Orgasm during late pregnancy: possible deleterious effect. Obstet Gynecol 1971;38:916.

22. Haesslein HC, Goodlin RC: Delivery of the tiny newborn. Am J Obstet Gynecol 1979;134:192.

23. Heionen OP, Slone D, Monson RR, et al: Cardiovascular birth defects and antenatal exposure to female sex hormone. N Engl J Med 1977;296:67.

24. Herron MA, Katz M, Creasy RK: Evaluation of a preterm birth prevention program: preliminary report. Obstet Gynecol 1982;59:452.

25. Howie RN, Liggins GC: Clinical trial of betamethasone therapy for prevention of respiratory distress in preterm infants, in Anderson A, Beard R, Brudenell JM, et al (eds): *Preterm Labor*. London, Royal College of Obstetricians and Gynecologists, 1977, p. 281.

26. Jacobs MM, Arias F: Maternal pulmonary edema resulting from betamimetic and glucocorticoid therapy. Obstet Gynecol 1980;55:56.

27. Johnson JW, Austin KL, Jones GS, et al: Efficacy of 17-α-hydroxy progesterone caproate in the prevention of premature labor. N Engl J Med 1975;293:675.

28. Kaas EH: Pregnancy, pyelonephritis and prematurity. Clin Obstet Gynecol 1970;13:239.

29. Kaufman R, Binder G, Gray P, et al: Upper genital tract changes associated with "in utero" exposure to diethylstilbestrol. Am J Obstet Gynecol 1977;128:51.

30. Kulovich MV, Hallman MB, Gluck L: The lung profile: I. Normal pregnancy. Am J Obstet Gynecol 1979;135:57.

31. Kulovich MV, Gluck L: The lung profile: II. Complicated pregnancy. Am J Obstet Gynecol 1979;135:64.

32. Lubchenco LO, Searls DT, Braie JV: Neonatal mortality rate: relationship to birth weight and gestational age. J Pediatr 1972;81:814.

33. Martin CV, Siassi B, Hon WH: Fetal heart rate patterns and neonatal death in low birthweight infants. Obstet Gynecol 1974;44:503.

34. Naeye RL: Coitus and associated amniotic-fluid infections. N Engl J Med 1979;301:1198.

35. Rush RW, Davey DA, Segal ML: The effect of pre-term delivery on perinatal mortality. Br J Obstet Gynaecol 1978;85:806.

36. Rush RW, Keirse MJNC, Howat P, et al: Contribution of pre-term delivery to perinatal mortality. Br Med J 1976;2:965.

37. Safarti P, Pageant G, Gauthier C: Le role de l'infection dans les avortements tardifs et les accouchements prematures. Can Med Assoc J 1968;13:1079.

38. Sher G, Statland BE, Freer BE, et al: Assessing fetal lung maturation by the Foam Stability Index test. Obstet Gynecol 1978;52:673.

39. Sher G, Startland BE, Knutzen VK: Evaluation of the small third-trimester fetus using the Foam Stability Index. Obstet Gynecol 1981;58:314.

40. Stewart Al, Turcan DM, Rawlings G, et al: Prognosis for infants weighing 1000 grams or less at birth. Arch Dis Child 1977;52:97.

41. TambyRaja RL, Atputharajah V, Salmon Y: Prevention of prematurity in twins. Aust NZ J Obstet Gynaecol 1978;18:179.

42. Torday J, Carson L, Lawson EE: Saturated phosphatidylcholine in amniotic fluid and prediction of the respiratory-distress syndrome. N Engl J Med 1979;301:1013.

43. Volpe JS: Perinatal hypoxic-ischemic brain injury. Pediatr Clin North Am 1976;23:383.

44. Weekes ARL, Flynn MJ: Engagement of the fetal head in primigravidas and its relationship to duration of gestation and time of onset of labor. Br J Obstet Gynaecol 1975;82:7.

45. Woods C, Bannerman RHO, Booth RT, et al: The prediction of premature labor by observation of the cervix and external tocography. Am J Obstet Gynecol 1965;91:396.

46. Zuckerman H, Reiss M, Rubinstein I: Inhibition of human premature labor by indomethacin. Obstet Gynecol 1974;44:787.

4

■ ■ ■

PREMATURE RUPTURE OF THE MEMBRANES

Fernando Arias and Edward G. Peskin

■ DEFINITION AND CHARACTERISTICS OF THE PROBLEM

Premature rupture of the fetal membranes (PROM) affects 2.7% to 17% of all pregnancies and in most cases happens spontaneously and has no apparent cause. The wide range in the incidence of PROM most probably reflects different definitions of the problem as well as true differences in its prevalence. In this chapter we will adopt the most common definition of PROM, that is, rupture of the fetal membranes occurring one or more hours before the initiation of labor.

When a pregnancy is at term or near term, PROM is usually followed within 24 hours by the spontaneous onset of labor. In a series[9] studied at University of California at Los Angeles, for example, labor started within 24 hours of PROM in 81% of patients with babies larger than 2500 grams, in 51% of patients with babies between 1000 and 2500 grams, and in only 26% of patients with babies weighing between 500 and 999 grams. Thus, for a patient with PROM, the chances of initiating spontaneous labor are directly related to the gestational age at the time of the rupture.

The contribution of preterm rupture of the membranes (PROM before 37 weeks of gesta-

tion) to the overall problem of preterm birth has not been adequately evaluated because most studies of the epidemiologic aspects of preterm birth do not separate patients with preterm labor from patients with preterm rupture of the membranes. This is unfortunate because these two problems have fundamental differences, and it is necessary to analyze them separately. In our own studies[1] preterm PROM was responsible for 34.9% of all preterm births.

■ MATERNAL AND FETAL PROBLEMS ASSOCIATED WITH PROM
Infection

The possibility of infection of the uterine cavity is the most important characteristic differentiating PROM from preterm labor. In fact, infection of mother and fetus occurs much more frequently in patients with PROM than in patients with preterm labor and intact membranes, and this increased risk for infection deeply influences the management of patients with PROM.

The occurrence of fetal and maternal infection following PROM seems to be greater in hospitals caring for low socioeconomic segments of the population than in institutions taking care of the affluent. The reason for this difference is not

63

clear, but it may depend on a decreased antibacterial activity in the amniotic fluid of the poor and undernourished.[22]

The risk of infection for the mother with PROM is less than the risk of infection for her fetus. In fact, only 5.1% of all women with PROM who have vaginal deliveries develop sepsis,[9] whereas 10% of their neonates show definite clinical infection. Maternal infectious morbidity increases five times when the patient is delivered by cesarean section. The difference in the prevalence of infection between mother and fetus probably results from the existence of more mature immunologic mechanisms in the mother. Maternal infection after PROM may be severe and has an overall mortality of 1 in 5400 cases.[14]

Infection and latent period. The incidence of infection in mother and fetus after PROM seems to be related to the duration of the latent period (time between rupture of the membranes and delivery of the fetus). Burchell,[4] for example, found that 1.7% of his patients developed fever within 24 hours after PROM, 7.5% between 24 and 48 hours, and 8.6% beyond 48 hours. In the UCLA series[9] the overall prevalence of chorioamnionitis, irrespective of infant weight or gestational age, was 2.7% before 12 hours of latent period, 6.3% between 12 and 24 hours, and 26.4% after 24 hours. If neutrophilic infiltration of the chorionic side of the placenta is taken as the index of infection,[19] 10% of PROM patients will have histologic evidence of infection 12 hours after rupture of the membranes, 30% in 24 hours, 45% in 48 hours, and 48% in 72 hours. However, the histologic criteria of infection does not necessarily correspond with culture-proven infection of mother or newborn. Some recent reports have found no increase in the incidence of infection with prolongation of the latent period.[18,24] Others have found improvement in both perinatal and maternal outcome in spite of the presence of chorioamnionitis.[7,12]

Infection and gestational age. The risk of infection after PROM is inversely related to the gestational age at the time of rupture. In the UCLA series[9] amnionitis (by histologic criteria) was present in 23.8% of all patients with PROM lasting more than 24 hours if the infant weight was 2500 grams or larger; in 31.2% if the baby weight was between 1000 and 2499 grams; and in 27.5% of the cases when the infant weight was less than 1000 grams. The data from the

Collaborative Perinatal Project[19] show that definite clinical infection of the neonate follows a similar pattern: the incidence of neonatal sepsis was 2.0% if the infant born after PROM was larger than 2500 grams; 4.8% if the infant's weight was between 2000 and 2500 grams; and 20% if the infant's weight was smaller than 2000 grams.

The higher incidence of chorioamnionitis and neonatal infection when PROM occurs in pregnancies remote from term may be the consequence of decreased antibacterial activity of the amniotic fluid,[17,22] a factor already mentioned in relation to the difference in prevalence of PROM among different socioeconomic classes. In fact, the antibacterial activity of the amniotic fluid is low in early pregnancy and increases with the advance in gestational age. Another factor is the impaired capacity of the preterm infant to fight infection.

Respiratory distress syndrome (RDS)

Several studies have concluded that hyaline membrane disease (HMD) is the greatest threat to the fetus when PROM occurs before term. For example, in the Yale–New Haven Hospital series[3] 29.8% of the perinatal deaths when PROM occurred before 36 weeks of gestation were directly caused by HMD, 14% were caused by complications of HMD, and 12.3% were caused by complications of the therapy used for HMD. This corresponds to a grand total of 56.1% of all deaths directly or indirectly caused by HMD. It is important to recognize that HMD, rather than sepsis, is the leading cause of neonatal mortality and morbidity associated with preterm PROM because this is in contradiction with the traditional concept that maternal and neonatal sepsis is the main problem and that it should be prevented by termination of pregnancy.

To further discredit undiscriminated termination of pregnancy as the best protocol for the management of patients with PROM, there is evidence that prolongation of the latent period has a beneficial effect on fetal lung maturation. Yoon and Harper[25] in a retrospective study found a 24.6% incidence of respiratory distress syndrome (RDS) among 138 infants weighing 1001 to 2165 grams who were delivered less than 12 hours after PROM. In contrast, RDS was present in only 12.5% of 48 infants of similar weight who were born more than 24 hours after membranes had ruptured. Bauer and Stern[2] in a prospective study found no cases of RDS in 10 premature infants born after more than 16 hours of latent period, whereas there were 4 cases of RDS in 7 infants born after a latent period of less than 16 hours. Richardson et al[16] found a 64% incidence of RDS in 42 neonates with an average gestational age of 32.4 weeks delivered less than 24 hours after PROM, whereas in 22 infants with a gestational age of 30.4 weeks and with PROM lasting more than 24 hours the incidence of RDS was 32%. In another study of 119 infants under 32 weeks of gestation born after PROM[3] it was found that the incidence of RDS decreased from 58% to 28% if the latent period was greater than 16 hours. However, there is one retrospective investigation in contradiction with the previously mentioned papers: Jones et al[10] reviewed 16,000 births and concluded that there was no association between decreased incidence of RDS and prolongation of the latent period after PROM.

Congenital abnormalities

An important fact that should be taken into consideration when planning strategies for the management of patients with PROM is the high incidence of major congenital malformations in babies born after PROM remote from term. In the Yale–New Haven series[3] 4 out of 20 non-RDS deaths were caused by severe congenital malformations. Likewise, the UCLA series[9] shows that 6 of 77 perinatal deaths (8%) in patients with PROM were caused by multiple fetal congenital abnormalities.

■ DIAGNOSIS OF PROM

The diagnosis of PROM is especially important in pregnancies remote from term. In fact, a false positive diagnosis of PROM in a patient at term or near term may lead to induction of labor. However, the morbidity associated with induction of labor in a term pregnancy is small when compared with the consequences of intervention when a false positive diagnosis of PROM is made early in gestation. The seven procedures described in this section are important in the diagnosis of PROM.

Visualization of amniotic fluid in the vagina

To examine the amniotic fluid, place a bedpan under the patient and have a bright light avail-able. Do not use any sprays or jellies. Place a sterile speculum in the vagina and observe for fluid. Amniotic fluid usually is colorless and may contain white flecks (vernix) near term. This fluid will often be yellowish in preterm gestations, brownish with meconium staining, and reddish brown in fetal death. If no fluid is immediately seen, have the patient cough or perform a Valsalva's maneuver and observe for a gush of fluid. Also compress the fundus of the uterus from the abdomen with your hand and observe if fluid comes out of the cervix. The finding of a vaginal pool of amniotic fluid or the direct observation of fluid coming out of the cervix makes a positive diagnosis of PROM.

Nitrazine Paper test

The procedure for Nitrazine paper testing is as follows: Take a sterile cotton-tipped applicator and touch it to the fluid present in the vagina. Place the secretions obtained on Nitrazine paper and compare the color of the paper to the standard chart to find out the fluid's pH. The vaginal pH is normally 4.5 to 5.5, whereas amniotic fluid usually has a pH of 7.0 to 7.5. The membranes probably are intact if the paper color remains yellow or changes to olive yellow (pH 5.0 to 5.5). They probably are ruptured if the paper turns blue (pH 7.0 or higher). Antiseptic solutions, urine, blood, and vaginal infections cause alteration of the vaginal pH and false readings with this test.

Fern test or arborization test

For the fern test a sample from the same fluid used for the Nitrazine test is placed on a glass slide and allowed to dry. The preparation is observed under the microscope to look for a crystallization pattern that resembles a fern. Ferning is a result of the drying out of salts contained in the amniotic fluid and is affected by the presence of blood or meconium. *The test may produce a high number of false positive results if the sample is obtained from the cervix instead of the vagina*. Cervical mucus forms a heavy and wide arborization pattern that may be accepted by the inexperienced as proof of PROM. The Nitrazine test is less accurate than the fern test in the diagnosis of PROM. The Nitrazine test gives 12.7% false negative and 16.2% false positive results, whereas ferning gives 4.8% false negative and 4.4% false positive results.[23] The diagnosis of PROM is very close to 100% reliable if the fluid found in the vagina gives positive Nitrazine and positive fern tests. In a minority of patients, however, visual inspection of the vagina along with Nitrazine and fern testing will be inadequate for establishing a positive diagnosis of PROM.

Ultrasound examination

Examination of the patient with real-time or B-scanning ultrasound is useful to evaluate the amount of amniotic fluid present inside the uterus. In patients with adequate clinical history of PROM but equivocal findings on pelvic examination (ie, no fluid seen, positive Nitrazine and negative ferning testing), if the ultrasound shows little or no fluid in the uterine cavity it should be assumed that PROM has occurred. On the contrary, equivocal clinical findings in the presence of a normal amount of fluid by ultrasound examination make the diagnosis of PROM very questionable. However, false positive ultrasonic diagnosis may occur in cases of oligohydramnios as well as false negative in cases of discrete amniotic fluid losses. The technique is useful only as an additional piece of information in questionable cases and must not be used as the primary means of diagnosis.

Injection of fluorescein into the amniotic cavity

Injection of fluorescein into the amniotic cavity is rarely indicated for the diagnosis of PROM. This invasive procedure is performed when the diagnosis of PROM cannot be confirmed with noninvasive techniques. Examples are patients complaining of persistent vaginal and vulvar wetting, with negative or equivocal Nitrazine and fern testing, and with a normal or slightly decreased amount of amniotic fluid by ultrasound. In these cases 1 or 2 cc of a sterile solution of 5% sodium fluorescein is injected into the amniotic cavity after localization of the placenta with real-time scanning. Fifteen minutes after the injection, the cervix and the vagina should be examined with a long-wave ultraviolet light. The detection of fluorescent material is equivalent to a positive diagnosis of PROM.[21] In many of these cases, however, PROM is the result of a high leak.

High leak is a term used to describe a loss of amniotic fluid caused by a tear in the membranes located above the lower uterine segment. In these cases it is possible to visualize an intact amniotic sac with an amnioscope introduced through the cervix. High leaks usually seal spontaneously, and they are not associated with the fetal and maternal complications occurring when the tear is in the proximity of the cervical opening. In the majority of cases the diagnosis of high leak can be made with noninvasive procedures, and only on rare occasions is it necessary to inject fluorescein into the amniotic sac or to perform amnioscopy to make a positive diagnosis. The majority of patients with high leaks have small losses of amniotic fluid, which usually decrease and eventually stop after a short period of observation. Serial ultrasound examinations will show a normal or slightly diminished amount of fluid in the amniotic cavity.

There is a rare condition in which unquestionable evidence of PROM is followed by the appearance of an intact amniotic sac at the time of labor. These cases of bag of waters rupturing twice are the consequence of accumulation of amniotic fluid between amnion and chorion ("chorionic cyst") with the fluid being leaked out the first time because of a rupture of only the amnion.[20] Initially the clinical picture is undistinguishable from PROM, but if the patient is observed for a few days after the initial gush of fluid, there is no further leakage and a normal amount of fluid is found by ultrasound. This is a benign condition since the true amniotic sac is left intact. In many cases, however, the rupture of a chorionic cyst is diagnosed as PROM, and iatrogenic intervention takes place.

Amnioscopy

Amnioscopy is another invasive diagnostic procedure that is rarely indicated in the diagnosis or management of patients with PROM. The procedure requires the presence of a soft and distensible cervix and consists of introducing a metallic or plastic narrow cone through the cervix for direct visualization of the membranes and the amniotic fluid. As in the injection of fluorescein into the amniotic cavity, amnioscopy may have a role in the diagnosis of high leaks. However, the procedure may cause premature rupture of the membranes in patients with intact membranes and may carry a large bacterial inoculum into the amniotic cavity in patients with PROM.

Diamine oxidase test

Diamine oxidase is an enzyme produced by the placental decidual cells, which enters the amniotic fluid but is absent from the vagina. Measurement of diamine oxidase by paper strips placed in contact with the vagina is an accurate way to diagnose PROM.[5] However, the test requires relatively elaborate laboratory procedures and is not ready for general use.

■ MANAGEMENT OF PATIENTS WITH PROM

There are few situations in obstetrics where individualization of patient management is as important as in the case of PROM. To avoid mistakes, the obstetrician should answer a sequence of questions focused on important aspects of the problem. The first question is as follows:

> **Are there signs or symptoms of intrauterine infection?**

A positive answer to this question indicates that management should be directed toward rapid termination of pregnancy without consideration as to the gestational age of the fetus. It also implies the initiation of aggressive antibiotic treatment. Maternal tachycardia (>100 beats per minute), maternal fever (>37.5° C), uterine tenderness, fetal tachycardia (>180 beats per minute), malodorous and purulent amniotic fluid, and elevation of the white blood cell count with a shift to the left are classic signs of developing or established chorioamnionitis. The presence of one or more of these signs in a patient with a history of several hours between rupture of the membranes and admission to the hospital makes positive a presumptive diagnosis of chorioamnionitis. It should be noted that positive cultures of blood or amniotic fluid are not necessary to establish a presumptive diagnosis of chorioamnionitis and that this diagnosis implies that initiation of an aggressive management program directed toward pregnancy termination. In some unfortunate instances, the patient may come to the hospital after chorioamnionitis has caused intrauterine fetal death, disseminated infection, and maternal septic shock.

If severe infection is present and delivery is not imminent, antibiotic treatment must be started after obtaining blood cultures and endocervical swabs for aerobic and anaerobic cultures. We use triple therapy with aqueous crystalline penicillin (4 million units by intravenous piggyback (IVPB) every 4 hours), gentamicin (3 mg/kg/day divided into three equal doses and given by IVPB every 8 hours) and clindamycin (300 mg by IVPB every four hours). With this antibiotic regimen we are presumptively treating infection by gram-negative bacteria and gram-positive cocci, which are the predominant culture isolates in cases of chorioamnionitis. Penicillin at this high dose will also cover anaerobes with the exception of *Bacteroides fragilis*, which is covered by clindamycin.

If there are no contraindications for vaginal delivery and if labor is not already in progress, the patient with chorioamnionitis should have labor induced with diluted intravenous oxytocin administered with a Harvard pump. If vaginal delivery is contraindicated (transverse lie, cephalopelvic disproportion, premature breech, etc) a loading dose of antibiotics (penicillin, 4 million units IVPB; gentamicin, 1 mg/kg IVPB; clindamycin, 300 mg IVPB) is given at least 1 hour before the cesarean section. The objective of this preoperative antibiotic administration is to obtain antibiotic tissue levels that may prevent colonization secondary to the bacterial spread that occurs during surgical manipulation of the infected uterus.

If intravenous oxytocin fails to produce cervical changes and vaginal delivery is not in sight after 12 hours of induction, the patient must be delivered by cesarean section. If the uterus bleeds poorly during surgery and there are thrombosed veins or myometrial abscesses, it is mandatory to proceed to a cesarean hysterectomy. During surgery, cultures of both surfaces of the placenta must be taken and repeated blood cultures must be obtained after emptying the uterus. These cultures are valuable for identification of the offending microorganism and evaluation of its antibiotic sensitivity.

If infection is not severe and delivery is anticipated to occur within 4 hours after the diagnosis of chorioamnionitis was made, initiation of antibiotic treatment may be postponed until the umbilical cord is clamped. In these cases the pediatrician will obtain material for cultures from the baby and will initiate antibiotic therapy that will be discontinued after 3 days if the cultures are negative. If the mother receives antibiotics before the cord is clamped, the value of the baby's cultures will be altered and most pediatricians will opt for a 10-day course of antibiotics.

If the answer to the first question is negative (no, there are no signs of intrauterine infection), one may start to consider an answer to the second question:

> **Is the mother at unusually high risk for the development of an infection?**

This is the time to meticulously review the past and present medical history of the mother in an effort to find out if there are factors making her highly susceptible to infection or there are circumstances making it unusually dangerous for her to develop an infection. Several of these factors and circumstances are the following:

1. Patient taking immunosuppressant drugs
   a. Glucocorticoids
   b. Azathioprine (Imuran)
   c. Antineoplastic agents
2. Patient with history of rheumatic heart disease
3. Patient who has insulin-dependent diabetes
4. Patient who has sickle cell disease
5. Patient with prosthetic valve in place following open heart surgery
6. Patient with IUD left inside the uterus during present pregnancy
7. Patient with infected Shirodkar or McDonald cerclages
8. Patient who has had several manual pelvic examinations since PROM occurred

If the mother belongs to one of the preceding groups, an adequate management is termination of pregnancy. Antibiotic *prophylaxis* is started immediately after cord clamping using cefoxitin, 1 gram IV every 6 hours for a total of 4 doses. If maternal cultures are positive, antibiotic administration must be continued for 5 to 10 days and appropriate changes made according to the bacteria being isolated and their antibiotic sensitivity. If the cultures are negative, antibiotics are discontinued. Prophylactic administration of antibiotics to patients with PROM does not change perinatal mortality. However, antibiotics reduce maternal febrile morbidity.[19]

If the answer to the question is negative (no, the patient is not at unusually high risk for developing infection), it will be necessary to move on to the following question:

> **Is this an abnormal fetus?**

Careful ultrasound examination should be performed in every patient with PROM, and occasionally a fetogram should be made, especially in pregnancies remote from term, to rule out the presence of gross congenital malformations. Microcephaly, hydrocephaly, and anencephaly are some defects that may be picked up. However, severe congenital defects, chromosomal abnormalities, and inborn errors of metabolism, will not be recognized with the use of ultrasound and x-ray.

If yes is the response to this question, the patient must be delivered. There is no reason to continue a pregnancy after PROM if the fetus has gross congenital abnormalities.

If the answer to the question is no, one must move on to the following question:

> **Is the pregnancy at more than 34 weeks of gestation and/or the fetal weight greater than 2000 grams?**

The answer to this question implies a careful evaluation of all the clinical information necessary to determine the duration of gestation (last menstrual period, early pelvic examination, time of positive pregnancy test, quickening, ultrasound dating, time when fetal heart was first heard by aural stethoscope, etc). For a detailed discussion about how to assess gestational age see Chapters 1 and 9. If the information available is insufficient to reach a conclusion, an ultrasound examination is indicated. In spite of the lack of accuracy of ultrasound examinations for determining gestational age in the third trimester of pregnancy, it is necessary to rely on the information provided by this examination unless there is a possibility of retarded or excessive fetal growth.

In many cases of PROM the estimation of fetal weight by ultrasound is difficult because the lack of fluid interferes with the resolution of the method and the accuracy of the measurements.

The obstetrician should use the clinical examination, the sonogram, and if necessary, the fetogram; the information provided by all these methods must be put together to make a decision about the fetal size.

If the answer is yes (fetus >34 weeks or >2000 grams), the patient must be delivered. There is no good reason to expose a mother and her fetus to the risk of infection when the chances of neonatal survival with good neurologic outcome are better than 97%. In these cases, and as long as there are no signs or symptoms of infection, one may wait for 24 to 48 hours after PROM before induction of labor, and a large majority of patients (about 80%) will spontaneously start laboring during this period. One exception may be patients who are closer to 34 than to 37 weeks of gestation and who show no spontaneous uterine activity during this waiting period. In these cases, if no signs of infection are present, the waiting period may be prolonged for more days until the patient starts to labor or show early signs of infection. In our experience, there is more maternal and fetal morbidity with prolonged and repeated inductions of labor than with prolongation of pregnancy and careful monitoring for early signs of infection.

If no is the answer to the question on gestational age and fetal weight, the patient is a candidate for expectant management. In some cases, however, further individualization of care can be provided by amniocentesis and amniotic fluid analysis. When fluid is obtained, it is possible to evaluate fetal lung maturation and to detect unrecognized intraamniotic colonization. For these purposes the amniotic fluid lecithin to spingomyelin (L/S) ratio is determined and the fluid is cultured (for details see Chapter 3). A Gram's stain (box below) is performed in a drop of centrifuged fluid. It is considered to be positive if bacteria are seen after 2 minutes of searching.[15] The Wright's stain (box below) is also useful when looking for neutrophils in the fluid. It seems that PROM patients with neutrophils in the fluid are at higher risk of infectious morbidity,[13] but there is controversy in this respect.[20] In the future, examination of the amniotic fluid with gas liquid chromatography[8] may

---

Gram's stain of amniotic fluid

1. Place one drop of centrifuged amniotic fluid on a glass slide. Heat fix. Allow to cool.
2. Flood slide with crystal violet. Allow to stain for 1 minute.
3. Wash with tap water.
4. Flood slide with iodine. Allow to stain 2 minutes.
5. Wash with tap water.
6. Decolorize slide with 95% alcohol (approximately 15 to 20 seconds).

Wright's stain of amniotic fluid

1. Place one drop of centrifuged amniotic fluid on a glass slide. Heat fix. Allow to cool.
2. Flood slide with Wright's stain and leave it on the slide for 2 minutes.
3. Add equal volume of buffer to slide.
4. Mix layers of stain and buffer by gently blowing on slide (an iridescent sheen should appear in 5 to 10 seconds).
5. Allow buffer to remain on slide for approximately 3 minutes.
6. Wash off stain-buffer mix with distilled water, wipe the back of the slide, and air dry.
7. Staining time may be modified to obtain a darker or lighter stain as desired.

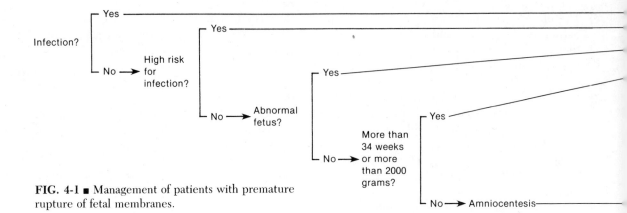

FIG. 4-1 ■ Management of patients with premature rupture of fetal membranes.

become the best method for the early diagnosis of bacterial colonization of the uterine cavity.

The majority of patients with PROM remote from term have little or no amniotic fluid left in the uterus, and transabdominal amniocentesis is unsuccessful in up to 30% of these patients despite attempts to reaccumulate fluid by placing the patient in Trendelenburg's position and despite the use of real-time ultrasound to guide the needle placement.

Finding a mature L/S ratio in uninfected patients with PROM far from term does not mean pregnancy must be terminated. Sometimes it is better to prolong intrauterine life in these patients with PROM and mature L/S and wait for spontaneous labor and cervical ripening than to proceed to prolonged, repeated, and often morbid attempts of induction.

The overall plan of management for patients with PROM is summarized in Fig. 4-1. Future developments most certainly will introduce modifications to that protocol.

■ EXPECTANT MANAGEMENT

The objective of expectant management in cases of PROM remote from term is to decrease perinatal mortality and morbidity without harmful maternal consequences. The rationale behind this approach is provided by an increasing amount of evidence indicating a decreased incidence of RDS with prolongation of the latent period after preterm PROM. The main risk of conservative management is that the longer the

membranes are ruptured, the greater the chances of intraamniotic infection. The only way to decrease the risk of being defeated by sepsis in our efforts to overcome RDS is by careful monitoring for signs and symptoms of infection in both mother and fetus during the period of expectant management.

The presence of spontaneous labor is not a contraindication for conservative therapy. If the patient is having regular uterine contractions at the time that the decision for expectant management is made, she should receive a beta mimetic agent. However, no heroic measures should be adopted to stop labor in patients with PROM, and our recommendation is never to use large doses of IV tocolytics for this purpose.

Digital pelvic examinations are not carried out during the period of expectant management. They increase the risk of maternal and fetal septic morbidity, and they are unnecessary in this phase of the problem. However, if the patient enters into the active phase of labor, pelvic examinations should be done to follow the course of labor, but they should be kept to a minimum.

At the time of admission, when a careful speculum examination is done for diagnostic purposes, an endocervical swab should be taken for routine and *Neisseria gonorrhea* cultures. The patient is then started on ampicillin, 500 mg orally four times per day, pending the result of the cultures. The use of ampicillin before the culture results are available is justified by the high incidence of beta streptococci colonization

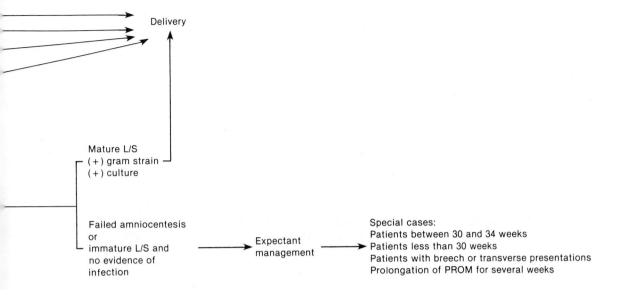

in patients with PROM and the severity of the neonatal infection with this particular organism. If the culture is negative (no pathogens are identified), ampicillin is discontinued. However, the growth of pathogenic organisms is an indication for antibiotic prophylaxis: If the culture grows more than 100,000 colonies of alpha or beta hemolytic streptococci, ampicillin administration should continue. If the cultures grow *Neisseria gonorrhea*, ampicillin is discontinued and the patient must receive aqueous procaine penicillin G, 4.8 million units intramuscularly, 30 minutes after 1 gram of oral probenecid. If the culture grows a mixed flora, but with predominance of *Escherichia coli*, ampicillin is discontinued and gentamicin, 3 mg/kg/day divided in three doses intramuscularly every 8 hours, should be used. The growth of other pathogenic bacteria in the cultures taken from the endocervix is an indication for treatment according to their sensitivity to the antibiotics that may be used in pregnant women.

Maternal temperature and pulse rate measurements are obtained every 4 hours and a white blood cell (WBC) count every 12 hours in patients under expectant management. Differential counts are obtained if there is a total increase of more than 5000 WBC. The patients are questioned every 12 hours about uterine contractions, chills, amount of vaginal leaking, and fetal movements and are examined to determine fetal heart rate, presence or absence of foul-smelling vaginal discharge, and uterine tenderness. They are restricted to bed rest with bathroom privileges. No pelvic examinations are carried out, and the patient is instructed to avoid douches, vaginal tampons, and tub bathing.

The following is a summary of expectant management protocol for certain patients with PROM:

1. Obtain endocervical swabs for routine and *Neisseria gonorrhea* cultures.
2. Start ampicillin, 500 mg four times daily, pending culture results.
3. *Do not do manual pelvic examination unless evaluation of cervical dilation is indicated.*
4. Restrict patient to bed rest with bathroom privileges.
5. Order regular diet.
6. Evaluate use of beta mimetics: Subcutaneous or oral administration depending on the characteristics of labor; medications to arrest labor should be discontinued after 24 hours (72 hours if the patient receives glucocorticoids).
7. Monitor as follows:
   a. Take maternal temperatures and pulse and fetal heart rate every 4 hours.
   b. Check WBC count every 12 hours. Obtain differential if WBC count rises 5000 or more.
   c. Check for uterine tenderness, foul-smelling vaginal discharge, amount of leaking, and fetal movements every 12 hours.

   d. Electronically monitor the fetus every
       24 hours if the fetus is in breech pre-
       sentation.
8. Administer betamethasone or dexamethasone if the infant's weight is less than 1000
   grams or the gestational age less than 28
   weeks.
9. Evaluate need for antibiotic treatment or
   antibiotic choice as soon as results of endocervical culture are available.

Further individualization of patient care is described for four subgroups of patients among
those selected for expectant therapy. With advances in our knowledge about PROM, it is possible that new subgroups will be created and
that some of the ones presently recognized will
disappear.

Patients between 30 and 34 weeks of gestation

The subgroup of patients between 30 and 34
weeks of gestation corresponds to infants with a
birth weight between 1200 and 2000 grams. The
overall survival rate of babies in this range of
gestational age and weight when managed in
adequate neonatal facilities is between 85% and
90%; in following observations, a similar percentage of the survivors (85% to 90%) are free
of any serious sequelae, including central nervous system damage. These percentages drop
precipitously in less sophisticated neonatal facilities. Thus there is a need for the establishment of systems for the transport of *the mother
with the infant in uterus* from small hospitals to
tertiary care centers.

Infants weighing between 1200 and 2000
grams are relatively close to physiologic lung
maturation in utero. Hence, a limited prolongation of the latent phase after PROM is probably required to decrease the incidence of respiratory difficulties in these infants during the
neonatal period. This means that administration
of beta mimetics to stop labor and prolong pregnancy is indicated for the first 24 hours after
PROM. Once this period is completed, the administration of labor inhibitors should be discontinued. However, no active intervention (induction of labor) should be carried out unless
signs of infection appear. Most patients in this
gestational age subgroup will go into spontaneous labor shortly after discontinuation of beta
mimetic agents.

Patients of less than 30 weeks of gestation

The birth weight of infants in the subgroup of
patients of less than 30 weeks of gestation is
under 1200 grams. The prognosis for these tiny
babies has improved considerably during the last
decade, and the overall perinatal survival rate
may be as high as 75% when the infant is managed within a neonatal intensive care unit. In
follow-up observation about 70% of the survivors
are neurologically intact. The *transport of the
mother with the fetus "in utero"* to a tertiary
center is of fundamental importance to the perinatal outcome of patients with PROM and less
than 30 weeks of gestation. In fact, infants in
this gestational age range have a very limited
chance of survival outside of a neonatal intensive
care unit.

In this subgroup a management assumption
has been that, since these fetuses are still quite
remote from the gestational age at which lung
maturation normally occurs, they do require
prolongation of the latent period as well as pharmacologic intervention to accelerate lung maturity. This assumption has been contradicted
by the work of Garites et al[6] demonstrating that
maternal glucocorticoid administration offers no
fetal or neonatal advantages in the management
of PROM. In our own study about PROM[11] we
found that glucocorticoids are of benefit for very
immature infants (birthweight less than 1000
grams) but they are not useful for larger babies.
Therefore our present policy is to give corticosteroids *only if the infant weight is less than 1000
grams* and the parents consent to their administration. Oral or subcutaneous administration
of a beta mimetic agent is maintained for 72
hours while the mother is treated with betamethasone or dexamethasone. In chapter 3
there is information related to the risks of maternal corticosteroid administration to induce fetal lung maturation. However, it is necessary to
emphasize two points about steroid therapy
which are pertinent to patients with PROM.
They are:

First, *glucocorticoid administration causes
drastic modifications in WBC and differential
count*. The elevation in WBC caused by corticosteroids is on the average 4000 cells with a
mild shift to the left and a decrease in monocyte
and lymphocyte count. These changes can easily
be mistaken as a sign of infection. In general, if

the patient becomes infected, the elevation in the WBC is greater than 4000 and the differential shows a more marked shift to the left with appearance of a significant number of bands.

Second, *glucocorticoids depress the immunologic response and impair the ability of the mother to fight infection*. This effect is significant and maternal infectious morbidity may be increased in mothers with PROM when they receive glucocorticoids.[6] However, the high risk of neonatal complications associated with RDS in the infant under 1000 grams justifies the use of corticosteroids in this situation.

The patient with breech or transverse presentation

Patients with PROM remote from term and with breech or transverse presentations are a special problem because of the risk of umbilical cord prolapse and because of problems associated with their delivery. In fact, apparent and occult cord prolapse frequently occurs in these patients during the latent phase of PROM. Therefore, they should be continuously electronically monitored during the first 24 hours after PROM and then at least 1 hour per day during the period of expectant management looking for variable decelerations indicating umbilical cord compression.

Vaginal delivery of preterm infants in breech and transverse presentations has an extremely high perinatal morbidity and mortality. Most of these cases must be delivered by low vertical cesarean section, a procedure that is associated with increased maternal morbidity. Finally, it must be remembered that the frequency of congenital abnormalities is greater in fetuses in other than vertex presentation and therefore one must screen for congenital malformations more carefully.

Prolongation of PROM for several weeks

Occasionally, the obstetrician is faced with a case in which PROM is prolonged several weeks without evidence of infection and with serial ultrasound examinations showing little or no amniotic fluid in the uterus. The question here is, how long may the pregnancy continue despite the lack of amniotic fluid? There are two factors indicating delivery. The first is the appearance of fetal distress. These patients must be monitored (nonstress testing) at least every week and

pregnancy must be terminated if spontaneous decelerations or variable decelerations, indicating cord compression, are present. The second is the development of musculoskeletal deformities. It seems that fetal malformations secondary to PROM will not appear before 4 weeks. Therefore, if PROM has been prolonged for more than 4 weeks, and repeated ultrasound examinations show no fluid in the uterus, the pregnancy should be terminated to avoid the formation of amniotic bands and the occurrence of musculoskeletal deformities.

■ REFERENCES

1. Arias F, Tomich P: Etiology and outcome of low birth weight and preterm infants. Obstet Gynecol 1982;60:277.
2. Bauer C, Stern L, Colle E: Prolonged rupture of membranes associated with a decreased incidence of respiratory distress syndrome. Pediatrics 1974;53:7.
3. Berkowitz RL, Bonta BW, Warshaw JE: The relationship between premature rupture of the membranes and the respiratory distress syndrome. Am J Obstet Gynecol 1976;124:712.
4. Burchell RC: Premature spontaneous rupture of the membranes. Am J Obstet Gynecol 1964;88:251.
5. Gahl WA, Kozina TS, Fuhrmann DD, et al: Diamine oxidase in the diagnosis of ruptured fetal membranes. Obstet Gynecol 1982;60:297.
6. Garite TS, Freeman RK, Linzey ME, et al: Prospective randomized study of corticosteroids in the management of premature rupture of membranes and the premature gestation. Am J Obstet Gynecol 1981;141:508.
7. Gibbs RS, Castillo MS, Rodgers PJ: Management of acute chorioamnionitis. Am J Obstet Gynecol 1980;136:709.
8. Gravett MG, Eschenbach DA, Spiegal C, et al: Rapid ddiagnosis of amniotic fluid infection by gas-liquid chromatography. N Engl J Med 1982;306:725.
9. Gunn GC, Mishell DR, Morton DG: Premature rupture of the fetal membranes. Am J Obstet Gynecol 1970;106:469.
10. Jones MD, Burd LI, Bowes WA Jr, et al: Failure of association of premature rupture of membranes with respiratory distress syndrome. N Eng J Med 1975;292:1253.
11. Knight AB, Tomich PG, Arias F: A comparison of prolongation of the latent period versus prolongation plus glucocorticoids in patients with preterm rupture of the membranes. Reprod Med, to be published.
12. Koh KS, Cham FH, Manfared AH, et al: The changing perinatal and maternal outcome in chorioamnionitis. Am J Obstet Gynecol 1979;53:730.
13. Larsen JW, Weis KR, Leniham JP, et al: Significance of neutrophils and bacteria in the amniotic fluid of patients in labor. Obstet Gynecol 1976;47:143.
14. Lebherz TB, Hellman LP, Madding R, et al: Double-blind study of premature rupture of the membranes. Am J Obstet Gynecol 1963;87:218.

15. Listwa HM, Dobek AS, Carpenter S, et al: The predictability of intrauterine infection by analysis of amniotic fluid. Obstet Gynecol 1976;48:31.

16. Richardson C, Pomerance JJ, Cunningham MD, et al: Acceleration of fetal lung maturation following prolonged rupture of the membranes. Am J Obstet Gynecol 1974;118:1115.

17. Schlievert P, Johnson W, Galask RP: Bacterial growth inhibition by amniotic fluid. V. Phosphate to zinc ratio as a predictor of bacterial growth inhibitory activity. Am J Obstet Gynecol 1976;125:899.

18. Schreiber J, Benedetti T: Conservative management of preterm rupture of the fetal membranes in a low socioeconomic population. Am J Obstet Gynecol 1980;136:92.

19. Shubeck F, Benson RC, Clark WW, et al: Fetal hazard after rupture of the membranes. Obstet Gynecol 1966;28:22.

20. Schuman W: Double sac with secondary rupture of the bag of waters during labor: a clinical entity, and its explanation from examination of the membranes. Am J Obstet Gynecol 1951;62:633.

21. Smith RP: A technique for the detection of rupture of the membranes. Obstet Gynecol 1976;48:172.

22. Tafari N, Ross SM, Naeye RL, et al: Failure of bacterial growth inhibition by amniotic fluid. Am J Obstet Gynecol 1977;128:187.

23. Tricomi V, Hall JE, Bittar A, et al: Arborization test for the detection of ruptured fetal membranes. Obstet Gynecol 1966;27:275.

24. Varner MW, Galask RP: Conservative management of premature rupture of the membranes. Am J Obstet Gynecol 1981;140:39.

25. Yoon J, Harper R: Observations on the relationship between duration of rupture of the membranes and the development of idiopathic respiratory distress syndrome. Pediatrics 1973;52:161.

5

■ ■ ■

ERYTHROBLASTOSIS FETALIS

Fernando Arias and Douglas C. Johnson

Before the discovery of the Rh system by Landsteiner in 1940, little was known about the etiology of erythroblastosis, a condition in which the fetus becomes edematous and often dies in the uterus from severe anemia and high output cardiac failure. After this discovery it was quickly learned that maternal Rh isoimmunization with placental transfer of IgG antibodies was the phenomenon responsible for the fetal red cell destruction. This was followed by the finding that spectrophotometric analysis of the amniotic fluid was an excellent index to measure the severity of the fetal anemia and by the realization that early delivery and intrauterine transfusions (IUTs) could be lifesaving maneuvers for the compromised fetus. Finally, it was found that the administration of anti-D immune globulin to mothers at risk is an extremely effective way of preventing the initial immune response causing Rh isoimmunization. The field has moved, therefore, from a stage of little knowledge about a serious disease in the early 1940s to a situation in which preventive measurements have made the occurrence of that problem a relatively rare event in the late 1970s.

■ ETIOLOGY

Erythroblastosis fetalis is a disease of the fetus and the newborn in which the infant's red blood cells are hemolyzed by maternal isoantibodies (antibodies capable of reacting with red cells from the same species but not with red cells of the individual producing the antibodies) that have been able to cross the placenta. The resulting anemia leads to fetal heart failure, massive edema (hydrops fetalis), and intrauterine death. It also may cause varied degrees of neonatal hyperbilirubinemia (hemolytic disease of the newborn). Approximately 97% of all cases of erythroblastosis fetalis are caused by maternal immunization against the Rh(D) antigen present in the fetal red cells. The remaining cases are caused by immunization against other fetal antigenic groups such as C, c, E, e, K, k, Fy^a, M, and Jk^a. Maternal isoimmunization may be a consequence of the transfusion or intramuscular administration of Rh positive blood to an Rh negative female, but in the overwhelming majority of cases it results from the passage of fetal Rh positive red cells into the bloodstream of Rh negative mothers in the course of pregnancy and especially at the time of delivery. In response to this immunologic stimulation the mother develops 19S and 7S antibodies, the latter being able to cross the placenta and destroy the fetal red cells.

■ PATHOPHYSIOLOGY

The inheritance of blood group antigens is, according to Mendelian laws and with the exception of the group X_ga (X-linked), autosomal and codominant (both alleles are expressed in

75

the heterozygous individual). According to the Fisher-Race "paired" gene theory, the Rh system is formed by six Rh genes, three carried on each chromosome. Each tri-gene complex (haplotype) is inherited from each parent as such with little or no crossing over. Three of the genes are dominant (C, D, E), and three are recessive (c, d, e); the most important is the D gene that confers to the individual the characteristic of being Rh positive. An Rh positive person may be homozygous (DD) or heterozygous (Dd), whereas an Rh negative individual may only be homozygous (dd). This has practical importance because a homozygous Rh positive father (DD), if mated with an Rh negative (dd) mother, passes to his offspring a dominant D gene regardless of which of the two paired genes is carried over to the child. As a result, the offspring is Rh positive in 100% of the cases. If the father is heterozygous (Dd), the chances of a child being Rh positive are only 50%. The distinction between homozygous and heterozygous Rh negative fathers is complicated by the fact that there is no antiserum against the d antigen, and therefore the prediction of heterozygosity or homozygosity has to be made using genotype frequency tables based on allelic frequency (Tables 5-1 and 5-2).

Some red cells react weakly with anti-D antibodies because they contain a gene that produces only a part of the D antigen. This variant is called *Du*, and it should be absent (Du negative) to consider a given individual as Rh negative. A third allele of C and c has also been identified, most commonly in association with D and e and has been called C^w. Some individuals have a rare state, termed *Rh-null* in which their red cells lack Rh antigen. The C and E Rh antigens may also in rare instances initiate the reactions leading to the production of erythroblastosis fetalis. Other antigens with similar potential are the K (Kell), Fy^a (Duffy), and Jk^a (Kidd) that usually cause isoimmunization via a previous blood transfusion rather than as a consequence of a previous pregnancy. An antigen frequently found in routine antenatal testing is the Lewis group (Le^a and Le^b). The Lewis antigens do not cause erythroblastosis fetalis and

TABLE 5-1 ■ Prevalence of Rh chromosome types in whites

Antigens	Frequency (%)
C D e	40
c d e	38
c D E	14
c D e	2.5
c d E	1.1
C d e	1.0
C D E	0.24
C d E	Very low

TABLE 5-2 ■ Genotype frequency table

C	D	E	c	e	Type	Not excluded	%	Homo/hetero (H)(h)
+	+	−	+	+	CDe/cde	CDe/cDe	32.0	h
						cDe/Cde	2.0	H
							0.1	h
							17.0	H
+	+	−	−	+	CDe/CDe	CDe/Cde	0.8	h
							12.0	H
+	+	+	+	+	CDe/cDE	CDe/Cde	1.0	jh
						cDE/Cde	0.3	h
							11.0	h
−	+	+	+	+	cDE/cde	cDE/cDe	1.0	H
						cDe/cdE	0.1	h
							2.0	H
−	+	+	+	−	cDE/cDE	cDE/cdE	0.3	h
							2.0	h
−	+	−	+	+	cDe/cde	cDe/cDe	0.1	H

differ from all the other red cell antigens in that they are not synthesized in the red cell membrane but are absorbed into it. There are other rare antigenic groups that may cause mild to severe erythroblastosis fetalis (see the review by Weinstein).[15]

During normal pregnancy fetal red cells cross the placenta in 5% of the patients during the first trimester and in 47% of the patients by the end of the third trimester.[4] In most of these cases the amount of fetal cells transferred to the mother is small and insufficient to produce a primary immune response. For this and other reasons the incidence of antepartum primary sensitization in the course of the first Rh incompatible pregnancy is less than 1%.[7] In the majority of cases maternal isoimmunization is the consequence of a fetal-maternal blood leakage happening at the time of delivery. Passage of fetal blood into the maternal circulation at the time of parturition is the rule rather than the exception, but only 10% to 15% of Rh negative mothers who have Rh positive husbands become sensitized after delivery. This low index of sensitization implies the existence of several factors influencing the probability of primary isoimmunization. One of these factors is the size of the inoculum; it is accepted that the greater the number of fetal cells entering the maternal circulation, the greater the possibility of maternal sensitization, although some mothers have been immunized with as little as 0.25 ml of fetal Rh positive cells. Another factor is the coexistence of ABO incompatibility between mother and fetus; if the mother is group O and the father A, B, or AB, the frequency of sensitization is decreased by 50% to 75% because the maternal anti-A or anti-B antibodies destroy the fetal red cells carrying the Rh antigen before they can elicit an immune response. Furthermore, 30% to 35% of Rh negative subjects are nonresponders (cannot be immunized) to the Rh positive antigen, a characteristic that seems to be genetically controlled but dependent to a certain extent on the amount of Rh positive blood injected into the maternal circulation.

If an immune response is elicited during pregnancy (incidence less than 1%) or after delivery (incidence 10% to 15%) in an Rh negative mother who carries an Rh positive baby, the initial maternal response will be the development of anti-Rh IgM antibodies with a molecular weight too large to cross through the placenta. Unfortunately, this is followed by the synthesis of anti-Rh IgG antibodies that crosses the placenta and sticks to the fetal red cells, accelerating their destruction in the infant's reticuloendothelial system. The time between the immunizing fetal-maternal bleeding and the initiation of the primary immune response is not exactly known and probably has some biologic variation, but it is several weeks before the first detectable anti-Rh antibody appears in the maternal serum. That is the reason prophylactic administration of anti-Rh globulin to the mother shortly after delivery inhibits the immune response. Even when the administration of anti-Rh globulin is delayed up to 2 weeks after transfusion of Rh-positive cells, the procedure is protective in 50% of the cases.

Maternal isoimmunization is usually detected during routine antenatal screening. The antibodies are assayed in saline solution, albumin, and with Coombs' serum.[8] Antibodies capable of agglutinating red cells suspended in saline solution in the cold (4° to 20° C) are complete (IgM) antibodies. This means that they are capable of bridging the minimal intercellular distance of 250 A that exists between red cells in solution. As mentioned before, IgM antibodies are not capable of crossing the placenta and do not produce erythroblastosis fetalis. Incomplete (IgG) antibodies, such as the anti-Rh antibody, are not capable of bridging the intercellular distance existing between erythrocytes. This distance results from the fact that red cells repel each other because of their negative surface charge or *zeta potential*. Therefore to produce red cell agglutination with incomplete antibodies it is necessary to reduce the zeta potential and decrease the intercellular distance. This is achieved in the laboratory by the addition of albumin to the suspending medium. Thus antibodies capable of agglutinating red cells at 37° C in the medium containing albumin are IgG and are important to the obstetrician because they are capable of crossing the placenta and causing fetal hemolytic disease. The Coombs' serum (containing antiglobulin antibodies) is, like albumin, capable of enhancing the agglutination of red cells coated with incomplete (IgG) antibodies or with complement.

Once Rh isoimmunity has been initiated, the individual may produce large amounts of antibodies (secondary response) in response to small amounts of fetal Rh positive blood leaked through the placenta in a subsequent pregnancy. The anti-Rh antibody crosses the placenta and attaches to the infant's red cells, making them susceptible to destruction by the reticuloendothelial system. Depending on the severity of the hemolysis, the clinical picture may include congestive heart failure, hepatomegaly, splenomegaly, peripheral edema, and placental hypertrophy. The marked hepatomegaly and splenomegaly present in erythroblastotic stillborns are a consequence not only of the development of large foci of compensatory extramedullary hematopoiesis but also of the accumulation of fluid because of congestive heart failure. If untreated, about 20% to 30% of fetuses affected by erythroblastosis die in uterus.

Kernicterus (bilirubin deposits in the basal nuclei of the brain) and jaundice are not components of erythroblastosis fetalis during intrauterine life, since accumulation of the pigment is prevented by its removal through the placental circulation and metabolism in the maternal liver. However, if the fetus is born alive, rapid increases in serum bilirubin and eventual tissue deposition will reflect the lack of functional capacity of the newborn liver to effectively handle the large amount of pigment released in the course of the brisk hemolytic process.

■ MANAGEMENT

In the management of erythroblastosis fetalis the obstetrician is usually faced with one of the two following situations: (1) the pregnant Rh negative nonimmunized patient or (2) the pregnant Rh negative immunized patient. These two groups of patients are managed differently.

Rh negative nonimmunized patient

The Rh negative nonimmunized group is formed by primigravida and multigravida patients who are Rh negative and do not have detectable isoantibodies in the initial prenatal evaluation. At this moment it is important to remember the following:

> Every Rh negative patient who has received anti-D immune globulin in a previous pregnancy should have antibody screening in all subsequent pregnancies.

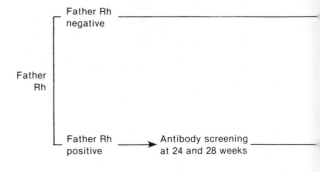

FIG. 5-1 ■ Management of the Rh-negative nonimmunized gravida.

As is discussed later, postpartum administration of anti-D immune globulin does not guarantee that isoimmunization is prevented in 100% of the cases. As a matter of fact, the search for maternal isoimmunization should not be restricted to Rh negative patients, and an antibody screening should also be obtained during the initial prenatal evaluation in Rh positive patients who have had previous blood transfusions, unexplained fetal losses, or infants with unexplained jaundice during the previous pregnancy.

If the pregnant patient is Rh negative and the antibody screening is negative, the problems for the obstetrician are (1) to assess the chances for the patient to become isoimmunized, (2) to take measures to detect isoimmunization if it actually occurs during the present pregnancy, and (3) to use adequate prophylaxis antepartum and in the immediate postpartum period.

To assess the possibility of isoimmunization in these patients, it is necessary to know the blood group and Rh classification of the father. If the father is Rh negative, the infant will be Rh negative, and there is no need for further testing. If the father is Rh positive, the infant has a 50% (if the father is heterozygous) to a 100% (if the father is homozygous) probability of being Rh positive, and the mother may become sensitized during pregnancy. As mentioned before, the chances for sensitization to occur before delivery are small (about 1%), and to detect its occur-

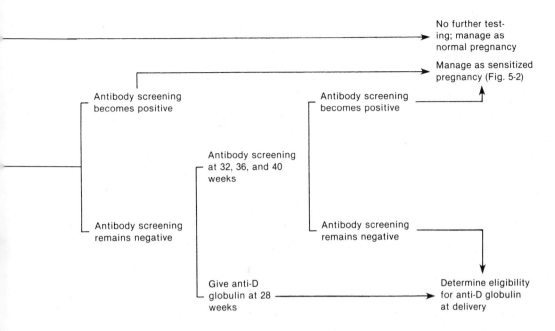

rence repeated antibody screening should be obtained at 24 and 28 weeks of gestation if anti-D immune globulin is given antepartum. If anti-D immune globulin is not given antepartum, antibody screening should also be obtained at 32, 36, and 40 weeks of gestation. If the antibody screening reveals the appearance of anti-D antibodies at any time during gestation, the patient should be managed as an Rh negative immunized pregnancy. If the antibody screening does not show evidence of isoimmunization, the patient should receive anti-D immune globulin at 28 weeks of gestation and postpartum. If anti-D immune globulin is not given antepartum, all the necessary steps should be taken at the time of delivery to determine the mother's eligibility for postpartum administration.

There are three points of discussion in the previous protocol for the management of the Rh negative nonimmunized gravida (Fig. 5-1). The first point has to do with the determination of the father's Rh genotype. The reason for the omission of this test from the protocol is that the finding of heterozygosity or homozygosity in the father does not alter the plan of management. In fact, even if the father is heterozygous, the mother is at risk of sensitization and should be screened during pregnancy, and receive anti-D globulin prophylaxis at 28 weeks.

The second point of discussion in the protocol has to do with the frequency of antibody screen-

ing testing. Since Rh isoimmunization is so rare during the antenatal period, the question arises about the need for antibody screening every 4 weeks. This frequency of testing is probably the most adequate to avoid missing the development of antibodies in the occasional patient who becomes immunized before delivery. The first immunized pregnancy may produce severe erythroblastosis,[6] and a poor fetal outcome may be the result of inadequate surveillance.

The third point of discussion concerns the antepartum administration of anti-D immune globulin. There is evidence that administration of anti-D immune globulin to Rh negative patients at 28 weeks of gestation decreases the incidence of third trimester immunization from 18 to 20 out of 1000 to 2 out of 1000 patients. After antepartum administration of anti-D immune globulin, the anti-D titer becomes positive, but it should not be greater than a trace at term. An anti-D titer of 1:1 or 1:2 at term most probably results from natural isoimmunization rather than from anti-D globulin administration.

It is not necessary to perform further Coombs' testing after administration of anti-D immune globulin at 28 weeks of gestation. At the time of antepartum administration the hospital blood bank should be notified that anti-D immune globulin has been administered to facilitate the interpretation of the patient's future antibody screening. A second dose of 300 μg of anti-D immune globulin should be given after delivery if the baby is Rh positive.

The problem with antepartum anti-D immune globulin administration is its cost-effectiveness. Many women receive one or two doses of a relatively expensive medication, and only a few benefit from it. However, in the present medicolegal climate, antepartum anti-D immune globulin administration is a procedure of choice.

In the Rh negative gravid who remains unsensitized (negative antibody screenings) during pregnancy or who receives anti-D immune globulin antepartum, eligibility for postpartum anti-D immune globulin is determined immediately after parturition. Anti-D immune globulin should be given under the following circumstances:

1. The infant is Rh-positive.
2. The direct Coombs' test on the umbilical cord blood is negative. This test reveals if the infant's red cells are covered by irregular antibodies.
3. A crossmatch between the anti-D immune globulin and the mother's red cells is compatible.

The usual dose of anti-D globulin is 300 μg. This amount of anti-D globulin is capable of neutralizing the antigenic potential of up to 30 ml of fetal blood (about 15 ml of fetal cells) and prevents Rh isoimmunization in 90% of the cases. In the other 10% of the cases anti-D globulin is ineffective, most probably as a consequence of undetected macrotransfusion of fetal cells into the mother and insufficient antigenic neutralization with the usual dose of anti-Rh globulin. A large fetal-maternal hemorrhage occurs in 1 out of every 300 to 500 deliveries, and it should be suspected with the birth of a pale baby, a fetal hemoglobulin concentration of less than 10 grams, abruptio placentae, midforceps operations, and traumatic deliveries. The clinical indicators of a large fetal-maternal hemorrhage are not completely reliable, and ideally the transfusion volume should be quantified with the use of the Betke-Kleihauer stain. This method is based on the fact that an acid solution (citric acid phosphate buffer pH 3.5) elutes the adult but not the fetal hemoglobin from the red cells; fetal erythrocytes appear in a smear stained dark red and surrounded by colorless "ghosts" that are adult erythrocytes without hemoglobin. This test can detect as little as 0.2 ml

of fetal blood diluted in 5 liters of maternal blood.

The Betke-Kleihauer test is useful only to evaluate *the volume of large fetal-maternal hemorrhages*. It is not useful and should not be used to determine the need for anti-D globulin administration. In fact, about 50% of Rh negative mothers who become sensitized have negative postpartum Betke-Kleihauer testing.[5] The Betke-Kleihauer test is somewhat difficult to perform and may produce false positive results as a consequence of multiple factors affecting the acid elution of hemoglobin from the red cells. Also, the presence of reticulocytes and adult red cells containing fetal hemoglobin may cause false positive results.

In the United States a crossmatch of the anti-D globulin against the mother's red cells is carried out before the administration of the anti-D globulin. This practice had its origin in the initial trials to determine the effectiveness of the treatment when there was a fear of causing hemolysis in the anti-D globulin recipient. Today it is known that the infusion of plasma containing antibodies incompatible with the recipient is innocuous and does not cause intravascular hemolysis. However, the important benefit of the anti-D globulin crossmatching is the ability of this test to detect a *large* fetal-maternal hemorrhage. In fact, if more than 20 ml of fetal blood has entered the maternal circulation, the anti-D globulin crossmatch becomes incompatible. Therefore this crossmatch test is used as a screening procedure to detect mothers who have had large fetal-maternal transfusions and who would not be protected by the administration of the usual 300 μg dose of anti-Rh globulin. Because of its simplicity, the anti-D globulin crossmatch is widely used in substitution of the Betke-Kleihauer stain to screen mothers in need of high anti-D globulin doses. However, the threshold sensitivity of the anti-D globulin crossmatch is high, and the Betke-Kleihauer test should be the procedure of choice to assess the volume of the fetal-maternal bleeding.

Anti-D globulin should also be given to all Rh negative women after spontaneous or induced abortions, after amniocentesis, and after ectopic pregnancies unless they are already sensitized. For this purpose a minidose of anti-D globulin containing 150 μg is available.

Anti-D globulin can be given any time up to

4 weeks after delivery. The maximal protective effect is obtained if the antibody is administered within 72 hours following delivery. There is nothing magic, however, in this standard timing for anti-D globulin administration. This limit was chosen arbitrarily in the original experiments carried out on male volunteers in which the value of anti-D in preventing Rh isoimmunization was proven. Other experiments have shown that administration of anti-D globulin several days and even weeks after delivery still has a protective effect although the efficiency of the protection is reduced. Therefore anti-D globulin should be given to any eligible Rh negative mother as soon as possible after delivery, but treatment should not be withheld if more than 72 hours have passed in the postpartum period. As mentioned before, the administration of anti-D globulin to eligible mothers after delivery decreases the incidence of Rh sensitization from 15% to 1% or 2%. The 1-in-10 failure rate is the result of undetected large fetal-maternal bleeding or isoimmunization occurring before delivery.

Rh negative immunized patient

This discussion concerns the management of pregnancy following the development of Rh isoimmunization. In the large majority of cases, immunization happened in a previous pregnancy, but occasionally it is the result of a previous transfusion of Rh negative blood or rarely of antepartum immunization. In any case, the unifying variables are that the patients are Rh negative and that anti-D antibodies are detected in the course of an antibody screening.

For management purposes the immunized Rh negative patients should be divided into two subgroups according to their past obstetric history. If there is a history of infants with erythroblastosis, either stillborns or neonates requiring intensive care, the present pregnancy should be managed with exclusive reliance on amniotic fluid analysis. If the past obstetric history is negative, maternal antibody titers play a role in the management of the problem. The reason for this division comes from a study at the Boston Lying-In Hospital[1] where it was found that immunized patients with titers remaining at or below 1:64 and with a negative past obstetric history had a 4% incidence of intrauterine death before 37 weeks. In contrast, patients with similar titers but with a history of delivering erythroblastotic infants had a 32% stillbirth rate before 37 weeks. When the titer was above 1:64, the patients with a negative history had a stillborn incidence of 17.2%, whereas those with a history of affected infants had a stillborn rate of 67.8%. Although there is a gross correlation between antibody titer and fetal outcome, in patients with similar

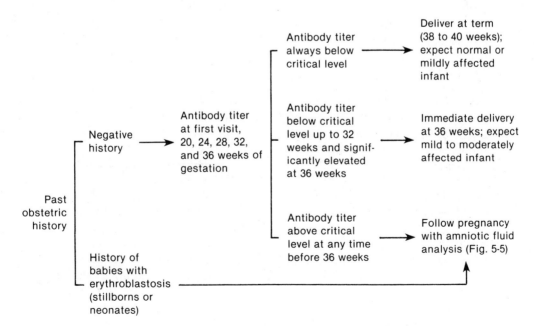

FIG. 5-2 ■ Management of the Rh-negative immunized gravida.

titers the past obstetric history is the predominant indicator of the outcome. Therefore patients with a history of infants with erythroblastosis should be managed on the basis of spectrophotometric analysis of the amniotic fluid even if their antibody titers do not exceed the critical level (Fig. 5-2).

Antibody titers. The concentration of anti-Rh antibodies in an immunized gravida is determined by a titration procedure in which progressively double dilutions of the maternal serum are incubated with Rh positive group 0 erythrocytes and agglutination used as the endpoint. There is a wide variation in antibody titers among different Rh immunized patients. In many of them, especially during the pregnancy immediately following the initiation of immunization, the concentration of antibodies is so low that they can only be detected in undiluted serum. In fact, maternal antibodies may not appear until late in the pregnancy following that which started the isoimmunization. The explanation for those cases of late appearance of antibodies is that fetal-maternal bleeding is more common in the later stages of gestation and that during the *first* affected pregnancy there is a good correlation between the secondary immune response and the amount and timing of fetal cell transfer into the maternal circulation. This correlation is completely lost during subsequent immunized pregnancies.

There are variations in antibody titers among different laboratories, and the obstetrician managing an immunized pregnancy should use the same laboratory for all the antibody titer determinations. For a maximal accuracy of the test, serum samples should be stored and the procedure repeated in the original sample every time that a titer is to be determined in a subsequent sample. Also, it is important to know the critical titer level associated with intrauterine death for the reporting laboratory. For example, this critical level is 1:16 in the Columbia-Presbyterian Medical Center,[7] 1:32 at the University of Louisville,[12] and 1:8 at Barnes Hospital. The critical level means that no death caused by erythroblastosis has occurred within 1 week of delivery when the titer was at that level or less.

An antibody titer should be obtained in the course of the first sensitized pregnancy at the first prenatal visit and repeated at 20, 24, 28, 32, and 36 weeks of gestation unless the following occurs:

1. The titer is found to be at the critical level or above in the initial evaluation.
2. The titer reaches or exceeds the critical level at any time during gestation.
3. There is a significant rise (two-tube dilution) in the titer between any two consecutive samples even if the upper dilution does not reach critical level (eg, an increase from 1:4 to 1:32 with a critical level of 1:64).

If any of these three conditions is fulfilled, there is no further use for antibody titers as an index to follow Rh immunized pregnancies. Further management is based on examination of the amniotic fluid except in those patients who have a titer that is negative or below the critical level up to 32 weeks of gestation and become positive or have a significant rise at 36 weeks. In these cases labor should be induced immediately and the pregnancy terminated rather than performing an amniocentesis. The birth of a mild to moderately affected baby should be anticipated. If the antibody titer remains under the critical level at all times up to 36 weeks of gestation, the patient should be delivered by elective induction of labor between 38 and 40 weeks, and the birth of a nonaffected (Rh negative) or mildly affected infant should be anticipated. The neonatologist should be notified in advance of the induction of an Rh negative immunized mother so that evaluation and treatment of the newborn can be carried out without delays.

Amniotic fluid analysis. In pregnancies affected by the presence in the maternal serum of any irregular antibody capable of producing erythroblastosis fetalis, spectrophotometric analysis of the amniotic fluid is a reliable method for evaluating the severity of the fetal hemolytic process and for determining the optimum time for IUT or for delivery of the infant. Amniotic fluid analysis becomes mandatory in the management of the Rh negative immunized gravida in the following cases:

1. When initial evaluation reveals an antibody titer above the critical level for the laboratory performing the analysis
2. When the critical level for the antibody titer is reached or exceeded at any time before 36 weeks of gestation
3. When there is a significant elevation (two-

tube dilution) in antibody titer even if it is below the critical level for the laboratory performing the analysis

4. In any immunized pregnancy in which the patient gives a history of a previous delivery of infants with moderate or severe erythroblastosis

In patients with initial high titers and in those with a poor obstetric history (categories 1 and 4 just listed) the first amniocentesis usually is carried out at 24 weeks of gestation. The reason is that IUT is technically difficult and gives poor results when carried out before 24 weeks. Patients without a poor obstetric history and with a titer initially low that increases in subsequent examinations (categories 2 and 3 just listed) should have the first amniocentesis immediately after the first appearance of a significantly high titer. If the first amniocentesis fails because of a bloody tap, the procedure should be repeated after 1 week. If amniocentesis is successful, the decision about when to repeat the procedure will be dictated by the results of the amniotic fluid analysis, as is discussed later.

Before performing an amniocentesis, the best site for the procedure should be determined using real-time ultrasound. The use of ultrasound has been instrumental in increasing close to 100% the success rate in obtaining adequate samples for amniotic fluid analysis. In fact, ultrasound allows identification of the placenta and delineation of the placental edges, and in the majority of cases amniocentesis can be performed safely and without blood contamination by selecting a tap site away from the placenta. The instrument is also helpful in showing "pockets" of fluid that may be reached by the clinician in patients with little fluid or with difficult placental localizations and can aid in measuring the distance from the skin to the pocket of fluid.

Once the tap site has been selected, the patient is instructed to empty her bladder, and the abdomen is prepared with aseptic technique using Betadine solution. The skin is anesthetized with 0.5 ml of 1% Carbocaine, and a 3½-inch 22-gauge disposable spinal needle is inserted to the depth previously determined with real-time ultrasound with a single thrust of the clinician's hand. Slow, hesitant thrusts usually give as a result either a tap failure or a bloody tap. Then the tip of the needle should be visualized with

the real-time ultrasound and advanced or withdrawn until it clearly reaches the middle of a pocket of fluid. About 5 to 10 ml of amniotic fluid are required for spectrophotometric analysis. The fluid should be kept in a brown bottle to protect it from exposure to the sunlight, which destroys some of the bilirubin and causes false low readings. The fluid is centrifuged at 4000 rpm for 20 minutes, filtered through a Whatman 2 filter, and analyzed in the spectrophotometer.

When normal amniotic fluid is examined in a spectrophotometer using water as a blank, the optical density (OD) readings between 350 and 650 nm form an almost straight line. If the amniotic fluid contains bilirubin, the OD readings will show a peak at 450 nm, and the size of the peak will be proportional to the amount of pigment in the fluid. Rather than using continuous scanning between 350 and 650 nm, the majority of laboratories measure the OD at 375, 450, and 525 nm. The results are plotted on a semilogarithmic paper, and a straight line is drawn between the readings at 375 and 525 nm. The difference between the point where the line crosses the 450 nm mark (expected value) and the actual reading at this wavelength is the delta OD 450 that is used by the clinician for patient management purposes (Fig. 5-3). When using amniotic fluid analysis in the management of sensitized Rh negative patients, it is important to remember several points.

Bilirubin content of normal amniotic fluid. Normal patients may show a small amount of bilirubin in the amniotic fluid that reaches a peak at 24 to 26 weeks of gestation and then decreases slowly until term.[11] It is exceptional to find a delta OD 450 value above 0.10 at 24 to 26 weeks resulting from bilirubin produced by a nonaffected baby. At this gestational age the value (0.10) falls within the low zone or zone 1 in Fig. 5-4 and should be followed by repeated amniocentesis 4 weeks later. If the infant is not affected, the delta OD 450 will show a considerable decrease in the subsequent amniocentesis.

Premature labor. Contractions are usually the rule following amniocentesis, but they often subside after 30 to 40 minutes. In rare cases contractions may continue and result in premature labor. Patients undergoing amniocentesis should be instructed to report if the contractions continue and become stronger several hours after

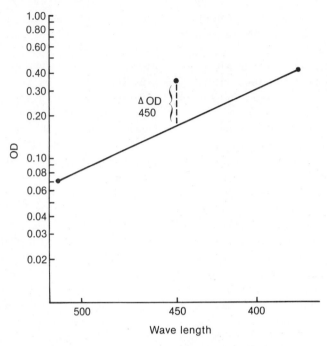

FIG. 5-3 ■ Example of calculation of the delta optical density (OD) 450. A line is drawn between the readings at 375 and 525 nm. The difference between the point where that line intersects the 450 nm mark and the actual reading of the fluid at that wavelength is the delta OD 450 value.

the procedure, and if that is the case, therapy with beta mimetics is indicated.

Bloody taps. Even if an amniocentesis is atraumatic and yields clear amniotic fluid, a small button of red cells is frequently found after centrifugation. However this is not a *bloody tap*, a term that is reserved for gross, visible contamination of the fluid with fetal or maternal blood. Bloody taps are becoming less common since the introduction of ultrasonic scanning before amniocentesis. In the large majority of cases the blood is maternal in origin, but it may be a mixture of maternal and fetal cells, especially in cases of transplacental amniocentesis. If fluid grossly contaminated with blood comes out of the needle after amniocentesis, the best thing to do is to let the fluid escape to see if spontaneous clearing occurs. If the hematocrit value after clearing is more than 5%, the OD 450 reading will be distorted and should not be used for patient management purposes. If the fluid is grossly contaminated, the chances of adequate spontaneous clearing are low, and the position of the needle must be assessed with real-time ultrasound. In these cases the tip of the needle frequently is found within the placenta (placen-

tal aspiration) rather than within the amniotic sac. If that is the case, adequate advancement of the needle will yield clear fluid.

When amniocentesis is carried out in a patient who is already immunized, there is no value in administering anti-D immune globulin after the tap. In contrast, administration of anti-D globulin is indicated in nonimmunized patients, especially if the tap was bloody.

Infection. Infection is a rare complication of amniocentesis. The resulting chorioamnionitis usually leads to preterm labor and results in preterm delivery. The most commonly found pathogen is *Staphylococcus epidermidis*, and the treatment is evacuation of the uterus. Adherence to aseptic technique is the key to the prevention of this problem.

Fetal distress. Occasionally after amniocentesis there are marked changes in fetal heart rate that may or may not be indicative of fetal distress. Electronic monitoring in the majority of these cases is characterized by the presence of variable decelerations and wide oscillations in baseline heart frequency. These changes usually disappear spontaneously within 1 or 2 hours after the procedure. However, if the tap has been bloody and especially if a sinusoidal pattern is observed after amniocentesis, there are reasons for concern; this pattern is frequently an indicator of fetal anemia, and if a good proportion of the red cells obtained with the procedure are of fetal origin, the possibility of fetal hemorrhage should be strongly considered.

Aspiration of urine. The best way to avoid aspiration of urine is to instruct the patient to empty her bladder immediately before amniocentesis. If there is any doubt that the liquid obtained is urine, a drop of it should be placed on a glass slide, smeared with a cotton tip, and observed with the microscope for ferning. Amniotic fluid ferns; urine does not. Also, the fluid may be checked for protein using an Albustix strip: the amniotic fluid has protein; normal urine does not.

Meconium-stained fluid. The peak absorption of meconium in amniotic fluid is similar to the Soret's band of hemoglobin (410 nm). As a consequence, meconium causes a marked rise in delta OD 450, and this change does not disappear after centrifugation. For this reason delta OD 450 values from meconium-stained specimens should not be used for patient management. If meconium is present in samples obtained at 24 to 28 weeks of gestation, it usually disappears over the next 2 to 3 weeks.

Polyhydramnios. Excessive production and accumulation of amniotic fluid are complications of erythroblastosis fetalis, usually indicating deterioration of the fetal status. In this situation the bilirubin content of the amniotic fluid becomes diluted, and a falsely low delta OD 450 value results that may be misleading when evaluating the severity of the disease. If polyhydramnios is suspected or diagnosed, the total volume of amniotic fluid should be determined using ^{51}Cr, Evans blue, or sodium paraaminohippurate, and the OD 450 value should be corrected for dilution. For example, a delta OD 450 value of 0.15 at 26 weeks of gestation (zone 2) in a patient with a total amniotic fluid volume of 2.5 liters is equivalent to a delta OD 450 of 0.6 (zone 3) when corrected for excessive volume (normal fluid volume at 26 weeks equals 675 ml).

Multiple gestation. If the immunized Rh negative mother has a multiple pregnancy, each fetus should be evaluated separately. In the most common case—twin pregnancy—both, neither, or only one of the twins may be affected and each one of the amniotic sacs should be aspi-

rated. For this purpose the help of real-time ultrasound is invaluable. It allows visualization of the membrane separating the sacs and its penetration by the needle if a single puncture is chosen as the procedure of choice. If each sac is to be entered using different puncture sites, 1 or 2 ml of indigo carmine must be injected into the sac entered first. The fluid obtained from the second sac must not contain any dye; if it does, the tip of the needle is probably still in the first sac.

Management based on delta OD 450 values. There are several methods for managing the immunized Rh negative patient using the delta OD 450 values obtained by spectrophotometric analysis of the fluid. A method commonly used is based on the work of Liley.[10] In his original description, Liley recorded the delta OD 450 of 101 immunized patients on semilogarithmic paper (gestational age in weeks in the ordinate, delta OD 450 values in the abscissa) and divided the graph into three zones (Fig. 5-4). The upper zone (3) corresponded to severely affected infants, the low zone (1) to nonaffected or mildly affected babies, and the middle zone (2) included both types of patients (severely and mildly affected).

If the amniotic fluid shows a delta OD 450 value in zone 1, there is no immediate danger of intrauterine fetal death, and the procedure should be repeated in 4 weeks. If the delta OD 450 values remain in zone 1 with amniocentesis carried out every 4 weeks, the patient should be delivered at term, and the birth of a nonaffected (Rh negative) or a mildly affected baby should be anticipated.

If at any time during gestation the amniotic fluid shows a delta OD 450 value in zone 2, the procedure should be repeated in 1 week, since values in this zone may correspond to moderate to severely affected infants. If the following amniocentesis shows a value in zone 1 (decreasing trend), there is no need for another tap before 4 weeks. If the following amniocentesis shows a delta OD 450 value that remains in zone 2 (horizontal trend), the procedure should be repeated in another week, and if further values remain in zone 2, the pregnancy should be terminated as soon as fetal lung maturation is reached (mature lecithin/sphingomyelin [L/S] ratio); the birth of a moderately affected infant should be anticipated.

If the initial amniotic fluid examination shows

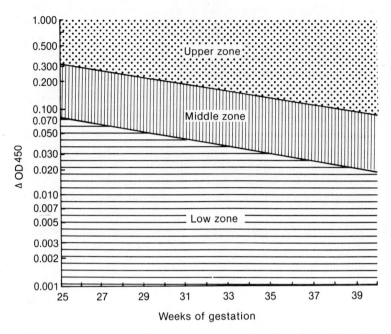

FIG. 5-4 ■ Management zones in Rh isoimmunization based on delta OD 450 values and gestational age. *Upper zone:* Hemoglobin less than 9 g/dl, delivery or transfusion urgent. *Middle zone:* Hemoglobin 9 to 12 g/dl, delivery at 36 to 37 weeks. *Low zone:* Not anemic, delivery at term.

a delta OD 450 in zone 3 or if any delta OD 450 value previously in zone 1 or 2 moves to zone 3 (rising trend), the infant may be in imminent danger of intrauterine death. In these cases amniocentesis should be repeated immediately, and the fluid L/S ratio should be determined. If the L/S ratio is mature, the infant should be delivered immediately. If the L/S ratio is immature, the mother should have an IUT or be treated with glucocorticoids and delivered 48 to 72 hours later. The decision about IUT versus glucocorticoids and delivery is not easy and depends to a large extent on the gestational age and weight of the infant, the expertise available for performing IUTs, and the ability of the nursery to manage compromised neonates. (This subject is discussed more later in this chapter). A summary of the management protocol using Liley's zones is shown in Fig. 5-5 and the list on p. 87.

The method of Robertson[14] is similar to the one previously described, is used in many places around the world, and is preferred by the authors of this chapter. It has the advantage over Liley's method of greater individualization of care by using amniocentesis intervals of 1, 2, 3,

and 4 weeks, depending on the delta od 450 value and the gestational age (Fig. 5-6).

Another method of fetal evaluation in erythroblastosis is that of Freda,[7] which uses the net value (not the delta value) of the OD at 450 nm. Freda correlated these absolute values with the bilirubin concentration in the fluid and the fetal status at birth (Table 5-3).

Early delivery and use of glucocorticoids. The classic approach to the management of sensitized Rh negative mothers was early delivery or IUT depending on the severity of the fetal hemolytic process. This has changed with the development of laboratory indexes to assess fetal lung maturation. Today it is possible to deliver affected babies when lung maturation is achieved rather than when an arbitrary gestational age has been reached. Also, it is possible to use drugs that accelerate the maturation of the infant's lungs and decrease the occurrence of neonatal respiratory distress syndrome (RDS).

Evaluation of the L/S ratio should be a part of the amniotic fluid analysis whenever the delta OD 450 value is in zone 3 and after 32 weeks of gestation if the value is in zone 2. In fact, if a zone 3 patient has an L/S ratio greater than 1.5

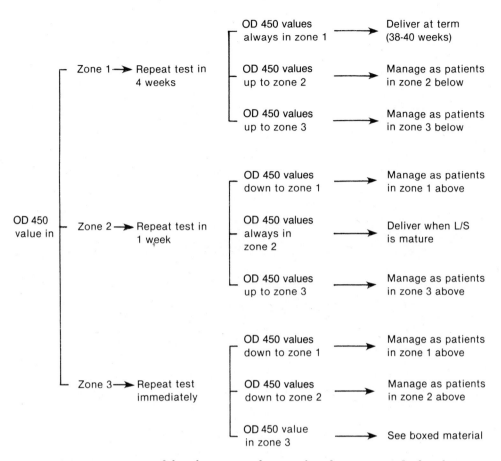

FIG. 5-5 ■ Management of the Rh immunized patient based on amniotic fluid analysis.

**Management of the Rh immunized patient with two consecutive
delta OD 450 values in zone 3**

FACTORS TO CONSIDER

1. Neonatal intensive care unit consistently saving without sequela more than 50% of new-borns weighing 800 to 1200 grams
2. Inexperienced clinician
3. Fetus in breech or transverse or with back anterior
4. Anterior placenta
5. Obese mother
6. Gestational age close to 30 weeks
7. Weight close to or above 1000 grams
8. Fetus has received glucocorticoids
9. OD 450 in high zone 3
10. Hydropic fetus

DECISION

If the answer to five or more of these factors is positive (yes), the infant should be delivered rather than submitted to IUT.

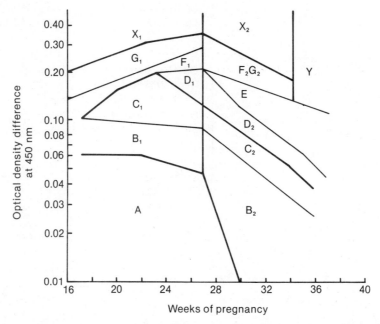

FIG. 5-6 ■ Management zones in Rh isoimmunization based on delta OD 450 values and gestational age, according to Robertson[14]: *A*, Repeat every 4 weeks and deliver at term; *B1* and *B2*, Repeat every 4 weeks and deliver at term; *C1*, Repeat every 3 weeks; *C2*, Repeat every 3 weeks and deliver at 39 weeks; *D1* and *D2*, Repeat every 2 weeks and deliver at 38 weeks; *E*, Repeat every week or every 2 weeks and deliver between 36 and 38 weeks; *F1*, Repeat every 2 weeks until delivery feasible; *F2*, *G1*, and *G2*, Repeat every 2 weeks until delivery feasible or intrauterine transfusion mandatory; *X1*, Intrauterine transfusion; *X2*, Immediate delivery or intrauterine transfusion; *Y*, Immediate delivery.

TABLE 5-3 ■ Net value of amniotic fluid OD 450 and fetal status

Freda's grade	Net OD 450 value	Bilirubin in the fluid (mg/dl)	Fetal status
1+	0.2 to 0.20	0 to 0.28	Normal or possibly affected
2+	0.2 to 0.34	0.28 to 0.46	Affected but not in jeopardy
3+	0.35 to 0.70	0.47 to 0.95	Distressed, probably in failure
4+	More than 0.70	More than 0.95	Impending fetal death

According to Freda VJ: Am J Obstet Gynecol 1965; 93:321.

or phosphatidyl glycerol (PG) is present in the amniotic fluid, the pregnancy should be terminated. In these patients the fetal mortality and morbidity caused by IUT is probably greater than that resulting from the delivery of the infant. Actually, the baby may not have RDS, or if affected by RDS, he may have only a mild to moderate form. For patients in zone 2, determination of the L/S ratio allows termination of pregnancy as soon as the fetus reaches lung maturity rather than when it reaches certain gestational age.

As discussed extensively in Chapter 3, evidence clearly indicates that maternal administration of glucocorticoids prevents the development of RDS in infants delivered before term, and this is a fact that may be used advantageously in the management of Rh sensitized pregnancies. All affected pregnant patients for whom the amniotic fluid analysis indicates the need for IUT or immediate delivery and the L/S ratio is immature should receive glucocorticoids if IUT cannot be performed. We use betamethasone (12 mg intramuscularly) daily in two consecutive days. Corticosteroid treatment must be followed by delivery even if the L/S ratio is still immature. Our own studies[2] have demonstrated that glucocorticoid treatment has little effect on the L/S ratio, and the studies by Caritis et al[3] have shown that RDS prevention occurs even if corticosteroids-treated erythroblastotic infants are delivered when they still have immature L/S ratios. Corticosteroids cause a decrease in delta OD 450 values[3] by a mechanism that may or may not be related to the hemolytic process. Therefore the obstetrician must avoid the false sense of security given by the drop in delta OD 450 values that follows glucocorticoid treatment and proceed to deliver the infant 24 hours after the second dose of betamethasone.

Intrauterine transfusion. Since its introduction in 1963, IUT has been instrumental in saving hundreds of infants affected by erythroblastosis fetalis. However, the indications for IUTs are becoming more narrow because of advances in antenatal and neonatal therapy. IUT is a procedure that carries a high risk of fetal death, and its results are deeply modified by variables such as the experience and skills of the clinician, the severity of the fetal disease, the placental implantation site, the obesity of the mother, and the fetal lie, among many other factors. It is not surprising therefore that a wide discrepancy exists among published results, with fetal death per procedure as high as 20% in some series[13] and as low as 2.2% in others.[9] Perhaps closer to reality is the 6.5% fetal mortality per procedure frequently quoted in the literature. The incidence of fetal death is per procedure and the majority of IUT-treated infants require three and often four procedures, raising the overall risk of fetal death because of the treatment to between 20% and 25%. However, there are some strong indications that with the use of real-time ultrasound the risks and complications of IUT may be substantially smaller.

It is because of the high risk of fetal death that the decision to adopt IUT as treatment for a given patient with erythroblastosis fetalis should be reserved for cases in which the risk of intrauterine death (if pregnancy continues) and the risk of neonatal death (if the fetus is delivered prematurely) are very high (box on p. 87). For example, this is the course of action for infants under 1000 grams or below 28 weeks of gestation with delta OD 450 values in the danger zone. In these cases the risk of intrauterine death is almost 100%, and the risk of neonatal death (in spite of the antenatal use of glucocorticoids) is higher than the 20% risk of fetal death using IUTs.

It is obvious from the previous discussion that the characteristics of the neonatal service are of fundamental importance in the decision of whether to deliver or to proceed to IUT treatment. In many neonatal intensive care units the chances of survival for a sick 28-weeks-of-gestation infant are better than the chances of success for a series of IUTs carried out by an obstetrician without a great deal of expertise in the procedure. In contrast, the same 28-weeks-of-gestation fetus has a better chance of survival if the pregnancy is managed with IUT by an individual with experience in the procedure than if delivered in a place where sophisticated neonatal care is not available. The obstetrician taking care of immunized Rh negative pregnant patients should know in detail the resources and referral routes available in the community for IUT treatment or intensive neonatal care or both. In these cases as well as in the majority of complicated pregnancies, it is important to remember that transfer of the mother before delivery to a tertiary care center is more conducive to a good fetal outcome than the transfer of a sick neonate.

■ REFERENCES

1. Allen FH, Diamond LK, Jones AR: Erythroblastosis fetalis: IX. Problems of stillbirth. N Engl J Med 1954; 251:453.
2. Arias F, Pineda J, Johnson LW: Changes in human amniotic fluid lecithin/sphyngomyelin ratio and dipalmitoyl/lecithin associated with maternal betamethasone therapy. Am J Obstet Gynecol 1979; 133:894.
3. Caritis SN, Mueller-Heubach E, Edelstone DI: Effect of betamethasone on analysis of amniotic fluid in the Rhesus-sensitized pregnancy. Am J Obstet Gynecol 1977; 127:529.
4. Clayton EM Jr, Feldhaus W, Phythyon JM, et al: Transplacental passage of fetal erythrocytes during pregnancy. Obstet Gynecol 1966; 28:194.
5. Cohen F, Zuelzer WW: Identification of blood groups antigens by immunofluorescence and its application to the detection of the transplacental passage of erythrocytes in mother and child. Vox Sang 1964; 9:75.
6. Erlandson ME, Huber JM: Severe erythroblastosis fetalis in first immunized pregnancies. Am J Obstet Gynecol 1964; 90:779.
7. Freda VJ: The Rh problem in obstetrics and a new concept of its management using amniocentesis and spectrophotometric scanning of amniotic fluid. Am J Obstet Gynecol 1965; 93:321.
8. Gorman JG: *The Role of Laboratory in Hemolytic Disease of the Newborn.* Philadelphia, Lea & Febiger, 1975, pp. 36 and 163-164.
9. Hamilton EG: Intrauterine transfusion: safeguard or peril. Obstet Gynecol 1977; 50:255.
10. Liley AW: Liquor amnii analysis in management of pregnancy complicated by Rhesus sensitization. Am J Obstet Gynecol 1961; 82:1359.
11. Queenan JT: Amniotic fluid analysis. Clin Obstet Gynecol 1971; 14:505.
12. Queenan JT: *Modern management of the Rh Problem.* New York, Harper and Row, Publishers, Inc., 1977, pp. 31-32.
13. Robertson EG, Brown A, Ellis MI, et al: Intrauterine fetal transfusion in the management of severe Rhesus isoimmunization. Br J Obstet Gynaecol 1976; 83:694.
14. Robertson JG: Management of patients with Rh isoimmunization based on amniotic fluid analysis. Am J Obstet Gynecol 1969; 103:713.
15. Weinstein L: Irregular antibodies causing hemolytic disease of the newborn. Obstet Gynecol Surv 1976; 31:581.

6

■ ■ ■

HYPERTENSION DURING PREGNANCY

Fernando Arias

■ DEFINITIONS AND CLASSIFICATION

When women who remain normotensive during gestation are compared with those who have elevated blood pressure, it is apparent that the hypertensive group has a significantly greater maternal and fetal mortality and morbidity.[5] In fact, although maternal hypertension is diagnosed in only about 7% of all deliveries (1.5% in private hospitals; up to 15% in public or university hospitals), it is associated with as much as 22% (mean value 12.5%) of all perinatal deaths and with about 30% of all maternal deaths occurring in the United States.

As determined by the Committee on Terminology, American College of Obstetricians and Gynecologists, there are four criteria for the diagnosis of hypertension in a pregnant woman, any one of which is an indication of the disease:

1. A sustained rise of 30 mm Hg or more in systolic blood pressure
2. A sustained rise of 15 mm Hg or more in diastolic blood pressure
3. A sustained systolic blood pressure of 140 mm Hg or more
4. A sustained diastolic blood pressure of 90 mm Hg or more

Sustained means on at least two different occasions at least 6 hours apart.

This definition of hypertension in pregnancy is controversial, especially in view of the findings of the Collaborative Perinatal Project, which showed a diastolic blood pressure above 85 mm Hg during pregnancy as abnormal.[9] At the present time, however, we must stick to the criteria of the American College of Obstetricians and Gynecologists (ACOG) to avoid the confusion derived from the use of different definitions.

The problem of hypertension in pregnancy is confused by the fact that pregnancy itself may induce hypertension in women who are normotensive before pregnancy and may aggravate the severity of the hypertension in women who are hypertensive before pregnancy. Also, the clinical and laboratory characteristics of hypertension peculiar to pregnancy are very difficult to differentiate from those of hypertension independent of pregnancy. As a consequence:

1. Severe pregnancy-induced or pregnancy-aggravated hypertension is frequently confused with other disease processes (thrombotic thrombocytopenic purpura, acute glomerulonephritis, chronic essential hypertension, etc.) occurring during pregnancy. This confusion may cause a dangerous delay in the establishment of appropriate treatment.

2. Diseases causing hypertension (brain tumors, pheochromocytoma, systemic lupus erythematosus, renovascular hypertension, etc.) may occur during pregnancy but are not diagnosed because their symptoms are similar to those of pregnancy-induced or pregnancy-aggravated hypertension. This type of confusion may also cause dangerous delays and iatrogenic problems.

The Committee on Terminology of ACOG has recognized these problems and developed a classification of hypertension during pregnancy. This classification is simple and makes a distinction between pregnancy-induced hypertension (group A), pregnancy-independent hypertension (group B), and pregnancy-aggravated hypertension (groups C and D). The classification is as follows:

A. Pregnancy-induced hypertension
   1. Preeclampsia
   2. Eclampsia
B. Chronic hypertension of whatever cause, but independent of pregnancy
C. Preeclampsia or eclampsia superimposed on chronic hypertension
D. Transient hypertension
E. Unclassified hypertensive disorders

The following definitions are given:

preeclampsia The development of hypertension in pregnancy (as defined previously) together with proteinuria (greater than 0.3 g/L in a 24-hour urine collection or greater than 1 g/L in a random sample) or generalized edema (general accumulation of fluid in the tissues with greater than 1+ pitting edema after 12 hours of rest in bed or a weight gain of 5 pounds or more in 1 week), or both after 20 weeks of gestation.

eclampsia The occurrence of convulsions in a patient with preeclampsia.

chronic hypertension of whatever cause The presence of sustained blood pressures of 140/90 mm Hg or higher before pregnancy or before 20 weeks of gestation.

preeclampsia or eclampsia superimposed on chronic hypertension The occurrence of preeclampsia or eclampsia in a woman with chronic hypertension. To make this diagnosis it is necessary to document a rise of 30 mm Hg or more in the diastolic blood pressure, together with proteinuria or generalized edema, or both.

transient hypertension The development of hypertension during pregnancy or the early puerperium in a previously normotensive woman whose pressure returns to normal within 10 days after delivery. There is no other evidence that preeclampsia is present.

unclassified hypertensive disorders Those in which there is not enough information for classification.

In this chapter the terms *preeclampsia* and *pregnancy-induced hypertension* will be used interchangeably. Most authors recognize that preeclampsia may be *mild* or *severe*, but there is considerable discussion about the advantages or disadvantages of adding to the classification an intermediate or *moderate* group. In this book we accept three degrees of severity (mild, moderate, and severe) according to the criteria shown in Table 6-1. The most important of the criteria for severity classification is the magnitude of the blood pressure elevation.

■ PREGNANCY-INDUCED HYPERTENSION
Pathophysiology

A complete review of the pathophysiology of preeclampsia and eclampsia is beyond the scope and goals of this book. However, certain selected pathophysiologic aspects require review at this time.

Vasospasm. Considerable evidence supports the view that hypertension in patients with preeclampsia is the consequence of increased arteriolar vasoconstriction. In fact, a great deal of research has been done to elucidate the mechanism of the vasospasm in the preeclamptic patient. The assumption is that by clarifying the cause of vasoconstriction the prevention and treatment of the disease will be found.

Vasospasm and its resulting hypertension are of fundamental importance in the pathogenesis of eclamptic seizures. In fact, cerebral blood perfusion is maintained at a constant level of about 55 ml/min/100 g of tissue despite variations in mean arterial pressure (MAP) and blood composition (Fig. 6-1). With increased severity of hypertension the upper level of autoregulation is reached, with production of a reactive vasospasm designed to limit the increase in tissue perfusion. This vasospasm may be severe enough to disrupt the endothelial capillary cell junctions, causing extravasation of blood cells and plasma fluid in the perivascular space. These pericapillary hemorrhages are the foci of abnormal electrical discharges, which may spread with production of seizures.

TABLE 6-1 ■ Severity classification of preeclampsia-eclampsia

Variable	Mild	Moderate	Severe
Diastolic blood pressure	90 to 100 mm Hg	100 to 110 mm Hg	Greater than 110 mm Hg
Convulsions	Absent	Absent	Present
Blindness	Absent	Absent	Present
Headaches	Minimal	Mild	Marked, persistent
Visual symptoms	Minimal	Mild	Marked, persistent
Oliguria	Absent	Absent	Present
Upper abdominal pain	Absent	Absent	Present
Fetal distress	Absent	Absent	Present
Fetal growth retardation	Absent	Absent	Present
Intravascular hemolysis	Absent	Absent	Present
Thrombocytopenia	Absent	Absent	Present
Blood urea nitrogen (BUN), creatinine, uric acid levels	Normal	Mildly elevated	Markedly elevated
Serum glutamic-oxaloacetic transaminase (SGOT), serum glutamic-pyruvic transaminase (SGPT), lactate dehydrogenase (LDH)	Normal	Mildly elevated	Markedly elevated

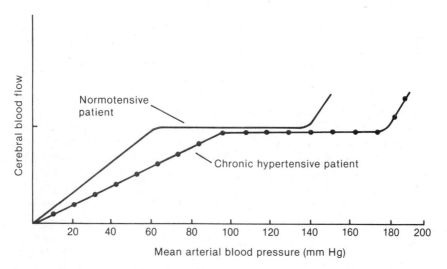

FIG. 6-1 ■ Representation of the relationship between cerebral blood flow and mean arterial blood pressure. Blood flow is kept constant within a wide range of mean blood pressure in both normotensive and hypertensive patients. However, patients with chronic hypertension have the lower and upper limits of autoregulation shifted to higher blood pressure values. (From Donaldson JO: *Neurology of pregnancy*. Philadelphia, WB Saunders Co, 1978, p. 216.)

The upper limit of cerebral perfusion pressure that may not be exceeded without causing arteriolar vasospasm, ischemia, and perivascular hemorrhage varies from one person to the other. Patients with chronic hypertension, for example, are capable of tolerating higher MAPs than patients without a previous history of hypertension. This explains why a young preeclamptic patient may convulse with systemic blood pressure values of 150/100 mm Hg while patients with chronic hypertension and superimposed preeclampsia may tolerate pressures as high as 220/150 mm Hg or more without convulsions. In the first patient a MAP of 116 mm Hg has exceeded the upper limit of autoregulation of the brain perfusion pressure, while in the second patient a MAP of 173 mm Hg is not large enough to reach that limit, which has become higher than usual through years of exposure to high blood pressure.

In conclusion, hypertension is a fundamental factor in the genesis of eclamptic seizures, and aggressive antihypertensive treatment must be a part of the management of the patient with severe pregnancy-induced hypertension.

Changes in intravascular volume. It is well known that the increase in intravascular volume that normally happens during gestation is reduced or completely absent in patients with preeclampsia and eclampsia. This limitation in blood volume expansion is probably the result of generalized vasoconstriction. The decrease in intravascular volume is predominantly of plasma volume, and as a result, the hemoglobin and hematocrit values rise as the severity of the disease progresses. After delivery, when the vasospasm disappears and the plasma volume increases, the hemoglobin and hematocrit values will decrease. Large postpartum drops in hemoglobin or hematocrit are almost always the consequence of excessive blood loss during delivery, of decreased vasospasm with secondary increase in plasma volume, or of a mixture of the two phenomena.

The limited intravascular volume expansion of the patient with preeclampsia-eclampsia leads to several management problems:

The problem of diuretics. Diuretics have been used in the past and continue to be used in the treatment of patients with pregnancy-induced hypertension. These medications will diminish an already depleted intravascular volume and aggravate the deficient uteroplacental perfusion present in preeclamptic patients. The deleterious effect of diuretics on the placental blood flow has been eloquently demonstrated by experiments showing that they decrease the placental clearance of dehydroepiandrosterone sulfate.[12a]

Some patients with pregnancy-induced hypertension have insidious sodium loss or are in negative sodium balance because of dietary manipulations. In these cases, administration of diuretics causes hyponatremia, which may be aggravated by oxytocin and water administration during the intrapartum period. Also, diuretics may cause neonatal thrombocytopenia and auditory nerve and renal dysfunction in the neonate.

Diuretics do not have a place in the therapy of preeclampsia and eclampsia except under very uncommon circumstances.

The problem of poor tolerance to blood loss and regional anesthesia. The limited intravascular volume expansion in patients with pregnancy-induced hypertension is the reason behind their poor tolerance to blood loss and to regional anesthesia. The first fact is exemplified by the patient with severe preeclampsia or eclampsia who goes into profound shock after cesarean section despite an average or below average blood loss during the operation. This happens because the average blood loss of 1000 ml during a cesarean section delivery correspond to about 35% to 40% of the blood volume in a pregnant woman with severe preeclampsia.

Profound shock may be seen in patients with severe pregnancy-induced hypertension not only as a consequence of blood loss but also as a consequence of regional anesthesia. The mechanisms of shock related to blood loss and to regional anesthesia are similar. In the case of blood loss during delivery the blood is lost to the outside; in the case of regional block the blood is lost to the capacitance vessels of the lower extremities as a consequence of the sympathetic-parasympathetic blockade. The hemodynamic effects of regional blocks may be avoided by elevating the lower extremities, avoiding compression of the return circulation by the pregnant uterus, and filling the intravascular compartment with water and electrolytes. However, it is better to avoid iatrogenic problems in unstable patients.

In our opinion, regional blocks (spinal and epidural anesthesia) are contraindicated in patients with *severe* pregnancy-induced hypertension.

The problem with the use of plasma volume expanders. Several communications in the literature suggest that administration of plasma volume expanders such as dextran or albumin may be of therapeutic value in preeclampsia. This mode of treatment attempts to correct the decreased intravascular volume, which is so important in the multiple-organ perfusion defect exhibited by these patients. In our opinion this therapy is inadequate because the decrease in plasma volume is secondary to vasoconstriction and cannot be adequately corrected unless the vasospasm is eliminated first.

Another reason to avoid the use of plasma volume expanders in preeclampsia is that their administration may cause pulmonary edema. In patients with *severe* preeclampsia or eclampsia—those cases in which the administration of albumin or dextran is frequently considered—the heart is working against a significantly increased afterload and may not respond adequately to a rapid increase in preload. Pulmonary edema may appear quickly if the administration of albumin is not adequately monitored with continuous measurements of pulmonary wedge pressure or central venous pressure. Furthermore, capillary damage with leakage of high molecular weight plasma components to the interstitial space is common in *severe* preeclampsia; in these cases pulmonary edema may be produced without elevation of the pulmonary wedge pressure (leaking capillaries). Pulmonary edema is a potentially lethal complication in patients with severe pregnancy-induced hypertension, and any therapy that increases the risk of pulmonary edema must be avoided.

Loss of resistance to angiotensin II and catecholamines

Women who remain normotensive during pregnancy show a progressive resistance to the pressor effect of catecholamines and angiotensin II throughout gestation. In contrast, patients destined to develop preeclampsia and eclampsia show a progressive decrease in their resistance to the pressor effects of these substances.[40] For example, a pregnant woman who remains normotensive during pregnancy will require an intravenous infusion of 12 to 14 ng/kg/min of angiotensin II to raise her diastolic blood pressure by 20 mm Hg when she is at 24 to 26 weeks of gestation. A patient of the same gestational age destined to develop pregnancy-induced hypertension will need less than 9 ng/kg/min and probably less than 8 ng/kg/min of angiotensin II to have a similar pressure response.[12] A pattern of decreased vascular resistance to the pressor effects of angiotensin II also exists in patients with chronic hypertension destined to develop superimposed preeclampsia or eclampsia (pregnancy-aggravated hypertension) as compared to patients with chronic hypertension who do not develop this complication.[13]

Since the abnormal vascular reactivity of the patient destined to develop pregnancy-induced or pregnancy-aggravated hypertension may be detected several weeks before the development of clinical signs and symptoms of the disease, vascular sensitivity to angiotensin II may be used as an early screening test. Early identification, in turn, allows the establishment of measures designed to prevent the appearance of the full-blown process. Unfortunately, angiotensin II sensitivity testing is far from being routine in the evaluation of pregnant women. An angiotensin II preparation for human use (Hypertensin) is not available in the United States, and even if the medication is obtained in Europe or South America, the test itself is invasive and time consuming and requires physician supervision.

Roll-over test. A noninvasive office procedure that correlates with angiotensin II sensitivity has been described.[11] This procedure, called the *roll-over test*, measures the pressor response of the pregnant woman to positional changes. For this purpose patients between 28 and 32 weeks of gestation are placed in the lateral recumbent position and the diastolic blood pressure is taken and recorded every 5 minutes for at least 15 minutes or until it is stable. At this point the patient is asked to change to the supine position (roll over), and the blood pressure is taken at 1 and 5 minutes. An increase in diastolic blood pressure of 20 mm Hg or more is considered abnormal (positive test). In the experience of the investigators who originally described the roll-over test 75% of primigravid patients with positive tests and 8% with negative tests developed pregnancy-induced hypertension.[11]

Similar results may be obtained with a less time-consuming modification of the test, which uses as an endpoint the pressor response obtained 1 minute after the positional change.[25] We also have found a significant difference in the pregnancy outcome of patients with positive and negative roll-over tests: 55% of the patients with positive and 17% of the patients with negative roll-over tests developed pregnancy-induced hypertension. The difference in outcome is greater if we consider that preeclampsia was *moderate* to *severe* in 10 of 19 patients with positive roll-over tests who developed preeclampsia but in only 3 of 19 patients with negative roll-over tests who developed the disease. In our opinion a negative roll-over test is reassuring, whereas a positive test has limited predictive value.

Coagulation abnormalities. The work of Pritchard et al[28] has conclusively demonstrated that coagulation abnormalities (in prothrombin time, thromboplastin time, platelet count, fibrinogen concentration, fibrinogen split products, protamine sulfate precipitation test) exist in only a minority of patients with *severe* forms of pregnancy-induced hypertension. This finding has important practical implications because the literature is rich in suggestions that disseminated intravascular coagulation is a fundamental etiopathogenic factor in preeclampsia, and this concept has led to the use of heparin in the treatment of the disease. This therapeutic modality should be strongly condemned: first, there is not a single controlled study showing that heparin administration modifies the course or improves the outcome of patients with preeclampsia, and second, the use of anticoagulants in patients with elevated arterial blood pressure is an open invitation to disastrous complications such as cerebral hemorrhage.

Morphologic changes. The organ that has been studied most intensively in preeclampsia is the kidney. The renal lesion in preeclampsia has been called *glomerular endotheliosis*,[38] and when evaluated by light microscopy it is indistinguishable from acute membranous glomerulonephritis. However, under the electron microscope it is apparent that the narrowing of the capillary lumen is not caused by swelling of the basal membrane but results from deposits of osmiophilic material between the basal membrane and the endothelial cells and from an increase in the cytoplasm of the endothelial and intercapillary cells. There is no change in the epithelial cells' foot processes, no proliferation of

intercapillary cells, and no alteration in the architecture of the renal medulla. The nature of the osmiophilic deposits has been elucidated with the help of immunofluorescent techniques, and it has been found that these deposits correspond to a material that reacts with antibodies against fibrinogen and fibrin. We have found a similar material in immunofluorescent studies of liver biopsies from patients with preeclampsia.[2]

When nulliparous patients who fulfill all the clinical criteria for the diagnosis of preeclampsia are submitted to kidney biopsy studies, only 70% of them show glomerular endotheliosis. Twenty-five percent of these women have chronic renal lesions, and in 5% of them no lesion will be found. If the same study is carried out in multiparous patients with a diagnosis of preeclampsia superimposed on chronic hypertension, the characteristic histologic lesion (with or without other renal pathology) will be found in only 14% of the cases. In this multiparous population nephrosclerosis will be present in 14% of the cases, chronic renal disease (including chronic pyelonephritis and chronic glomerulonephritis) will be present in 21% of the cases, and no renal lesion will be found in 53% of the patients.[23]

There are some practical implications in these facts about the histology of preeclampsia and eclampsia. First, the difficulties and complications associated with kidney biopsy during pregnancy make tissue diagnosis of the disease far from being routine. The consequence is confusion in attempts to rigorously interpret information obtained from populations selected on clinical criteria. Second, it is important to recognize that in multiparous patients a tissue diagnosis of preeclampsia is positive in only 1 of every 10 patients. Therefore the existence of chronic renal disease must be strongly considered in every multiparous patient who develops the hypertension-edema-proteinuria syndrome, and an adequate workup must be carried out.

Diagnosis

Excessive body weight gain. Excessive body weight gain and edema are no longer considered clear signs of preeclampsia. Large increases in body weight as well as edema of hands, face, or both are common in normal pregnancy; in fact, the incidence of preeclampsia is similar in the presence or in the absence of generalized edema. This is reflected in the results of the Collaborative Perinatal Project,[9] which found that there was no correlation between excessive body weight gain and poor perinatal outcome. However, a positive correlation was found between excessive weight gain during pregnancy and infant size at birth; thus the greater the gain, the heavier the infant. Therefore the inclusion of excessive weight gain or edema in the definition of preeclampsia seems to be no longer appropriate.

There is no evidence that the imposition of measures to limit weight gain during pregnancy (such as low salt diet or the use of diuretics) improves the outcome of gestation or prevents the development of preeclampsia. These measures may cause harm to both mother and fetus, and their use must be condemned.

Blood pressure elevation. Hypertension is the most important clinical sign of preeclampsia because it reflects the severity of the arterial vasospasm. Unfortunately, mistakes are frequently made because of defects in technique or lack of consistency in the methods used for blood pressure measurements. A common error is to take the blood pressure of an obese patient with a regular-size cuff. This causes higher readings and generates unnecessary alarm, testing, and consultation. Another common error in blood pressure evaluation during pregnancy is not to use the same maternal position in repeated measurements. The blood pressure in each prenatal visit is usually taken with the patient in the sitting position. If an abnormally high blood pressure reading is obtained, the measurement is repeated with the patient in the lateral recumbent or supine position. It is not surprising that in most cases the second blood pressure reading is different from the first. In the pregnant woman, blood pressure values are always lower in the lateral recumbent than in the sitting position, and they may be higher or lower in the supine than in the sitting position. A common result of this mistake is that the high blood pressure value is disregarded and diagnosis and treatment are delayed. An abnormally high blood pressure measurement in a pregnant woman must be verified by repeating the measurement with the woman in the same position.

Another error in blood pressure measurements is the use of different endpoints to measure the diastolic blood pressure. Some observers use the change in the quality of sound, while others use the cessation of sound as the indicator for diastolic blood pressure. The point of cessation of sound is the best index and must always be used for this purpose. It is not uncommon, however, for the cessation of sound not to occur in pregnant women; in these cases the point where the sound changes and becomes dull and muffled should be recorded as the diastolic blood pressure. In this case some sign must be used to indicate to a second observer that there was a variation in the routine procedure for blood pressure assessment so that if a repeated evaluation is necessary it can be carried out using a similar technique.

Page and Christianson[24] have emphasized the importance of mean arterial pressure (MAP) during the second trimester as a predictor of the development of preeclampsia, and there is evidence that if a patient exhibits both a high MAP during the second trimester (more than 85 mm Hg) and a positive roll-over test, the chances of developing preeclampsia are greater than 95%.[26] MAP is obtained by adding the systolic blood pressure to twice the diastolic blood pressure, then dividing the product by three:

$$MAP = \frac{Systolic + 2 \ (Diastolic)}{3}$$

To obtain the MAP of the second trimester all the blood pressure values obtained during this time are converted to MAPs and averaged.

Proteinuria. Proteinuria is a sign of preeclampsia that usually follows excessive body weight gain and the appearance of hypertension. The proteinuria of preeclampsia is *nonselective*, corresponding to a mixture of several proteins of different molecular weight.

The proteinuria of preeclampsia occurs in the absence of either a nephritic (red cells, red cell casts) or a nephrotic (birefringent lipids, wax casts) urinary sediment. The urinary sediment in preeclampsia is usually benign and unrevealing and in most cases shows an abundance of fine and coarse granular casts. The presence of a nephritic or nephrotic type of urinary sediment in a patient with signs and symptoms of preeclampsia must alert the clinician to the possibility of a disease independent of pregnancy causing the picture of pregnancy-induced hypertension.

Proteinuria is extremely valuable as a prognostic sign in preeclampsia. Frequent monitoring of the amount of protein excreted in the urine must be a part of the evaluation of patients with pregnancy-induced hypertension, and a significant increase in proteinuria means that the disease has taken a turn for the worst.

Vasospasm. Clinical evidence of the presence of vasospasm and its severity may be obtained by ophthalmologic examination, which must be a part of the initial and subsequent evaluation of the patient with pregnancy-induced hypertension. The most common findings in patients with *moderate* or *severe* forms of pregnancy-induced hypertension are an increase in the vein to artery ratio (normal, 4:3) and segmental vasospasm. Patients with *mild* preeclampsia usually have a negative funduscopic examination.

Examinations of the optic fundi in pregnant patients with hypertension is also important because it may suggest the presence of maternal hypertensive disease independent of pregnancy. For example, papilledema is not a common finding in preeclampsia, and its existence suggests the possibility of a brain tumor causing increases in intracranial pressure and secondary hypertension. Similarly, the presence of hemorrhages, exudates, or extensive arteriolar changes will point to the presence of chronic hypertension, and the presence of microaneurysms will indicate the existence of diabetes.

Other signs and symptoms of preeclampsia. *Headaches* are usually present in moderate to severe forms of preeclampsia, but they also may appear in the primigravid patient before other indications of overt disease. The pain may be frontal or occipital, may be pulsatile or dull, may be simultaneous with visual symptoms, and may frequently be intense, especially when preceding the onset of convulsions.

Epigastric or right upper quadrant pain is also common in patients with moderate or severe forms of the disease but may also happen before the onset of obvious signs or symptoms of preeclampsia. This complaint is frequently attributed to indigestion or to gallbladder disease and is treated with antacids and antispasmodics. When epigastric or right upper quadrant pain appears in patients with severe hypertension, it is frequently a forerunner of convulsions and is commonly accompanied by marked alterations in SGOT, SGPT, and LDH values.

The visual symptom usually appearing first in patients who are going to develop preeclampsia is a transient perception of bright or black spots in front of their eyes (scotomas). This may progress to sudden but transient lack of ability to focus the eyes, blurred vision, and in severe cases, complete blindness. In most patients complaining of visual symptoms ophthalmologic examination reveals only vasospasm, indicating that they originate in the occipital brain cortex rather than in the retina. We have observed several patients with cortical blindness appearing in the course of pregnancy-induced hypertension and have been amazed by the speed of their visual recovery following termination of pregnancy.

Brisk deep tendon reflexes are a common finding in preeclamptic patients. They are evidence of abnormal central nervous system irritability and in severe cases occur simultaneously with clonus and twitching of fingers and toes. We have never seen the onset of seizures in preeclamptic patients not showing signs of excessive nervous system irritability.

Laboratory findings in preeclampsia. The laboratory is usually unrevealing in cases of mild preeclampsia, but it shows multiple findings in moderate or severe forms of the disease. The laboratory changes reflect the effects of the disease on the kidney, liver, and fetoplacental unit and, in some cases, the presence of hematologic abnormalities.

Laboratory changes reflecting altered renal function. In severe preeclampsia there are elevations in serum creatinine, BUN, and uric acid levels; decreases in creatinine clearance; proteinuria; and changes in the urinary sediment. The elevation in serum creatinine level almost never exceeds 1.3 to 1.4 mg/dl (upper limit of normal during pregnancy is 0.8 mg/dl). The elevation of BUN in preeclampsia rarely exceeds 20 to 25 mg/dl (upper limit of normal in pregnancy is 15 mg/dl) in the absence of complications. The endogenous creatinine clearance is usually at the normal nonpregnant level. It is important to remember that a creatinine clearance of 100 ml/min, which is completely normal outside of pregnancy, is abnormal during gestation, when the lower limit of normal is 130 ml/min.

Many have postulated that serum uric acid elevation is a specific laboratory finding in preeclampsia. However, there is a high degree of overlapping among the values found in normal pregnancy, mild preeclampsia, severe preeclampsia, and eclampsia.[18] Serum uric acid levels normally decrease at the beginning of pregnancy, remain low during the second trimester, and slowly increase during the third trimester, nearly reaching nonpregnant levels at term.

In most cases of mild or moderate preeclampsia, serum uric acid levels are indistinguishable from those obtained in normotensive patients at term. They are markedly elevated only in association with severe forms of preeclampsia, which is similar to what happens to the BUN and creatinine values.

Other changes in renal laboratory parameters, such as proteinuria and alterations in the urinary sediment, were considered before and will not be repeated here.

Laboratory changes reflecting altered liver function. Patients with mild forms of preeclampsia show little or no alteration in hepatic enzyme levels, but in severe preeclampsia marked elevations in SGPT, SGOT, and LDH are commonly found. The elevation in LDH is usually made at the expense of isoenzyme 5 (liver) unless the disease is complicated with hemolytic anemia, in which case the electrophoretic pattern will show elevation of fractions 1,2 (red cell) and 5. After termination of pregnancy, SGPT and SGOT levels rapidly start to decrease and in most cases reach normal levels by the fifth postpartum day. LDH falls more slowly, and normal values are reached by the eighth to tenth postpartum day.

Laboratory changes reflecting hematologic abnormalities. The only hematologic change that may be observed in patients with mild or moderate preeclampsia is an elevation of hemoglobin and hematocrit caused by the decrease in plasma volume and the vasospasm characteristic of the disease. In some patients with severe preeclampsia it is possible to observe other hematologic abnormalities, the most common being thrombocytopenia. Pritchard et al,[28] for example, found 26% of 91 eclamptic patients with platelet counts below 150,000; 17% with platelet counts below 100,000; and only 3% with platelet counts below 50,000. Typically, plasma fibrinogen concentration is elevated, and it is extremely unusual to find a fibrinogen concentration below 200 mg/dl unless the clinical course is complicated by abruptio placentae.

Another laboratory value that may be abnormal in the preeclamptic patient is the thrombin time, which is likely to be prolonged in about 50% of the patients with severe forms of preeclampsia. This alteration is peculiar, since it occurs in the presence of normal levels of fibrinogen and normal levels of fibrinogen split products.

Laboratory changes reflecting abnormal fetoplacental function. A common finding in women with moderate or severe preeclampsia is a biparietal diameter corresponding to 2 to 4 weeks less than the gestational age, suggesting intrauterine growth retardation. Urinary and plasma estriol values, as well as human placental lactogen (HPL) values, may be normal or low in preeclampsia. Low values are usually found in situations where fetal danger is evident as a result of the severity of the maternal disease, but frequently they are falsely positive. Normal values may be seen despite maternal and fetal compromise. In our opinion, estriol determinations have little value in the management of patients with preeclampsia.

Determination of fetal reactivity (nonstress test [NST]) and contraction stress testing (CST) are useful when a quick evaluation of the fetal status is considered necessary. However, it is important to recognize that the use of these tests in patients with preeclampsia offers possibilities for serious mistakes. The commonly accepted 8-day interval after a negative NST or CST (where fetal demise is highly improbable) has no validity in the presence of an unstable or rapidly deteriorating maternal situation. Another common source of error is the dictum: *positive testing = fetal distress = cesarean section delivery.* In fact, a significant percentage (between 35% and 50%) of fetuses with positive oxytocin challenge testing will be capable of tolerating labor without distress, and if all positive tests are confirmed by direct intrapartum monitoring, a number of unnecessary cesarean sections will be avoided.

Diagnostic difficulties. There are few diagnostic difficulties in cases of mild preeclampsia. The problem in mild cases is the reluctance of the physician to accept the diagnosis and the inappropriate management of the disease.

Unfortunately, the most serious diagnostic problems are found in cases of severe preeclampsia. As mentioned in the introduction to this chapter, mistakes are made because signs and symptoms of preeclampsia may be produced by pregnancy-independent diseases such as systemic lupus erythematosus, brain tumors, and kidney lesions. A more common error is to diagnose hepatitis, gallbladder disease, idiopathic hemolytic anemia, thrombotic thrombocytopenic purpura, brain tumor, nephrosis, glomerulonephritis, or epilepsy in patients with severe preeclampsia.

There are no easy rules to follow to avoid mistakes in the diagnosis of pregnancy-induced versus pregnancy-independent hypertension, but the following suggestions may be of some value:

1. Severe preeclampsia is not common in multiparous patients. Each multiparous patient with severe hypertension must be suspected to have pregnancy-independent hypertension and must have a minimal workup, including antinuclear antibodies (ANA) titer, potassium determination in plasma and, if low, in the urine, and a 6-week postpartum, rapid sequence intravenous pyelogram (IVP).

2. The earlier in gestation severe hypertension occurs, the greater the possibility of its being caused by a pregnancy-independent event.

3. If pregnancy is terminated by cesarean section in a patient with severe hypertension, the surgeon should carefully palpate the kidneys, adrenal glands, and periaortic region during the procedure. During explorations carried out at the time of cesarean sections, we have found a large kidney tumor (hypernephroma), a large cyst (lymphangioma) compressing the aorta just above its bifurcation, adrenal tumors, and more frequently, small, scarred kidneys of chronic pyelonephritis indicating pregnancy-independent causes of hypertension.

4. Hypertension is the key element in the differential diagnosis. Hepatitis, gallbladder stones, idiopathic thrombocytopenic purpura, epilepsy, and many other diseases that may appear during pregnancy do not have hypertension as one of their manifestations. In contrast, every time a bizarre clinical condition appears during pregnancy it must be suspected of being caused by preeclampsia if hypertension is present.

Management

Once a diagnosis of preeclampsia is established, the patient must be admitted to the hospital. There is no place for outpatient treatment of preeclampsia.

The first and most important question to be answered when the clinician is confronted with the management of a patient with preeclampsia is:

What is the severity of the disease?

Success in the management of the preeclamptic patient depends on our accuracy in answering this question. The question can only be answered in one of three ways, which correspond to the different degrees of severity of preeclampsia (mild, moderate, and severe).

Severe cases. If the answer to the question is that the patient has severe preeclampsia or eclampsia, the management will consist of (1) termination of pregnancy, (2) administration of magnesium sulfate, and (3) administration of hydralazine.

Termination of pregnancy. Termination of pregnancy is the consequence of a fact established throughout multiple observations of patients with this problem: *the only specific treatment of severe preeclampsia is termination of pregnancy.* Failure to remember this cardinal rule and reluctance to terminate pregnancy, usually because of an early gestational age, was one of the most common physician errors found in a study in Los Angeles[17] of maternal mortality caused by preeclampsia. This study found the most common physician errors in the management of preeclampsia-eclampsia to be the following:

1. Underestimation of the severity of the disease
2. Overconfidence in drugs that mask symptoms but do not impede the progress of the disease (diuretics, sedatives, antihypertensives)
3. Failure to use antihypertensive drugs to combat extreme elevations of blood pressure
4. Reluctance to terminate the pregnancy

In most cases of severe preeclampsia, pregnancy may be terminated by induction of labor with intravenous oxytocin. This procedure (see box on p. 101) is frequently successful even in

Protocol for the use of oxytocin in induction of labor

PREPARATION

Add 10 units of oxytocin to a plastic bag containing 250 ml of 5% dextrose in water (D_5W). This yields a solution containing 40 mU of oxytocin per milliliter.

ADMINISTRATION

Electronic monitoring is a prerequisite for oxytocin administration. Oxytocin should be given IV via piggyback port using a Harvard pump. The pumps come calibrated to deliver a certain volume of solution depending on the size of the syringe used with the instrument. The infusion should be started at no more than 1 mU/min and should not be increased more than twice the previous rate or at intervals less than 15 minutes. The infusion should not be increased if there are more than four contractions in 10 minutes. The situation must be reevaluated if a dose of 18 mU/min is reached and fails to induce labor.

SIDE EFFECTS

Oxytocin infusion should be immediately discontinued if:
1. There are signs of fetal distress on the electronic monitor.
2. The uterine tonus is elevated, and there is poor relaxation between contractions.
3. The interval between contractions is less than 90 seconds. In these cases the patient should be turned to her side, oxygen administered by mask, and if there are no contraindications, 250 μg of terbutaline sulfate (0.25 ml) should be given subcutaneously.

cases where the cervix appears firm and closed. Another method of inducing labor that is becoming increasingly popular for patients with unripened cervix is the application of 2.5 mg of prostaglandin E_2 (PGE_2) in the posterior vaginal fornix.[36] Induction must be carefully monitored, since fetal distress is common during labor in these patients. Appearance of fetal distress or failure of induction requires termination by cesarean section.

Magnesium sulfate. The objective of magnesium sulfate ($MgSO_4$) administration is to prevent eclamptic seizures. The effect of magnesium sulfate on the central nervous system does not account for its anticonvulsive effect. The cerebrospinal fluid Mg^{++} concentration is independent and significantly higher (2.4 mEq/L) than the plasma concentration and increases very slowly despite therapeutic plasma levels. Mg^{++} is a peripheral anticonvulsant because of its ability to block neuromuscular transmission by decreasing the amount of acetylcholine released in response to nerve action potential. Therefore the arrest or prevention of eclamptic seizures with magnesium sulfate does not modify the progression of the brain lesions causing the seizures. Treatment or prevention of eclamptic seizures with other medications acting directly on the brain cells (diazepam [Valium], phenytoin [Dilantin], phenobarbital) is also symptomatic because none of these drugs interferes with the cause of the abnormal electric discharge. Definitive treatment of eclamptic seizures is achieved only by termination of pregnancy.

The best maternal and fetal outcomes in patients with severe preeclampsia and eclampsia have been obtained through therapeutic regimens using magnesium sulfate.[29,42] Other protocols using different types of anticonvulsants require comparison of their results against those obtained with magnesium sulfate before they may claim superiority and are adopted for routine clinical use.

An intravenous dose of 4 grams of magnesium sulfate causes an immediate elevation of the normal Mg^{++} level (1.6 to 2.1 mEq/L) to about 7 to 9 mEq/L. Intracellular transfer of the ion and elimination by the kidney will cause a drop in plasma concentration to 4 to 5 mEq/L approximately 1 hour after injection. At this elevated plasma level about one third of the Mg^{++} is protein bound, and its renal clearance is very similar to the glomerular filtration rate. We administer magnesium sulfate by continuous intravenous infusion for the prevention and treatment of eclamptic seizures (see box below). In other medical centers intramuscular administration is preferred (see box on p. 103). In most cases of eclampsia the initial loading dose of magnesium sulfate (both the intravenous and the intramuscular forms) is enough to arrest convulsions. It is rare for a patient to convulse again after the loading dose. In these cases we give 125 to 250 mg of Amytal Sodium injected very slowly IV to obtain complete control of the convulsive state.

Magnesium sulfate is not an innocuous drug, and it is necessary to monitor carefully those patients who are receiving the medication to prevent the occurrence of serious side effects. The clinical variables to monitor are urinary output, patellar reflex, and respiratory rate.

Monitoring of the urinary output is extremely important because Mg^{++} is eliminated by the urine and urine production is frequently decreased in patients with severe preeclampsia, a situation that may lead to the accumulation of Mg^{++} and the production of respiratory and car-

diac arrest. A urinary output of at least 30 ml/hr is a necessary prerequisite for the continuous administration of magnesium sulfate.

Monitoring the patellar reflex is also important because its disappearance is the first sign of impending toxicity. The patellar reflex usually disappears when plasma Mg^{++} concentration reaches 8 to 10 mEq/L. In this case the administration of the drug must be discontinued until the patellar reflex is obtained. If this is not done, the plasma levels will continue increasing until they reach a point (more than 12 mEq/L) at which there will be a decrease in respiratory rate that may progress to respiratory paralysis. Pritchard[27] has observed that administration of furosemide to a patient with impaired renal function caused by preeclampsia did not prevent Mg^{++} accumulation to toxic levels despite the increase in urine flow observed after administration of the diuretic. Obviously the increase in urinary output was not equivalent to improved renal function or to improved ability to excrete Mg^{++}.

An excess of Ca^{++} will increase the amount of acetylcholine liberated by the action potentials at the neuromuscular junction. Thus if re-

Guidelines for intravenous magnesium sulfate administration in the prevention and treatment of convulsions in patients with pregnancy-induced hypertension

LOADING DOSE

Give 20 ml of 20% magnesium sulfate (4 grams) IV over a 15- to 20-minute period. If 20% magnesium sulfate is not available, mix 8 ml of 50% magnesium sulfate and 12 ml of sterile water.

MAINTENANCE DOSE

Add 20 grams of magnesium sulfate (four 10 ml ampules of 50% solution) to 1000 ml of D_5W and give by continuous intravenous infusion at a rate of 100 ml/hr (2.0 g/hr). If the amount of magnesium sulfate given is less than that required to maintain adequate serum magnesium levels (6 to 8 mEq/L), the rate of administration must be increased. Continue magnesium sulfate administration for 24 hours postpartum.

MONITORING FOR MAGNESIUM TOXICITY

Every hour monitor:
  Urine output (should be at least 30 ml/hr)
  Deep tendon reflexes (should be present)
  Respiration rate (should exceed 14/min)
Any decrease in these indexes makes it mandatory to reevaluate the rate of magnesium sulfate administration.

spiratory depression is induced by the administration of magnesium sulfate, calcium gluconate, 10 ml of a 10% solution given by slow (over 3 minutes) intravenous injection, is the logical antidote.

Magnesium sulfate may also be harmful to the fetus. Maternal Mg^{++} rapidly equilibrates with fetal plasma, and the concentrations in both compartments are very similar. Respiratory depression and hyporeflexia have been observed in newborns delivered when the mother is undergoing intravenous magnesium sulfate therapy. It seems that this problem does not occur or is significantly less frequent if magnesium sulfate is given IM. The reason for this difference in fetal outcome between intravenous and intramuscular magnesium sulfate is unknown, but most probably it is the consequence of higher maternal and fetal plasma levels in patients receiving intravenous therapy.

Magnesium sulfate decreases beat-to-beat variability as seen by electronic monitoring of the fetal heart rate. It is important to remember that the effect of Mg^{++} on variability is not marked and that decreased or absent variability is a sign of fetal distress in patients with preeclampsia who are receiving magnesium sulfate treatment.

Magnesium sulfate acts synergistically with the muscle-relaxant drugs used for general anesthesia. Obstetric anesthesiologists are aware of this fact and prescribe a smaller dosage of muscle-relaxant medications to patients undergoing magnesium sulfate therapy who will be given general anesthetics.

Hydralazine. The objective of hydralazine administration is to decrease marked elevations of blood pressure. This helps to prevent seizures and diminish the likelihood of cerebral hemorrhage and left ventricular failure. As stated at the beginning of this chapter, a large amount of clinical and laboratory research suggests the following steps in the pathogenesis of hypertensive intracranial bleeding:

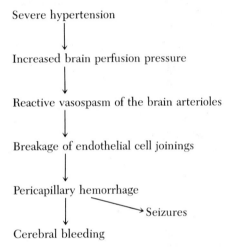

Guidelines for intramuscular magnesium sulfate administration for the treatment and prevention of convulsions in patients with pregnancy-induced hypertension

LOADING DOSE (IV, ONLY FOR PATIENTS WITH ECLAMPSIA)

Administer 4 grams of magnesium sulfate IV in 3- to 5-minute period. Use 8 ml of 50% magnesium sulfate solution diluted with 12 ml of sterile water, or 20 ml of a 20% solution.

LOADING DOSE (IM)

Administer 10 grams of magnesium sulfate IM. Give 10 ml of 50% solution deeply in the upper, outer quadrant of *each* buttock using a 3-inch, 20-gauge needle. The intramuscular dose should immediately follow the intravenous loading dose in patients with convulsions. *Patients without convulsions receive only the intramuscular loading dose.*

MAINTENANCE DOSE

Give 5 grams (10 ml of 50% solution) deep by IM in alternate buttocks every 4 hours if (1) the patellar reflex is present, (2) the urine output has been at least 100 ml during the preceding 4 hours, and (3) the respiration rate is normal (at least 14/min). Continue maintenance dose until 24 hours postpartum.

Guidelines for the use of hydralazine in patients with pregnancy-induced hypertension

INTERMITTENT INTRAVENOUS ADMINISTRATION

If the diastolic blood pressure exceeds 110 mm Hg, give 5 mg of hydralazine by intravenous push. Measure the blood pressure every 5 minutes thereafter. If the diastolic blood pressure does not decrease to the desired range (90 to 100 mm Hg), advance in 5 mg increments every 15 to 20 minutes until a therapeutic response is obtained or a dose of 20 mg is given.

CONTINUOUS FETAL MONITORING

Hydralazine may reduce the placental blood flow, and continuous electronic fetal monitoring is mandatory during hydralazine therapy in undelivered patients.

According to this scheme, administration of a hypotensive agent is of fundamental importance to prevent seizures and cerebrovascular accidents in patients with preeclampsia. The medication used for this purpose is hydralazine, which acts directly on the arteriolar smooth muscle and decreases blood pressure by reducing peripheral vascular resistance. The blood pressure response to intravenous hydralazine is almost immediate and does not have the dramatic characteristics observed with diazoxide. As shown in the box above, we use hydralazine in repeated intravenous boluses.

The most serious side effect of hydralazine administration is decreased uteroplacental perfusion. Late decelerations of the fetal heart rate are frequently observed after hydralazine therapy in patients who previously had a normal electronic fetal monitoring trace. It is also possible to observe the recovery from the abnormal monitoring pattern after hydralazine is discontinued and the blood pressure is allowed to rise. This complication happens more often if there is a pronounced drop in diastolic blood pressure, usually below 80 mm Hg. For this reason, electronic monitoring of the fetus is mandatory when hydralazine is used in preeclampsia, and the amount and frequency of hydralazine administration must be conditioned by both the maternal and the *fetal* response.

Other antihypertensive agents. Other antihypertensive agents are not superior to hydralazine in the management of the preeclamptic patient and may have serious disadvantages. Methyldopa, an excellent drug for therapy of chronic hypertension, requires several hours between administration and full effect; for this reason it is not adequate in situations where a quick response to treatment is necessary. Reserpine may cause nasal stuffiness in the newborn—a rather serious problem because of the obligatory nasal breathing condition of the neonate. Diazoxide is a very powerful medication causing a dramatic drop in blood pressure a few seconds after its administration. At least one maternal death has been reported in a patient with preeclampsia who went into profound, irreversible shock after diazoxide administration.[16] Diazoxide also causes fetal and maternal hyperglycemia, arrests uterine contractions, and causes marked sodium and water retention. Sodium nitroprusside is an excellent medication for obtaining a gradual decrease of elevated blood pressure levels, but the cyanide generated by its metabolism may be as harmful for the human fetus as it has been shown to be for the sheep fetus.

• • •

It is clear that the management of severe preeclampsia using (1) termination of pregnancy, (2) administration of magnesium sulfate, and (3) administration of hydralazine involves not only a series of positive actions but also continuous adherence to some "what not to do" principles, which are summarized in the box on p. 105.

Moderate cases. If the answer to the initial question—what is the severity of the disease—is that the patient under consideration has *moderate* preeclampsia, the next step will be the

---

What *not* to do in the management of patients with severe pregnancy-induced hypertension

DO NOT GIVE DIURETICS

In the majority of cases anuria and oliguria are indications for prompt pregnancy termination and not for diuretic therapy.

DO NOT GIVE DIAZEPAM

Diazepam accumulates in the fetus, causing respiratory depression at birth.

DO NOT GIVE DIAZOXIDE, SODIUM NITROPRUSSIDE, OR RESERPINE

All these antihypertensive agents may have harmful effects on the fetus, and the indications for their use during pregnancy are very limited.

DO NOT GIVE HEPARIN

The danger of anticoagulation in the presence of hypertension (intracranial bleeding) is very high. There is no evidence that heparin improves the outcome of patients with severe pregnancy-induced hypertension.

---

assessment of gestational age and fetal lung maturation. There are several clinical and laboratory means of assessing gestational age (Chapter 7), and they should be used in the patient with moderate preeclampsia to determine if the pregnancy is close to term (36 or more weeks of gestation) or remote from term (less than 36 weeks of gestation). If the pregnancy is close to term, steps should be taken for immediate pregnancy termination. There is no good reason to continue pregnancy in a situation where the infant and the mother have close to a 100% chance of good outcome if delivery is accomplished.

If the pregnancy is at less than 36 weeks of gestation (remote from term), the chances for a good fetal outcome decrease because of the rising incidence of respiratory distress syndrome and other stigmas of prematurity. Preeclampsia is one obstetric situation causing fetal stress and acceleration of fetal lung maturation, and a good number of preterm infants born to mothers with preeclampsia have adequate lung maturation. However, the chances of this happening decrease precipitously at gestational ages less than 36 weeks.

Management of the patient with moderate preeclampsia at less than 36 weeks of gestation will depend on the clinical and laboratory observation of the patient during the 24 to 48 hours following admission to the hospital. This period of observation is better carried out in an intensive care area. An NST (followed by a CST if necessary) is performed, as well as maternal laboratory evaluation, including tests for serum creatinine, BUN, uric acid, SGOT, LDH, and platelet count. These data will be used to reassess the question of severity. Frequent (every 4 hours) measurements of blood pressure, urinary output, qualitative proteinuria, and neurologic signs and symptoms will be carried out. If at any time during the period of observation the clinical and laboratory indexes indicate that the patient's condition is worse than initially evaluated, is deteriorating, or is not improving, the patient must be delivered without consideration of gestational age or status of fetal lung maturation.

Fortunately most patients admitted with *moderate* preeclampsia at less than 36 weeks of gestation improve quickly with bed rest in the hospital, their diastolic blood pressure decreases to the *mild* range (90 to 100 mm Hg), there is an increase in urinary output, and there is amelioration of headaches, visual symptoms, and nervous system irritability. If this occurs, the classification of the patient changes to *mild* preeclampsia and she should be entered into a *chronic care program*, to be described later.

Mild cases. If the answer to the initial question—what is the severity of the disease—is that the patient under consideration has *mild* preeclampsia, the next step (similar to that for the patient with moderate preeclampsia) will be an assessment of gestational age and/or fetal lung maturation. If the patient has *mild* preeclampsia, the main criterion to determine her management is gestational age because if the pregnancy is close to term there is no reason for prolongation of pregnancy. Thus if the patient is at 36 or more weeks of gestation, the pregnancy must be terminated. However, in mild preeclampsia there is not the sense of urgency in terminating the pregnancy that exists in the case of severe or moderate preeclampsia. In *mild* cases induction of labor by intravenous oxytocin administration may be repeated on alternate days unless the patient becomes moderately or severely hypertensive. Amniotomy should not be performed in the initial attempts to induce labor to avoid the complications associated with this procedure.

If the patient with mild preeclampsia is at less than 36 weeks of gestation, she should be entered into a *chronic care program*. The rationale behind chronic care is that in-hospital limitation of the patient's physical activity is an effective way of slowing the progression of the disease and gains the time necessary to achieve a degree of fetal maturity more compatible with a good pregnancy outcome.

The keys to success in chronic care of preeclamptic patients are (1) strict selection criteria for admission of patients to chronic care and (2) careful monitoring for signs and symptoms of aggravation of the disease.

Selection is a problem of the utmost importance. Only patients with mild preeclampsia or patients with stable moderate preeclampsia at less than 36 weeks of gestation are to be admitted into a chronic care program. No attempts should be made to prolong gestation in patients with preeclampsia of any severity who are at term or who have adequate fetal lung maturation, nor should attempts be made in patients with severe or moderate preeclampsia who do not improve after a 24-hour period of observation or who are at more than 36 weeks of gestation.

Monitoring of both mother and fetus is the other key to success. Maternal monitoring consists of the following:

1. Measurement of blood pressure four times per day

2. Measurement of total body weight every other day
3. Measurement of qualitative urinary protein excretion with Albustix in the first urine specimen produced every morning
4. Measurement of endogenous creatinine clearance every week
5. Measurement of serum biochemical profile (SMA-18) twice per week
6. Daily questioning of the patient about fetal movements, development of scotomas or headaches, or presence of epigastric or right upper quadrant pain

Fetal monitoring is carried out as follows:

1. The fetal biparietal diameter should be measured on admission to the hospital and every 3 weeks thereafter.
2. Fetal reactivity determination (NST) should be carried out every week and more frequently if the mother complains of decreased fetal movement or if there is a clinical or sonographic suggestion of retarded fetal growth.
3. Only rarely is determination of the lecithin/sphingomyelin (L/S) ratio in amniotic fluid necessary, since the decision to deliver or not depends on maternal and fetal deterioration rather than on maturity of the fetal lungs.

During the chronic care program:

1. The patient should not receive any medication different from the vitamin and iron supplements she was receiving preceding her admission to the hospital. It must be emphasized that *no diuretics or antihypertensive drugs are to be given*. Objections to the use of diuretics were stated before. With respect to antihypertensives, if the blood pressure of a preeclamptic patient in chronic care rises to a point where treatment with antihypertensives is necessary, the patient needs to be delivered.
2. There is no dietary sodium restriction. Patients should eat the regular hospital diet (about 2500 calories per day), and neither decreased or increased sodium intake should be encouraged.
3. Strict bed rest is not necessary, and there is no limitation on physical activity. In-hospital activity, however, is much less than outpatient activity, and most of the patients

will spend a majority of their time lying in bed.

4. The preeclamptic patient under chronic care must remain in the hospital until delivered.

The decision to deliver a patient who is in chronic care depends on maternal and fetal deterioration. The most important variable affecting that decision is the maternal blood pressure. Elevation of the blood pressure to a moderate range (between 100 and 110 mm Hg diastolic) is the most common indication for delivery. Unfortunately, a commonly used alternative is to give antihypertensive medications and try to prolong the pregnancy for a few more days or weeks. This alternative must be vigorously rejected: antihypertensive medications for preeclamptic patients should be given only in the labor room, simultaneously with magnesium sulfate, while preparing for pregnancy termination. Trying to deal with a deteriorating condition using antihypertensive medication and avoiding delivery is an open invitation to disaster.

Excessive body weight gain; elevation of BUN, creatinine, or uric acid levels; decreased creatinine clearance; and increased proteinuria are not indications for delivery unless they occur concomitantly with elevated diastolic blood pressure. The truth of the matter is that these alterations usually appear as the hypertension worsens. Among these signs, proteinuria is an important sign of deteriorating renal function and is second only to hypertension as an index of worsening of the disease. A summary of the overall plan of management of patients with uncomplicated preeclampsia is shown in Fig. 6-2.

Complicated forms

Preeclampsia complicated by thrombocytopenia and hemolytic anemia. When an abnormally low platelet count (less than 100,000/mm³) is seen in a severely preeclamptic patient, it is important to look at the blood smear for evidence of red cell fragmentation and obtain a serum haptoglobin determination. If fragmented red cells are seen in the smear and serum haptoglobin is absent, the patient has preeclampsia with hematologic complications. In these cases red cell and platelet destruction results from their passage through small vessels partially obliterated with fibrin deposits.

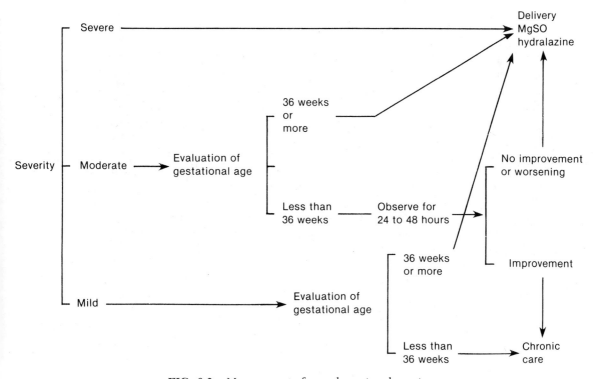

FIG. 6-2 ■ Management of preeclampsia-eclampsia.

The diagnostic problem in some of these patients is to differentiate between thrombotic thrombocytopenic purpura (TTP) and preeclampsia with hematologic complications. In most cases it is impossible to establish this distinction antepartum, since the clinical, laboratory, and histologic characteristics of both processes are equal. Frequently, however, the obstetrician and the internal medicine consultant fall into the trap of diagnosing TTP and start a course of useless medical therapy and dangerous procrastination. In our opinion every hypertensive pregnant patient with hematologic complications must be managed as if the process were induced by pregnancy, and this implies termination of pregnancy. In most of cases the patient will improve rapidly after delivery. If TTP is present, hemolysis and neurologic symptoms will not be modified by termination of pregnancy. The plan of management must include the following:

1. Induction of labor with intravenous oxytocin or vaginal PGE_2 must be initiated immediately unless there is a contraindication for vaginal delivery. We prefer to see changes in the cervix shortly after induction. If vaginal delivery is not in sight 12 hours after initiation of induction, we prefer to terminate gestation by cesarean section.

2. Platelets and coagulation factors are not given unless the platelet count is below 20,000/mm³ and the patient is bleeding from venipuncture sites. If a platelet transfusion is necessary, each unit of platelets transfused will raise the count by about 10,000/mm³/M². Since the objective is to raise the count to about 50,000/mm³, the transfusion of 10 units of platelets will achieve that goal in the majority of cases. The survival of the transfused platelets in a presumably nonimmunized recipient will depend on the severity of the disease and the speed of the recovery after pregnancy termination. The platelet count will remain low the 3 initial postpartum days but will rapidly increase afterward. Very high platelet counts (more than 600,000/mm³) are not uncommon by the seventh or eighth day. Unless the patient is bleeding or shows continuous deterioration, there is no need to repeat the platelet counts at intervals shorter than 24 hours.

3. Packed red cells are transfused if the hematocrit drops below 30%. This occurs very frequently in the immediate postpartum period, mostly as a consequence of vasodilation, hemodilution, and blood loss during delivery, rather than as a result of increased intensity of the hemolytic process.

4. Quite frequently these patients are oliguric, and there is a need to insert a central venous pressure (CVP) line to monitor the administration of intravenous fluids. Subclavian lines are contraindicated in the preeclamptic patient with thrombocytopenia because of the high risk of internal bleeding and hemomediastinum. If a CVP line is necessary, it should be inserted using the internal jugular or peripheral veins.

Preeclampsia complicated by electrolyte imbalance. Electrolyte disturbances in the preeclamptic patient are almost always the consequence of dietary salt restriction combined with the use of diuretics. Hyponatremia and hyperkalemia are the alterations most commonly found.

It is important to notice that only in exceptional cases does hyponatremia in preeclamptic patients become symptomatic or reach levels below 110 mEq/L. However, the sodium deficit should be corrected even if there are no symptoms in order to prevent the occurrence of postpartum circulatory collapse (see later discussion). The first step in the correction of hyponatremia is to calculate the approximate total sodium deficit, which usually is in the vicinity of 300 to 500 mEq. The following illustrates how to make the calculations:

Normal sodium concentration	140 mEq/L
Patient's sodium concentration	129 mEq/L
Deficit	11 mEq/L
Total body water (approximately 60% of body weight in kilogram)	45 Liters
Total sodium deficit = 45×11	495 mEq

No attempt must be made to obtain full correction of the sodium deficit. We usually administer enough sodium, in the form of 3% NaCl solution, to compensate for about 50% of the total deficit. In our hypothetical case 500 ml of 3% NaCl (containing 256 mEq of sodium) will be given at a rate of 100 ml/hr. Plasma sodium will be measured after the infusion, and if it is 135 mEq/L or more, there is no need for further hypertonic saline administration.

Hyperkalemia in these cases is usually not severe and rarely exceeds 5.5 mEq/L. In most cases it will be corrected, provoking intracellular mobilization of potassium ion with the administration of 45 mEq of sodium bicarbonate ($NaHCO_3$) dissolved in 1000 ml of 5% dextrose in normal saline solution given parallel, and in a different IV line, to the 3% NaCl solution, over a period of 3 to 4 hours.

The fear of circulatory overload with the use of 3% NaCl frequently leads the obstetrician to attempt sodium deficit corrections using ½ normal, or 0.9% saline solutions. This is not adequate in situations where a relatively rapid achievement of electrolyte balance is desired.

Preeclampsia complicated by pulmonary edema. Pulmonary edema is not a common complication of preeclampsia-eclampsia. In the Los Angeles County study[17] pulmonary edema was the cause of death in 3 of 67 eclamptic patients. In most of the cases reported in the literature the complication occurs before labor and delivery and is characterized by profound respiratory distress, severe hypoxemia, and diffuse rales on auscultation of the lungs.

There are clinical differences when pulmonary edema occurs in a patient with known organic heart disease and when it complicates the course of preeclampsia. Most cases of pulmonary edema in preeclamptic patients occur in young women without a previous history of heart disease, with normal electrocardiograms, and without cardiomegaly on radiographic or echographic examination of the heart. Also, the course of the disease in the preeclamptic patient is characterized by its slow response to therapy. The reason for these differences is that increased capillary permeability (noncardiogenic pulmonary edema) is the fundamental etiopathogenic factor in preeclampsia. There are some cases, however, in which pulmonary edema in preeclampsia is associated with fluid overload and left ventricular failure. Since the only way to adequately understand the pathophysiology of a given situation is through the use of a Swan-Ganz cath-

eter and measurements of the pulmonary wedge pressure, this should be the first step in the management of a preeclamptic patient with pulmonary edema.

If the pulmonary capillary pressure is high (more than 20 mm Hg), pump failure and fluid overload are the major etiologic factors and rapid digitalization and intravenous administration of furosemide will be the cornerstones of treatment. If the pulmonary wedge pressure is normal or below normal, leaking capillaries with diffusion of high-protein fluid into the alveoli is the reason behind the problem; in this case, therapeutic priority should be given to providing adequate respiratory support and to termination of pregnancy.

If it is not feasible to insert a Swan-Ganz catheter, a CVP line may be used. CVP measurements in this situation are not as reliable as pulmonary wedge pressure measurements. A CVP greater than 15 cm H_2O suggests pump failure and fluid overload, and a normal or subnormal CVP indicates that the cause of the problem is leaking capillaries. The Swan-Ganz or CVP measurements will also be valuable in monitoring the effects of therapy.

Pulmonary edema in preeclamptic individuals is an indication for termination of pregnancy. Delivery should be carried out after hemodynamic stabilization in the patient with primary pump failure and immediately after establishing respiratory support in the patient with leaking capillaries. In the first case (pump failure), digitalization, diuresis with furosemide, and normalization of pulmonary wedge pressure must precede delivery to avoid the deleterious effects of the acute hemodynamic changes happening in parturition. In the second case (leaking capillaries), the chances of maternal survival will depend primarily on the obstetrician's ability to affect the basic disease process by means of pregnancy termination.

Preeclampsia complicated by postpartum circulatory collapse. Occasionally patients with severe preeclampsia develop profound shock following vaginal or, more commonly, cesarean section delivery. If not rapidly corrected, this serious complication may lead to maternal death, acute tubular necrosis, and panhypopituitarism (Sheehan's syndrome).

Postpartum circulatory collapse usually occurs

within the first hour after cesarean section, but it may happen any time within the first 24 hours postpartum. The patient with moderate or severe hypertension who was agitated and hyperactive before delivery becomes hypotensive, tachycardic, clammy, and pale, and the urinary output is minimal or nonexistent. There is a rapid respiratory rate and the chest x-ray film may show diffuse bilateral infiltrates (shock lung).

Unfortunately there is no adequate explanation for the events leading to postpartum circulatory collapse in the preeclamptic patient. Electrolyte disturbances, particularly hyponatremia (ranging from 108 to 126 mEq/L) was found in eight cases where plasma sodium was measured[41]; potassium ion level was elevated (5.1 and 6.2 mEq/L) in two cases where it was measured. These findings are the basis for recommending correction of sodium and potassium deficits in patients with severe preeclampsia before delivery. Hypovolemia is another component of postpartum circulatory collapse.

Patients with severe preeclampsia and normal hematocrit and hemoglobin before delivery may develop postpartum hypovolemia despite what was estimated to be a usual or less than usual blood loss during delivery. The explanation for this is a combination of the following facts:

1. Antepartum hemoglobin and hematocrit in the preeclamptic are misleading. They frequently are within the normal range as a result of vasoconstriction and decreased plasma volume and do not reflect the real red cell concentration.
2. Since the total intravascular volume is markedly decreased in severe preeclampsia, the usual blood loss during delivery corresponds to a significant percentage of the patient's blood volume.
3. When the preoperative hematocrit and hemoglobin of patients undergoing cesarean section are within normal limits, operative blood losses are usually replaced with crystalloid solutions, bringing further hemodilution.
4. Some of the vasospasm existing before delivery subsides after delivery, and the newly available intravascular space is filled up with the crystalloid solutions given IV or by mobilization of interstitial fluid, causing further hemodilution.

The net result of the combination of these factors is that a preeclamptic patient with, for example, a preoperative hematocrit of 35% may have a postpartum hematocrit of 18% and all the signs and symptoms of severe cardiovascular collapse. It is also possible that other factors, such as pump failure and adrenal insufficiency, may play a role in the genesis of this problem.

The management of the preeclamptic patient who develops postpartum circulatory collapse is similar to the management of the obstetric patient in hypovolemic shock, which is described in detail in Chapter 15.

Preeclampsia complicated by renal failure. Oliguria is not uncommon in patients with moderate or severe preeclampsia. In most cases oliguria resolves after delivery, but in a few instances it may progress to anuria, acute tubular necrosis, bilateral cortical necrosis, and maternal death. In fact, 7 of the 67 maternal deaths related to toxemia in the Los Angeles County study were caused by renal failure.[17]

Renal complications are more common in preeclamptic patients with abruptio placentae than in other patients with severe preeclampsia. The latter frequently develop oliguria, but it rarely progresses to severe renal damage; in contrast, severe renal disease is the predominant cause of maternal death in patients with abruptio placentae.

The most common situation occurs when patients with moderate or severe preeclampsia show decreased urinary output (less than 30 ml/hr) at the time of labor. Usually this can be corrected, at least temporarily, by increasing the rate of intravenous fluid administration. Occasionally, however, the patient does not respond to this treatment and the oliguria becomes more marked. If the patient seems to be far from delivery, pregnancy should be terminated by cesarean section. Operative delivery is quickly followed by normalization of the urinary output, most probably as a result of decreased renal vasospasm and increased renal blood flow following cessation of the placental circulation and redistribution of the cardiac output. If the patient is relatively close to vaginal delivery (in normal labor, with 6 or more cm of cervical dilation), we maintain a rapid administration of intravenous fluids (about 150 ml/hr) and medicate the patient with 10 to 20 mg of intravenous furosemide. This usually results in adequate urinary output for the next 2 or 3 hours, which should be enough time for the patient to deliver vaginally. Once the patient delivers, the urinary output usually continues within normal limits without additional diuretic therapy.

The decision whether to deliver by cesarean section or to treat with intravenous fluids and diuretics when managing an oliguric-anuric preeclamptic patient is not easy. Both diuretic administration and cesarean section delivery have fetal and maternal iatrogenic potential. However, reestablishment of adequate urinary output is a very important priority. The longer the state of oliguria-anuria persists, the greater the possibility that the patient will develop severe or irreversible renal damage.

We prefer furosemide to mannitol in the treatment of the oliguric preeclamptic patient who is close to vaginal delivery. The reason for this preference is that in severe preeclampsia-eclampsia there is a significant degree of capillary damage and the mannitol may leak out from the intravascular space where it is needed to exert its osmotic effect, thus making the response to this medication not as predictable as the response to furosemide.

The management of the preeclamptic patient with abruptio placentae who develops anuria is identical to the management of the obstetric patient in acute renal failure, as described in Chapter 13.

Preeclampsia complicated by hepatic rupture. The liver is involved in the multiple organ defects that characterize severe preeclampsia.[2,23] In the majority of cases this involvement is shown by elevations of SGOT, SGPT, and LDH. There are a few cases, however, where the liver lesion has unusual severity and culminates in hepatic rupture. In the Los Angeles County series hepatic involvement was the cause of death in 10 of 67 maternal deaths related to eclampsia.[17]

The majority of preeclamptic patients with severe hepatic involvement complain of epigastric or upper right quadrant pain several days before the onset of more serious symptoms. The pain is frequently disregarded as unimportant or is confused with a minor gastrointestinal ailment. In fact, most patients with preeclampsia and severe hepatic lesions have been treated with ant-

acids for their "indigestion." Some other patients develop mild jaundice and are frequently diagnosed as having "hepatitis" or "gallbladder stones" until the evolution of the disease clearly demonstrates the presence of preeclampsia.

Hepatic rupture may occur antepartum or postpartum, and in both cases the signs and symptoms are those of profound circulatory collapse. The presence of peritoneal irritation signs and the progressive hypovolemia soon will point to massive intraabdominal bleeding as the cause of the problem. If the patient has not yet delivered, the pregnancy must be terminated immediately. At the time of the laparotomy the tear on the liver is almost always found on the diaphragmatic aspect of the right lobe. It frequently coexists with subcapsular petechiae and/or subcapsular hematomas.

The prognosis for preeclamptic patients with liver rupture is ominous. Attempts to approximate surgically the tear with sutures or to carry out a partial hepatectomy are usually followed by extension of the laceration, more bleeding, consumption coagulopathy, patient's exsanguination, and death. In these cases the least manipulation of the hepatic tissue will be rewarded with the best results. The bleeding hepatic surface should be covered with Avitene, Oxycel, or Gelfoam and then packed with surgical sponges placed above the hemostatic agent. One of the extremes of the sponges should be brought outside throughout the abdominal incision to facilitate removal in the second or third postoperative day.

The reason why simple, gentle packing may be lifesaving while attempts to suture may make the situation worse has to do with the nature of the lesion causing hepatic rupture. The situation in preeclampsia is different from traumatic liver rupture when the parenchyma is healthy and surgical approximation of the tear may be carried out without provoking additional bleeding. In preeclampsia, as illustrated by Sheehan and Lynch,[35] the hepatic tissue is diffusely affected by a hemorrhagic process that starts as periportal bleeding, continues with the formation of hematomas under Glisson's capsule, is followed by coalescence of the hematomas, and culminates in rupture of the capsule and massive intraabdominal hemorrhage. Any surgical suture placed on this abnormal tissue will cause further bleeding and further separation of the tissue.

If the preeclamptic patient with liver rupture survives surgery, she must be intensively monitored; careful attention must be given to adequate replacement of blood products and electrolytes during the postoperative period.

Preeclampsia complicated by abruptio placentae. About 7% of all patients with eclampsia will have premature separation of the placenta. Abruptio placentae is less frequent in preeclampsia and often an unexpected finding at the time of delivery. The management of abruptio placentae in preeclamptic patients is no different from the management under other circumstances and is described in Chapter 15.

Preeclampsia complicated by cerebral hemorrhage. Intracranial bleeding is the leading cause of death in preeclampsia. In the Los Angeles County series 21 of 67 maternal deaths related to eclampsia (31%) were caused by cerebral hemorrhage.[17] Underestimation of the severity of the disease, extended treatment as outpatients, failure to use antihypertensive drugs to treat extreme elevations of blood pressure, and discharge from the hospital before obtaining adequate control of the hypertension were the most frequent physician errors found in the analysis of those deaths.

In the majority of cases the pregnant hypertensive patient with brain bleeding is admitted to the hospital in coma following the onset of headaches and convulsions at home. The diagnosis is suggested by the deepening stupor and the presence of motor and sensory deficits and becomes highly probable if focal neurologic signs, such as unilateral pupil dilation, are present. The diagnosis is confirmed by computerized tomography of the brain (CAT scanning) or by lumbar puncture showing hemorrhagic cerebrospinal fluid. The prognosis is very poor, and recovery is the exception rather than the rule. In most cases coma becomes more profound, respiratory paralysis appears, and finally, the electroencephalogram shows lack of electrical activity in the brain.

Severe occipital or temporal headaches are a symptom of great importance in patients with severe preeclampsia because they frequently precede the onset of convulsions and coma. Severe headaches usually occur in patients with inadequate blood pressure control, and they are an indication for aggressive treatment with hypotensive agents. This is a situation where maternal life is at risk, and if the blood pressure cannot be brought under control with intravenous hydralazine, it is necessary to use diazoxide despite its potential iatrogenic effects.

Sometimes the fetus remains alive in the uterus of a comatose mother with intracranial bleeding. If the pregnancy is viable, the fetus should be removed quickly to avoid hypoxia, which will become severe with further maternal deterioration.

Preeclampsia complicated by visual disturbances. Blindness may occur in patients with severe preeclampsia and eclampsia and may persist for several days, although quick recovery after delivery is the rule. In most cases, examination of the eyegrounds does not show severe retinopathy, since the problem usually is caused by multiple microhemorrhages and microinfarcts occurring in the cortex of the occipital lobe of the brain. The cortical origin of blindness in the patient with preeclampsia makes this symptom equivalent to a seizure, and this patient should be diagnosed as having eclampsia and treated as such.

The fundoscopic examination of patients with preeclampsia usually does not reveal more than focal and generalized vasospasm and, in some cases, retinal edema, which frequently is missed in the examination *because it begins in the periphery of the retina.* The appearance of papilledema in a patient with severe preeclampsia or eclampsia is highly unusual and demands a reevaluation of the situation to rule out the possibility of a brain tumor imitating the signs and symptoms of the disease induced by pregnancy. Diplopia is a symptom that may occur in patients with preeclampsia and is caused by functional impairment of the sixth cranial nerve pair. In some rare cases the symptoms become more marked, and it is possible to find sixth nerve paralysis. This finding usually requires CAT scanning to rule out the existence of a tumor close to the brainstem area. Like most lesions caused by preeclampsia, sixth nerve paralysis improves after delivery and eventually disappears several weeks later.

Long-term prognosis of pregnancy-induced hypertension

Frequently the obstetrician is asked about the prognosis for future pregnancies and about the possibility of developing chronic high blood pressure by patients who had preeclampsia or eclampsia. Another common question from patients who had pregnancy-induced hypertension concerns their risk of developing hypertension if oral contraceptives are used for family planning. Finally, another question has to do with the risk of developing preeclampsia for the patient who becomes hypertensive while taking birth control pills.

With respect to the prognosis for future pregnancies and the possibilities of developing chronic hypertension later in life, the best answers are provided by the studies of Chesley.[4,5] This investigator has periodically reexamined women with eclampsia for periods up to 44 years and compared their subsequent reproductive performance and the development of chronic hypertension with control women matched by race and age. He found that the remote prognosis differs significantly when nulliparous and multiparous patients are compared. I have discussed before in this chapter how the diagnosis of preeclampsia-eclampsia is frequently in error in multiparous patients who have a predominance of chronic hypertension and chronic renal disease. Therefore Chesley's finding that multiparous patients who develop eclampsia have a higher incidence of hypertension in later life, an increased annual death rate, and a greater proportion of deaths resulting from cardiovascular disease than nulliparous patients with eclampsia is not surprising.

With respect to the risk of hypertension in future pregnancies, Chesley found that 33.8% of 151 women having eclampsia as nulliparas developed hypertension in later pregnancies. In about 40% of these cases hypertension was mild, and only 8% of the women had severe preeclampsia or recurrent eclampsia. He also found that 50% of women with eclampsia as multiparas developed hypertension in later pregnancies.

Chesley also found some adverse factors useful in predicting the probability of recurrence of preeclampsia-eclampsia in nulliparous patients who had eclampsia.

1. *Hypertension persisting throughout the tenth day after delivery.* If hypertension is still present on the tenth postpartum day, the possibility of recurrence is 59%, compared to 21% in women whose blood pressure is back to normal at that time ($p < .001$).

2. *Obesity.* If the weight of the patient in pounds divided by the height in inches is 2.2 or greater 6 weeks after delivery, the recurrence rate of preeclampsia-eclampsia will be 70%, compared with 27% for thinner women ($p < .001$).

3. *Onset of preeclampsia before the thirty-sixth week of gestation.* If preeclampsia starts before 36 weeks of gestation, the chances of recurrence are 56%, compared with 27% if preeclampsia was of late onset ($p < .01$).

4. *Average systolic pressure above 160 mm Hg during eclampsia.* If the average systolic pressure was greater than 160 mm Hg during eclampsia, the probability of recurrence is 46%, compared with 27% in patients with lower pressures ($p < .01$).

Chesley also found that the likelihood of recurrence of preeclampsia increases with the number of adverse factors. Seven percent of patients with no factors, 25% of patients with one factor, 56% of patients with two factors, and 78% of patients with three or four factors will develop hypertension in future pregnancies.

With respect to the ultimate development of chronic hypertension, Chesley demonstrated that women who have eclampsia as nulliparas do not develop chronic hypertension more frequently than do normal controls. In contrast, women who have eclampsia as multiparas will have a higher prevalence of hypertension later in life than will normotensive controls.

The question of the risk of oral contraceptive–induced hypertension in women who had preeclampsia-eclampsia has been answered by Pritchard and Pritchard.[30] They compared the incidence of hypertension in 200 nulligravid women and in 180 primiparous women who recently had pregnancy-induced hypertension while all of them were taking mestranol, 50 μg, plus norethindrone, 1 mg, for family planning purposes. He found that nine of the women previously hypertensive during pregnancy and five of the nulligravidas developed diastolic blood pressures exceeding 90 mm Hg during the initial 3 months of oral contraceptive use. After the first 3 months the incidence of diastolic blood pressure evaluation was similar for both groups. Interestingly enough, the absence of hypertension while using oral contraceptives did not preclude the subsequent development of hypertension during pregnancy in women from both groups. These results indicate that if hypertension occurs during the first pregnancy and reappears during the first 3 months of oral contraceptive use the patient most likely has chronic vascular disease. These researchers also concluded that the frequency and severity of oral contraceptive hypertension are not great enough to preclude the use of this medication in women who have had preeclampsia-eclampsia during their first pregnancy.

The last question, what will the blood pressure response be during pregnancy in women who developed oral contraceptive–induced hypertension before pregnancy, has not been answered yet by prospective, controlled studies.

■ CHRONIC HYPERTENSION IN PREGNANCY

Pregnancy-independent hypertension is present in 25% to 50% of all the cases of hypertension during pregnancy. According to the ACOG definition, to establish a diagnosis of chronic hypertension during pregnancy it is necessary to have either of the following:

1. Clear documentation of hypertension (140/90 mm Hg or above) before pregnancy
2. Discovery of hypertension before 20 weeks of gestation

Unfortunately a significant number of gravidas with chronic hypertension start their prenatal care after 20 weeks of gestation, and in many of them it is not possible to document the presence of hypertension outside of pregnancy. To make the situation worse these patients are normotensive in midpregnancy and become hypertensive in the last trimester, making the differential diagnosis with preeclampsia quite difficult.

The large majority of pregnant women with chronic hypertension have essential hypertension.[39] Occasionally the hypertension is a consequence of renal disease, especially chronic glomerulonephritis and chronic pyelonephritis.

The overwhelming majority of pregnant patients with chronic hypertension belong to the mild group when classified by severity criteria (Table 6-2). This fact is to a certain extent unfortunate because it generates a false sense of security in the obstetrician who assumes that *mild* means good prognosis for pregnancy and that there is no difference between the prenatal care of these patients and the care of nonhypertensive gravidas. The reality is that mild chronic hypertension is associated with increased perinatal mortality, preterm deliveries, intrauterine growth retardation, and antepartum and intrapartum fetal distress. Our studies of patients with mild chronic hypertension in pregnancy[1,3] have found 3.8% incidence of stillbirth, 15.3% incidence of premature labor, 16.6% incidence of intrauterine growth retardation, and 25.8% incidence of antepartum or intrapartum fetal distress. These figures are in general agreement with others previously reported in the literature. Thus the classification of pregnant women with chronic hypertension as *mild* does not imply that a superficial surveillance of the maternal and fetal status is all that is necessary. Every patient with mild chronic hypertension is at high risk for a poor pregnancy outcome and requires careful follow-up during gestation.

There are no good figures about maternal mortality in chronic hypertension and pregnancy. It is well known, however, that these patients frequently (9% to 11%) develop abruptio placentae.[6] Since abruptio placentae is a complication with significant mortality, it is logical

TABLE 6-2 ■ Severity classification of chronic hypertension in pregnancy

Degree	Diastolic pressure (mm Hg)	Optic fundus grade*	Left ventricular hypertrophy	Renal damage
Mild	100	0-I	None	None
Moderate	100-120	0-II	None or left ventricular strain	None or few abnormalities
Severe	>120	III-IV	Yes	Yes
Complicated	Evidence of severe vascular lesion (nephroangiosclerosis, angina pectoris, congestive failure, stroke), superimposed toxemia, or renal failure			

*Keith-Wagener-Barker classification.

to assume that mothers with chronic hypertension have a higher mortality than nonhypertensive gravidas. Also, patients with chronic hypertension in pregnancy may have an aggravation of the hypertension in the third trimester, which may lead to intracranial bleeding and left ventricular failure.

A similar lack of information exists about maternal morbidity in chronic hypertension. However, because of the high frequency of fetal problems, cesarean section is common in hypertensive gravidas, and this increases the maternal morbidity.

Management of chronic hypertension in pregnancy

The management of pregnant patients with chronic hypertension requires proper diagnosis, workup, classification of severity, and decisions regarding treatment.

Diagnosis. It is necessary to remember that, by definition, the diagnosis of chronic hypertension in pregnancy is possible only if an abnormal blood pressure (140/90 mm Hg or above) is found before 20 weeks of gestation or if there is a clear documentation of hypertension before pregnancy. There are many cases in which neither of these conditions is fulfilled and the diagnosis cannot be made despite strong clinical suspicions. Situations also exist where a false positive diagnosis is made as a consequence of measuring the blood pressure in an obese patient with a small cuff. Also, sometimes patients are erroneously classified as having chronic hypertension because they had recurrent intrapartum hypertension in several pregnancies, but there is no documentation of hypertension at the beginning of pregnancy or outside of gestation.

A common differential diagnosis problem exists when patients with chronic hypertension develop aggravation of their hypertension at the end of gestation. The problem is to differentiate if this situation corresponds to aggravation of the chronic hypertension or to superimposition of preeclampsia. This differential diagnosis is difficult and has little value for the patient's management. It is the *severity* rather than the *origin* of the hypertension that must determine management, especially the decision about early delivery.

Workup. The most important elements in the evaluation of the pregnant patient with chronic hypertension are the medical and obstetric history and the physical examination. The large majority of these women have mild essential hypertension and do not require extensive laboratory testing.

In the majority of patients the workup should be limited to an electrocardiogram (necessary to evaluate the severity of the disease); a serum biochemical profile (SMA-18), which includes determination of electrolytes and nitrogen products; and a urine culture for the detection of asymptomatic bacteriuria. Creatinine clearance testing is ordered *only* if the serum creatinine concentration is at or above the upper limit for pregnancy (0.8 mg/dl). Quantitative urinary protein determination and analysis of the urinary sediment are carried out *only* if the patient shows 2+ or more albuminuria in qualitative spot checks. ANA titers are ordered if there is some possibility of autoimmune disease. Urinary electrolyte tests are ordered if there is a frank abnormality in serum electrolyte levels.

Very rarely do pregnant hypertensive patients require more extensive evaluation. However, if the hypertension is severe or is accompanied by unusual signs and symptoms, the patient may require determination of urinary and plasma catecholamine levels, measurement of plasma renin activity, a rapid-sequence intravenous pyelogram, a chest x-ray film, and eventually renal arteriogram and renal biopsy.

Severity classification. Following diagnosis, the severity of the hypertension has to be established, and this involves examination of the optic fundi, evaluation of renal function, and assessment of left ventricular size (Table 6-2). Assignment of a degree of severity depends on the level of diastolic blood pressure and the existence or absence of target organ damage.

Classification of the pregnant woman with chronic hypertension by severity criteria accomplishes two main objectives:

1. *To establish a prognosis.* There is significant agreement among clinicians and some data[7] supporting the hypothesis that the greater the severity of the hypertension, the worse the pregnancy outcome and the greater the possibility of fetomaternal complications.
2. *To make a decision about the need for antihypertensive therapy during pregnancy.* If the patient is classified as moderately or

severely hypertensive, the need for treatment is clear. If the patient has complicated hypertension, a consideration should be given to the possibility of therapeutic abortion. If the patient has mild hypertension, there is a debate about the need for treatment and it will be necessary to be more discriminating in the risk analysis, as discussed later.

Classification of patients by severity also helps to introduce order in the analysis of this problem and facilitate retrospective and prospective interpretations of data.

To treat or not to treat. Both common sense and some evidence from the literature[19] support the concept that treatment of chronic hypertension during pregnancy is useful in moderate and severe cases. The decision about treatment becomes controversial in the case of pregnant patients with mild chronic hypertension. There are several controlled studies[6,20,32] of antihypertensive treatment for patients with mild hypertension and pregnancy, and all indicate that treatment is associated with better pregnancy outcome. At the same time, there is a natural reluctance to initiate treatment in patients who frequently are normotensive at the time of the initial evaluation. In my opinion the following pregnant patients with mild chronic hypertension require treatment:

1. Patients with diastolic blood pressure above 85 mm Hg or MAP of 95 mm Hg or more after 12 weeks' gestation as determined by repeated observations at least 6 hours apart
2. Patients with a history of severe hypertension in a previous pregnancy
3. Patients with a history of abruptio placentae
4. Patients with a history of stillbirth or unexplained neonatal death
5. Patients with a history of previous delivery of a small for gestational age baby
6. Patients older than 35 years
7. Very obese patients

Patients in these categories represent most of the heavy contributors to perinatal and maternal morbidity. Other pregnant patients with mild hypertension should be treated only if their blood pressure exceeds the normal limits. Further studies are necessary in this respect.

When to treat and how to treat. Treatment should be initiated early in pregnancy, as soon as the diagnosis and the indication for treatment have been established. The studies of Leather et al[20] and Redman et al[32] have shown a significant decrease in the number of midtrimester abortions in treated patients as compared with untreated controls. The possibility exists that blood pressure reduction late in gestation may impair the uteroplacental perfusion and affect fetal growth and well-being. However, the study of Redman et al[32] shows that treatment started late in gestation caused no harm to patients. Treatment, therefore, should not be denied to patients with chronic hypertension who have an indication for treatment even if it is late in gestation.

The first-choice drug for the treatment of chronic hypertension in *nonpregnant* patients is a diuretic. *This is not true in the case of the pregnant patient with hypertension.* There is evidence that patients with chronic hypertension with or without superimposed preeclampsia have decreased intravascular volume and that when the expansion of intravascular volume fails to reach normal levels the fetal outcome is poor.[1,37] Therefore administraion of diuretics to pregnant patients with hypertension without knowledge of the stage of expansion of their intravascular volume is a serious mistake.

In another study[3] it was shown that pregnant patients with hypertension who were treated with a combination of drugs including diuretics had a significant reduction in creatinine clearance when compared with nontreated controls, suggesting that their intravascular volume was depleted. This depletion of plasma volume in diuretic-treated pregnant patients may be the explanation for the significant difference in fetal outcome between treated and untreated patients who developed aggravation of the hypertension. The worse outcome of the treated group suggests that, by decreasing plasma volume, diuretics have generated a labile fetal homeostasis. The obstetrician should assume that *all* pregnant patients with chronic hypertension have a limited capacity to expand their intravascular volume and therefore should avoid using diuretics. Also, diuretics should be discontinued if the patient was taking them before the beginning of her prenatal care.

The first-choice medication for the treatment of chronic hypertension in the pregnant patient has been methyldopa (Aldomet). This is the only antihypertensive medication that has been submitted to controlled trials during pregnancy[20,32] and has been shown to have beneficial effects. Methyldopa causes dilation of both the arterial side of the circulation and the capacitance vessels, thereby allowing increases in intravascular volume to occur. Also, renal blood flow is maintained during methyldopa administration, and this property makes it the drug of choice in patients with actual or potential limitations in kidney function. Methyldopa reaches a maximum effect in 4 to 6 hours with a total duration of action of about 8 hours. These pharmacokinetics make the medication of little use when rapid effects should be obtained and determines its use every 6 or 8 hours (three or four times daily) for maximum therapeutic efficiency. The drug is primarily excreted in the urine and may accumulate in patients with severe impairment of renal function.

We usually start patients with 250 mg of methyldopa three times a day and increase the amount of medication up to a total of 2 g/day according to their response. The most common side effect of methyldopa is postural hypotension, which subsides rather quickly with a decrease in the amount of medication. Excessive sedation and depression are occasionally seen. Positive Coombs' testing and hemolytic anemia are uncommon complications of methyldopa therapy.

In some pregnant patients continuous administration of methyldopa causes salt and water retention, manifested clinically by increase in body weight beyond that expected for pregnancy alone, edema, and hemodilution (low hematocrit, low serum creatinine concentration, low BUN, low serum uric acid level). This situation may progress to a point where "rebound" hypertension caused by excessive intravascular volume expansion is observed. In these cases hydrochlorothiazide should be added to the treatment using an initial dose of 25 mg/day, which may be increased to 50 mg/day if necessary. Diuresis, decrease in edema fluid, lowering of the blood pressure, and decrease in body weight will result from adding a diuretic to the treatment if the clinical picture was a consequence of unopposed methyldopa action.

In some other patients administration of methyldopa up to 2 g/day is insufficient to achieve an adequate degree of blood pressure control, that is, diastolic blood pressure measurements consistently below 80 mm Hg in the second trimester of pregnancy. In these cases we add hydralazine to the therapeutic regimen. Hydralazine is a nonadrenergic vasodilator that acts directly on the smooth muscle fibers of the arterial side of the circulation. The onset of action occurs rapidly after ingestion and reaches a peak in 3 to 4 hours, with a total duration of action of about 6 hours. We give hydralazine, 40 to 200 mg, orally in four divided doses. The medication causes an increase in cardiac output, tachycardia, and salt and water retention. Hydralazine is rapidly acetylated in the liver in a reaction in which the rate is genetically determined. Slow acetylators respond to relatively small doses of medication with significant decreases in blood pressure, whereas the fast acetylator is relatively resistant to the hypotensive effect of the drug. Hydralazine lupus is limited in its occurrence to slow acetylators and usually responds to discontinuation of the medication. The appearance of positive ANA titers in pregnant patients with chronic hypertension treated with hydralazine is rare.

Propranolol, a beta blocker, may soon become the drug of choice for the treatment of pregnant women with chronic hypertension. In fact, studies on the hemodynamics of mild chronic hypertension in pregnancy[22] have shown that hyperkinetic circulation caused by hyperactivity of the sympathetic system is a significant component of the problem. This observation provides strong theoretical grounds for the use of beta blockers in treating pregnant patients with chronic hypertension. Also, there is abundant literature[8,10,31,34] about the excellent outcome of pregnant hypertensive patients treated with beta blockers. This information is in contrast with some other papers,[14,15,21,33] mostly case reports, where it is argued that maternal propranolol administration may have adverse effects on the fetus.

We have been using propranolol for the treatment of pregnant patients with mild chronic hypertension for several years, and have been comparing their outcome with that of patients treated with methyldopa or hydralazine. Preliminary observations in more than 20 patients suggest that propranolol is a very effective drug for the treatment of this condition with virtually no side effects. We start treatment once the patient enters the second trimester without showing significant spontaneous decrease in diastolic blood pressure (usually between 14 and 20 weeks of gestation), using a dose of 20 mg three times daily. If the patient is going to respond to the medication, a significant decrease in blood pressure is usually seen in 48 to 72 hours. The initial dose is adjusted up or down according to the blood pressure response and the side effects (sleepiness, drowsiness). We have never used more than 160 mg of propranolol a day to adequately control a patient's blood pressure. The medication is discontinued when the patient goes into labor and restarted in the postpartum period if necessary. We have not yet seen any fetal complications. All pregnancies have gone to term and produced adequate for gestational age infants. Naturally a larger series of patients is necessary before the beneficial results of the treatment can be firmly established.

Most pregnant patients with chronic hypertension can maintain adequate blood pressure control with the use of propranolol, methyldopa, hydralazine, and occasionally thiazide diuretics. Pregnant patients with chronic hypertension who are unresponsive to these medications most probably should not be pregnant, but if they are, it will be necessary to use more potent antihypertensive agents whose effects on the fetus are unknown and potentially dangerous.

Follow-up of the pregnant patient with chronic hypertension. There is no substitute for frequent clinical observations in the follow-up of pregnant patients with chronic hypertension. It has been shown[3] that laboratory evaluation of these patients is disappointing, with a very high number of false positive and false negative results.

The pregnant patient with chronic hypertension should be seen in the prenatal clinic every 2 weeks until she reaches 36 weeks of gestation and then every week until the end of her pregnancy. The critical points to monitor during the prenatal visits are as follows:

1. Blood pressure
2. Uterine growth
3. Fetal movements
4. Renal function
5. Maternal weight

The levels of blood pressure are a critical index. If the diastolic blood pressure starts to fall at the beginning of the second trimester, this is an indication of decreased peripheral vascular resistance, expanded intravascular volume, and possibly a good outcome. If the diastolic pressure remains unaltered, above 80 mm Hg well into the second trimester, this is an indication of increased peripheral vascular resistance, a forecast of future complications, and an indication for initiation of therapy. The levels of blood pressure are also an indication of the response to therapy, and every effort should be made to repeat them at every prenatal visit with the same instruments and under the same conditions.

As mentioned in Chapter 18, evaluation of the growth of the uterus and assessment of fetal movements are important clinical indicators of fetal well-being. We see very little point in obtaining ultrasound measurements every 3 or 4 weeks in pregnant patients with well-controlled chronic hypertension if the uterus is growing adequately during gestation. The chances of finding ultrasonic evidence of growth retardation in these cases are minimal. Similarly, there is little or no need to obtain weekly or biweekly estriol or HPL determinations in these patients if the uterus is growing well, if the mother perceives no change in fetal movements, and if the blood pressure remains normal.

Pregnant patients with chronic hypertension are frequently followed with monthly or bimonthly creatinine clearance tests and quantitative urinary protein determinations to assess their renal function during pregnancy. This is a waste of time and money and a common source of errors. There is no need to order a creatinine clearance test and proceed to 24-hour urine collections (usually cumbersome and in most cases incomplete) in pregnant patients with chronic hypertension whose serum creatinine level is 0.7 mg/dl or less. The finding of this serum creatinine level indicates that an increase in glomerular filtration rate has occurred and that the creatinine clearance, if correctly measured, will be above nonpregnant levels.

It is also a waste of money and time to order quantitative urinary protein determination in pregnant patients with chronic hypertension who do not show 2+ or more protein in the qualitative analysis of a random specimen obtained during the prenatal visit. Measurement of serum creatinine early in pregnancy and two or three more times during gestation and monitoring of albuminuria twice per week by examination of the first urine voided in the morning with Albustix strips are the two tests that should be employed to monitor renal function during pregnancy in patients with stable chronic hypertension. Only if there is an alteration in these tests will it be necessary to carry out more precise evaluations. Also, it is exceptional for a patient to show significant deterioration of renal function during pregnancy without exhibiting concomitant aggravation of the hypertension.

Monitoring maternal weight is also important in the prenatal follow-up of patients with chronic hypertension. We are concerned about extreme deviations, that is, too much weight gain or too little or no weight gain, but our preoccupation with the latter (too little or no weight gain) should be greater than with the first. In fact, the pregnant patient with chronic hypertension who does not gain weight during pregnancy is at high risk of intrauterine growth retardation and fetal problems; in contrast, too much weight gain may be normal and predictive of the birth of a large baby. Excessive weight gain may also be a consequence of unopposed methyldopa action or the first sign of superimposed preeclampsia.

With respect to laboratory evaluation of the fetoplacental unit in the chronic hypertensive gravid, our recommendations follow:

1. *Ultrasound* should be ordered one time between 18 and 24 weeks of gestation to confirm the dates, localize the placenta, and have a baseline biparietal diameter. Future ultrasonic measurements of the fetal head should be obtained only if there are clinical signs (inadequate maternal weight gain, inadequate uterine fundus growth) suggesting fetal growth retardation.
2. *Fetal reactivity determination* (nonstress test [NST]) should be carried out if there are clinical and ultrasonic suggestions of growth retardation, if there is a sudden deterioration of the maternal status, if the mother reports decreased or absent fetal movements, or if the patient has a history of one or more stillbirths.
3. *Estriol and HPL determinations* may be carried out if any of the indications for fetal reactivity determination are present. HPL seems to be a better test than estriol in the monitoring of chronic hypertension. How-

ever, both tests have a high number of false positive and false negative results and cannot substitute for adequate clinical observation.
4. Occasionally determination of *fetal pulmonary maturity* is necessary in patients with chronic hypertension, and in this case amniocentesis and measurement of the L/S ratio should be carried out. In the majority of pregnant patients with chronic hypertension early delivery is a product of either fetal or maternal deterioration, and the L/S ratio will not change the plan of management.

When and how to deliver the pregnant patient with chronic hypertension. The large majority of patients who remain stable during the prenatal period will develop spontaneous labor and will deliver at term. Cesarean section delivery will be necessary for obstetric indications or for intrapartum fetal distress. Fetal or maternal deterioration may require termination of pregnancy before term.

■ **REFERENCES**

1. Arias F: Expansion of intravascular volume and fetal outcome in patients with chronic hypertension and pregnancy. Am J Obstet Gynecol 1975;123:610.
2. Arias F, Mancilla-Jimenez R: Hepatic fibrinogen deposits in preeclampsia. immunofluorescent evidence. N Engl J Med 1976;295:578.
3. AriasF, Zamora J: Antihypertensive treatment and pregnancy outcome in patients with mild chronic hypertension. Obstet Gynecol 1979;53:489.
4. Chesley LC: Eclampsia: the remote prognosis. Semin Perinatol 1978;2:99.
5. Chesley LC: *Hypertensive Disorders in Pregnancy.* New York, Appleton-Century Crofts, 1978, p. 2.
6. Dickman WJ: Essential hypertension and pregnancy. Surg Clin North Am 1953;33:27.
7. Dunlop JCH: Chronic hypertension and perinatal mortality. Proc R Soc Med 1966;59:838.
8. Eliahou HE, Silverberg DS, Reisin E, et al: Propranolol for the treatment of hypertension in pregnancy. Br J Obstet Gynaecol 1978;85:431.
9. Friedman EA, Neff RK: *Pregnancy Hypertension*, Littleton, Mass., Publishing Sciences Group, 1977, p. 236.
10. Gallery EDM, Saunders DM, Hynyor SN, et al: Randomized comparison of methyldopa and oxprenolol for treatment of hypertension in pregnancy. Br Med J 1979; 1:1591.
11. Gant NF, Chand S, Whorley RJ, et al: A clinical test useful for predicting the development of acute hypertension in pregnancy. Am J Obstet Gynecol 1974;120:1.
12. Gant NF, Daley GL, Chand S: A study of angiotensin II pressor response throughout primigravid pregnancy. J Clin Invest 1973;52:2684.

12a. Gant NF, Madden JD, Siiteri PK, et al: The metabolic clearance rate of dehydroisoandrosterone sulfate. Am J Obstet Gynecol 1975;123:159.

13. Gant NF, Whalley P, Chand S, et al: A prospective study of angiotensin II pressor responsiveness in pregnancies complicated by chronic essential hypertension. Am J Obstet Gynecol 1977;127:369.

14. Gladstone GR, Gersony WM: Propanolol administration during pregnancy: effects on the fetus. J Pediatr 1975; 86:962.

15. Habib A, McCarthy JS: Effects on the neonate of propanolol administered during pregnancy. J Pediatr 1977; 91:808.

16. Henrich WL, Cronin R, Miller PD, et al: Hypotensive sequelae of Diazoxide and hydralazone therapy. JAMA 1977;237:264.

17. Hibbard LT: Maternal mortality due to acute toxemia. Obstet Gynecol 1973;42:263.

18. Hill LM: Metabolism of uric acid in normal and toxemic pregnancy. Mayo Clin Proc 1978;53:743.

19. Kincaid-Smith P, Bullen H, Mills J: Prolonged use of methyl-dopa in severe hypertension of pregnancy. Br Med J 1966;1:274.

20. Leather HM, Humpreys DM, Baker PB, et al: A controlled trial of hypotensive agents in hypertension in pregnancy. Lancet 1968;1:488.

21. Lieberman BA, Stirrat GM, Cohen SI, et al: The possible adverse effect of propanolol on the fetus in pregnancies complicated by severe hypertension. Br J Obstet Gynaecol 1978;85:678.

22. Lim YL, Walters WAW: Hemodynamics of mild hypertension in pregnancy. Br J Obstet Gynaecol 1979; 86:198.

23. McCartney CP: Pathological anatomy of acute hypertension of pregnancy. Circulation 1964;30(suppl. 2):37.

24. Page EW, Cristianson R: The importance of mean arterial pressure in the middle trimester upon the outcome of pregnancy. Am J Obstet Gynecol 1976;125:740.

25. Peck TM: A simple test for predicting pregnancy-induced hypertension. Obstet Gynecol 1977;50:615.

26. Phelan JP: Enhanced prediction of pregnancy-induced hypertension by combining supine pressor test with mean arterial pressure of middle trimester. Am J Obstet Gynecol 1977;129:397.

27. Pritchard JA: Management of severe preeclampsia and eclampsia. Semin Perinatol 1978;2:83.

28. Pritchard JA, Cunningham FG, Mason RA: Coagulation changes in eclampsia: their frequency and pathogenesis. Am J Obstet Gynecol 1976;124:855.

29. Pritchard JA, Pritchard SA: Standardized treatment of 154 consecutive cases of eclampsia. Am J Obstet Gynecol 1975;123:543.

30. Pritchard JA, Pritchard SA: Blood pressure response to estrogen-progestin oral contraceptive after pregnancy-induced hypertension. Am J Obstet Gynecol 1977; 129:733.

31. Pruyn SC, Phelan JP, Buchanan GC: Long-term propanolol therapy in pregnancy: maternal and fetal outcome. Am J Obstet Gynecol 1979;135:485.

32. Redman CWG, Beilin LJ, Bonnar J, et al: Fetal outcome in a trial of antihypertensive treatment in pregnancy. Lancet 1976;2:753.

33. Reed RL, Cheney CB, Fearon RE, et al: Propanolol therapy throughout pregnancy: a case report. Anesth Anal 1974;53:214.

34. Rubin PC: Beta-blockers in pregnancy. N Engl J Med 1981;305:1323.

35. Sheehan HL, Lynch JB: *Pathology of Toxemia in Pregnancy*. Edinburgh, Churchill Livingstone, 1973, pp. 328-490.

36. Sheppard JH, Bennett MJ, Laurence D, et al: Prostaglandin vaginal suppositories: a simple and safe approach to the induction of labor. Obstet Gynecol 1981; 58:596.

37. Soffronoff EC, Kaufman BM, Connaughton JF: Intravascular volume determinations and fetal outcome in hypertensive diseases of pregnancy. Am J Obstet Gynecol 1977;127:4.

38. Spargo B, McCartney CP, Winemiller R: Glomerular capillary endotheliosis in toxemia of pregnancy. Arch Pathol 1959;68:593.

39. Sullivan JM: Blood pressure in pregnancy. Prog Cardiovasc Dis 1974;16:375.

40. Talledo OE, Chesley LC, Zuspan FP: Renin-angiotensin system in normal and toxemic pregnancies. III. Differential sensitivity to angiotensin II and norepinephrine in toxemia of pregnancy. Am J Obstet Gynecol 1968; 100:218.

41. Tatum HJ, Mule JG: Puerperal vasomotor collapse in patients with toxemia of pregnancy: a new concept of the etiology and a rational plan of treatment. Am J Obstet Gynecol 1956;71:492.

42. Zuspan FP, Ward MC: Improved fetal salvage in eclampsia. Obstet Gynecol 1965;26:893.

7

■ ■ ■

DIABETES AND PREGNANCY

D. Michael Nelson

Before the time of generalized insulin availability, pregnancy in women with diabetes was a rare event and was associated with a high maternal mortality and an even higher perinatal morbidity and mortality. With usage of insulin now commonplace, maternal mortality for the pregnant patient with diabetes is only slightly higher than that of the nondiabetic patient. In addition, improved perinatal and neonatal care has led to marked improvements in the outcome for infants of mothers with diabetes. In spite of this, perinatal morbidity remains high; mortality for infants of diabetic patients with vascular complications is approximately 20%.[26]

Diabetes mellitus can be defined as a state of carbohydrate intolerance resulting from inadequacy of insulin secretion or ineffectiveness of insulin action. This imbalance between insulin supply and demand leads to abnormal metabolism of carbohydrates, fats, and proteins. This altered metabolic state is made worse during gestation because the pregnant state results in changes in carbohydrate, fat, and protein metabolism that can aggravate the existing diabetes or may uncover latent diabetes in patients with a genetic predisposition to the disease.

■ METABOLISM

The developing fetus is continuously draining substrates normally available to the mother, especially glucose, its major energy source. Since the glucose level of the fetus is normally 10% to 20% less than that of the mother, this differential concentration enhances the transfer of glucose from mother to fetus. A glucose transfer, called *facilitated diffusion*, also takes place, but this is independent of both the maternal and fetal insulin levels.

In contrast to glucose, amino acids are actively transported across the placenta to the fetal circulation. This is especially true of gluconeogenic aminoacids such as alanine. This active placental transfer of amino acids deprives the maternal liver of a major gluconeogenic source and creates the need for another source to meet the metabolic demands of the mother. As a result, there is an acceleration of maternal lipolysis with an attendant increase in circulating levels of free fatty acids and triglycerides along with a predisposition to ketogenesis. The higher maternal levels of fat breakdown products normally are not reflected in the fetal circulation, since the placenta is relatively impermeable to both triglycerides and free fatty acids. However, ketone bodies are an exception to this rule, since they can cross the placenta and serve as an energy source for the fetus.

In early normal pregnancy the metabolic demands of a developing fetus lead to a metabolic state in the mother characterized by the presence of (1) fasting hypoglycemia with a resultant decrease in circulating insulin levels, (2) hypoaminoacidemia (especially hypoalaninemia), and (3) accelerated lipolysis with a predisposition to ketosis, made worse with fasting.

In the second half of pregnancy the nutritional demands of an even more rapidly growing fetus continue to be an important factor in determining the metabolic status of the mother. However, fetal demands for both glucose and amino acids are highest at term,[63] and it has been estimated that fetal glucose consumption per kilogram is about twice as high as in an adult (6 mg/kg/minute compared to 2 to 3 mg/kg/ minute). Also, in the latter half of pregnancy several factors leading to a state of relative insulin resistance develop peak activities. Primary among these is the increasing synthesis and secretion of the hormone human placental lactogen (HPL) that appears in the maternal circulation in the first trimester of pregnancy but does not reach peak concentration until 34 weeks of gestation. HPL acts as a peripheral antagonist to the metabolic action of insulin. Because of this antagonism, increased levels of insulin must be secreted by the pancreas to maintain normoglycemia. Beta cell hypertrophy and hyperinsulinemia characteristic of the last trimester of pregnancy thus ensue. Other factors that contribute to the insulin resistance of the last trimester of pregnancy include enhanced degradation of insulin by the kidney, higher insulinase activity of the placenta, and increased circulating levels of potentially diabetogenic steroids (eg, cortisol, progesterone, estrogen).

In the third trimester of pregnancy the normal metabolic state of the pregnant patient is characterized by (1) insulin resistance, (2) hyperinsulinemia, and (3) a persistent tendency for fasting hypoglycemia and postprandial hyperglycemia. Despite these marked metabolic changes, the normal average blood glucose level stays within a rather narrowly defined range throughout the day and throughout the pregnancy, even in the presence of mixed meals during a 24-hour period. The normal fasting blood sugar level in the nondiabetic patient is 65 ± 9 mg/dl, whereas the mean daily nonfasting level is 80 ± 10 mg/dl.[68] Postprandial elevations never exceed 140 mg/dl.[12]

The normal oral glucose tolerance test (GTT) in pregnancy reflects the metabolic state of the pregnant patient by showing (1) lower fasting values; (2) a peak elevation in blood sugar level at 1 hour, generally higher than in the nonpregnant patient; and (3) a fall in blood sugar level 2 and 3 hours after carbohydrate load that often lags behind that of nonpregnant patients. This latter metabolic state is the result of the slower absorption and decreased motility of the gastrointestinal (GI) tract in pregnancy. A lack of awareness about these changes in the GTT during pregnancy may lead to mistakes in diagnosis. For example, although a fasting blood sugar level of 110 mg/dl is considered normal for a nonpregnant patient, it is markedly abnormal during pregnancy. Also, pregnant patients may be submitted to unnecessary treatment because a 2-hour postprandial blood sugar level seems elevated by nonpregnant standards.

■ DIAGNOSIS
Screening for diabetes

The diagnosis of diabetes in the pregnant woman is self-evident in patients who had abnormal carbohydrate metabolism before pregnancy and required diet and insulin to maintain metabolic control. In these individuals the task is primarily to determine what exacerbation of the diabetic state is imposed by pregnancy and to alter management appropriately. However, the physiologic changes that occur during pregnancy may cause a patient with a genetic predisposition to diabetes to first evidence signs of abnormal carbohydrate metabolism when pregnant (gestational diabetes). The increased risk for perinatal morbidity and mortality associated with undiagnosed gestational diabetes has led O'Sullivan and colleagues[62] to recommend that all expectant mothers be screened for abnormal carbohydrate metabolism at their initial prenatal visit and again at approximately 30 weeks of gestation. Failure to do this might lead to overlooking as many as 25% of patients with gestational diabetes. The suggested screening test consists of providing 50 grams of oral glucose to a patient who does not need to be fasting but who should not have eaten within 2 hours of the test. A blood sugar level is then obtained 1 hour following the ingestion of the carbohydrate load. If the blood sugar level is greater than 130 for whole blood or 150 for plasma, the screen is considered positive; the patient should then be subjected to a 3-hour oral GTT. If the screen is negative, the patient should be screened again at 30 weeks of gestation when the diabetic po-

Risk factors requiring diabetic screening

1. Obesity (>200 pounds or >15% of nonpregnant ideal body weight)
2. Positive family history of diabetes (sibling or parent)
3. History of stillbirth
4. History of delivery or a large infant (>4000 grams)
5. Glucosuria
6. History of unexplained neonatal death
7. History of congenital anomaly
8. History of prematurity
9. History of preeclampsia as a multipara
10. Polyhydramnios
11. History of traumatic delivery with associated neurologic disorder in the infant
12. Poor reproductive history (>3 spontaneous abortions in the first or second trimester)
13. Chronic hypertension
14. Recurrent severe moniliasis
15. Recurrent urinary tract infections
16. Age >30 years
17. History of diabetes in a previous pregnancy

tential of pregnancy is nearing a maximum. According to O'Sullivan,[62] this screening test has a 70% sensitivity rate and is 87% specific.

Another screening test is the fasting and the 2-hour postprandial plasma glucose levels. If both values are normal (fasting plasma glucose level below 100 mg/dl and 2-hour postprandial below 140 mg/dl), the screen is considered negative; if only one value is above normal limits, a GTT should be obtained; if both values are abnormal, there is no need for a GTT, since the diagnosis of gestational diabetes has been made.

Oral GTT

Some patients are at high risk for diabetes during pregnancy (see box above) and should be screened directly with a GTT, the most sensitive diagnostic method for diabetes. Among these patients are the following:

1. Obese patients (the largest high-risk group). Since obesity outside of pregnancy is a well-known insulin-resistant state, all pregnant patients weighing more than 200 pounds (90 kg) or more than 15% of their ideal body weight should be screened with a GTT.
2. Patients with a family history of diabetes.[91] It is impossible to predict exactly what percentage of the offspring of a diabetic pa-

tient will develop diabetes, since multiple genes appear to be involved. However, estimates indicate that about 1 out of each 14 persons who have a diabetic parent evidences abnormal glucose tolerance.

3. Patients with glucosuria. If glucosuria is marked or if there are clear clinical suggestions that the patient has overt diabetes, the GTT should be avoided and a fasting blood sugar level should be determined. If the fasting blood sugar value is frankly abnormal, more than 130 mg/dl, there is no need to perform the GTT to confirm the diagnosis; in fact, it may be dangerous to do so. If the fasting blood sugar level is normal or close to normal, a GTT is indicated.
4. Patients over 30 years of age. Those patients who are over 30 years of age have an increased risk for carbohydrate intolerance when compared with their younger counterparts.[30]

Whether an oral GTT is better than the intravenous test for detecting significant abnormal glucose tolerance is somewhat controversial. The oral test is more practical for outpatients and is better at estimating the efficiency of glucose disposal in patients with mild abnormalities of glucose tolerance.[59] In addition, intestinal factors appear to have an effect on normal insulin response,[52] and oral glucose ingestion represents the normal route for carbohydrate absorption. It should be pointed out, however, that the intravenous test is useful in patients with GI disorders that may make the results of the oral test misleading.

A patient scheduled for an oral GTT should be instructed to eat a high carbohydrate diet for at least 3 days before the test, since diet alteration can alter insulin binding and action.[41] The recommended 200-gram minimal carbohydrate in the diet can be conveniently assured if the patient eats a candy bar daily for the 3 days before the test. She should come the day of the test after fasting overnight. A fasting blood sugar level should then be drawn, and a glucose load consisting of approximately 100 grams (1.75 gm/kg ideal body weight) of glucose dissolved in 200 to 400 ml of water should be ingested within a 5-minute period. Blood sugar levels are drawn 1, 2, and 3 hours later. Concomitant urine spot checks are carried out to detect glucosuria and to determine an approximate renal threshold for glucose.

Normal values for the oral GTT in pregnancy are given for plasma and whole blood glucose determinations in Table 7-1. The original study[61] describing normal values for the oral GTT during pregnancy used whole blood for glucose determinations, but today plasma glucose determinations, which are approximately 14% higher than whole blood, are used in most institutions. The following two points should be made: (1) a metabolic inhibitor of glycolysis, such as sodium fluoride, should be present in the tubes used for

collecting blood samples to avoid falsely low values; and (2) venous rather than capillary blood samples should be obtained, since the latter generally yields a higher (about 15%) value when used for glucose determinations.

A patient is considered to have an abnormal GTT if two or more values are elevated. If only one value is high, the test is considered normal. Patients in the high-risk groups (see box on p. 123) should have a GTT done as early in pregnancy as possible, and if they have a normal glucose tolerance curve, the test should be repeated at 30 weeks of gestation. At this gestational age the diabetogenic effect of pregnancy is near its peak, and the chances of a positive result from the GTT are higher. If an oral GTT is "borderline," a repeat examination to confirm the diagnosis is indicated. A diagnosis of gestational diabetes should not be made unless there is a clear indication that abnormal carbohydrate metabolism exists, since the social implications of labeling a person as having diabetes may be long-standing (eg, when the patient is purchasing life insurance).

Intravenous GTT

If an intravenous GTT is to be performed, 0.5 gram of glucose per kilogram of ideal body weight is administered IV in 2 minutes or less. Blood glucose determinations are made before the injection and at 15-minute intervals for the following hour. These five plasma sugar determinations (fasting plus four values after a glucose injection) are used to construct a graph. The time taken for the blood or plasma glucose level to fall to half of its value is used to calculate the absolute glucose disappearance rate (K). K values of 1.5 mg/minute or below are indicative of abnormal glucose tolerance.[6]

Renal glucosuria

Some patients have a normal GTT but have a low renal threshold allowing glucose to appear in the urine in several urine spot checks. They are considered to have renal glucosuria. It has been estimated that glucosuria occurs in as many as 10% of pregnant women at some time during pregnancy[87]; thus glucosuria in pregnancy is not diagnostic of diabetes. Glucosuria appears frequently during pregnancy because there is an increase in the glomerular filtration rate, which is not accompanied by a proportional increase

TABLE 7-1 ■ Normal glucose values for the oral GTT in pregnancy

Time	Whole blood	Plasma	Plasma (pregnant)	Plasma (nonpregnant)
Fasting	90	100	100	110
1 hour	165	200	190	170
2 hours	145	150	165	130
3 hours	125	130	145	110

Data compiled from Barnes Hospital (plasma, pregnant and nonpregnant); Gabbe SG, Mestman JH, Freeman RK, et al: Am J Obstet Gynecol 1978; 129:723 (plasma); O'Sullivan JB, Mahan CM, Charles D, et al: Am J Obstet Gynecol 1973; 116:895 (whole blood).

in proximal tubular reabsorption of glucose.[89] The average renal threshold in the pregnant patient is 155 ± 17 mg/dl by the third to fourth month of pregnancy, compared to 197 ± 6.5 mg/dl in the nonpregnant patient.[8] Glucosuria has been found more frequently in nulliparous patients; 2.8% of these patients in the second trimester and 43% in the third trimester will have glucosuria during the course of a 2-hour GTT.[97] A wide variation in quantitative excretion can occur, and sugar may be present in the urine with blood sugar levels as low as 70 to 100 mg/dl. The only way to determine if a pregnancy-associated glucosuria is pathologic is (1) to determine blood sugar levels after exposure to a carbohydrate load and (2) to estimate the total carbohydrate losses caused by the glucosuria.

Women with renal glucosuria during pregnancy are at a high risk for premature delivery (25% incidence), according to Chen et al,[7] and for the development of fetal macrosomia (7% incidence compared with 1.6% in the general population). In some cases renal glucosuria during pregnancy is a manifestation of renal tubular damage caused by chronic pyelonephritis. These patients frequently exhibit asymptomatic bacteriuria and may develop acute pyelonephritis.

Management of patients with renal glucosuria includes (1) a GTT to rule out gestational diabetes as soon as the glucosuria is noted and again when the diabetogenic effects of pregnancy become maximal at about 30 weeks of gestation, (2) frequent urine cultures to detect asymptomatic bacteriuria, and (3) an increased number of meals with less calories per meal to lessen the swings in the blood sugar level created by less frequent meals with high caloric content.

Whether a diet with a specified number of calories is needed depends largely on the amount of carbohydrate losses in the urine. Patients with renal glucosuria may lose as much as 100 grams of glucose per day in the urine, may have ketonuria during fasting, or may gain too little weight during gestation. These patients should receive dietary instructions and a diet essentially like that of the gestational diabetic patient to assure adequate nutrition.

■ CLASSIFICATION

Nonpregnant diabetic patients are classified into two large groups. Type I or insulin-dependent diabetic patients (IDDM) do not produce insulin and depend on exogenous insulin administration for their normal metabolic functions. They are ketosis prone and usually develop the disease during their childhood and adolescence. Type II or noninsulin-dependent diabetic patients (NIDDM) have adequate and occasionally exaggerated endogenous insulin production, are not ketosis prone, and usually develop the disease during their adult life. They are further divided into (1) nonobese NIDDM and (2) obese NIDDM. Although many type II diabetic patients are in insulin therapy, their clinical course is stable, and they must remain classified as NIDDM. Type II constitutes 90% to 95% of all diabetic patients.

Pregnant diabetic patients are classified differently than nonpregnant individuals. There are several systems to classify pregnant diabetic patients, but the most commonly used is the White's classification.

White's classification

After the diagnosis of diabetes is established, the pregnant patient is usually classified into one of a series of groups originally formulated by White.[90] This classification, which takes into account the time of onset of diabetes, the duration of the disease, and the presence of vascular complications, is useful for establishing a prognosis of the perinatal outcome and to a smaller extent for determining management (Table 7-2).

Patients assigned to Class A, also called *gestational diabetic patients*, exhibit an abnormal GTT but have a normal fasting blood sugar level. Their inadequate insulin response to a glucose load during pregnancy generally returns to normal by the sixth postpartum week, if not sooner. Class A patients with an abnormal fasting blood sugar level are managed like Class B patients and usually require insulin.

Patients are assigned to Class B or C on the basis of their age at onset, duration of the disease, and if they do not have demonstrable vascular complications. Class D patients who may or may not have vascular complications have been subclassified as follows: D_1 patients who have diabetes before age 10; D_2 patients who have had diabetes longer than 20 years; D_3 patients with benign retinopathy (retinal vein dilation, exudates, and microaneurysms); D_4 patients with calcified leg vessels; and D_5 patients with associated hypertension. Class E requires

TABLE 7-2 ■ White's classification of pregnant diabetic patients

Class	Onset	Duration	Vascular complication
A	Pregnancy	Gestation	None
B	After 20 years of age	Less than 10 years	None
C	Between 10 and 19 years of age	10 to 19 years	None
D_1	Less than 10 years of age	Greater than 20 years	Benign retinopathy
D_2			Calcified leg vessels
D_3			Hypertension
D_4			
D_5			
E*			
F	Any	Any	Nephropathy
H	Any	Any	Heart disease
R	Any	Any	Proliferative retinopathy

*No longer sought as a diagnosis.

the presence of pelvic calcifications and is no longer used as a classification. Class F patients have decreased creatinine clearance and proteinuria indicative of diabetic nephropathy. Class G has been dropped in the most recent update of White's classification.[92] Class H includes patients with arteriosclerosis, including coronary artery disease. Class R patients have proliferative retinopathy and exhibit newly formed vessels extending into the vitreous.

White's classification of diabetes in pregnancy not only has too many groups but it fails to recognize the considerable overlap that exists among patients with different severity of problems and similar age of onset and duration of the disease. For example, two patients in Class B may be completely different in the stability or lack of stability of their disease and may differ radically in the number of hospitalizations needed during pregnancy to achieve adequate metabolic control.

Marble's classification

Marble[50] has described a classification of abnormal carbohydrate metabolism commonly used in nonpregnant patients. The usefulness of this classification in management and prognosis during pregnancy has not been studied; its groups are presented here for definition purposes only.

prediabetes State in which there is a strong genetic predisposition to diabetes (eg, offspring of two diabetic parents).

latent diabetes Abnormality of glucose tolerance revealed after a period of stress (pregnancy, febrile illness) or after administration of steroids.

chemical diabetes Abnormal response to a glucose load occurring without stress and with fasting blood sugar levels within normal limits.

overt diabetes Generally symptomatic (ie, polyphagia, polydipsia, polyuria), and its presence is evident by abnormal fasting and random blood sugar levels. It is divided into juvenile-onset and maturity-onset diabetes.

Our classification

In our opinion, a classification system with *management* implications has to be simple and should recognize the existence of different degrees of stability among diabetic patients. Therefore we suggest that the following classification, already suggested for nonpregnant diabetic patients,[22] should be used for management purposes:

1. Gestational diabetic patients (noninsulin-dependent)
2. Stable insulin-dependent diabetic patients
3. Unstable insulin-dependent diabetic patients
4. Insulin-dependent diabetic patients with end-organ damage

gestational diabetic patient   Has an inadequate response to a glucose load during pregnancy and normal fasting blood sugar levels (White's Class A).

stable insulin-dependent diabetic patient   May correspond to White's Class B, C, or D. These patients require insulin, but they are easy to control, have no tendency to ketoacidosis, and follow a predictable course of insulin requirement during pregnancy.

unstable insulin-dependent diabetic patient   May correspond to White's Class B, C, or D. She requires insulin and is difficult to regulate. She has wide swings in blood sugar levels despite well-titrated insulin dosages and well-controlled caloric intake. She shows wide variations in blood sugar values on successive days, despite similar food intake and stable insulin dosage. She is prone to ketoacidosis, hypoglycemia, and Somogyi's phenomenon and usually requires multiple hospital admissions during pregnancy for blood sugar control and treatment of complications (eg, infections, hypertension).

insulin-dependent diabetic patient with end-organ damage   May be in White's Class D but usually corresponds to White's Classes F, H, and R. This patient has microvascular or macrovascular lesions, follows an unstable clinical course, and needs careful monitoring and treatment of affected end organs.

Each of these groups requires a different plan of management and has a different perinatal outcome.

■ MANAGEMENT

The management of all pregnant diabetic patients is aimed at (1) achieving a metabolic state similar to that normally present in pregnancies of nondiabetic patients, (2) avoiding iatrogenic prematurity, (3) detecting intrauterine distress before fetal demise, and (4) eliminating maternal complications.

General measures for all pregnant diabetic patients

Classification. By referring to her past medical history and laboratory data (ECG, creatinine clearance, blood studies, ophthalmologic examination), the obstetrician must classify the patient into the appropriate category of White's scheme or our scheme for pregnant diabetic patients. This is important because each group has a certain perinatal mortality and presents specific management problems.

Dating. Accurate estimation of gestational age is mandatory and should include serial ultrasonography.

Urine cultures. A urine culture and sensitivity test must be obtained not only at the initial visit but at 4- and 6-week intervals to rule out asymptomatic bacteriuria.

Ophthalmoscopic examination. In the first office visit an ophthalmoscopic examination with dilation of the pupils should be performed to detect the presence or absence of diabetic retinopathy. Patients with a history of proliferative retinopathy and photocoagulation treatment do not need this examination, since the diagnosis of end-organ damage is evident.

Renal function. A baseline serum creatinine determination is necessary to assess renal function. If the result is abnormal (greater than 0.8 mg/dl), a creatinine clearance must be ordered. The renal function must be assessed every 4 weeks.

Patient education. The diabetic patient must be educated thoroughly in the importance and logic behind designing a diet, the effects of insulin, the signs of hypoglycemia and hyperglycemia, the diabetogenic effects of pregnancy, and the importance of eating regular meals. She should be aware of the effects of good versus poor control on perinatal morbidity and mortality. In addition, family members should be instructed, particularly for symptoms of hypoglycemic reactions. Patients using insulin for the first time need instruction on proper insulin administration and syringe and insulin care. A "dog tag" indicating that the patient has diabetes is recommended. Surprisingly, patients who have had diabetes for many years also need education about diabetes and pregnancy. They may not be aware of the different, more stringent control that is mandatory during pregnancy and often resist changes in their usual therapeutic regimen, especially dietary changes. The patient with end-organ damage should be informed about her poor prognosis (eg, limited life span) and the need to consider long-term planning for her infant. Discussion about the diabetic patient's suitability for pregnancy should occur before conception, ideally when she visits the physician for advice about contraception.

Urine checks. Urine testing is inadequate for blood sugar level control during pregnancy.

Some patients may have negative urine sugar values with blood sugar levels over 200 mg/dl. More often, urinary sugar values may be positive with normal blood sugar levels because of the low renal threshold of pregnancy.

Blood sugar checks. Blood sugar testing with visually read strips (Chemstrip) or with electronic devices (Glucometer, Accucheck, Visidex, Glucoscan II) is the method of choice for blood sugar monitoring during pregnancy. Patients should be instructed in self-glucose monitoring and ideally in record keeping of their blood glucose values in a graph form.

Routine prenatal laboratory studies. Serum biochemical profile (SMA-18), serology (VDRL), blood cell count (CBC), blood group, Rh and antibody screen, and gonorrhea culture must be performed along with a Papanicolaou smear.

Gestational diabetic patients

The primary goal in the management of a gestational diabetic patient is the achievement of normal blood sugar levels for pregnancy, which in the nondiabetic patient remain within a rather narrow range throughout gestation, despite mixed, irregularly timed meals. Strict dietary control is the key to a successful management.

Calorie intake. Calorie intake is aimed at supplying an adequate number of calories for the needs of pregnancy and simultaneously achieving normoglycemia. Usually a diet containing 30 kcal/kg of actual body weight or 35 to 40 kcal/kg of ideal body weight provides the necessary base. This caloric intake may be reduced to 25 or 20 kcal/kg of actual body weight or even less in the markedly obese gestational diabetic patient as long as the patient does not show marked ketonuria in urine tests carried out four times per day. In general, however, severe calorie restriction with weight loss is to be avoided because of the possibility of ketogenesis associated with this situation.

Calorie distribution and fiber in the diet. The diet should include 40% to 45% carbohydrate in the total caloric intake. Concentrated sweets with their associated marked swings in blood sugar levels should be avoided in favor of more complex starches. Multiple metabolic changes occur in response to changing any patient's diet, and a recent review by Mann[49] indicates improved carbohydrate metabolism in patients ingesting carbohydrate-rich diets with higher contents of unabsorbable plant polysaccharides such as pectin and cellulose. Whether or not pregnant diabetic patients benefit from such dietary manipulation remains unproven, but the morbidity should be minimal if a high fiber diet is instituted in an attempt to achieve improved glucose tolerance. Protein intake should equal 2 g/kg (100 to 200 g/day) and should provide about 25% to 30% of total caloric intake. The remaining 25% to 30% of the calories should be in the form of fat (45 to 60 grams).

Weight gain. The goal for total weight gain is the same in the nonobese gestational diabetic patient as in a nondiabetic pregnant patient. The caloric intake previously suggested usually provides for adequate weight gain. A total weight gain of 24 pounds (10.8 kg) is recommended by the Committee on Maternal Nutrition of the National Research Council although an average weight gain of 27.5 pounds (12.4 kg) was associated with the least perinatal mortality, toxemia, and prematurity in a study by Hytten and Thompson.[36] In the obese diabetic patient a smaller increase or no increase in body weight is reasonable as long as the patient does not show ketonuria.

Number of meals per day. The number of meals should be flexible and determined by the blood sugar levels at various times during the day along with the life-style of the patient. In general, six meals, including three regular meals (each providing two ninths of the total daily caloric intake) along with mid-morning, mid-afternoon, and nighttime snacks (each providing one ninth of the daily caloric intake), are theoretically the most beneficial in supplying a constant amount of calories throughout the day. However, a four-meal regimen with breakfast supplying 25% of the total daily caloric intake, lunch 30%, dinner 30%, and a bedtime snack 15% (with at least 25 grams of carbohydrate) may be more functional in a patient who finds the six-meal regimen unworkable. In addition to encouraging patients to follow their diets, the obstetrician should advise them to take supplemental vitamins and avoid alcohol.

The obstetrician should see the gestational diabetic patient every other week until the last month of gestation when weekly visits begin. A record of the patient's fasting blood sugar levels should be examined at each visit. In addition, it is wise to check blood sugar levels obtained periodically (once or twice weekly) at 11 AM, 4 PM, and 9 PM. Also, urine spot checks for acetone and glucose are excellent indicators of the success of dietary management. The presence of urinary ketones in the absence of glucosuria indicates inadequate caloric intake and use of fatty acids for energy generation purposes. If acetonuria appears, dietary manipulation should be effected to eliminate the ketones. Ketonuria during pregnancy has been associated with decreased intelligence in infants when examined several years later,[9] although recent studies question this result.[10,57] The addition of a bedtime snack including 25 grams of carbohydrate (eg, a glass of milk) often is all that is needed to eliminate any ketonuria present in the fasting urine spot check. Marked increases in glucosuria with or without the presence of ketones are generally indicative of *inadequate metabolic control* and demand immediate evaluation of blood sugar levels.

If the fasting blood sugar level becomes abnormal (100 mg/dl or more in two or more consecutive checks), the woman should be reclassified as an insulin-dependent stable diabetic patient and managed with insulin. If the fasting blood sugar level remains normal, it is useful to monitor the 1-hour postprandial blood sugar level that should be under 140 mg/dl. Occasionally, patients are found with normal fasting blood sugar levels but with less than optimal control throughout the day. In these cases the first movement is toward dietary modification aimed at spreading the caloric intake and avoiding marked postprandial hyperglycemia. If these measures fail, the woman should also be reclassified as an insulin-dependent stable diabetic patient and managed with insulin. In this situation the administration of 10 to 15 units of NPH insulin before breakfast, with or without regular insulin, usually improves mean daily blood sugar values to satisfactory levels.

Women with a history of requiring insulin in a previous pregnancy or with a history of previous stillbirth should be managed as insulin-dependent stable diabetic patients. In addition, any gestational diabetic patient who is older than 25 years is probably benefited by the use of insulin during her pregnancy. In a prospective study of insulin treatment of gestational diabetic patients, no improvement in perinatal outcome was noted.[60] A later retrospective study by O'Sullivan and colleagues[62] showed an improved fetal salvage in gestational diabetic patients treated with insulin if they were older than 25 years.

The obstetrician should never use oral hypoglycemic agents in an attempt to correct alterations in fasting blood sugar levels or marked postprandial elevations in the gestational diabetic patient. These drugs are contraindicated in the management of pregnant diabetic patients because they can induce fetal hyperinsulinemia and neonatal hypoglycemia.[2] The latter can be prolonged, especially with long half-life hypoglycemic agents (eg, chlorpropamide with half-life equals 37 hours). In addition, oral hypoglyecmic agents may be teratogenic and can cause hyperbilirubinemia by competing with bilirubin for albumin-binding sites.

Stable insulin-dependent diabetic patients

The primary goals in the treatment of insulin-dependent diabetic patients are (1) to have a glucose metabolism as close to physiologic as possible and (2) to deliver a normal infant at term with minimal if any neonatal problems. The major challenge implied by these goals includes maintaining the mean maternal glucose levels below 100 mg/dl and avoiding anomalies, macrosomia, and premature intervention in the pregnancy.

The question that must be addressed early in assigning these goals is whether or not normoglycemia improves the perinatal outcome in the pregnancy of a diabetic patient. In 1972 a retrospective study by Karlsson and Kjellmer[38] was one of the first pieces of evidence suggesting an affirmative answer. Mean blood sugar levels in the last 8 weeks of pregnancy of greater than 150 mg%, 100 to 150 mg%, and less than 100 mg% were associated with perinatal mortalities of 24%, 15%, and 4%, respectively.

Terms such as *tight*, *strict*, and *rigid* have been used by various authors to describe their approach to achieve normoglycemia in the pregnant diabetic patient. In one recent study of rigid glucose control versus perinatal outcome,[46] the conclusion was that maternal hyperglycemia exceeding a mean preprandial of 172 mg/dl was to be avoided but that levels of less than or equal to 115 mg/dl (ie, rigid control) were unnecessary for a successful perinatal outcome. However, only 14% of the 120 patients in this study had a mean less than or equal to 115 mg% so that rigid control was attempted but not achieved. In addition, macrosomia, delivery before term, and other neonatal morbidity remained high in this study. Conversely, Roversi et al[73] reported success in lowering perinatal morbidity and mortality using a "maximal tolerated dose" of insulin, to the point of near hypoglycemia.

The goal in managing the pregnant diabetic patient is to obtain a physiologic glucose profile, the implication being that diabetic patients must have glucose levels that are normal for any pregnancy. The potential risks to the mother with this approach include ketosis and hypoglycemic reactions; the potential benefits lie primarily in reducing infant morbidity by reducing fetal hyperinsulinemia and thus macrosomia[33] with its associated complications (eg, hypoglycemia, birth injury). That maternal glucose control can influence these factors has been suggested by studies in which cord C-peptide levels[83] and maternal hemoglobin A_{1c} levels[93] have been measured and correlated with perinatal outcome and by studies suggesting an effect of fetal hyperinsulinism on fetal growth.[33] Coustan et al[13] have reported that more babies can be delivered vaginally at term if glucose control is optimal.

To achieve adequate metabolic control of stable insulin-dependent diabetic patients throughout gestation, a combination of dietetic measures and insulin is necessary. Diet is as important to these patients as to the gestational diabetic woman. Unfortunately, the role of insulin in metabolic control is usually overemphasized, whereas the role of diet is not emphasized enough. The result is that these patients are usually careful and capable of handling their insulin but pay little attention to their meal composition and planning. They need a diet designed to provide them with an adequate number of calories, and the obstetrician should repeatedly emphasize the importance of diet in their metabolic control.

Stable insulin-dependent diabetic patients usually follow a rather predictable course during pregnancy. In the first half of pregnancy they may require about one third less insulin than when not pregnant. This is the result of the glucose and amino acid drain from the maternal circulation induced by the developing fetus. The nausea and vomiting commonly accompanying early pregnancy also reduce the available caloric ingestion. From about 20 to 24 weeks of gestation the insulin requirements begin to increase, and the amount of exogenous insulin required to overcome the resistance factors associated with pregnancy is between 38% and 98% higher than that required when not pregnant, depending on the patient's endogenous insulin stores.[70]

The insulin requirements for stable insulin-dependent diabetic patients are determined shortly after the first prenatal visit when the woman is admitted to the hospital for tests. A heparin lock or a short intravenous plastic catheter with a catheter plug is placed in a peripheral vein and used for blood sampling immediately before each meal, 2 hours after each meal, just before bedtime, and at 2 AM for as long as she stays in the hospital. Blood sugar values obtained before meals provide inadequate information about glucose levels, since they ignore completely the postprandial state and thus the time when hyperglycemia is most likely. The catheter is filled with a solution of heparin to avoid obstruction of the lumen between samplings. In this way a 24-hour blood sugar profile is built, and modifications in dietary intake or insulin dosage are carried out to correct the abnormalities found in the profile. A characteristic of stable patients is that the abnormalities of their blood sugar profiles are usually modified with minimal dietary or insulin dosage manipulation.

The initial hospitalization, soon after the first prenatal visit, not only allows a glucose profile to be constructed but just as important allows time for intensive education about the effects of pregnancy on diabetes while baseline studies of the heart, kidney, and eye are being performed. Close observation for hypoglycemic reactions and extreme insulin sensitivity is also made. The obvious disadvantage to in-hospital determination of insulin requirements is that people, tending to be more sedentary when hospitalized, are not performing their usual activities, and their daily exogenous insulin requirements may thus be overestimated. This drawback may be partly overcome by encouraging the patient to go off the floor where her room is located as well as arranging for recreational or physical therapy activities to simulate her caloric expenditure at home or work. Another measure to counteract the sedentary life in the hospital is to decrease the insulin dosage by 10% to 20% at the time of discharge. The total insulin required daily is determined by the amount needed to keep blood sugar levels within a desired range. *The goal of metabolic control during pregnancy is to keep mean daily blood sugar levels below 100 mg/dl without creating ketonuria or symptomatic hypoglycemia. For this purpose the fasting blood sugar level should be under 100 mg/dl, and the immediate postprandial blood sugar level (within 1 hour of meals) should be under 140 mg/dl.* With this type of control, urinary glucose is usually negative in the fasting state and before meals, except in patients with an extremely low renal threshold.

A complication of this rigorous control is the tendency to develop hypoglycemia, especially at night.[27,68] This is associated with maternal morbidity (eg, coma or seizure), and one study showed a two-fold to threefold increase in fetal mortality with severe maternal hypoglycemia.[1] Hypoglycemic episodes, especially nighttime hypoglycemia, can be difficult to detect, and they require both patient and family education about the symptoms. Nocturnal sweating, nightmares, seizures, difficulty of arousal, loss of consciousness, and excessive fatigue on awakening suggest nocturnal hypoglycemia. Fortunately, the stable patient tolerates rigorous control without frequent or severe hypoglycemic episodes although they are frequent in the unstable diabetic patient.

No preset formula for insulin administration is applicable to all diabetic patients during pregnancy. Most insulin-dependent stable diabetic patients require twice-daily dosages of combinations of short- and intermediate-acting insulins, especially by the end of pregnancy. Exceptions to this rule include some White's Class B diabetic patients for whom a single dose of intermediate-acting insulin (10 to 15 units NPH), with or without regular insulin, may yield satisfactory control.

Regular insulin is the preferred short-acting insulin preparation. After subcutaneous injection, its effect begins within 15 minutes, peak action occurs approximately 4 hours later, and total duration of the drug's effect is approximately 6 to 8 hours (Table 7-3). NPH is the preferred intermediate-acting insulin preparation, since unlike other forms of intermediate-acting insulins, it can be mixed in the same syringe with regular insulin, and the combination

TABLE 7-3 ■ Pharmacokinetics of insulin preparations given subcutaneously

Type of insulin	Beginning of action (hours)	Peak of action (hours)	Duration of effect (hours)
Regular	¼	4 to 6	6 to 8
NPH	3	8 to 12	18 to 24
Semilente	½	4 to 6	12 to 16
Lente	3	8 to 12	18 to 28

can be given as one injection. After a subcutaneous injection, the effect of NPH insulin begins in 3 hours, the peak action is 8 to 12 hours later, and the total duration of the effect is 18 to 24 hours. The pharmacokinetics of other forms of insulin (lente, semilente) are shown in Table 7-3. The morning dosage of regular insulin is largely determined by the noontime preprandial blood sugar value, whereas the morning dosage of NPH is determined by both the noontime postprandial and the evening preprandial blood sugar levels. The afternoon dosage of regular insulin is primarily determined by the evening meal postprandial blood sugar level and the blood sugar level before bedtime. The next day's 2 AM blood sugar level and the next morning's fasting blood sugar level primarily determine the afternoon quantity of NPH needed.

The following general guidelines can be used when ordering insulin dosages: (1) the AM dose usually consists of a 2:1 ratio of NPH to regular insulin, (2) the PM dose usually requires a 1:1 ratio of NPH and regular insulin, and (3) approximately two thirds of the total daily insulin requirements should be given in the AM dose with about one third in the PM dose. Once a rough estimate of the patient's insulin requirements is achieved, it is possible to fine tune the dosages based on fasting and postprandial glucose levels. If these doses remain unsatisfactory, they should be increased by approximately 20% and the situation reevaluated 2 to 3 days later before changing diet or insulin again.

Even in pregnant diabetic patients belonging to the stable group, there is no place for the use of "sliding scales" based on urinary or blood sugar concentrations. In fact, the amount of insulin to be given depends not only on the blood sugar level but also on other factors such as how long it has been from the last meal or snack, how long to the next meal or snack, time of day or night the blood sugar value was obtained, and the patient's sensitivity to insulin. For example, a sliding scale order to give 10 units of regular insulin for each 50 mg above 150 mg/dl may cause a severe hypoglycemic reaction when executed in a patient who had a blood sugar level of 160 at 11 PM. However, the same amount of insulin may be insufficient if given to a patient who has the same blood sugar concentration (160 mg/dl) in the fasting state.

After the initial in-hospital evaluation with regulation of insulin requirements, stable insulin-dependent diabetic patients should be seen on a weekly or every-other-week basis. At that time the obstetrician can review the daily record of urine spot checks (fasting, before meals, after meals, and bedtime), evaluate uterine growth, measure weight gain, and check a fasting and 2-hour postprandial blood sugar value. The urine spot checks are useful for detecting ketonuria and estimating urinary carbohydrate losses. However, glucosuria correlates poorly with blood sugar levels and should not be used for evaluation of diabetic control. The presence of glucosuria or ketonuria suggests the need for using more reliable methods for assessing glucose regulation. Urine collections taken every 24 hours for total glucose losses and ketone excretion are more sensitive indexes of diabetic control and can be used in combination with more frequent evaluations of fasting, preprandial, and postprandial blood sugar levels to guide insulin dosage alterations.

Intensive monitoring of blood sugar levels can be accomplished on an outpatient basis. Mintz et al[55] and Jovanovic et al[37] have described good results with patients taught to evaluate their blood sugar levels at home using glucose oxidase indicator papers (Dextrostix) in combination with a colorimetric analyzer to read the results. Patients are instructed to check the fasting blood sugar level and one postprandial sugar level daily and to check the blood sugar level before and after meals and at nighttime (six measurements) 1 day per week. Insulin administration can then be fine tuned to the desired preprandial and postprandial blood glucose range of 60 to 120 mg%. The obvious advantage of this approach is better glucose control without hospitalization. This home evaluation usually leads to greater

patient enthusiasm, a prerequisite for the management to be successful. The outpatient cost of such a program, however, is not small with Dextrostix at 40 cents each strip and reflectance meters about $500. If the patient cannot afford to buy a blood glucose electronic monitoring device, an adequate alternative may be to use visually read reagent strips (Chemstrip).

Hemoglobin (Hb) A_{1c} is a glycosylated form of Hb that normally composes 3% to 6% of the Hb of nondiabetic patients. Recent studies in nonpregnant patients indicate that Hb A_{1c} represents an integration of mean blood sugar levels over the previous weeks and hence is a measure of diabetic control over a period of about 60 days.[40] Further studies of pregnant women indicate that an abnormal Hb A_{1c} determination is a valuable test for identifying the patient who is poorly controlled (eg, mean blood sugar levels of greater than 200 mg/dl), but normal A_{1c} levels do not distinguish between patients with physiologic control (mean blood sugar levels less than 100/dl) and patients with higher blood sugar levels (eg, 100 to 150 mg/dl). Hb A_{1c} levels are also significantly increased if the patient is anemic. Hb A_{1c} levels are a poor screening test for gestational diabetes but may have some value in suggesting the presence of a congenital anomaly, since in one study[45] higher than normal levels of Hb A_{1c} were associated with an increased risk of an anomaly. However, further studies must document this potential use.

Unstable insulin-dependent diabetic patients

Shortly after the first prenatal visit, unstable or brittle insulin-dependent diabetic patients should be admitted to the hospital for assessment of their blood sugar profile with determinations made every 2 hours. These patients generally exhibit a profile characterized by sharp variations in glucose values with hypoglycemia intermixed with hyperglycemia. In general, these patients have a tendency to symptomatic hypoglycemia during the night and sharp elevations during the day, especially after meals.

Commonly, they have completely different blood sugar profiles on successive days, despite receiving the same amount of insulin and the same caloric intake. They also have a marked tendency to exhibit the Somogyi phenomenon. Because of this, they sometimes are controlled more easily by cutting their insulin dosage to half and then gradually increasing it. In some unstable patients there is marked insulin resistance, whereas in others the time of onset and the peak action of both regular and NPH insulin do not follow the predictable pattern observed in the stable patient.

The management of these brittle patients should include identification of possible causes of instability different from pregnancy itself. Too often it is assumed that the correlation between insulin dosage and the elevation of blood glucose values is direct and unaffected by other variables. The result of this approach is repeated episodes of hypoglycemia, poor metabolic control, prolonged hospitalization, and a disheartening lack of compliance on the patient's part. In our experience, the most common causes of instability unrelated to pregnancy are included in the discussions that follow.

Somogyi phenomenon. Somogyi phenomenon occurs frequently in the pregnant, brittle diabetic patient. It consists of a rebound hyperglycemia following a hypoglycemic reaction. Commonly, the blood sugar level is measured at the time of the hyperglycemia, and the patient is erroneously treated with increases in insulin dosage. Management of the problem consists of decreasing the insulin dosage until the hypoglycemic episodes disappear. This should be followed by a gradual dosage increase for control of the hyperglycemic peaks. An every 2-hour, 24-hour glucose profile is quite useful in suggesting the presence of this phenomenon.

Dietary compliance. Lack of dietary compliance is a common and unfortunately difficult-to-correct cause of metabolic instability in the pregnant diabetic patient. The role of the dietitian in these cases is paramount and is much more than simply formulating the allowed substitutions in an American Diabetes Association diet. The dietitian should obtain a dietary history, prepare a diet with the prescribed caloric intake and food composition, and by repeated questioning learn about the patient's food preferences and dislikes to design a meal plan that the patient may follow. To be successful a dietitian must obtain the patient's acceptance of the diet and reemphasize the need for accurate measuring of food. A common dietary problem in some unstable pregnant diabetic patients is the eating of pastries and sweets. The sugar that they contain is quickly absorbed from the GI tract, overwhelming the ability of the injected insulin to mobilize glucose into cells, resulting in sharp swings in blood sugar values. Control can often be established in such patients by minor alterations in habits without changes in insulin dosages.

Insulin antibodies. The serum of an average insulin-treated diabetic patient binds up to 10 units of insulin per liter. This binding depends on the presence in the serum of antiinsulin antibodies that are generated because of immunologic stimulation by the bovine and porcine insulins used for most diabetes treatment. These proteins are similar but not antigenically identical to human insulin, and eventually the body reacts to their administration with an antibody response. In some unstable patients insulin binding by antibodies may be 10 to 100 times that found in stable patients. If insulin antibodies are markedly increased in a given patient and this seems the best explanation for her instability, she should be switched to a "single peak" pork insulin or to human insulin, since beef insulin is the most important antigenic stimulator.

End-organ insensitivity. It has become apparent that a great deal of responsibility for the phenomenon of insulin resistance should be assigned to a decrease in number or affinity of insulin receptors located in the cell membrane of target tissues. This seems to be the case in the insulin resistance associated with obesity in which it has been possible to demonstrate not only decreases in receptor number per adipocyte but a decrease in the affinity of these receptors for insulin. It is possible that the increase in adipocyte size and number that normally occurs during pregnancy causes a decrease in insulin receptor density, generating an important factor in the insulin resistance of pregnancy. If this is the case, caloric restriction and weight loss should result in an increase in receptor density and a decrease in insulin resistance. Unfortunately, there is no easy way to establish the diagnosis of end-organ insensitivity to insulin, and no studies are available to indicate if caloric restriction and weight loss during pregnancy are beneficial in improving insulin sensitivity and thus metabolic control. However, a recent study[10] suggests that pregnant obese diabetic patients can be managed on low calorie (eg, 1000 kcal) diets without adversely affecting the neonatal outcome.

Problems at the injection site. Insulin resistance may be present because the administered insulin is being absorbed erratically or is being degraded at its subcutaneous injection site. The rate of insulin absorption is more rapid when the site of injection is the arm rather than the leg, and rotating injection sites may yield enough alterations of absorption time to complicate management. In addition, certain unstable diabetic patients exhibit marked insulin degradation when the hormone is given subcutaneously, creating an insulin-resistant status not present when insulin is given IM or IV.[64]

Drugs that interfere with insulin action. Another factor to be considered in insulin-resistant patients is the possibility of antiinsulin effects from other medications that the patient may be taking. Propranolol used as an antihypertensive can impair hepatic glycogenolysis. Ethanol on the other hand can impair gluconeogenesis. Diuretics (eg, furosemide, thiazides) have also been associated with hyperglycemia. Corticosteroids decrease peripheral glucose use and increase gluconeogenesis, both effects antagonizing insulin's action.

Prognostic signs in the pregnant diabetic patient. Pedersen and Pedersen[67] have outlined what they call *prognostically bad signs in pregnancy* that if present will adversely affect fetal prognosis by increasing perinatal mortality fourfold above that characteristic for a given diabetic class of patients. Included among these "bad signs" are the following:

pyelonephritis Diagnosed by clinical signs, fever (39° C), and positive urine culture.
precoma Diabetic ketoacidosis with HCO_3^- less than 10 mEq/L.
acidosis HCO_3^- levels between 10 and 17 mEq/L.
severe toxemia Presence of two of the following:
1. Blood pressure of 150/100 for 5 days before delivery.
2. Albuminuria 0.1% (1 gram protein per liter) for 24 hours before delivery.
3. Severe edema or weight gain greater than 45 pounds (20 kg).
mild toxemia Presence of two of the following:
1. Blood pressure 140/90 for 3 days before delivery.
2. Proteinuria 0.05% (500 mg protein per liter) for 24 hours before delivery.
3. Moderate edema or weight gain greater than 34 pounds (15 kg).

neglectors Patients who fail to follow recommended treatment regimens, irrespective of etiology for noncompliance (eg, low intelligence, late first attendance, lack of proper information).

A primary goal in scheduling frequent clinic visits and close observation in the antenatal period is to detect or prevent the prognostically bad signs. Urinary tract infection should be looked for to avoid the pyelonephritis that may result if bacteriuria is left undetected. Elevation of blood pressure with or without proteinuria should be treated aggressively with in-hospital monitoring and bed rest. As many as 25% of diabetic patients developed hypertensive complications during pregnancy in one large series.[26] Even mild diabetic ketoacidosis requires hospitalization to reestablish adequate control. Severe vomiting, infections, acute illness, and surgery require reevaluation of diabetic control and thus hospitalization. Patients who miss clinic appointments should be contacted by telephone and encouraged to attend, and arrangements should be made with employers or social service workers to maximize compliance.

Insulin-dependent diabetic patients with end-organ damage

Insulin-dependent diabetic patients with end-organ damage usually have had diabetes for several years, have minimal or no endogenous insulin production, and exhibit problems in metabolic control similar to unstable diabetic patients. They constitute a special group because the presence of end-organ damage adds further complexities to their care during and outside of pregnancy. The cases most frequently seen in pregnant patients are those with diabetic retinopathy, diabetic nephropathy, and ischemic heart disease.

Diabetic retinopathy. Patients with diabetic retinopathy can be divided into two types: those with *background retinopathy* (microaneurysms, exudates) and those with *proliferative retinopathy*. Patients in the first group may belong to either the stable or unstable categories mentioned before and should be managed accordingly, since the end-organ disease they exhibit does not alter their management.[72] Patients with proliferative retinopathy were previously considered at such high risk that therapeutic abortion was the rule. Recent developments with retinal photocoagulation techniques, however, have led to the recommendation that pregnancy can be undertaken in patients with this vascular complication of diabetes.[32] In a recent study pregnancy was not associated with any increased risk to the mother for visual loss or retinal changes. In fact, the *only* direct relationship of ocular complications in pregnant patients with proliferative retinopathy was that of the total duration of diabetes before pregnancy.[35]

Advice to the pregnant diabetic patient with proliferative retinopathy should include information that existing lesions may progress making photocoagulation necessary during pregnancy or in the postpartum period. The need for pregnancy termination by cesarean section should be pointed out, since catastrophic vitreous hemorrhage may result from expulsive efforts associated with natural childbirth. Finally, the potential for blindness at some point in the future mandates that these patients consider that long-term child care may become necessary. Ideally, such counseling should be given before conception but at least in the first trimester.

Diabetic nephropathy. The pregnant patient with diabetic nephropathy is usually hypertensive and may have background or proliferative retinopathy. Existing kidney damage may cause one or several problems during pregnancy. *Water retention* with edema may become extremely uncomfortable. These patients are usually taking large doses of furosemide before pregnancy to avoid accumulation of edema fluid, and if this is the case, the medication should be continued during pregnancy to avoid massive accumulation of sodium and water. *Hypertension* usually requires treatment with methyldopa, hydralazine, or other antihypertensive agents, and both hydralazine and methyldopa may worsen the patient's problem with water retention. Hypertension usually becomes aggravated during the third trimester. *Urinary tract infections* are common and may be associated with chronic pyelonephritis or neurogenic bladder. Occasionally, these patients develop *acute pyelonephritis* or *necrotizing papillitis*, thereby worsening their already compromised kidney function.

Ischemic heart disease. Pregnancy in diabetic patients with ischemic heart disease, White's Class H, is uncommon. A recent review of the subject described 12 patients, 8 of whom died in pregnancy.[80] The ill effects of hypoglycemia in such patients (catecholamine release resulting

in induced tachycardia, increased demands on the myocardium, and possibly arrhythmias) make blood sugar control extremely challenging. During labor, hypertension and tachycardia may result from inadequate pain relief causing excessive demands on cardiac function. Swan-Ganz catheter monitoring is necessary to direct intrapartum management. Advice about abortion and contraception, including sterilization, is paramount in providing optimal care for these patients.

■ **ANTEPARTUM EVALUATION OF THE FETUS IN THE PREGNANT DIABETIC PATIENT**

Antepartum monitoring of fetal well-being is aimed at preventing intrauterine deaths and determining when pregnancy termination should be considered.

Serial ultrasound is an indispensable adjunct to present-day management of the pregnant diabetic patient. The information to be gained from serial ultrasound examinations includes (1) accurate dating so that the estimated date of confinement can be assigned with confidence, (2) observation of the pattern of fetal growth so that developing macrosomia or intrauterine growth retardation can be detected, and (3) detection of gross congenital anomalies such as anencephaly or hydrocephaly.

Scheduling of the initial ultrasound examination should optimally coincide with a gestational age of approximately 16 weeks so that major anomalies can be detected at a time when abortion is a safe option. Repeat examinations should then occur at 4-week intervals to confirm dating and to follow fetal growth. All types of pregnant diabetic patients should have the benefit of serial ultrasound for fetal evaluation.

Estriol assays of both plasma and urine have been extensively studied in high-risk pregnancies in attempts to outline a reasonable protocol to evaluate the presence of fetal distress. Goebelsman et al[29] suggested that 24-hour urinary estriol measurements are useful as an adjunct to the management of the diabetic patient. *Daily* urinary estriol assays in combination with urine creatinine determinations were recommended, since many significant falls in urinary E_3 values are missed in patients undergoing only biweekly estriol determinations. A subsequent study[17] indicated that unconjugated plasma estriol assay was the most predictive test among the presently available estriol assays in managing the pregnant diabetic patient. Because there is a great variability in plasma estriol levels (unconjugated or total),[4] a "normal range" for uncomplicated pregnancies and especially for pregnant diabetic patients is difficult to determine with confidence. Hence if estriol assays are used in the management of the pregnant diabetic patient, the obstetrician should look at changes in estriol levels in the individual rather than at changes in estriol levels in relation to a "normal population" of pregnant patients.

Because of the problems just discussed, several authors have suggested that estriol assays are not useful in managing the pregnant diabetic patient, particularly if such assays are not done daily,[19,79] and we fully agree with this opinion. However, others have recommended the use of unconjugated plasma estriol assays in managing the pregnant diabetic patient if the following criteria can be met: (1) baseline estriol values can be established for the patient' (2) estriol values are measured from 32 weeks of gestation on a *daily* basis by a reliable laboratory that can provide results within 12 hours; and (3) serial ultrasound data are available to indicate the pattern of fetal growth and pinpoint the gestational age accurately.

If these criteria can be met, a drop of 35% in estriol values, compared to the previously established "normal" value for the particular patient being evaluated, would indicate the need for further assessment of fetal well-being by a nonstress test (NST) with or without an oxytocin challenge test. Using this approach, Schmidt et al[79] identified two acidotic infants within 2 days of reactive nonstress testing. In conclusion, the use of estriol determinations in managing diabetic patients is indicated only if strict criteria, as just outlined, can be achieved. Otherwise, the estriol assay can lead to unnecessary and premature intervention.

HPL is of no use in the management of pregnant diabetic patients. HPL levels are proportional to placental mass, and since large placentas are associated with Classes A, B, and C diabetic patients, this explains the frequent occurrence of higher than normal HPL values in pregnant diabetic women.

Placental hypoplasia may develop secondary to vascular disease in diabetic patients with vascular complications. Absence of the expected rise in insulin requirements in the second half of pregnancy or the development of a fall in insulin requirements near term suggests placental insufficiency that may be reflected also in a decrease in HPL production. However, this correlation (HPL equals placental insufficiency) is extremely insensitive, and management of a pregnant diabetic patient cannot depend on HPL levels for estimating uteroplacental insufficiency.

Fetal activity recording for 30-minute periods in the morning, afternoon, and evening is a simple method for day-to-day assessment of fetal well-being.[65,77] Marked reductions in fetal activity (less than 10 movements in a 12-hour period) suggest the need for more sensitive methods of fetal evaluation.

An *NST* is easily performed but does require appropriate monitoring equipment, a satisfactory tracing for evaluation, and some cost to the patient (in time if not money). A reactive NST is a good indication of fetal well-being for at least 1 week,[69] providing the maternal condition is stable. A nonreactive NST, however, is not predictive and thus requires performance of a contraction stress test (CST) to more clearly define the possibility of fetal distress.

The *CST*, either spontaneous or with the aid of intravenous oxytocin, is valuable in determining fetal jeopardy. In a large series by Gabbe et al,[25] none of 211 Class A diabetic patients who had a negative CST suffered intrauterine fetal death within 1 week of the examination. A positive CST was associated with increased incidence of perinatal mortality, prematurity, respiratory distress syndrome (RDS), and reduced birth weight.

Thus either a reactive NST or a negative CST indicates that the pregnancy of a diabetic patient can be continued for 1 more week with reassurance that fetal demise is unlikely. This assumes adequate control of maternal glucose metabolism during the prolongation period, since the predictive value of both tests is based on the premise that the maternal condition is stable.

Gestational diabetic patients should be followed from 36 weeks to term with NSTs. NSTs (and CSTs if indicated) should begin at 34 weeks of gestation for stable insulin dependent diabetic patients and as early as 28 weeks of gestation for unstable insulin dependent diabetic pregnant women.

Amniotic fluid analysis is discussed in Chapter 3 so that only a brief consideration of lecithin/sphingomyelin (L/S) ratios pertinent to the management of diabetic patients is presented here. Amniocentesis should be done by 37 to 38 weeks in all pregnant insulin-dependent diabetic patients, although maternal or fetal indications may dictate earlier evaluation. Two points should be made concerning amniotic fluid analysis in diabetic patients. The first point is that although L/S ratios greater than 2.0 are associated with infrequent (5%) development of RDS in the nondiabetic populations, this may not be true for the infant of a diabetic patient. Reports of L/S ratios in diabetic patients indicate that from 6% to 27% of patients with L/S ratios greater than or equal to 2.0 develop hyaline membrane disease.[21] Fortunately, most of these are in the mild to moderate category with few neonatal deaths. Conversely, Gabbe et al[24] found no difference between infants of diabetic and nondiabetic patients in regard to development of RDS if the L/S ratio was 2.0 or greater. They point out that the studies reporting a difference are poorly controlled and have limited numbers of patients. In addition, intrapartum asphyxia and neonatal acidosis with their destabilizing effect on lung surfactant may be important factors in RDS development in the infant of a diabetic mother. Route of delivery may also be important in explaining RDS development, since diabetic patients undergo cesarean-section delivery more often than nondiabetic patients and RDS is more frequent in patients who have cesarean section.[56] A recent review[48] on the subject of L/S ratios in diabetic patients points out the problems existing in using this test to predict RDS in infants of diabetic mothers. Recent studies of other phospholipids (eg, phosphatidyl glycerol) may help to determine which patients with L/S ratios greater than 2.0 are at risk for developing RDS. It seems that the absence of phosphatidyl glycerol in fluid from diabetic patients is associated with a higher probability of RDS despite a mature L/S ratio,[14] and thus elective delivery of an infant of a diabetic mother should be dependent on the presence of phosphatidyl glycerol instead of the L/S ratio alone.

A second point to be considered regarding

amniotic fluid analysis is the observation that the normal rise in L/S ratio does not occur at the same gestational age in patients with diabetes when compared to nondiabetic patients. Delayed maturation was noted in patients in Classes A, B, and C, whereas early maturation was noted in Classes D, F, and R.[16,28] The mechanism for the delay in lung maturation in Classes A, B, and C diabetic patients remains speculative. It is possible that the normal sequence of cortisol production, receptor interaction, and phospholipid enzyme stimulation with resultant surfactant synthesis is antagonized at the cellular level by the higher circulating insulin levels often present in infants of diabetic mothers. Another speculation suggests that fetal hyperinsulinism may reduce glycerol-3-phosphate and dihydroxyacetone phosphate production and thus impair surfactant synthesis by substrate depletion.[86]

Management of diabetic patients must take into account the different timing of increased lecithin synthesis in diabetic patients. This points out the absolute necessity of amniocentesis for documenting pulmonary maturity before preterm or "elective" term delivery in the absence of fetal or maternal deterioration. In addition, rigid attention must be paid to avoid intrapartum asphyxia and neonatal acidosis during labor in the diabetic patient. In the absence of deterioration of fetoplacental function, delivery should be delayed until an L/S ratio of at least 2.0 (preferably 2.5 to 3.0) is accompanied by the presence of a phosphatidyl glycerol spot on chromatographic analysis of amniotic fluid.

■ TIMING OF DELIVERY

A liberal policy of hospitalization should be exercised at all times for pregnant diabetic patients. When the patient is near term, she should be hospitalized in a perinatal center with a neonatal intensive care nursery staffed with personnel familiar with the complications associated with the infant of a diabetic mother and with adequate monitoring facilities for antepartum evaluation of both the mother and the fetoplacental unit. Several factors determine the optimal time for delivery: (1) the increased risk of intrauterine death in all but Class A patients beyond 36 weeks of gestation, (2) the presence of absence of maternal complications, (3) the presence or absence of intrauterine fetal distress, (4) the degree of metabolic control achieved during pregnancy and the presence of signs indicating that control is deteriorating. Emphasis must be placed on the fact that "routine" preterm delivery of the infant of a diabetic mother is no longer tenable.

The *gestational diabetic patient* with a normal fasting blood sugar level may be delivered at term without increasing the risk of intrauterine death.[25] However, this excludes those patients who develop preeclampsia or pyelonephritis and those who have delivered a stillbirth in the past. Class A patients should be hospitalized if the diabetic control is not optimal, maternal complications develop, or there is evidence of fetal distress. Ideally, Class A patients scheduled for planned delivery (ie, induction or cesarean section) should be hospitalized 3 to 4 days earlier for bed rest, fetal evaluation, and stabilization of diabetic control. They can be delivered vaginally providing fetal weight is not excessive (ie, less than 4000 grams), clinical pelvimetry is adequate, and intrapartum monitoring facilities are available for detecting signs of fetal distress. Spontaneous labor is preferred, but induction may become necessary because of maternal or fetal reasons or for those patients who do not develop spontaneous labor by 40 weeks of gestation.

Determining the optimal time for delivery of insulin-dependent diabetic patients is based primarily on three factors: (1) fetal well-being, (2) lung maturation, and (3) presence of maternal complications. A just discussed, prime determinants of fetal well-being include a reactive NST and a negative CST. In the presence of either, the pregnancy can be carried to term (38 to 40 weeks of gestation) with little chance of fetal demise. Only anecdotal reports of a fetal demise within 1 week of a negative CST are reported in the literature. In most centers estriol measurements are not used in determining fetal well-being.

In the presence of a reactive NST or a negative CST, the prime determinant of delivery is the presence of mature fetal lungs. The aim is to achieve a mature L/S ratio and a positive phosphatidyl glycerol spot in the chromatographic analysis of amniotic fluid. Occasionally, however, amniotic fluid analysis indicating pulmonary maturity should not be the only determinant for time of delivery if the maternal and fetal status

remain stable. Neonates delivered before term experience a higher incidence of hyperbilirubinemia, hypoglycemia, and hypocalcemia. The lungs are only one among several organ systems that need adequate time for maturity to avoid neonatal complications.

If fetal reactivity is absent and the CST is positive, immediate amniotic fluid analysis should be performed. If the L/S ratio proves to be less than 1.5, delivery should be delayed and the patient should be placed on strict bed rest while tight metabolic control and daily contraction stress testing is continued. If the L/S ratio is in the range of 1.5 to 1.9, delivery should be seriously considered. Other factors to be considered include the presence of phosphatidyl glycerol, maternal medical stability, the presence of meconium, growth retardation by ultrasound, and the absence of fetal reactivity. If a good neonatal intensive care unit is available, delivery of this group of infants (L/S ratio 1.5 to 1.9) evidencing signs of fetal distress in utero will usually be beneficial. If the L/S proves to be greater than 2.0 in combination with a positive CST, a plan for delivery should be immediately instituted. The presence of amniotic fluid phosphatidyl glycerol, irrespective of the L/S ratio, makes the possibility of RDS unlikely.

Management of pregnant diabetic patients at the time of delivery

Vaginal delivery can be attempted in a diabetic patient who is in spontaneous labor or undergoing induction if the following criteria are met:

1. Clinical pelvimetry is adequate
2. The infant is in vertex presentation
3. Adequate fetal monitoring equipment is available for the intrapartum period
4. Fetal weight is estimated to be less than 4000 grams
5. No sign of fetal distress appears intrapartum

If cephalopelvic disproportion, malpresentation, inadequate monitoring facilities, macrosomia, or evidence of fetal distress is present, cesarean section is the safest method of delivery.

Induction of labor with intravenous oxytocin can be attempted in diabetic patients if a favorable cervix is present, as suggested by Bishop scoring. If an unripe cervix is present, serial inductions can be undertaken provided that good metabolic control is maintained throughout the induction period and no sign of fetal distress develops. Rarely, however, will unstable diabetic patients benefit from the stress presented by serial inductions. Thus a liberal policy of cesarean-section delivery should be practiced in these patients if they fail to progress after an adequate trial of induction.

If cesarean-section delivery becomes necessary, general anesthesia as compared to spinal anesthesia appears to provide a more normal acid-base state during delivery of the infant.[15] In addition, careful consideration should be given to the kind of skin incision to be made at the time of surgery. As many diabetic patients are obese, a transverse incision optimizes wound healing and tends to avoid many of the complications associated with wound dehiscence and infection.

Insulin and glucose control during labor

Physiologic control of blood sugar levels in diabetic patients is the goal throughout pregnancy, and delivery is no exception. Good control of blood sugar levels immediately before and during labor can potentially avoid the excessive fetal insulin secretion causing the neonatal hypoglycemia so frequent in infants of diabetic mothers.[47] At the same time ketosis is to be avoided, since this shows that inadequate carbohydrate is being supplied to fulfill the energy requirements of the mother.

A liberal policy of hospitalization should be exercised for diabetic patients scheduled for either induction or cesarean section so that delivery occurs in patients optimally controlled in the immediate antepartum period. Patients should continue on their diet and insulin dosages as previously outlined, but they should fast after midnight the day preceding delivery. A measurement of blood glucose should be obtained in the early morning on the day of attempted delivery. In addition, some of the same blood sample should be tested at the bedside using glucose oxidase impregnated papers (Dextrostix) and analyzed with a glucose analyzer. The result obtained from this procedure can be compared with the laboratory determination of glucose to verify the accuracy of the bedside technique. Generally, glucose values within 15% of the true glucose determination by standard laboratory techniques can be expected. Patients who are

in spontaneous labor should also have immediate determination of blood glucose, but in addition, a careful history of insulin administration and meals eaten that day should be obtained.

A large-bore intravenous cannula should be placed for administration of 5% dextrose, usually in a balanced salt solution, at a rate that provides between 5 and 10 grams of glucose per hour. The administration of intravenous fluids is aimed at providing carbohydrate and water to avoid the ketonuria and dehydration associated with fasting. This also helps to avoid the development of intrapartum acidosis, reduces the potential for neonatal hypoglycemia, and maintains a normal intravascular volume, thus minimizing the risk of maternal hypotension.

Regular insulin can be administered by a constant infusion pump connected intravenous piggyback into the main line. An initial intravenous bolus of regular insulin (0.02 to 0.05 units/kg) can be given if the need is suggested from the patient's fasting blood glucose determination. A solution of regular insulin for constant infusion can be prepared by adding 25 units of regular insulin to 500 ml of normal saline solution (see box on p. 140). This results in a solution containing 1 unit/20 ml. The initial setting for the hourly intravenous piggyback infusion of regular insulin is determined somewhat empirically and is based on frequent blood glucose determinations in the early part of its administration. Most people are controlled with hourly intravenous insulin rates equaling 0.25 to 2.0 units/hour,[96] but others may need up to 10 to 20 units/hour, especially if insulin antibodies are present. A rapid rate of glucose administration to the diabetic mother must be avoided, since it predisposes the infant to the development of neonatal hyperglycemia.[47]

Adjustment of the dextrose and insulin infusions depends on blood sugar determinations made frequently (every 20 to 30 minutes) soon after beginning the infusions. Blood can be obtained from a heparin lock for analysis at the bedside using Dextrostix and a glucose analyzer as previously described. The goal in management is to keep the blood sugar values in a range of 60 to 100 mg/dl while avoiding ketonuria. The total hourly fluid intake, including the dextrose infusion, insulin solution, and Pitocin diluent if induction is attempted, should approximate 75 to 150 ml/hour (see box on p. 140). Patients with cardiac or renal disease should receive lower

---

Intravenous insulin administration

PREPARATION OF INSULIN SOLUTION
25 units regular insulin plus
500 ml normal saline solution equal 1 unit/20 ml

USUAL STARTING DOSE
0.25 to 2.0 units/hour (5 to 40 ml/hour)

TOTAL FLUID INTAKE DURING LABOR
Main intravenous plus insulin solution plus oxytocin diluent equal 75 to 150 ml/hour
    (D_5W)   (IVPB)   (if induction)

---

amounts of fluid and may benefit from the placement of a central venous catheter for closer monitoring of their fluid status. Once the initial regulation of blood glucose and fluid intake is accomplished, blood glucose determinations can be less frequent (eg, every 1 to 2 hours).

Other variables to be followed closely during the course of labor include urine spot checks for glucose and ketones, serum electrolytes, and intake and output. Development of ketonuria indicates an inadequate supply of carbohydrates, insulin, or both. A flow sheet that includes this information along with blood sugar determinations, record of medications given, vital signs, and fetal heart rate patterns, helps to organize the rather large bulk of data generated by the close monitoring of a diabetic patient in labor.

If an attempt at induction fails on a given day, the insulin and dextrose infusions may be discontinued on the night of the failed induction and the patient's diet resumed simultaneously. Blood sugar determinations 3 to 4 hours after the evening meal may be used to determine the amount of regular insulin necessary for the patient overnight. Care must be taken not to overestimate these needs and cause iatrogenic hypoglycemia. The patient's normal diet and previous daily insulin dosages can be resumed the day after failed induction, assuming that a repeated induction is not attempted.

■ MANAGEMENT OF THE PUERPERIUM

Close attention must be paid to the immediate postpartum blood glucose levels whether delivery was accomplished vaginally or abdominally. With removal of the placenta, an important

source of peripheral insulin antagonism is eliminated. The half-life of HPL is short, approximately 20 to 30 minutes. The vast majority of peripheral insulin antagonism derived from this peptide is gone within 2 to 3 hours after delivery. Thus the patient is subjected to development of hypoglycemia unless adjustments are effected in insulin administration immediately postpartum.

To avoid the development of hypoglycemia after delivery the glucose infusion should be continued, but the intravenous administration of insulin should be discontinued. Blood sugar levels should be obtained frequently until a rising or stable glucose level is documented. If the patient does not need to be fasting, the intravenous glucose solution can then also be stopped. The amount of insulin to be administered subsequently is determined by frequent checks on blood sugar levels. Sliding scales must be avoided.

If the infant is mature, breast-feeding is permitted in the diabetic patient. If the mother is breast-feeding, her caloric intake must be supplemented usually with 600 to 800 kcal/day. The increased caloric intake requires adjustment of insulin dosages that must be individualized during and after the breast-feeding period.

■ THE INFANT OF THE DIABETIC MOTHER

Neonatal complications in the infant of the diabetic mother (IDM) can be arbitrarily grouped into two categories: (1) those associated with prematurity and (2) those resulting from a pregnancy complicated by diabetes.

Robert and colleagues[71] have estimated the

risk for RDS in infants of diabetic mothers to be sixfold higher than for infants delivered of non-diabetic patients. This higher incidence of RDS is corrected for gestational age and takes into account the higher probability of developing RDS in infants delivered by cesarean section without preceding labor. Hyperbilirubinemia is more frequent in preterm infants, since maturation of the liver glucuronyl transferase responsible for bilirubin conjugation and excretion is often lacking. Feeding difficulties and apneic episodes are more common in preterm infants, and the infants of diabetic mothers are no exception.

A primary neonatal complication related to diabetes is the frequent appearance of neonatal hypoglycemia (blood sugar level less than 30 mg%). Infants with symptoms of hypoglycemia often appear quiet and lethargic but may instead become apneic, cyanotic, tachypneic, or may evidence seizure activity. Peak incidence of hypoglycemia is 1½ to 2 hours after delivery. Its development is related to a blunted glucagon secretion response to normal physiologic stimuli.[95] The theory suggesting that maternal hyperglycemia results in specific fetal beta cell hyperplasia with resultant hypoglycemia[86] after birth has been recently questioned.[54] No matter what the mechanism, the high risk for hypoglycemia mandates that a glucose determination is to be done immediately after birth on the infant of the diabetic mother. If either a glucose level of greater than or equal to 150 mg% or less than or equal to 30 mg% is present, an intravenous glucose infusion should be started at a rate of 6 mg/kg/minute. Early oral feeding is desirable; intravenous boluses of glucose are not, since reactive hypoglycemia is a frequent consequence of such treatment. Hypoglycemic episodes can be especially difficult to treat when oral hypoglycemic agents are used to control maternal glucose because of their prolonged half-life.

Other neonatal complications include polycythemia, hyperviscosity, thrombosis (especially of the renal vein), hypocalcemia, hypomagnesemia, and macrosomia. Polycythemia is diagnosed by a central hematocrit level greater than or equal to 65%. Infants with polycythemia often appear plethoric and are in a hyperviscosity state requiring partial exchange transfusion. A recent study[94] suggests that elevated erythropoietin in infants born to diabetic mothers is the reason

for polycythemia. Abnormalities in mineral metabolism (eg, Mg^{++}, Ca^{++}) may be related to functional hypoparathyroidism in the infant. Additional discussion of neonatal care and long-term outcome of infants of diabetic mothers is presented by Oh.[58]

Macrosomia is a primary reason for the increased cesarean-section delivery of infants of diabetic mothers and also an important factor in the higher incidence of traumatic delivery. Birth injuries frequently associated with vaginal delivery of macrosomic infants include phrenic nerve paralysis, shoulder dystocia, clavicular fracture, Erb's palsy, pneumothorax, and injuries to the head and neck.

Congenital anomalies with *major* malformations are found more commonly among infants of diabetic mothers. The range reported in the literature is 5% to 9%[25,34,39,66] compared to about 2% for the general population. Included among the congenital anomalies frequently seen in infants of diabetic mothers are (1) the caudal regression syndrome and vertebral dysplasia[3,76]; (2) anencephaly and meningomyelocele[20]; (3) cardiovascular abnormalities including transposition of the great vessels, ventricular septal defect, and coarctation of the aorta[74]; (4) anal atresia[82]; and (5) ureteral duplication and renal agenesis.[43] Mills et al[53] have used a developmental morphologic approach to show that malformations in infants of diabetic mothers occur before the seventh gestational week. This finding implies that diabetic control before conception and early in gestation is the key to reducing the high incidence of anomalies occurring in infants of diabetic patients.

Maternal ketonuria and hypoglycemia are complications that appear sometimes during treatment of pregnant diabetic patients and have been associated with neonatal morbidity. Infants of mothers with ketonuria during pregnancy have been found to have a decreased IQ when tested several years later.[85] However, the large prospective study of over 53,000 pregnancies from the Collaborative Perinatal Study of the National Institute of Neurological and Communicative Disorders and Stroke could not demonstrate that maternal acetonuria adversely affected psychomotor or IQ development in their children. Naeye[57] has found evidence indicating that diabetic mothers who were ketotic during pregnancy have infants with an excess of neurologic abnormalities and low IQs more as a result of amniotic fluid bacterial infections and their complications than because of the maternal ketosis. Although the fetus may be able to withstand severe maternal hypoglycemia without dying,[75] Drew and colleagues[18] found maternal hypoglycemia to be associated with an increased frequency of congenital anomalies of genital organs and with clubfoot.

The infant of either a diabetic mother or a diabetic father is at higher risk for developing diabetes than infants born to nondiabetic parents. Though the exact figures predicting this higher risk remain unknown, a reasonable estimate is that about 9% of such infants develop diabetes themselves.[81]

The severity of the maternal disease and the presence of vascular complications have always been factors in determining the perinatal prognosis for the infant of a diabetic mother. A compilation of data presented by Gabbe[23] reports perinatal mortality in treated Class A patients to be 1.6% and thus comparable to that of the nondiabetic population. However, Class A patients who remained undiagnosed or untreated continued to have a perinatal mortality as high as 10%.[25] The perinatal mortality is higher for other classes: Class B patients have a 4.8% mortality; Class C, 7.9%, Class D, 10%, and Classes F, H, and R, 18.6%. Although the mortality remains high, the present figures represent a considerable improvement when compared to the results of 20 years ago.

■ MATERNAL COMPLICATIONS IN DIABETES AND PREGNANCY

Several complications of pregnancy, though not unique to the diabetic patient, develop more often in that individual than in the normal pregnant patient. Preeclampsia has a fourfold increased frequency in the diabetic patient, even in the absence of preexisting vascular disease.[44] Infections (especially wound and urinary tract) develop more often in the diabetic patient. Pyelonephritis in particular was observed in 6% of diabetic patients compared to about 2% in nondiabetic patients.[67] Postpartum hemorrhage also occurs more frequently in the diabetic patient. This may be related to antepartum overdistention of the uterus secondary to polyhydramnios (complicating 25% of pregnancies involving diabetes) and to macrosomia.

Information on the effects of pregnancy on the vascular complications of diabetes is limited. Proliferative retinopathy is of particular concern, since there is evidence that this lesion may deteriorate during pregnancy, resulting in blindness[51] or leading to the need for photocoagulation.[32,35]

Whether pregnancy affects the ultimate course of diabetic nephropathy is unclear. Although kidney function can deteriorate during pregnancy, it is generally felt that clinical and laboratory measurements of renal function return to their prepregnancy level after termination of the pregnancy.[66] If pyelonephritis or preeclampsia develop, however, kidney function can be permanently worsened.

Class H patients represent the group with the highest probability of maternal mortality during pregnancy. Only one of four patients described by Hare and White[31] survived pregnancy. Whether pregnancy per se influences the development of coronary artery disease in affected patients remains unknown. In the absence of arteriosclerotic disease, maternal mortality in diabetic patients is infrequent, especially in comparison to the era before insulin usage. The increased risk to maternal well-being presented by proliferative retinopathy, renal failure, or severe coronary artery disease makes patients affected with these problems prime candidates for therapeutic abortion.

Diabetic ketoacidosis

Diabetic keotacidosis is a serious complication that develops when a relatively severe insulin deficiency leads to abnormal carbohydrate, fat, and protein metabolism. The deficiency usually is a consequence of one or both of two situations: (1) failure to supply adequate exogenous insulin to satisfactorily complement the patient's own inadequate insulin production and (2) appearance of an increased insulin demand created by stressful situations. The former situation appears in cases of dietary indiscretions or when compliance with insulin regimen is poor. The latter situation can develop when the diabetic patients is exposed to infection, injury, or surgery.

The deficiency in insulin supply leads to hyperglycemia, hyperosmolality, and metabolic acidosis. Hyperglycemia causes osmotic diuresis with resultant losses of large amounts of water, sodium, and potassium. Increases in fatty acid mobilization in combination with liver oxidation result in ketone body formation, including beta hydroxybutyrate, acetoacetic acid, and acetone. These compounds aggravate the developing metabolic acidosis directly but also worsen the dehydration by making the patient nauseated and causing her to vomit.

Patients with ketoacidosis may have chief complaints of vomiting, hyperpnea, abdominal pain, weakness, rapid weight loss, or in severe cases mental obtundation. Rapid bedside evaluation to rule out the diagnosis includes obtaining (1) urine for analysis of glucose and ketones, (2) arterial blood gases, (3) blood glucose and electrolyte levels, and (4) a measurement of serum ketones. Although the patient's history may offer strong suspicions for the presence of ketoacidosis, the diagnosis is established by the presence of large glucosuria and ketonuria, acidotic arterial blood pH, and significant ketonemia. Ketonemia can be determined at the bedside by taking a commercially available nitroprusside-containing tablet (Acetest), crushing it, and adding a drop of fresh serum to the crushed tablet. If ketonemia is present, a purple color will appear after 2 minutes. Ketonemia in the absence of glucosuria should raise the possibility of starvation ketosis or insulin overdosage. These possibilities can be rapidly evaluated at the bedside determining the approximate level of blood glucose with Dextrostix. The pregnant patient with nondiabetic ketoacidosis does not have a markedly elevated blood glucose, even in the presence of marked glucosuria and ketonuria. However, blood glucose levels of 200 or more, when coupled with ketonuria and acidosis, indicate the presence of diabetic ketoacidosis.

Although the serum electrolyte status of the patient is not a key to the diagnosis of ketoacidosis, it is an important indicator of the degree of salt loss and the magnitude of the acidosis. The bicarbonate concentration in a normal pregnant patient is lower than that in a nonpregnant patient as a result of the loss of carbon dioxide that accompanies the hyperventilation of pregnancy. Thus when ketoacidosis develops, the bicarbonate concentration is more markedly reduced in the pregnant than in the nonpregnant patient receiving a similar acidotic insult. Hyponatremia is usually present, and the serum sodium suggests a sodium loss that is more apparent than real if hemodilution is taken into account. The potassium is often normal or even high, since potassium movement from the intracellular to the extracellular space induced by diuresis is made worse with acidosis. Total body potassium is decreased in the patient with ketoacidosis, thus making potassium supplementation a necessity. In addition, hypophosphatemia is common in diabetic ketoacidosis and usually becomes apparent 4 to 12 hours after instituting therapy. Phosphorus supplementation is recommended to replenish erythrocyte 2,3-diphosphoglycerate and improve oxygen delivery to the tissues.[42]

Treatment of the patient with ketoacidosis is aimed at restoring total body fluid and electrolyte deficits, eliminating the ketogenesis and acidosis, reducing hyperglycemia, and restoring normal carbohydrate metabolism. Insulin administration along with electrolytes containing intravenous fluids provide the necessary base for achieving these goals. In a normotensive patient, the initial intravenous fluids should be 0.45% saline solution run at a rate of 500 to 1000 ml/hour. Normal saline solution should be used in hypotensive or oliguric patients. At the same time rapid-acting insulin should be administered by the intravenous piggyback route by constant infusion at a rate of 5 to 8 units/hour. The insulin-containing solution can be mixed by putting 50 units of regular insulin into 500 ml of 0.45% saline, yielding a solution of 1 unit/10 ml fluid. If the blood glucose level fails to decline by approximately 30% in the first 2 to 3 hours, insulin administration should be increased to twice the previous level. The rate of total intravenous fluid administration is usually decreased after 2 to 3 hours, at which time potassium supplements should be added to the fluids. Potassium should be added earlier if the initial blood potassium is reported to be below normal, since this indicates severe total body potassium depletion. With the correction of the acidosis underway, life-threatening hypokalemia may develop as the result of potassium shifting back into the cells. No more than 40 mEq/hour of potassium should be administered without continuous ECG monitoring, since life-threatening cardiac arrhythmias may otherwise go unnoticed.

Administration of bicarbonate should be reserved for specific situations including the following: (1) pH less than 7.1, (2) serum bicarbonate less than 5 mEq/L, or (3) comatose state.

These situations warrant treatment on the basis that central nervous system depression and myocardial contractility are reduced in the face of severe acidosis. In all other situations, restoration of normal carbohydrate metabolism is accompanied by bicarbonate generation, thus restoring a normal pH. If bicarbonate is needed, 1 or 2 ampules (44 or 88 mEq) should be *added* to a *hypotonic* solution for infusion. The bicarbonate should *not* be given by intravenous push. The pH should be checked 2 to 3 hours later. If the pH is still below 7.25, more bicarbonate may be given. Also, a central venous pressure catheter should be placed in patients with evidence of renal or cardiac impairment. A Foley catheter should be placed in comatose patients and in those unable to produce urine in a 3- to 4-hour period. However, routine insertion of a Foley catheter is probably not necessary, for it exposes the patient to increased risks of urinary tract infection.

Once therapy with fluids and insulin has begun and the patient has been stabilized, further evaluation should be directed toward the identification of precipitating factors for the acute episode. Since infection is a common precipitating factor in the development of ketoacidosis, a chest x-ray film with shielding, sputum for Gram stain, white blood count with differential, blood cultures, and spinal tap should also be taken. A urine specimen should be obtained for culture and sensitivity, microscopic examination, and Gram stain. Aggressive antibiotic treatment should be instituted if evidence suggestive of infection is found.

The following testing schedule should be observed: blood sugar levels repeated hourly, urine spot checks hourly, serum ketones every 2 to 4 hours, arterial blood gases every 4 hours, and electrolyte concentrations every 2 to 4 hours. A flow sheet including the measurements just mentioned is a functional way to collate the large volume of data accumulated as a result of treatment of a patient with ketoacidosis.

When a downward trend is established in blood glucose levels, fluid administration should be changed to solutions containing 5% dextrose to avoid the development of hypoglycemia and to provide adequate carbohydrate substrates to replenish the liver glycogen stores that ultimately serve as the protector against ketogenesis.

The goals in the acute management of a patient with ketoacidosis include (1) restoration of the normal glycemia of pregnancy, (2) restoration of total body fluid losses, usually indicated by return of weight to previous levels, (3) return of normal electrolyte levels, and (4) elimination of ketone bodies from blood and urine. When these goals have been achieved, the patient can be returned to her diet, and an insulin dosage can be reinstituted for long-term therapy.

Preterm labor

Management of preterm labor in the pregnant diabetic patient is especially difficult. As discussed in Chapter 3, beta mimetic agents (eg, terbutaline, ritodrine) have been used with success in attempts to arrest premature uterine muscle activity.[5,78,84] These agents have not been used in a controlled study of preterm labor in diabetic patients. Their use in this group is limited by the fact that the beta mimetic action of these drugs antagonizes the endogenous release of maternal insulin and causes accelerated lipolysis and increased glycogenolysis, making blood glucose regulation difficult.

Corticosteroids have been used in attempts to accelerate fetal lung maturation in nondiabetic patients at risk of imminent preterm delivery, also discussed in Chapter 3. Use of these potent insulin antagonists in the diabetic patient is also limited, but a small series of infants born of diabetic mothers has been reported to have benefited from their use.[88] Maternal glucose control can suffer greatly, however, and some evidence suggests that corticosteroids may impair fetal insulin release and produce fetal islet degeneration.[11] Nonetheless, the risks associated with beta mimetic and glucocorticoid administration need to be weighed against the neonatal hazards when the infant of a diabetic mother is delivered before term. Temporary difficulties in managing blood sugar levels may be acceptable in these circumstances.

Premature rupture of the membranes

Premature rupture of the membranes is discussed in Chapter 4 in detail. This complication of pregnancy is an especially difficult problem in diabetic patients. The first question to be asked in any case of premature rupture of the membranes is whether or not the patient is at increased risk for developing an infection and if it does develop, whether or not the patient is at an increased risk for unusual severity of the disease. For the diabetic patient the answer is affirmative. Thus in all but rare instances premature rupture of the membranes in a diabetic patient should be managed with plans calling for delivery.

■ REFERENCES

1. Abell DA, Beischer NA, Papas AJ, et al: The association between abnormal glucose tolerance (hyperglycemia and hypoglycemia) and estriol excretion in pregnancy. Am J Obstet Gynecol 1976;124:388.

2. Adam PAJ, Schwarts R: Should oral hypoglycemic agents be used in pediatric and pregnant patients? Pediatrics 1968;42:819.

3. Assemany SR, Muzzo S, Gardner LI: Syndrome of phocomelic diabetic embryopathy (caudal dysplasia). Am J Dis Child 1972;123:489.

4. Bashore RA, Westbake JR: Plasma unconjugated estriol values in high-risk pregnancy. Am J Obstet Gynecol 1977;128:371.

5. Borberg C, Gillmer MDG, Beard RW, et al: Metabolic effects of betasympathomimetic drugs and dexamethasone in normal and diabetic pregnancy. Br J Obstet Gynaecol 1978;85:184.

6. Camerini-Davalos RA, Caulfield JB, Rees SB: Preliminary observations on subjects with prediabetes. Diabetes 1963;12:508.

7. Chen WW, Sese L, Tantakasen P, et al: Pregnancy associated with renal glucosuria. Obstet Gynecol 1976; 47:37.

8. Christensen PJ: Tubular reabsorption of glucose during pregnancy. Scand J Clin Lab Invest 1958;10:364.

9. Churchhill JA, Berendes, HW, Nemore J: Neurophysiological deficits in children of diabetic mothers. Am J Obstet Gynecol 1969;105:257.

10. Coetzee EJ, Jackson WPU, Berman PA: Ketonuria in pregnancy—with special reference to calorie-restricted food intake in obese diabetics. Diabetes 1980;29:177.

11. Colle E, Goldman H: Effect of glucocorticoids on insulin release from human fetal islets. Diabetes 1976;25(suppl. 1):359.

12. Cousins L, Rigg L, Hollingsworth D, et al: The 24-hour excursion and diurnal rhythm of glucose, insulin and C-peptide in normal pregnancy. Am J Obstet Gynecol 1980;136:483.

13. Coustan DR, Berkowitz RL, Hobbins JC: Tight metabolic control of overt diabetes in pregnancy. Am J Med 1980;68:845.

14. Cunningham MD, Desai NS, Thompson SA, et al: Amniotic fluid phosphatidyl glycerol in diabetic pregnancies. Am J Obstet Gynecol 1978;131:719.

15. Data S, Brown WU: Acid-base status in diabetic mothers and their infants following general or spinal anesthesia for cesarean section. Anesthesiology 1977;47:272.

16. Dingh EJ, Mejia A, Zuspan FP: Studies of human amniotic fluid in normal, diabetic and drug-abuse pregnancy. Am J Obstet Gynecol 1974;119:623.

17. Distler W, Gabbe SG, Freeman RK, et al: Estriol in pregnancy: V. Unconjugated and total plasma estriol levels in comparison to 24-hour urinary estriol and creatinine excretion in the management of diabetic pregnancies. Am J Obstet Gynecol 1978;130:424.

18. Drew JH, Abell DA, Beischer NA: Congenital malformations, abnormal glucose tolerance and estriol excretion in pregnancy. Obstet Gynecol 1978;51:129.

19. Duenhoelter JH, Whalley PJ, McDonald PC: An analysis of the utility of plasma immunoreactive estrogen measurements in determining delivery time of gravidas with a fetus considered at high risk. Am J Obstet Gynecol 1976;125:889.

20. Farquhar JW: Prognosis for babies born to diabetic mothers in Edinburgh. Arch Dis Child 1969;44:36.

21. Farrel PM, Avery ME: Hyaline membrane disease. Am Rev Respir Dis 1975;111:657.

22. Flood TM: Diet and diabetes mellitus. Hosp Pract, February 1979, pp. 61-69.

23. Gabbe SG: Application of scientific rationale to the management of the pregnant diabetic. Semin Perinatol 1978;2:361.

24. Gabbe SG, Lowensohn RI, Mestman, JH, et al: Lecithin/sphyngomyelin ratio in pregnancies complicated by diabetes mellitus. Am J Obstet Gynecol 1975;128:757.

25. Gabbe SG, Mestman JH, Freeman RK, et al: Management and outcome of class A diabetes mellitus. Am J Obstet Gynecol 1977;127:465.

26. Gabbe SG, Mestman JH, Freeman RK, et al: Management and outcome of pregnancy in diabetes mellitus, class B to R. Am J Obstet Gynecol 1978;129:723.

27. Gillmer MDG, Oakley NW, Brooke FM, et al: Metabolic profiles in pregnancy. Isr J Med Sci 1975;11:601.

28. Gluck L, Kulovich MV: Lecithin/sphyngomyelin ratios in amniotic fluid in normal and abnormal pregnancy. Am J Obstet Gynecol 1973;115:539.

29. Goebelsman U, Freeman RK, Mestman JH, et al: Estriol in pregnancy: II. Daily urinary estriol in the management of the pregnant diabetic woman. Am J Obstet Gynecol 1973;115:795.

30. Granat M, Sharf MM, Cooper A: Glucose intolerance during pregnancy: I. A reappraisal of alleged screening criteria. Obstet Gynecol 1979;53:157.

31. Hare JW, White P: Pregnancy in diabetes complicated by vascular disease. Diabetes 1977;26:953.

32. Hercules BL, Wozwncroft M, Gayed II, et al: Peripheral retinal ablation in the treatment of proliferative diabetic retinopathy during pregnancy. Br J Ophthalmol 1980; 64:87.

33. Hill DE: Effect of insulin on fetal growth. Semin Perinatol 1978;2:317.

34. Holms L, Driscroll SG, Atkins L: Etiologic heterogeneity of neural tube defects. N Engl J Med 1976; 294:365.

35. Horvat M, Maclean H, Goldberg L, et al: Diabetic retinopathy in pregnancy: a 12-year prospective survey. Br J Ophthalmol 1980;64:398-403.

36. Hytten FE, Thompson MA: Maternal physiologic adjustments, in National Academy of Sciences, Committee on Maternal Nutrition: Maternal Nutrition and the Course of Pregnancy. Washington, D.C., The Academy, 1970.

37. Jovanovic J, Peterson CM, Saxena BB, et al: Feasibility of maintaining normal glucose profiles in insulin-dependent pregnant diabetic women. Am J Med 1980; 68:105.

38. Karlsson K, Kjellmer I: The outcome of diabetic pregnancies in relation to the mother's blood sugar level. Am J Obstet Gynecol 1972;112:213.

39. Kitzmiller JL, Cloherty JP, Younger MD, et al: Diabetic pregnancy and perinatal morbidity. Am J Obstet Gynecol 1978;131:560.

40. Kjaergaard JJ, Ditzel J: Hemoglobin A₁c as an index of long-term blood glucose regulation in diabetic pregnancy. Diabetes 1979;28:694.

41. Kolterman OG, Greenfield M, Reaven GM, et al: Effect of high carbohydrate diet on insulin binding to adipocytes and on insulin action in vivo in man. Diabetes 1979;28:731.

42. Kreisberg RA: Diabetes ketoacidosis: new concepts and trends in pathogenesis and treatment. Ann Intern Med 1978;88:681.

43. Kucera J: Rate and type of congenital anomalies among offspring of diabetic women. J Reprod Med 1979;7:61.

44. Kyle GC: Diabetes and pregnancy. Ann Intern Med 1963;59(suppl. 3):15.

45. Leslie RDG, John PN, Pyke DA, et al: Hemoglobin A₁ in diabetic pregnancy. Lancet 1978;2:958.

46. Leveno KJ, Hauth JC, Gilstrap LC, et al: Appraisal of "rigid" blood glucose control during pregnancy in the overtly diabetic woman. Am J Obstet Gynecol 1979;135:853.

47. Light IJ, Keenan WJ, and Sutherland JM: Maternal intravenous glucose administration as a cause of hypoglycemia in the infant of the diabetic mother. Am J Obstet Gynecol 1972;113:345.

48. Lowensohn RI, Gabbe SG: The value of lecithin/sphingomyelin ratios in diabetes: a critical review. Am J Obstet Gynecol 1979;134:702.

49. Mann JI: Diet and diabetes. Diabetologia 1980;18:89.

50. Marble A: Early stages of the diabetic state: definitions and concepts, in Camerini-Davalos RA, Cole HS (eds): *Advances in Diabetes*. New York, Academic Press, Inc., 1970, p. 255.

51. Marble A, White P, Bradley RF: *Joslin's Diabetes Mellitus*. Philadelphia, Lea & Febinger, 1971, pp. 581-598.

52. McIntyre N, Holdsworth CD, Turner DS: Intestinal factors in the control of insulin secretion. J Clin Endocrinol Metab 1965;25:1317.

53. Mills JC, Baker L, Guldman AS: Malformations in infants of diabetic mothers occur before the seventh gestational week: implications for treatment. Diabetes 1979;28:292.

54. Milner RDG, Wirdnam PK, Tsanadas J: Quantitative morphology of B, A, D, and PP cells in infants of diabetic mothers. Diabetes 1981;30:271.

55. Mintz DH, Skyler JS, Chez RA: Diabetes mellitus and pregnancy. Diabetes Care 1978;1:49.

56. Mueller-Huebach E, Caritis SN, Edelstone DI, et al: Lecithin/sphyngomyelin ratio in amniotic fluid and its value for the prediction of neonatal respiratory distress syndrome in pregnant women. Am J Obstet Gynecol 1978;130:28.

57. Naeye RL, Chez RA: Effects of maternal acetonuria and low pregnancy weight gain on children's psychomotor development. Am J Obstet Gynecol 1981;139:189.

58. Oh W: Neonatal care and long-term outcome of infants of diabetic mothers, in, Merkatz IR, Adam P (eds): *The diabetic pregnancy: a perinatal perspective*. New York, Grune and Stratton, Inc., 1979, pp. 195-205.

59. Olefsky JM, Farquhar JW, Reaven GM: Do the oral and intravenous glucose tolerance tests provide similar diagnostic information in the patients with chemical diabetes mellitus? Diabetes 1972;22:202.

60. O'Sullivan JB, Gellis SS, Dandrow RV, et al: The potential diabetic and her treatment in pregnancy. Obstet Gynecol 1966;27:683.

61. O'Sullivan JB, Mahan CM: Criteria for the oral glucose tolerance test in pregnancy. Diabetes 1964;13:278.

62. O'Sullivan JB, Mahan CM, Charles D, et al: Screening criteria for high-risk gestational diabetic patients. Am J Obstet Gynecol 1973;116:895.

63. Page EW: Human fetal nutrition and growth. Am J Obstet Gynecol 1969;104:378.

64. Paulsen EP, Courtney JW, Duckworth WC: Insulin resistance caused by massive degradation of subcutaneous insulin. Diabetes 1979;28:640.

65. Pearson JR, Weaver JB: Fetal activity and fetal wellbeing: an evaluation. Br Med J 1976;1:1305.

66. Pedersen J: *The pregnant diabetic and her newborn*. Copenhagen, Munsgaard, 1977, pp. 191-196.

67. Pedersen J, Pedersen LM: Prognosis of the outcome of pregnancy in diabetes: a new classification. Acta Endocrinol 1965;50:70.

68. Persson B, Lunell NO: Metabolic control in diabetic pregnancy. Am J Obstet Gynecol 1975;122:737.

69. Richard P, Schiffrin BS, Goupil F, et al: Nonstressed fetal heart rate monitoring in the antepartum period. Am J Obstet Gynecol 1976;126:699.

70. Rigg L, Cousins L, Hollingsworth D, et al: Effects of exogenous insulin on excursions and diurnal rhythm of plasma glucose in pregnant diabetic patients with and without residual B-cell function. Am J Obstet Gynecol 1980;136:537.

71. Robert MF, Neff RD, Hubbell JP, et al: Association between maternal diabetes and the respiratory distress syndrome in the newborn. N Engl J Med 1976;294:357.

72. Rodman HM, Singerman LJ, Aiello LM, et al: Diabetic retinopathy and its relationship to pregnancy, in Merkatz IR, Adam PA (eds): *The Diabetic Pregnancy: a Perinatal Perspective*. New York, Grune and Stratton, Inc., 1979, pp. 73-91.

73. Roversi GD, Gargiulo M, Nicolini U, et al: A new approach to the treatment of diabetic pregnant women: report of 479 cases seen from 1963 to 1975. Am J Obstet Gynecol 1979;135:567.

74. Rowland TW, Hubbell JP, Nodas AS: Congenital heart disease in infants of diabetic mothers. J Pediatr 1973; 83:815.

75. Rubens R, Carilier A, Thiery M, et al: Pregnancy complicated by insulinoma. Br J Obstet Gynaecol 1977;84:543.

76. Rusnak SL, Driscoll SG: Congenital spinal anomalies in infants of diabetic mothers. Pediatrics 1966;35:989.

77. Sadovsky E, Yaffe H: Daily fetal movement recording and fetal prognosis. Obstet Gynecol 1973;41:845.

78. Schilthuis MS, Aarnoudse JG: Fetal death associated with severe ritodrine induced ketoacidosis. Lancet 1980;1:1145.

79. Schmidt PL, Thorneycroft IH, Goebelsmann U: Fetal distress following a reactive nonstress test. Am J Obstet Gynecol 1980;136:960.

80. Silfen SL, Wapner RJ, Gabbe SG: Maternal outcome in class H diabetes mellitus. Obstet Gynecol 1980;55:749.

81. Simpson JL: Genetics of diabetes mellitus and anomalies in offspring of diabetic mothers. Semin Perinatol 1978;2:383.

82. Smith DW: *Recognizable Patterns of Human Malformation: Genetic, Embryologic and Clinical Aspects*, Philadelphia, WB Saunders, Co., 1970, p. 5.

83. Sosenko ER, Kitzmiller JL, Loo SW, et al: The infant of the diabetic mother: correlation of increased cord C-peptide levels with macrosomia and hypoglycemia. N Engl J Med 1979;301:859.

84. Steel JM, Parboosingh J: Insulin requirements in pregnant diabetics with premature labour controlled by ritodrine. Br Med J 1970;1:880.

85. Stehbens JA, Baker GL, Kitchell M: Outcome at ages 1, 3, 5 years of children born to diabetic women. Am J Obstet Gynecol 1977;127:408.

86. Stubbs WA, Stubbs SM: Hyperinsulinism, diabetes mellitus, and respiratory distress of the newborn: a common link? Lancet 1978;1:308.

87. Sutherland HW, Stowers JM, McKenzie C: Simplifying the clinical problem of glucosuria in pregnancy. Lancet 1970;1:1069.

88. Sutton C: Practical approach to problems of the parturient diabetic in developing countries. Br Med J 1977;2:1069.

89. Welsh GW: The mechanisms of renal glycosuria in pregnancy. Diabetes 1960;9:363.

90. White P: Pregnancy complicating diabetes. Am J Med 1949;7:609.

91. WhiteP: Childhood diabetes: its course and influence on the second and third generations. Diabetes 1960; 9:345.

92. White P: Classification of obstetric diabetes. Am J Obstet Gynecol 1978;130:228.

93. Widness JA, Schwartz HC, Thompson D, et al: Glycohemoglobin (Hb A_{1c}): a predictor of birth weight in infants of diabetic mothers. J Pediatr 1978;92:8.

94. Widness JA, Susa JB, Garcia JF, et al: Increased erythropoiesis and elevated erythropoietin in infants born to diabetic mothers. Diabetes 1981;30:271.

95. Williams PR, Sperling MA, Racasa Z: Blunting of spontaneous and alanine-stimulated glucagon secretion in newborn infants of diabetic mothers. Am J Obstet Gynecol 1979;133:51.

96. Yeast JD, Porreco RP, Ginsberg HN: The use of continuous insulin infusion for the peripartum management of pregnant diabetic women. Am J Obstet Gynecol 1978;131:861.

97. Zerowitz H, Newhouse S: Renal glycosuria in normoglycemic glycosuric pregnancy: a quantitative study. Metabolism 1973;22:755.

8

■ ■ ■

INTRAUTERINE GROWTH
RETARDATION

Elliott K. Main

Intrauterine growth retardation (IUGR) is an important and particularly challenging problem for modern obstetricians. It is a cause of significant perinatal morbidity and mortality and may have profound postnatal sequelae. Depending on the definition used, IUGR affects 2% to 10% of all pregnancies. Further, it is estimated that IUGR accounts for as much as 25% of all perinatal morbidity and mortality. One third of all infants less than 2500 grams at birth are growth retarded.[79] Unfortunately, the diagnosis of IUGR is difficult and often elusive until birth. In most modern series, fewer than 50% of all small for gestational age (SGA) infants have been diagnosed prenatally.

Many advances have been made in recent years in diagnosis, risk assessment, and management of IUGR. These advances are reviewed together with some concepts of etiology, neonatal problems, and long-term follow-up care.

■ DEFINITION

It was not until the late 1950s and early 1960s that pediatricians and then obstetricians began to identify a group of low birth weight babies (less than 2500 grams at birth) that was not truly premature (born before 37 weeks of gestation). Different investigators coined their own terms to refer to this condition, and the following syn-

onyms proliferated: IUGR, SGA, small for dates, chronic fetal distress, fetal malnutrition, and dysmaturity. The identification of this group of babies was based on the development of norms for newborn weight, head circumference, and length at varying gestational ages and on the widespread use of Dubowitz and other examinations for rapid and accurate estimates of gestational age in the newborn.

For a newborn to be classified as IUGR most studies require the infant weight to be below the 10th percentile or less than 2 SDs from the mean weight for gestational age. The most commonly used reference chart in the United States is the Colorado Growth Chart developed in Denver by Lubchenco et al.[54] However, babies born in Denver at over 5000 feet in altitude do weigh significantly less than infants born at sea level. In fact, the 10th percentile in the Colorado chart corresponds to about the 3rd or 4th percentile of weights of infants born at sea level.[83] Other birth weight standards are from Baltimore, Chapel Hill, Montreal, Portland, and the Collaborative Perinatal Project that involved 12 hospitals throughout the United States.

There are several problems beside altitude with all the studies just mentioned except the collaborative study. Only one study actually examined the infant's maturity, whereas the others used the date of the last menstrual period with or without additional corroborative information from the obstetric history to establish gestational age. Naeye and Dixon,[58] using the computerized data on 48,239 single births from the Collaborative Perinatal Project, identified two other important biases. First, they found that the estimation of gestational age is often incorrect by a 1- or 2-month interval because of bleeding patterns following conception. Second, all the growth charts include data on infants who subsequently died, many of whom were growth retarded and hence distort the normal curve. They then constructed a growth chart eliminating the monthly clusters and the data from nonsurvivors and found that the mean weight for each week of gestation was quite comparable to other sea level studies. Most important, this method allowed them to reduce the standard errors (hence shrink the normal range), especially for the preterm infants. Naeye's and Dixon's study is in agreement with both animal data and other human studies and demonstrates that most placental disorders, as well as maternal caloric deprivation, exert their largest effect late in the third trimester, which is also the time when normal growth tapers off leading to a relatively wide range for normalcy at term. Preterm infants have had fewer extrinsic effects on their fetal growth pattern and therefore should have a narrower weight range.

Another problem with using population growth standards to identify individual retardation is that they fail to diagnose infants who are genetically determined to have a birth weight large for gestational age (LGA) but who suffer the influences of a limiting intrauterine environment and are born, for example, at the 20th percentile. These infants were afflicted with IUGR and in fact may develop the common neonatal sequelae. Similarly, infants genetically small are automatically included in the high-risk group without being at increased risk. Turner[82] demonstrated that if standard growth charts were used, the diagnosis of IUGR in one half of these babies would be missed. One alternative approach may be to use the well-known phenomenon of concordance of sibling birth weight. Examining sibships of 54 children who had a firm diagnosis of rubella embryopathy, Turner found that although 41% of affected infants fell below the 10th percentile (Colorado Growth Chart),

80% fell below 2 SDs of the corrected mean birth weights of their siblings.

Overall, the percentile birth weight charts are quick and easy to use and give uniformity to the diagnosis. If the practitioner understands the limitations of this diagnostic tool, exceptions can be better identified and a chart can be chosen to fit the altitude of the patient population. For most areas, however, Naeye's curve seems to eliminate many significant biases. Identification and definition of growth retardation in utero require different terminology and are reviewed in the section on diagnosis.

■ ETIOLOGY

In most reviews there are long lists of potential causes of IUGR. A large number of these are quite rare or the product of case reports and therefore have limited usefulness to the practitioner. A more useful approach for evaluating IUGR is to identify a time span at a hospital and examine all the SGA infants born in that period. Relative incidences and severity of risks can then be calculated. Four large studies have used this approach.[25,50,65,78] They examined over 17,000 deliveries and found 830 IUGR infants. In only 50% of these infants could maternal diseases, maternal drug addiction, or obstetric complications be identified. The similarity of the results of each of these four studies is striking. A large and recent survey is from Galbraith et al in Kingston, Ontario.[25] They presented a series of 8030 births over a 4-year period with 395 cases (4.9%) of IUGR not attributable to congenital anomalies. They were able to identify risk factors in previous and present pregnancies that are useful in isolating segments of the population requiring further perinatal study. These factors are presented in detail along with the relative incidences of IUGR for each subcategory in Table 8-1.

Etiologies for growth retardation have been categorized in a number of ways.[68] A useful approach is to look at the source of the insult (intrinsic versus extrinsic) and at the recipient of the deficit (fetus, placenta, or both). Intrinsic defects arise in the fetus, whereas the extrinsic environmental influences usually attack both fetus and placenta. Furthermore, a specific group of diseases involves a decrease in fetoplacental perfusion.

Pediatricians have noted two basic types of

TABLE 8-1 ■ Incidence of IUGR in relation to different risk factors

	Percent incidence* of IUGR in present pregnancy
Complications occurring in previous pregnancies	
IUGR	20
Recurrent abortion	11
Fetal death	9.4
Neonatal death	9.4
Preterm	9
Congenital anomalies	8
Maternal medical complications	
Mild to moderate hypertension	12
Severe hypertension	44
Nephritis	21
Urinary tract infection	8
Cardiopulmonary disease	15
Complications occurring in present pregnancy	
Mild to moderate toxemia	10.5
Severe toxemia	31
First trimester bleeding	8
First trimester bleeding with recurrence	11
Second trimester bleeding	8
Second trimester bleeding with recurrence	12
Third trimester bleeding	11
Multiple pregnancy	21
Preterm delivery	11

Modified from Galbraith RS, Karchmar EJ, Piercy WN, Am J Obstet Gynecol 1979;133:281.
*Percent of present pregnancies that will result in IUGR if the factor was or is present.

IUGR babies: (1) *symmetrically* small babies who are proportional in all body measurements and have few problems in the perinatal period and (2) *asymmetrically* retarded babies whose soft tissues are wasted, whose liver size is markedly reduced, and who have disproportionate anthropomorphic measurements—the head is preserved and the body is starved. These babies are at high risk in the perinatal period.

Diseases producing inadequate uteroplacental blood flow are the causes of asymmetric retardation, whereas all the other intrinsic and extrinsic influences lead to symmetric retardation (see box on p. 151). As in any biologic process,

there is overlapping between classifications, but in IUGR the fit is actually quite close.

The importance of this classification is increased by the ability to identify distinctive growth patterns in utero. By using ultrasonic measurements of the fetal head, obstetricians have noted two types of abnormal growth patterns.[10] The *low growth profile* pattern shows measurements for the fetal head that are chronically below 2 SDs from the mean values obtained in a normal population (Fig. 8-1) but grow in a somewhat parallel manner. In contrast, the *late flattening* pattern shows normal fetal head growth during the first 30 to 34 weeks of gestation but little or no growth during the following weeks (Fig. 8-2). These patterns correlate with the symmetric and asymmetric types of growth retardation respectively.

Most series in developed nations have shown that the asymmetric form of IUGR is the most prevalent, and 70% to 90% of all SGA infants are this type. Perhaps the index of suspicion for growth retardation is lower when the neonate is proportionally smaller, and a number of these symmetric IUGR infants go unrecognized. Conversely, in developing countries from 20% to 40% of infants are low birth weight (less than 2500 grams); most are born at term (80%) and the majority are symmetric.[8]

Causes of symmetric growth retardation

Genetic. A compelling evidence of genetic influences on suboptimal fetal growth is that sisters of women who had IUGR infants also tend to have SGA infants. In the famous series of Ounsted and Ounsted[64] the siblings of SGA probands were all small; in fact, the mothers themselves tended to be small at their own birth.

In general, single gene mutations do not affect fetal size nearly as consistently as chromosomal disorders.[42] For example, phenylketonuric (PKU) infants born to homozygous mothers are almost universally growth retarded, whereas homozygous infants born to heterozygous parents are mixed.[69] Other syndromes commonly associated with SGA infants include Cornelia De Lange, osteogenesis imperfecta, and familial dysautonomia.[42]

IUGR is a common finding in most chromosomal abnormalities with the exception of Klinefelter's and the XXX and XXXX syndromes. Growth arrest is most accentuated in trisomy 18

Etiology of IUGR

Symmetric	Asymmetric
Frequency: 10% to 30% Ultrasound: low growth profile Basic pathology: intrinsic or environmental insult	Frequency: 70% to 90% Ultrasound: late flattening Basic pathology: placental insufficiency

Symmetric

CHROMOSOMAL ANOMALIES

Trisomy 18 and D
Down's syndrome
Cri du chat
Turner's syndrome

GENETIC SYNDROMES

Phenylketonuria
Familial dysautonomia
Cornelia de Lange
Osteogenesis imperfecta
Aminoaciduria
Progeria

CONGENITAL ABNORMALITIES

Microcephaly
Single umbilical artery
Multiple anomalies (Potter's, etc.)
Congenital heart disease

INTRAUTERINE INFECTIONS

Rubella
Toxoplasmosis
Herpes
Syphilis
Cytomegalovirus

SEVERE MALNUTRITION

Famine
Gastric bypass surgery
Severe folate deficiency

RADIATION

MATERNAL HABITS

Ethanol
Tobacco
Heroin
Methadone

MATERNAL MEDICATION

Antimetabolites
Alkylating agents
Coumadin
Steroids
Propranolol

MATERNAL HYPOXIC DISEASE

Cyanotic congenital heart disease
Hemoglobinopathies
Severe asthma
High altitude

Asymmetric

MATERNAL VASCULAR DISEASE

Toxemia
Chronic hypertension
Collagen vascular disease
Advanced stage diabetes
Hemoglobinopathies

MULTIPLE PREGNANCIES

Discordant twins
Transfusion syndrome

PLACENTAL MALFORMATIONS

Abnormal insertion
Hemangiomas
Multiple infarcts

THIRD TRIMESTER BLEEDING

Placenta previa
Unknown origin

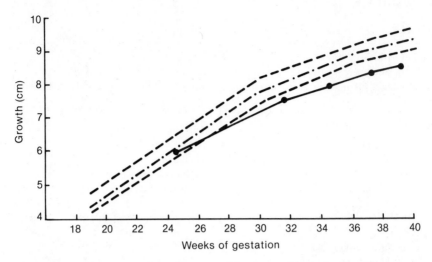

FIG. 8-1 ■ Ultrasonic low growth profile type of fetal growth retardation. Characteristically there is continuous growth of the fetal biparietal diameter, but the growth curve remains below the 10th percentile of normal.

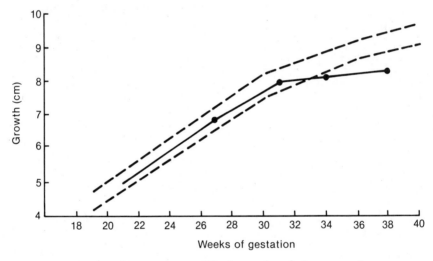

FIG. 8-2 ■ Ultrasonic late flattening type of fetal growth retardation. In these patients the fetal biparietal diameter growth ceases completely, usually after 32 or 34 weeks of gestation.

and D and is a common finding in Down's and Turner's syndromes. The actual mechanism of growth arrest remains speculative, but it is clearly part of an intrinsic continuum of developmental failure, abortion, stillbirth, early neonatal death, childhood failure to thrive, and markedly diminished life span.[42]

An increased frequency of congenital malformations has long been noted in infants with IUGR. This increase occurs entirely within the symmetric group and can range as high as 33%[48] as shown in the following material.*

Pattern of retardation		Number and percent of malformed babies
Symmetric	24	8 (33%)
Asymmetric	94	3 (3.2%)
TOTAL	118	11 (9.3%)

*From Kurjak A, Latin V, Polak J: J Perinat Med 1978; 6:102.

Asymmetric infants have an overall malformation rate of 3% to 4% that is consistent with that found in the general population. The biggest association of IUGR is with defects of the central nervous system (CNS) and Potter's syndrome. A large percentage of infants with one umbilical artery have IUGR. Every symmetrically retarded infant needs to be screened carefully for the presence of congenital anomalies.

Intrauterine infection. It was not until the rubella epidemics of 1963 that solid data showed that intrauterine viral infection led to growth retardation. Infection and disease, however, are not necessarily synonymous. For example, although it is clear that cytomegalovirus (CMV) can cause obvious IUGR, it is equally evident that 90% of babies infected in utero and shedding the virus at birth appear perfectly normal in the neonatal period and are adequate for gestational age (AGA).[44] There is less clear evidence that other TORCH agents can cause IUGR. Herpes, toxoplasmosis, and syphilis are all suspected of being related to IUGR, but the association is difficult to prove. Symmetrically retarded infants should be screened for hepatosplenomegaly, jaundice, hemolytic anemia, petechia, thrombocytopenia, signs of acute CNS involvement, signs of chronic CNS involvement (microcephaly, cerebral atrophy, or intracranial calcifications), myocarditis, and pneumonitis. In nonepidemic years infections represent a rare cause of IUGR and carry a particularly poor prognosis.

Severe maternal malnutrition. No topic has so much controversy and vested emotions as the relation between maternal nutrition and birth weight. The two most famous observational studies date back to World War II. The 18-month siege of Leningrad provided conditions of extreme hardship.[2] The diet consisted mainly of bread and water, and thousands died of starvation. In the first half of 1942 average birth weight fell 530 grams, and the incidence of infants with birth weights less than 2500 grams was 49%. During the siege the women were exposed to a number of other severe strains. The possible contribution of excessive physical exercise, lack of rest, and constant nervous tension cannot be easily assessed.

In the Dutch "famine winter" of 1944 to 1945 food deprivation occurred in a sharply demar-

cated time period and was accompanied by fewer and less severe privations of other kinds.[75] Birth records reveal a decline in birth weights to a nadir after 20 weeks of famine and an immediate rise after the end of the famine. Further analysis of the data shows that the greatest risk of low birth weight was in mothers exposed in the second half of pregnancy, whereas in the first 20 weeks of gestation the fetus seemed well protected.

Observational surveys have provided little valid information, however, as poor nutrition is generally found together with many other causes of growth retardation that cannot be easily separated. In a recent review, Stein et al[76] examined eight *controlled* studies carried out during the last decade. The best that they could conclude was that among women at risk of delivering SGA infants, prenatal nutritional supplementation can lead to only a modest rise in birth weight of about 50 grams. The rise in birth weight seemed to be proportional to the woman's baseline nutritional status: a starved person benefits most; a heavier woman is unlikely to have any benefit. In practice this means that a mother needs to suffer severe malnutrition before the fetus loses weight.

One clinical situation that occurs fairly often is the patient who has had a gastrointestinal bypass procedure for morbid obesity. Studies of pregnancies in these women have shown that 20% to 40% of their babies are SGA. Further, in one large series, 92% of babies were lighter than any previous term infant born before the bypass.[39] Maternal hypoalbuminemia correlates well with IUGR. Although serum albumin levels are reduced during normal pregnancies (by as much as 20% in second trimester), mothers who had a gastrointestinal bypass had even lower levels: over 60% had albumin concentrations below 3.5 g/dl, and when these levels fell below 3.0 g/dl, there was a high prevalence of SGA babies.[39] This relation is further supported by the work of Stein[74] who examined protein depletion in mothers of low birth weight infants and found an increasing incidence of IUGR with decreasing serum albumin. Thus a pregnant woman with a markedly reduced serum albumin (less than 2.5) requires intensive evaluation for IUGR, and a mother with a moderate reduction (less than 3.0) should be watched closely.

Radiation. Radiation exposure to the extent of causing significant decrements in fetal growth or development is rare with modern safeguarded equipment and a high suspicion of pregnancy. Nearly all radiation injuries to the fetus come from therapeutic, not diagnostic radiology. Like chromosomal anomalies, radiation injury to the fetus leads to a spectrum of problems: spontaneous abortions, congenital abnormalities, reduced birth weight, and impaired postnatal function, all seeming to form a continuum. For fetal growth to be significantly affected by radiation, the insult needs to be at the time of most rapid division of cells, which is in the first trimester. The ultrasonic growth pattern when seen is the "low growth profile." Although most authors warn that there may not be a threshold for radiation effects, none have seen any malformation at fetal doses less than 25 rads. Several argue for a 10-rad "cutoff" (usual fetal dose in typical barium enema study is 1.3 rads), but all agree that radiation exposure should be kept at an absolute minimum during pregnancy.[1]

Maternal habits. Maternal addictive habits have been clearly associated with reduced fetal growth. A large body of literature has implicated cigarette smoking with statistically significant reduction of newborn weight of 150 to 400 grams, and heavy smoking has been linked to frank IUGR.[40] Others have noted increased maternal blood levels of carboxyhemoglobin, acute decreases in intravillous blood flow in the placenta after smoking, and depressed fetal breathing movements. Finally, a study from India[46] suggests that tobacco chewing gravidas are at great risk for stillbirth and growth retardation, meaning that nicotine alone may be a culprit as well as carboxyhemoglobin.

A "fetal alcohol syndrome" has recently been identified.[41] In one series of 76 cases of alcoholic embryopathy IUGR was the most common feature occurring in 91% of these infants. The effect seems to be dose dependent with noticeable effects even when 1 ounce of absolute alcohol is consumed per day.[34]

Heroin-addicted mothers also have a documented high incidence of IUGR in the range of 25% to 35%.[88] The mechanism is unclear, but several studies have indicated that the reduction in cell growth is not secondary to poor nutrition as had been postulated. Animal studies also implicate chronic morphine administration as a

cause of SGA infants.[40] The use of methadone can reduce this high incidence of IUGR, but such a solution can lead to additional problems. Although the incidence of growth retardation may be lowered by at least one third in methadone-treated gravidas, neonatal withdrawal symptoms are typically more severe.[91]

Maternal medication. A group of medications that would be expected to be associated with IUGR is cancer chemotherapeutic agents. DNA inhibitors, such as cytosine arabinoside and 6-thioguanine, and folic acid antagonists (aminopterin and methotrexate) have all been associated with symmetric growth retardation.

Anticonvulsants as a group are probably associated with a syndrome like fetal alcohol syndrome, although the most incriminating evidence points to phenytoin (Dilantin). This area is quite controversial in the pediatric literature.[33,72,77]

Coumadin, particularly in the first trimester, is associated with a series of birth defects and growth retardation.[71] In fact, this is a recurring pattern in teratology; drugs causing malformations can lead to stunted growth even at lower dosages and shorter durations.

There are reports linking propranolol, a beta-blocking agent, to growth retardation.[27] This has been suggested in humans and in rats and may be dose dependent. Placental weights have been reduced by up to 30%. It is tempting to speculate that the beta blocking agent leads to increased uterine vascular tone and hence less uteroplacental perfusion, although this has yet to be demonstrated.

Maternal hypoxic disease. Most pregnancies complicated by maternal congenital heart disease with right-to-left shunting and cyanosis result in growth retarded infants.[67] The most common example is tetralogy of Fallot. Eisenmenger's syndrome, especially with significant pulmonary hypertension, leads to IUGR if the mother and fetus survive.[28] Outcome is directly proportional to arterial oxygen saturation and to the degree of polycythemia.[67] Likewise, severe asthma has been reported to be associated with SGA babies.

Anemia from any etiology, especially if severe, can lead to relative hypoxia and hence to IUGR. Hemoglobinopathies, particularly sickle cell disease, can lead to IUGR through several mechanisms. Patients with sickle cell disease usually have severe anemia, and their red cells have reduced oxygen-carrying capacity because of the abnormal hemoglobin. In addition, sickle cell disease primarily involves the capillary beds so that the placenta is a prime target. The end result is a mixed type of IUGR with symmetric retardation as a result of hypoxia or asymmetric retardation if the sickling has been significant and placental vasculature is altered.

The effects of environmental hypoxia are well known. For example, decreased birth weights and placental weights have been demonstrated in studies from the Andes[47] and higher elevations in Colorado.[55]

Causes of asymmetric growth retardation

Maternal vascular disease. Chronic hypertensive vascular disease is clearly the most common identifiable cause of IUGR. In Low and Galbraith's survey of 3428 sequential deliveries, mothers with chronic hypertension and chronic renal disease had a 30% incidence of SGA babies.[50] Similarly, gravidas with severe preeclampsia gave birth to IUGR infants in 46% of their pregnancies. The autopsy study by Naeye[57] showed best that infants of hypertensive mothers are asymmetrically growth retarded. He found striking decreases in the weights of the liver, thymus, and pancreas, and confirming previous observations the organs least affected were the brain, heart, and kidney. Any vascular disease that affects the kidney, whether immunologic (eg, collagen vascular disease such as systemic lupus erythematous) or metabolic (diabetic nephropathy), often similarly affects the uteroplacental circulation. These patients are also at high risk for asymmetric growth retardation.

Placenta abruptio and placenta previa. Premature separation of the placenta and placenta previa have often been associated wtih suboptimal fetal growth. Hibbard and Jeffcoate[35] in their large series of abruptions noted that 81% of their infants were below the mean weight for gestational age. Varma[84] followed a group of patients with placenta previa using serial ultrasound and found that one third of the pregnancies with significant previa resulted in SGA births. Further, he was able to predict this suboptimal growth by serial ultrasonography in 22 out of 24 affected infants.

Multiple gestation. Multiple gestation is associated with a high incidence of growth retardation of one or more of the infants. In the series by Galbraith et al[25] 21% of multiple gestations resulted in IUGR births. Factors involved included one twin having a suboptimal implantation site, placental crowding, and vascular anastomosis in the placental bed (twin-twin transfusion syndrome). Studies examining perinatal and long-term outcome of discordant twins have found problems similar to those of singleton IUGR. All multiple gestations need to be followed closely with ultrasound to detect as early as possible any discordant growth pattern indicative of the development of IUGR in one of the fetuses.

Placental abnormalities. In a large study[70] of 6500 consecutive placentas, four types of gross placental abnormalities were identified in association with SGA babies:

1. Abnormal insertion of the cord (velamentous, battledore) occurs in approximately 1.5% to 2.0% of the population, and if this anomaly is present, the fetus has at least twice the usual risk of IUGR.
2. Hemangiomas of the placenta, particularly of the sinus type, may lead (rarely) to a large arteriovenous shunt and hence to growth retardation.
3. Diffuse multiple infarcts when grossly covering 40% to 50% of the placental surface area are associated with poor fetal growth.
4. Twin-twin transfusion syndrome in monochorionic placentas with major arteriovenous shunt can lead (rarely) to marked stunting of one twin, fetal wastage, and neonatal problems.

Molteni et al[56] in Denver examined 2000 placentas and calculated fetoplacental (F/P) weight ratios. The ratio rises consistently through gestation from approximately 5 at 30 weeks to 7.5 at 40 weeks. SGA infants had a consistently lower F/P ratio, suggesting that the fetus had outgrown the placenta. When this occurs, especially when the F/P ratio is larger than 10.0, there is high risk of fetal distress or low Apgar scoring.

■ DIAGNOSIS

Prenatal recognition of fetal growth retardation enables the obstetrician to focus resources on the gravida at risk in an attempt to reduce the chances of intrauterine death. Further, intensive obstetric care can be provided to minimize the incidence of intrapartum asphyxia, and neonatologists can be alerted to the delivery of a high-risk infant. The fact that prenatal diagnosis and management have an impact on perinatal morbidity and mortality is best shown in one of the few comparison studies between infants diagnosed and undiagnosed antepartum. Tejani and Mann[78] critically examined 148 SGA infants out a total 3798 births. Fifty-one of these pregnancies were identified antepartum (diagnostic rate 34%), and the perinatal mortality was 20 out of 1000 births in this group. The remaining unidentified 97 SGA infants had a mortality of 103 out of 1000: 8 of these 10 deaths were intrauterine, and all but one occurred at or after 37 weeks of gestation. In contrast, there were no stillbirths in the group that was identified prenatally.

All available diagnostic methods—clinical, hormonal, and ultrasonic—have major weaknesses. Most are highly nonspecific with a large number of false positive results; thus they identify as at risk a significant number of normal pregnancies, causing not only a swamping of perinatal facilities and budgets but also leading to early intervention and thus iatrogenic harm. The present methods are also inexact and miss many pregnancies that end in IUGR babies. The best results are obtained with advanced ultrasonographic techniques, such as measurements of the fetal head circumference, the head/abdomen ratio, or the total intrauterine volume.

Clinical diagnosis

In the past, physicians approached the task of diagnosis of IUGR armed only with a tape measure and with the patient's history. These tools still remain as the most important route for identification of pregnancies at risk for IUGR and for selection of patients for more refined testing. Estimation of fetal weight by abdominal palpation is notoriously inaccurate, and this is accentuated as weight decreases below 2500 grams.[63] Fundal height is also a poor indicator of gestational age.[5] The value of fundal measurements, however, comes from the delineation of fetal *growth*. Previous criticism of this measurement centered on its purported high rate of false positives and false negatives. In Tejani and Mann's series[78] of 148 pregnancies with IUGR, 58% of the affected babies had "inadequate" (not defined) uterine growth. Others have found even poorer predictability. Conversely, one study[30] noted that only 10% of the patients referred because of a uterus small for dates ended with an IUGR infant at birth. This is a common finding at many perinatal centers and is usually related to poor dating.

The poor results with fundal height measurements are not surprising in view of the lack of a systematic approach to measurement and interpretation. Two recent studies use uterine size in a serious manner. They both examined a series of "normal" patients with good dates and constructed a normal curve for fundal growth. Then they used the method prospectively for the diagnosis of fetal growth abnormalities with surprisingly good results. Belizan et al[9] in Argentina were able to identify 38 out of 44 (86%) fetuses whose birth weights were under the 10th percentile (local norms). Further, there was only a 10% false positive rate, probably because a prerequisite for entry into the study was a firmly established date of last menstrual period. The second study by Westin[87] in Sweden examined serial changes in maternal weight, girth, and fundal height. Fundal height was the most sensitive indicator (ie, smallest coefficient of variation) for the identification of conditions such as growth retardation, infants large for dates, and twins. Also, 44% of pregnancies with inadequate fundal height (2 cm or more below the mean) resulted in IUGR babies. Fundal measurements greater than 2 cm above the mean effectively ruled out asymmetric IUGR. Fully 75% of all SGA infants were diagnosed by this method. Thus it appears that when fundal height is used with a chart of norms for gestational age, it can be a reasonably sensitive indicator of the need for more intensive evaluation.

Decreased maternal weight gain during pregnancy is another controversial clinical sign. One of the findings of the Collaborative Perinatal Study[59] was an association between maternal weight loss or failure to gain weight and low birth weight infants. In addition, the data from famines and less severe forms of starvation have demonstrated that maternal malnutrition can be passed on to the fetus. Tejani and Mann[78] found poor weight gain (less than 15 pounds) in 20% of their SGA pregnancies. However, this may not be significantly higher than expected. In Low and Galbraith's series[50] this association was not observed with 182 SGA infants. The average weight gain in pregnancy was 20 pounds (9 kg), and only three patients gained less than 5 pounds (2.3 kg). British investigators[24] have found that women with a low weight before pregnancy (less than 110 pounds [50 kg]) are nearly four times as likely to have an SGA infant than women weighing greater than 140 pounds (63 kg). This risk is exacerbated by smoking. The petite smoker runs seven times the risk of IUGR. Studies correlating maternal pregnant height and weight with fetal size seem to indicate a genetic limitation on intrauterine growth.

Maternal history is probably the most important screening tool. As seen in Table 8-1, mothers with significant medical or obstetric problems are at particularly high risk for asymmetric IUGR. Toxemia, chronic hypertension, chronic renal failure, and insulin-dependent diabetes (less than Class D) are the most frequent examples. Multiple pregnancies and third trimester bleeding are also important conditions associated with SGA infants. Previous obstetric performance is important, and gravidas with a history of one or more SGA infants are at increased risk, whereas those with a history of an LGA baby are at nearly no risk. When a gravida has any of these conditions, she should be followed clinically, and if poor fundal growth or poor weight gain occur, she is at high risk for having an SGA infant and requires sonographic follow-up care.

The list of conditions associated with symmetric growth retardation was reviewed in the section on etiology. As this type of growth retardation is less common and the perinatal period usually passes without incident, the data are usually valuable only in retrospect for identifying a reason for an infant's small size. Overall, it must be remembered that in 50% of IUGR babies no significant medical or obstetric risk factors can be identified, thus indicating the limitations of the history.

Nowhere in obstetrics is estimation of gestational age by history and early examination as important as in suspected growth retardation; though serial ultrasound can help in this regard, good early clinical dating is indispensable.

Diagnosis by ultrasound

Ultrasonography has emerged as the most reliable and accurate method for the prenatal diagnosis of IUGR. The first approach developed was to measure serially the fetal biparietal diameter (BPD). Campbell and Dewhurst[11] in 1971 found that 82% of growth retarded fetuses had BPD growth rates below the 10th percentile. This method had a false negative rate of approximately 20%. Further, 17% of normal pregnancies exhibited subnormal growth. Though clearly an improvement over any other screening or diagnostic test, available BPD measurements still lacked the desired accuracy.

Campbell and Dewhurst also identified two distinct ultrasonic fetal growth patterns. In the "late flattening" pattern (Fig. 8-1) there was reduced or absent BPD growth only in the last portion of pregnancy. These babies were asymmetrically small with preserved heads and wasted bodies. The second pattern was that of "reduced growth profile" (Fig. 8-2) and corresponded to symmetrically growth-retarded fetuses.

Two major problems arise with using BPDs for the diagnosis of IUGR. It is well known that BPD growth tapers off in late normal pregnancies. After 36 weeks, mean growth is approximately 1.4 mm per week. This is less than the average reported standard error for BPD measurement of 1.5 to 2.0 mm. Also, late in pregnancy the fetal head is beginning to undergo a molding process as it dips into the pelvis. Therefore interpretation of late flattening patterns requires several weeks of observation to minimize artifactual influences. The other concern arises from the theoretical basis of growth retardation. In the asymmetric (late flattening) type, body fat and liver stores are depleted first, leading to a disproportion between head and body size. The focus of fetal metabolism is to preserve brain perfusion and head growth at all costs. Ironically, head size is the variable that is followed for ultrasonic diagnosis.

With these concerns it is no surprise that several other investigators have not done well using the BPD for the antenatal diagnosis of IUGR. Queenan et al[66] in Louisville could only identify 56% of growth retarded fetuses in a high-risk series. Arias,[3] looking at the outcome of abnormal BPD growth, found that only 43% went on to deliver SGA infants. Crane et al[18] also looking at growth arrest, found a similar outcome—50% (5 out of 10) delivered babies with IUGR by pediatric criteria. Crane and Arias also found that the timing of BPD growth arrest was important, and when it happened before 36 weeks, there was a strong relation to IUGR at birth, especially if associated with maternal high-risk factors. Conversely, when the growth arrest began at or after 36 weeks—late onset—it was a poor predictor of birth weight below the 10th percentile.

Several groups have been examining refinements of their ultrasonic measurements to eliminate the false positives and negatives encountered with the use of serial fetal BPDs. Since neonatal weight is the criteria for diagnosis, investigators have attempted to use ultrasound to estimate fetal weight, although it has long been recognized that the BPD correlates poorly with body weight, especially when pathologic states are considered. The best constructed curve to date for forecasting fetal weight with ultrasound uses measurements of the abdominal circumference at the level of the umbilical vein in combination with BPD.[86] Using these two measurements with a computer-generated table, fetal weight can be estimated within 106 grams (1 SD) if the fetus weighs less than 3000 grams. In large fetuses the error with this method may be considerable.

A more sophisticated (and technically difficult) measurement is the ratio of head to abdominal circumference (H/A ratio). Fetal abdominal circumference is measured at the level of the umbilical vein that beside being a easily observable landmark gives an estimation of fetal liver mass. Head circumference values are obtained at the level of the thalami or the corpus callosum and give an estimate of brain size. The H/A ratio (Fig. 8-3) compares the most preserved fetal organ (the brain) and the most compromised (the liver) in cases of asymmetric growth retardation. A further advantage of using the head circumference rather than the BPD in calculating the H/A ratio is that by using two measurements (biparietal and longitudinal diameters) the effect of head molding caused by malpresentation (transverse, breech), oligohydramnios, and early engagement of the fetal head is minimized.

Campbell and Thoms[12] developed the H/A ratio as a clinical tool in the diagnosis of asymmetric IUGR. They examined 568 normal pregnancies with good dates and developed a normal curve. Then from a group of patients referred because of (1) poor fundal growth, (2) medical or obstetric complications, or (3) a fall below the 5th percentile in BPD, they were able to identify

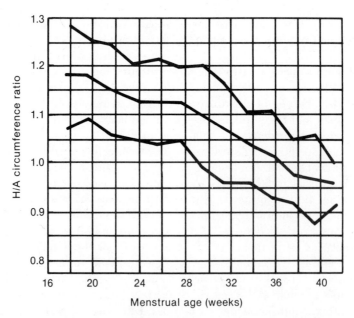

FIG. 8-3 ■ Head/abdomen circumference (H/A) ratio at different gestational ages. The midline corresponds to the mean value and the upper and lower lines to 1 SD above and below the mean. Babies with asymmetric growth retardation tend to have H/A ratios above the upper line. Infants symmetrically retarded usually have normal H/A ratios.

31 fetuses who later were diagnosed as SGA. Twenty-two of the 31 had H/A ratios above the 95th percentile and clinically were wasted, suffered intrapartum distress, and were felt to have other stigmata of asymmetric IUGR. The other 9 infants were symmetrically retarded.

Crane and Kopta[16] at Barnes Hospital recently validated Campbell's normal curve for his population and then prospectively studied patients referred for suspicion of IUGR. Twenty-six patients were referred for clinical signs and histories suggestive of IUGR and had BPDs smaller than expected for their dates. The H/A ratio was used to distinguish between the two possible diagnoses—error in dating or true IUGR—and the ultrasound findings were found to correlate perfectly with the pediatric diagnosis. However, in another study, Crane and Kopta[17] questioned the validity of the "brain sparing" concept in asymmetric IUGR, since antropometric measurements (including head circumference) failed to distinguish symmetric from asymmetric growth retarded newborns. However, H/A ratios are useful in eliminating two major shortcomings of biparietal measurements. First, they can eliminate false positive diagnoses based on technical problems such as intrauterine molding with flattening of the fetal skull. Second, a single positive H/A ratio measurement makes the diagnosis of asymmetric IUGR possible; this is important when the growth discrepancy is not suspected until the third trimester, since to document suboptimal growth a second BPD measurement would take 2 to 3 weeks longer.

A somewhat different approach is to estimate the total volume of the intrauterine contents (TIUV). Since in growth retardation the placenta is usually small and often there is oligohydramnios, the distinction between a normal and an abnormal intrauterine volume is somewhat clearer. An equation to calculate this volume from the three diameters (longitudinal, transverse, and anteroposterior) of an idealized ellipsoid was reported in 1977 and 1978.[30,37] In over 3 years of working with this method the investigators found that no patient with a normal intrauterine volume delivered an IUGR infant. Likewise, they had exceptionally few patients with an abnormal TIUV who delivered normal weight babies. There is a "gray zone" in this method (-1 to $1\frac{1}{2}$ SD) in which the risk of delivering an IUGR infant is approximately 33%.

Oligohydramnios by itself can lead to a low TIUV, but it can be distinguished from real asymmetric IUGR by direct fetal measurements such as the H/A ratio. A more significant difficulty with TIUV is the all too common problem of poor dating. If the patient is off several weeks on her estimated gestational age (a fact that is quite common in suspected IUGR), this method may give a falsely abnormal value. Dating needs to be secured by another method—most commonly by serial cephalometry. Measurement of TIUV is evidently rapid and associated with a low rate of false negative results. Furthermore, the diagnosis of IUGR can usually be ruled out with one visit, making this an attractive screening evaluation. It is not as yet widely used, and we have no experience with it.

Diagnosis by endocrine evaluation

Estriol. Maternal estriol represents the end product of a long series of metabolic interactions in the fetoplacental unit. The fetal adrenal, the site of a key step in this chain (the synthesis of dehydroepiandrosterone), has been found to be markedly atrophic in newborns with asymmetric IUGR.[57] IUGR infants also have lower levels of dehydroepiandrosterone sulfate and 16-hydroxy-pregnenolone in their serum and urine than AGA infants in control groups,[80] and these steroids are the main precursors of estriol. The exact reasons for these reduced levels are unclear. Though it is generally accepted that estriol production is proportioned to fetal size, there is probably also a component related in an unknown manner to "chronic malnutrition."

In actual clinical practice, estriol levels are not as useful for evaluating fetal well-being as originally hoped. While several small studies have shown good correlation in selected populations in which 60% to 90% of at-risk patients who go on to have IUGR infants have subnormal 24-hour urinary estradiol excretions,[26] other much larger series have shown higher incidences of normal estriol values in patients with IUGR.[7] Furthermore, the false positive rates of estriol as a general screening test can be as high as 80%.[7] In general, however, the lower the urinary estriol excretion the greater the chance that a distressed IUGR infant is involved. Some authors feel, conversely, that a normal urinary estriol (though not ruling out IUGR) at least suggests that the infant is compensating reasonably well.

Human placental lactogen (HPL). The measurement of hormones of placental origin for the diagnosis of IUGR is attractive because one major etiology for IUGR is felt to be placental insufficiency. Spellacy,[73] who has done considerable research in this area, has reviewed the literature and found nine reports in which decreased levels of HPL were found in most patients delivering infants with IUGR. However, other investigators have found low HPL levels in only a minority of patients delivering SGA babies, typically in mothers with hypertension.[43]

In summary, estriol and HPL determinations are a poor substitute (and a poor complement) to clinical observation and biophysical testing in the screening, diagnosis, and evaluation of IUGR fetuses. Presently they are being supplanted by ultrasonography and electronic monitoring of the fetus.

Dehydroepiandrosterone sulfate (DHEA-S) loading test. A theoretically attractive method for the dynamic testing of the fetoplacental unit is loading the mother with DHEA-S and quantifying its transformation to estradiol (E_2, "placental function") and estriol (E_4, "fetal function"). Tulchinsky et al,[81] in a small series of high-risk patients, found this test useful in identifying false positive estriols and hence bringing more precision to the diagnosis of antepartum fetal distress. Theoretically, DHEA-S loading opens the possibility of distinguishing placental from fetal causes of IUGR. However, despite the fact that the DHEA-S loading test was described several years ago, no information is available about its usefulness in cases of IUGR.

■ ANTEPARTUM MANAGEMENT OF PATIENTS AT RISK OR SUSPECTED OF IUGR

One of the most common situations the obstetrician faces in his or her practice in relation to the problem of fetal growth retardation is how to manage patients *at risk* of fetal growth retardation. In these cases there are no indications that IUGR is present. The patient may have chronic hypertension, chronic renal disease, or cardiac disease and be at high risk for IUGR and fetal death but not have given any indication that this is actually happening. Another situation involves what to do in cases in which IUGR is *suspected*. In these cases the patient who may

be at high risk for fetal growth retardation but usually is not, is showing some signs (discrepancy between BPD and dates, lack of uterine growth) indicating the possibility of retarded fetal growth.

Patients at risk of IUGR

Patients at risk of IUGR belong to one or several of the groups shown in Table 8-1. The most common cases are patients with chronic hypertension, those with a history of delivering an IUGR infant, or those with chronic renal or cardiopulmonary disease. They may come to the obstetrician early or late in pregnancy, and they may not have a clear recollection of their last menstrual period. In any case, the obstetrician should follow a plan of fetal surveillance that allows early recognition of abnormalities of growth.

The first step in the management of the patient at risk of IUGR is to establish, on the basis of clinical examination, if the pregnancy is under or beyond 20 weeks of gestation. This first step is important because if the patient has not reached 20 weeks of gestation (uterus below the umbilicus, fetal heart not audible with aural stethoscope), the obstetrician by serial physical examinations may obtain information to corroborate the patient's estimation of the duration of her pregnancy or to determine the gestational age if the patient is uncertain of her dates. If the pregnancy is less than 20 weeks, the patient should be examined at adequate intervals, and the expected date of confinement should be firmly established by the time the gestation reaches 20 weeks. The next step is to follow the patient with ultrasound measurements of the fetal BPD every 4 weeks. If the BPD increases normally with the progression of pregnancy, the possibilities of IUGR are minimal, and the gestation should continue to term or until termination is indicated for other reasons. If the BPD growth is less than expected in any of the serial measurements, the patient becomes *suspect* of IUGR.

If the patient at risk for IUGR is seen first when the gestation is beyond 20 weeks (uterus above umbilicus, fetal heart heard with aural stethoscope), an ultrasonic measurement of the fetal BPD must be obtained within the following 10 days. If the BPD agrees with the patient's dates, she should be followed with serial BPD

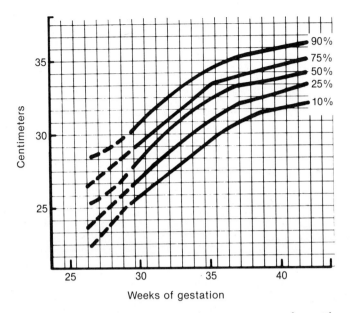

FIG. 8-4 ■ Fetal head circumference growth in relation to gestational age. This measurement is particularly important to identify abnormal biparietal diameter measurements resulting from molding of the fetal head.

measurements similarly to the patients described in the previous paragraphs.

The management of the patient at risk of IUGR who comes for evaluation after 20 weeks of gestation is more complex if the initial ultrasound evaluation shows a BPD smaller than expected for the patient's dates or if the patient has no dates. In these cases the first step is to rule out the possibility of a technical error in the ultrasound measurement, a possibility that has to be considered in cases of abnormal fetal presentations such as breech or transverse lie and in vertex presentations when the fetal head is deeply engaged in the maternal pelvis. When the fetal head is molded, there is an increase in the anteroposterior diameter and a reduction in the BPD. This situation is easily recognized by examining the ultrasound results and can be corrected by measuring both the transverse and the anteroposterior diameters of the fetal head and calculating the head circumference, which should be within normal percentiles for the gestational age. Technical problems in obtaining good BPDs are the most common reason for the referral of low-risk patients suspected of IUGR to perinatal centers. Fig. 8-4 shows the normal values for the fetal head circumference at different gestational ages.

If there are technical problems making inaccurate the BPD measurements, the patient should have repeated BPDs as indicated in Fig. 8-5. If no technical problems are present and the BPD is of good quality, the next step is to rule out the presence of congenital malformations. In fact, congenital abnormalities and intrauterine infections are common causes of growth retardation and must be searched for routinely in every patient suspected of IUGR, especially when this suspicion appears early in pregnancy.

If a congenital abnormality causing IUGR is detected by ultrasound or by any other diagnostic test, the management should be individualized depending on the nature of the anomaly and the chances for intrauterine therapy or for successful correction in the neonatal period. If no abnormalities are detected, IUGR must be suspected.

Patients suspected of carrying an IUGR fetus

From a practical viewpoint IUGR should be suspected only in pregnancies that are beyond 20 weeks of gestation. This does not mean that a fetus of 20 weeks or less may not be growth retarded. Growth retardation in the first half of

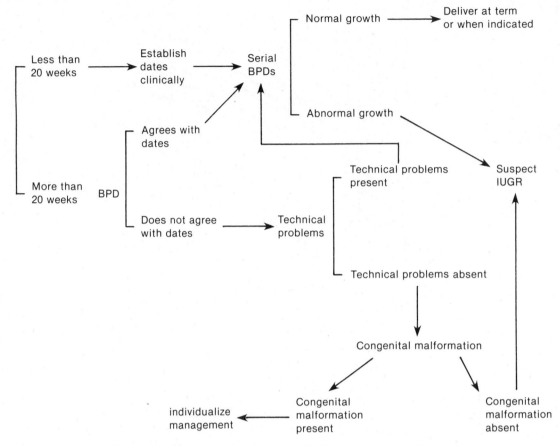

FIG. 8-5 ■ Management of the patient *at risk* of intrauterine growth retardation.

pregnancy is usually the result of congenital malformations or intrauterine infections and in most cases is followed by an early pregnancy loss. The following discussion on the management of patients suspected of IUGR deals exclusively with pregnancies that are in their second half.

The patient at high risk for an IUGR infant is often in a clinical situation such as a discrepancy between the clinical and the ultrasonic evaluation of the gestational age that converts the patient from being *at high risk* for IUGR to being *suspected* of IUGR. However, most of the gravidas who are referred to ultrasound laboratories because of suspected IUGR are patients without high-risk factors in whom the clinical suspicion of IUGR usually results from a lack of adequate uterine growth in repeated prenatal examinations. Most of these cases are patients too obese or too thin, nulliparas with strong abdominal walls, multiparas with flaccid anterior abdominal muscles, or patients with breech or transverse presentations in which clinical measurement of

the uterine growth is open to serious error.

Since the incidence of IUGR is much larger in a population at risk than in normal gravidas, the main question to be answered in the management of a patient suspected of carrying an IUGR infant is the following:

> **Are there any historical, medical, or obstetric factors that make this patient at high risk for IUGR?**

If the answer to the question is no, the test to order is a simple measurement of the fetal BPD. If the BPD agrees with the patient's dates, the patient should be followed with serial BPD measurements. In the overwhelming majority of cases serial BPDs show adequate fetal growth. Only in a few cases the fetus of a patient at low risk for IUGR shows an abnormal BPD growth pattern. In this case the patient should have an

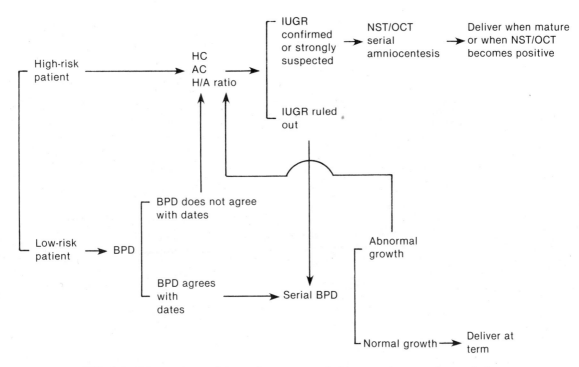

FIG. 8-6 ■ Management of the patient *suspected* of intrauterine growth retardation.

ultrasonic measurement of the H/A circumference ratio.

If the answer to the question is yes (the patient has risk factors for IUGR), the mother should be referred to the ultrasound laboratory for determination of the H/A ratio. This measurement is not a routine procedure and should be requested only in situations such as the following: (1) patients at high-risk for fetal growth retardation and with clinical indicators that IUGR may already be present; (2) patients showing abnormal BPD growth in serial measurements; (3) patients with excellent dates and BPD measurements smaller than dates. If the result of the H/A circumference ratio is above normal limits (Fig. 8-3), asymmetric growth retardation is present, and the fetus must be carefully monitored to prevent antepartum fetal death and to determine the appropriate delivery time. More about this later in this chapter. If the result of the H/A ratio is normal, the fetal growth should be followed clinically and with serial BPDs: normal fetal growth is prognostic of the delivery of an AGA infant; subnormal fetal growth requires repetition of the H/A ratio to rule out the presence of asymmetric IUGR.

If the H/A ratio is normal, the fetus may be normal or may have symmetric growth retardation. Babies with symmetric growth retardation most probably have an incidence of perinatal complications not greater than normal babies, but until this fact is more clearly established, they must be monitored similarly to an asymmetric IUGR fetus. If the H/A ratio is below normal limits, the possibility of microcephaly or the existence of a large fetal abdomen must be considered. A flow-sheet diagram of how to manage patients suspected of carrying an IUGR infant may be found in Fig. 8-6.

Pregnancies with asymmetric IUGR infants

When asymmetric IUGR is diagnosed (abnormal H/A ratio), all the perinatal resources should be focused on these patients in an efficient manner. Weekly nonstress tests (NSTs) are performed. If the fetus is not reactive, an oxytocin challenge test (OCT) must be performed. If the NST is reactive or the OCT is negative, the testing must be repeated at weekly intervals. In our experience, given the chronic nature of the condition, this frequency has been quite adequate. However, an underlying assumption is that the maternal medical condition is stable.

With continued negative NSTs/OCTs, amniocentesis to assess fetal lung maturation should start at 36 weeks and continue on a weekly basis. Delivery is carried out if the shake test or the Foam Stability Index (FSI) is positive, the L/S ratio is greater than 2.0, or meconium is present. Early delivery is recommended because of the rising risk of stillbirth as term approaches. Even in those patients who do well throughout pregnancy (ie, repeated negative NSTs/OCTs), there is a high rate of intrapartum fetal distress and an increased rate of cesarean section (20% to 25%).

Management of an IUGR pregnancy that develops a nonreactive NST and a positive OCT is a difficult problem. At 34 or more weeks the risk of respiratory distress syndrome (RDS) in an IUGR infant is less than the risk of intrauterine death if there is a positive OCT and a nonreactive NST, and delivery must be accomplished without evaluation of the fetal lung maturity. If the pregnancy is less than 32 weeks, an amniocentesis should be done and tests of fetal lung maturation obtained immediately. If the shake test or the FSI test is positive or the lecithin/sphingomyelin (L/S) ratio is greater than 1.5, there is little to be gained by further intrauterine life, and delivery is effected. Some authors feel that cesarean section without a trial of labor is indicated in this high-risk group.[14] Others lament over the high false positive rates for OCTs (25% to 50%) and argue that a carefully monitored labor with scalp pHs and liberal cesarean section do not add to the neonatal morbidity.[83] This has been our experience, and we are hesitant to recommend an abdominal delivery on the basis of only a positive OCT without a trial of labor first.

If the OCT is positive, the shake test is negative, the FSI test is intermediate, and the L/S ratio is less than 1.5, there is the difficult position of weighing the risk of fetal demise versus neonatal immaturity. Various factors need to be analyzed in reaching a judgment.

1. *What corroborative evidence is there of fetal distress?* A positive OCT is considerably more ominous in the presence of other indicators of fetal ill health, such as an abnormal fetal biophysical profile. Also, low estriol or HPL values or meconium in the amniotic fluid, in combination with a positive OCT, demand delivery.

2. *How stable are the mother's medical and obstetric problems?* If maternal toxemia or chronic high blood pressure are not controllable, or if cyanotic heart disease is worsening, the risk of intrauterine demise is quite high, and these maternal factors may demand delivery on their own.

3. *Are there any reassuring aspects in the stress test?* The OCT tracing needs to be reexamined carefully to ascertain the correctness of the diagnosis and to look for more subtle signs of fetal health such as beat-to-beat variability and reactivity to fetal motion. When these are present, the significance of late decelerations is reduced.

4. *What is the real risk of RDS for this newborn?* It is well known that there is early maturation of pulmonary surfactant in SGA fetuses. Further, several studies have shown that RDS occurs less commonly and is less morbid in preterm SGA infants even with L/S ratios below 2.0.[6] Finally, it seems that the shake test and the FSI are more reliable than the L/S ratio in determining the pulmonary maturity of the IUGR fetus.

5. Finally, *what are the capabilities of your newborn nursery?* If it has a neonatal intensive care unit capable of handling sick preterm infants with good results, the risks of continued intrauterine life may be higher than those of immediate delivery. If the hospital has only a routine nursery, referral to a perinatal center is indicated.

If after examining all these questions the risk of delivery seems higher than that of intrauterine death, the following protocol must be followed: the mother should be hospitalized, kept in bed in the lateral position, and given an intravenous infusion of glucose. There is reasonable evidence that these procedures at least temporarily improve estriol secretion and by inference uteroplacental blood flow is also improved.[6] We feel that this procedure can buy a short period of time to allow for the action of glucocorticoids in maturing the fetal lungs. The prompt and dramatic fall in serum or urinary estriol values that follows the use of steroids should be remembered. Hypertensive disorders that account for a large number of these high-risk patients may be relative contraindications to corticosteroids according to Liggins and Howie.[49] Other authors,[60] however, have used glucocorticoids without reproducing the increase in fetal demise, and Liggins has since narrowed his contraindication to severe hypertension with proteinuria larger than 5 grams per day. We use steroids in IUGR pregnancies only in carefully selected and monitored patients. In summary, it would be rare to delay delivery of a distressed IUGR infant. In fact, we would recommend amniocentesis only in the young infant (less than 32 weeks) and would move toward delivery in all others.

Pregnancies with symmetric IUGR infants

A management plan for symmetric growth retardation is not well established. The diagnosis is usually missed during pregnancy and requires a combination of excellent dates, low growth profile in serial fetal BPD measurements, and normal H/A ratio. Even if the patient has serial sonograms indicationg low growth profile, the tendency is to reassign the gestational age rather than to diagnose symmetric growth retardation. Only when the pregnancy has excellent clinical dating is there reasonable hope for prenatal discovery. In several small series of symmetrically retarded babies there has been no increase in the usual perinatal problems, such as fetal distress and asphyxia, except as related to congenital anomalies. In fact, most of the labors seem to "sparkle." Thus many authors feel that no additional monitoring is needed during pregnancy in these cases and that no special consideration needs to be given to the labor and delivery. As this has not been proven, in the rare instance that a symmetrically retarded patient is identified, we follow with serial NSTs and perform extra testing only if the NST is nonreactive. There is no attempt to deliver before term. Symmetric growth retardation should make the clinician suspect congenital anomalies. This is especially true if the pregnancy is complicated by diabetes.

Resources are fairly well-conserved with this protocol, and false positives and negatives are kept to a minimum. This is important to preserve the usually limited perinatal budget and to minimize iatrogenic harm to otherwise healthy pregnancies.

■ INTRAPARTUM MANAGEMENT OF THE SUSPECTED IUGR FETUS

The management of labor and delivery is a critical aspect of the obstetric care of the SGA baby, since intrapartum asphyxia is the most common and serious problem of these infants. In fact, excluding congenital defects, asphyxia is the major cause of antenatal and early neonatal death and a common precursor for many subsequent newborn complications.

The fully grown term fetus has a large capacity to withstand labor partially because of its generous energy reserve. In the IUGR fetus the liver and placental glycogen stores and subcutaneous adipose tissues are markedly depleted. With hypoxia, these reserves are used rapidly with progression to anaerobic metabolism and metabolic acidosis. Low et al[52] in a detailed study of acid-base changes in growth retarded babies during labor, found cord pH and lactate levels suggesting moderate to severe acidosis in fully 48% of 31 infants. Preterm SGA babies are at high risk for severe metabolic acidosis.

Fetal monitor tracings suggesting fetal distress (unfortunately not well defined) have been found in 30% to 35% of IUGR pregnancies by a number of authors.[14,52,61] All studies have also found an increased number of low 5-minute Apgar scores in IUGR infants. With such a high incidence of intrapartum asphyxia leading to immediate neonatal consequences (hypoxic brain damage, meconium aspiration, hypoglycemia, seizures) and also long-term consequences (learning and behavioral difficulties), the intrapartum period in the IUGR infant should be managed aggressively. Early amniotomy with internal fetal monitoring is important. Because of the known lack of fetal reserve, even mild to moderate electronic monitoring signs of fetal distress should be followed with fetal scalp pH sampling. Such a trial of labor results in 20% to 30% incidence of cesarean section but with the end result of healthier babies in the nurseries. The second stage of labor, with its well-known association with fetal acidosis,[89] needs to be kept to a minimum. Measures to shorten its course, such as generous and early episiotomy, outlet forceps, and proper coaching in bearing down are to be encouraged. Cord blood gases should be measured at the time of delivery to help the obstetrician and the pediatrician determine the degree of fetal hypoxia.

Anesthesia and analgesia during labor in IUGR pregnancies, like other high-risk situations, generate difficult questions. CNS depressant drugs like meperidine or diazepam should be avoided. Similarly, there is good evidence that local anesthetics bind more tightly to the fetal brain in the presence of acidosis, so that many feel that paracervical blocks are undesirable. Regional anesthesia such as epidural blocks should be used cautiously. Even after proper loading of the gravida's vascular system with a large volume of lactated Ringer's solution, there is a risk of maternal hypotension. Further, it is well known that epidural anesthesia is associated with longer second stages of labor, although there is some evidence that the epidural-related prolonged second stage does not lead as quickly to acidosis.[90] The same inability to bear down effectively and cause descent of the head leads to less diminution of placental perfusion and hence less acidosis.

Clearly, the best anesthesia is psychoprophylactic breathing exercises. If a mother is decompensating and hyperventilating, the compensatory maternal metabolic acidosis is not in the interest of the fetus. Some compromises may need to be made. Competent perinatal staff members need to be present at the moment of delivery to offer maximal resuscitative efforts.

■ NEONATAL CONSIDERATIONS

Identification of an SGA infant at birth is accomplished largely through the use of weight-for-gestational-age charts as discussed earlier. Physical examination of asymmetrically retarded infants reveals marked soft tissue wasting. Their skin is loose, thin, and often dry and cracked. The abdomen is scaphoid, they have protuberant ribs, and the muscle mass is reduced. This is easily seen over cheeks, arms, buttocks, and thighs. The combination of wrinkled skin and wasted musculature may make the face quite expressive. Even those infants who are SGA without evident soft tissue wasting have reduced subcutaneous fat as measured by double skin thickness.

The umbilical cord is limp, thin, and often meconium stained. Infants not depressed by asphyxia or hypoglycemia seem more vigorous and active than other infants of the same weight. In fact, quiet IUGR infants demand careful watching not only for metabolic abnormalities but for potentially catastrophic apneic spells. Asymmetrically retarded infants have relative sparing of their head circumference when plotted against gestational norms. The symmetrically retarded infant needs to be rigorously examined for signs of intrauterine infection (hepatosplenomegaly, rashes, cardiac and neurologic abnormalities) and congenital anomalies. The placenta needs careful inspection for infarctions, fibrin deposition, cord insertion, and presence of arteriovenous malformations and should be sent to pathology for microscopic evaluation. A good placental pathologist can be helpful in determining the etiology of the growth retardation. A single umbilical artery requires careful search for other abnormalities.

The neonatal course for SGA infants is quite different from that of preterm AGA infants. Because of the relative maturity of most organ systems, there are fewer problems with diseases of immaturity such as hyaline membrane disease and hyperbilirubinemia of the newborn.

The lungs of an IUGR infant have quite different characteristics from those of a normal preterm baby. It is well known from Gluck's and Kulovich's[29] work that SGA infants show accelerated maturation of their L/S ratio. Further, this group of infants has a high rate of false negative L/S ratios (ie, they fail to develop or have only mild RDS despite an immature ratio).[31] Beside early production of surfactant, perhaps stimulated by high endogenous steroid levels caused by chronic fetal distress, researchers have noted changes in the mechanical properties of the lungs. Dahms et al[19] have found increased compliance and elevated crying vital capacity. These changes may be related to increased surfactant in the alveolus or to changes in the structure of the elastic tissues of the newborn lung.

The neonatal complications of IUGR infants can be organized into the following three major areas:

1. Morbidity related to perinatal asphyxia and fetal distress (meconium aspiration syndrome, persistent fetal circulation, and hypoxic encephalopathy).
2. Morbidity related to metabolic aberrations secondary to long-standing intrauterine stresses (hypoglycemia, hypocalcemia, hyperviscosity, hyperglycemia, and hypothermia).

3. Morbidity related to specific etiologic factors for growth retardation (congenital malformations, congenital infections, chromosomal malformations).

It cannot be overstressed that the delivery room management of an IUGR newborn may minimize or even eliminate significant neonatal sequelae. The adequate treatment of hypoxia, clearance of meconium, and identification of hypoglycemia will not only shorten the infant's intensive care nursery stay, but will also improve his long-term prognosis.

Asphyxia-related disorders

Meconium aspiration syndrome. Meconium aspiration syndrome is a major cause of mortality and morbidity for IUGR infants. However, by using proper resuscitative techniques the meconium aspiration syndrome can be almost 100% eliminated. Because of this opportunity for prevention, the management of meconium at delivery is presented in detail.

The ability to pass meconium represents a maturational milestone of the fetal gut, but since it is also associated with hypoxic insults, it is not surprising that it is commonly present at SGA deliveries. Meconium aspiration syndrome is often quite severe and difficult to treat. Meconium is not only a highly caustic agent, but it is also an excellent culture media. The clinical picture is one of progressive "stiffening" (loss of compliance) of the lungs, hypoxia, return to fetal circulation, and recurrent air leaks. Pneumothorax, pneumomediastinum, pneumopericardium, and pulmonary interstitial emphysema are frequent complications of the aspiration syndrome as particulate matter acts in a ball-valve manner to cause alveolar "blowouts."

Gregory et al[32] have demonstrated the effectiveness of direct laryngeal visualization and tracheal suctioning in the moments immediately following delivery. The Denver group[13] has further emphasized nasopharyngeal suctioning at the time of delivery of the head, reducing the incidence of meconium aspiration syndrome to zero at its large medical center. The following protocol is based largely on these two studies:

1. The mother is instructed to absolutely cease pushing at the moment of delivery of the head. With the thorax compressed and the infant unable to take in a breath, the obstetrician uses either bulb or DeLee suction to meticulously clear the oropharynx and nasopharynx of mucous and meconium fluid. If the oropharynx is empty, there will be nothing for the infant to aspirate with his first breaths.

2. Delivery is then effected, the cord quickly clamped, and the infant placed in head-dependent position under a radiant warmer. The cords are directly visualized with a laryngoscope, and an endotracheal tube is passed into the trachea. Suction is applied directly to the tube, either with the mouth or with mechanical suction devices. The tube is withdrawn as suction is continued (particulate meconium too large to pass through the tube can be removed quite effectively in this manner). The procedure is repeated until no meconium is obtained. To minimize tracheal trauma, the procedure should be performed by trained personnel. However, as obstetricians encounter meconium so frequently (8% of all deliveries), they should become expert in the technique of neonatal intubation.

Infants who have only thin serous "tea" meconium and are vigorous at birth need only thorough oropharyngeal suctioning. Every infant with thick meconium demands direct tracheal suctioning. It is only with routine intubation that meconium aspiration can be eliminated. Over 10% of infants with no meconium seen at the cords have returns from intubation.[32]

3. Intubation and tracheal suctioning often induce vagal slowing of the heart, and the infant may actually lose Apgar points during the initial phase of resuscitation. Positive pressure ventilation is to be avoided if at all possible until all meconium is cleared. Particulate matter in the bronchial tube is retrievable, but in the small airways it is not. An iatrogenically low 1-minute Apgar score is acceptable, since after suctioning is completed (usually no later than 2 to 3 minutes), oxygenation and stimulation rapidly revive the infant.

4. Adjunctive therapy in the first 15 minutes of life, such as postural drainage and chest physiotherapy, is quite productive. Likewise, a DeLee catheter should be passed and the stomach contents emptied. The fetus often swallows large amounts of meconium in utero and can regurgitate and secondarily aspirate these contents after birth.

5. A similar protocol can be followed after cesarean section. Thorough suctioning with ei-

ther DeLee or bulb is performed at the moment of delivery of the head through the uterine incision. Suctioning is continued as the cord is clamped and the infant handed to the pediatrician.

Our results and that of others[13] using this preventive approach have been excellent.

Persistent fetal circulation. Persistent fetal circulation is a frequent complication of severe hypoxia and/or acidosis. It can develop after meconium aspiration or after intrapartum asphyxia. The pathophysiology includes a return to the fetal blood flow pattern in combination with marked pulmonary vasoconstriction. Signs include cardiomegaly, hypoxia with less severe hypercarbia, pulmonary hypertension, and right-to-left shunting without evidence of intrinsic heart disease. Treatment revolves around correcting the acidosis, adequate ventilation, and the use of vasodilators such as tolazoline (Priscoline) that are active on the pulmonary bed.

Hypoxic ischemic encephalopathy. Hypoxic ischemic encephalopathy is a nonspecific diagnosis used to describe a variety of neurologic symptoms occurring after perinatal asphyxial episodes. The actual injury may range from cerebral edema to periventricular bleeding and other forms of intracranial hemorrhage to nonspecific asphyxial injury. The symptomatology is general—irritability, twitching, apnea, and convulsions—and can be mimicked by several metabolic disorders (hypoglycemia, hypocalcemia, hypoxia, hyperviscosity, and sepsis). Treatment is supportive and symptomatic. Intracranial hemorrhage is discussed more fully in Chapter 3.

Metabolic aberrations

Hypoglycemia. Hypoglycemia is perhaps the most common neonatal problem in IUGR infants. The condition is related to lack of liver glycogen and fat tissue energy stores. The incidence of hypoglycemia approaches 25% in term SGA infants and is much higher (about 67%) in IUGR and preterm infants.[25] The most widely used definition is a blood sugar level below 30 mg/dl, the lower limit of normal for all age groups. The symptoms are nonspecific: jitteriness, twitching, apnea, tachypnea, and occasionally convulsions.

Blood glucose levels should be monitored in the first 2 hours of life and then every 2 to 4 hours (depending on values) for the first day of life. Dextrostix are quite useful and accurate for screening as long as values are above 40 mg/dl. Determinations below 40 mg/dl are not accurate and need confirmation. Early feeding, either oral or intravenous, has been shown to minimize or prevent hypoglycemia.[53]

An additional important component of neonatal hypoglycemia appears to be a deficiency of the liver gluconeogenic enzymes. In refractory cases it may be necessary to use glucocorticoids to induce gluconeogenesis pharmacologically.[62]

Hypocalcemia. Hypocalcemia, particularly first day hypocalcemia, is quite common in low birth weight infants and is felt to be related to several factors such as relative hypoparathyroidism, asphyxia-related increase in calcitonin level, increased phosphorus level secondary to tissue destruction and decreased excretion, and finally to decreased oral calcium intake in sick infants.[4] The most important factor does not appear to be intrauterine malnutrition but rather perinatal asphyxia. Symptoms are nearly identical to those of hypoglycemia. Attention should also be paid to magnesium homeostasis in cases of refractory hypocalcemia.

Polycythemia/hyperviscosity syndrome. Polycythemia is defined as a central hematocrit in excess of 65% or a hemoglobin concentration greater than 22 g/dl. It occurs in 18% of IUGR infants.[62] Polycythemia is felt to be secondary to a chronic hypoxic stimulation of the erythropoietic system together with a redistribution of blood volume from the placenta to the fetus. The clinical problems with polycythemia in the newborn relate to the following:

1. Increased destruction of red blood cells resulting in hyperbilirubinemia
2. Volume overload leading to congestive heart failure and pulmonary edema
3. Hyperviscosity

Clinical manifestations of hyperviscosity are a result of sludging of blood in the capillary circulation of various organs. Symptoms include twitching to seizures (CNS), pulmonary infarcts and hemorrhage (lung), digital infarcts (peripheral circulation), and necrotizing enterocolitis (mesenteric vascular bed). Treatment of the syndrome involves partial exchange transfusion with plasma or albumin replacing blood.

Hypothermia. Hypothermia is related to the

decreased layer of insulating fat and to the lack of readily usable energy stores to maintain central core temperature. These characteristics underline the importance of artificial warmth in the first hours of life.

Long-term prognosis of the IUGR infant

A hostile intrauterine environment can clearly lead to a number of neonatal problems, some of which can be fatal. Today a large proportion of IUGR infants survive the neonatal period, and attention is then focused on their long-term growth and development. The question is whether IUGR infants suffer permanently or if the fetal insult can be corrected by good quality of postnatal life.

The first follow-up studies of low birth weight infants born during the 1950s and 1960s found a significant incidence of poor growth and neurologic and developmental sequelae. Most experimental animals, if starved in the prenatal period, generally grow up to be small adults no matter how intensive the postnatal period of rehabilitation.[20] However, recent studies have demonstrated a much improved outcome.

A nearly universal finding is that SGA babies as a group remain smaller than their AGA cohorts at follow-up examinations. However, some recent studies show "catch-up" growth—an initial acceleration in growth of all measurements (weight, length, head circumference). This growth is in addition to the already extremely rapid growth in the first 6 months of life. Several years later, 20% to 30% of infants will remain at less than the 30th percentile in weight, but only 10% to 20% will be over the 50th percentile.[22,36,51] Catch-up growth occurs, but it is not complete.

Several studies have looked for characteristics that may help to distinguish between those babies who will remain growth stunted and those who will move into more normal growth ranges. Fitzhardinge and Steven[22] in a prospective 4-year follow-up of 96 full-term SGA infants found that if growth was to catch up, the acceleration had to occur in the first 6 months. Further, the degree of initial growth failure did not have predictive value. Infants less than 60% of the mean birth weight, the most severely affected babies (ie, less than 1900 grams at term), grew as well as their less markedly afflicted cohorts.

Another approach to prognosis is to identify the type of IUGR. Holmes et al[38] examined a group of infants for body composition and used "ponderal index" (weight for length ratio) that gives results roughly comparable to asymmetric (low ponderal index) and symmetric (normal ponderal index) growth retardation. The rate of postnatal growth was directly related to the index at birth. Those with a low ponderal index had the highest velocity of weight gain. In other words, the skinniest, most wasted babies grow the fastest after birth. In perhaps the most important study, Fancourt et al[21] followed a series of infants who had serial prenatal sonographs. Infants whose growth retardation had an onset before 34 weeks of gestation were much more likely to remain below the 10th percentile at 4 years of age than babies whose BPD began to slow after 34 weeks. This again supports a difference between symmetric and asymmetric growth retardation.

Another finding of interest is retardation of bone age. In the IUGR fetus development of epiphysis and bone age are delayed.[22] The difference between height age and bone age persists through the duration of follow-up studies (4 to 6 years). This could indicate either a defect in skeletal maturation that may be partly responsible for the slow growth in height, or it may signify that these children have a longer potential growth span and may eventually achieve a similar final height to their peers.

A major concern extrapolated from animal studies is that chronic intrauterine deprivation could lead to a permanent decrease in brain cell number. Like the physical growth findings, early follow-up studies for neurologic sequelae found a higher incidence of major problems in SGA babies than the more recent investigations have found. Koops[45] recently reviewed the literature on neurologic sequelae. A number of studies show that babies with congenital infections and anomalies (especially if there is CNS involvement) have a significant incidence of major neurologic problems later in life. Fitzhardinge and Steven[23] studied a group of term SGA infants who did not have the above congenital problems and found only a 1% incidence of motor deficits and a 6% incidence of seizures. However, minimal cerebral dysfunction (hyperactivity, decreased attention span, learning difficulties, poor coordination) was diagnosed in 25%. Speech defects were also present in 33% of boys and 26% of girls tested. Significantly, all the infants with spasticity or seizures had sustained severe neonatal asphyxia, once again underlining the additive effects of IUGR and hypoxia.

Fancourt et al[21] in their follow-up of abnormal ultrasound growth patterns found a mean development quotient depressed by nearly 10 points in infants whose growth failure had a very early onset when compared to either late onset or normal control. In contrast, several recent studies[15,85] have found equal or even improved outcome in less than 36-week SGA babies (without congenital defects) when compared to preterm AGA babies.

Overall, asymmetric SGA infants at term are at significant risk for *minor* developmental problems, whereas babies with asphyxia at birth or symmetric retardation may have more major neurologic problems in their childhood. Further, the length of the insult seems more important than the severity in both somatic growth and neurologic development. In all the studies it is difficult to separate the effect of being IUGR from hypoxia during labor and delivery, and from effects such as neonatal hypoglycemia and hyperviscosity. The best prognosis then is for the late asymmetrically retarded infant who grows rapidly in the first months of life. The worst prognosis is for the symmetrically retarded baby in association with congenital infection or anomaly.

■ REFERENCES

1. American College of Radiology: Diagnostic x-rays are no cause for abortion but caution is advised. JAMA 1976;236:2269.
2. Anatov AN: Children born during the seige of Leningrad in 1942. J Pediatr 1947;30:250.
3. Arias F: The diagnosis and management of intrauterine growth retardation. Obstet Gynecol 1977;49:293.
4. Bard H: Neonatal problems of infants with intrauterine growth retardation. J Reprod Med 1978;26:359.
5. Beazley JM, Underhill RA: Fallacy of fundal height. Br Med J 1970;4:404.
6. Beischer NA, Abell DA, Drew JH: Management of fetal growth retardation. Med J Aust 1977;2:641.
7. Beischer NA, Brown JB: Current status of estrogen assays in obstetrics and gynecology. Obstet Gynecol Surv 1972;27:303.
8. Belizan JM, Lechtig A, Villar J: Distribution of low-birth weight infants in developing countries. Am J Obstet Gynecol 1978;132:704.
9. Belizan JM, Villar J, Nardin JC, et al: Diagnosis of intrauterine growth retardation by a simple clinical method: measurement of uterine height. Am J Obstet Gynecol 1978;131:643.
10. Campbell S: Fetal growth. Clin Obstet Gynecol 1974;1:41.
11. Campbell S, Dewhurst CJ: Diagnosis of the small-for-dates fetus by serial ultrasound cephalometry. Lancet 1971;2:1002.
12. Campbell S, Thoms A: Ultrasonic measurement of the fetal head to abdominal circumference ratio in the assessment of growth retardation. Br J Obstet Gynaecol 1977;84:165.
13. Carson BS, Losey RW, Bowes WA, et al: Combined obstetric and pediatric approach to prevent meconium aspiration syndrome. Am J Obstet Gynecol 1976;126:712.
14. Cetrulo CL, Freeman R: Bioelectric evaluation in intrauterine growth retardation. Clin Obstet Gynecol 1977;20:1979.
15. Churchill JA, Masland RL, Naylov AA, et al: The etiology of cerebral palsy in preterm infants. Dev Med Child Neurol 1974;16:143.
16. Crane JP, Kopta MM: Prediction of intrauterine growth retardation via ultrasonically measured head/abdomen circumference ratios. Obstet Gynecol 1979;54:597.
17. Crane JP, Kopta MM: Comparative newborn antropometric measurements in symmetrical vs. asymmetrical growth retardation, in *Society for Gynecological Investigation Abstracts*, 27th annual meeting, Denver, 1980, p. 106.
18. Crane JP, Kopta MM, Welt SI, et al: Abnormal fetal growth patterns—ultrasonic diagnosis and management. Obstet Gynecol 1977;50:205.
19. Dahms BB, Krauss AN, Auld PAM: Pulmonary function in dysmature infants. J Pediatr 1974;84:434.
20. Drillen CM: The small-for-date infant: etiology and prognosis. Pediatr Clin North Am 1970;17:9.
21. Fancourt R, Campbell S, Harvey D, et al: Follow-up study of small-for-date babies. Br Med J 1976;1:1435.
22. Fitzhardinge PM, Steven EM: The small-for-date infant. I. Later growth patterns. Pediatrics 1972;49:671.
23. Fitzhardinge PM, Steven EM: The small-for-date infant. II. Neurological and intellectual sequelae. Pediatrics 1972;50:50.
24. Fredrick J, Adelstein P: Factors associated with low birth weight of infants delivered at term. Br J Obstet Gynaecol 1978;85:1.
25. Galbraith RS, Karchmar EJ, Piercy WN, et al: The clinical prediction of intrauterine growth retardation. Am J Obstet Gynecol 1979;133:281.
26. Galbraith RS, Low JA, Boston RW: Maternal urinary estriol excretion pattern in patients with chronic fetal insufficiency. Am J Obstet Gynecol 1970;106:302.
27. Gladstone GR, Hordof A, Gersony WM: Propranolol administration during pregnancy: effects on the fetus. J Pediatr 1975;86:967.
28. Gleicher N, Midwall J, Hochberger D, et al: Eisenmenger's syndrome and pregnancy. Obstet Gynecol Surv 1979;34:721.
29. Gluck K, Kulovich MV: Lecithin/sphyngomyelin ratio in amniotic fluid in normal and abnormal pregnancy. Am J Obstet Gynecol 1973;115:539.
30. Gohari P, Berkowitz RL, Hobbins JC: Prediction of intrauterine growth retardation by determination of total intrauterine volume. Am J Obstet Gynecol 1977;127:255.

31. Gould JB, Gluck L, Kulovich MV: The relationship between accelerated pulmonary maturity and accelerated neurologic maturity in certain chronically stressed pregnancies. Am J Obstet Gynecol 1977;127:181.

32. Gregory GA, Gooding CA, Phibbs RH, et al: Meconium aspiration in infants: a prospective study. J Pediatr 1974;85:848.

33. Hanson JW, Smith DW: The fetal hydantoin syndrome. J Pediatr 1975;87:285.

34. Hanson JW, Steissguth AP, Smith DW: The effects of moderate alcohol consumption during pregnancy on fetal growth and morphogenesis. J Pediatr 1978;92:457.

35. Hibbard BM, Jeffcoate TNA: Abruptio placentae. Obstet Gynecol 1966;27:185.

36. Hill DE: Physical growth and development after intrauterine growth retardation. J Reprod Med 1978;21:335.

37. Hobbins JC, Berkowitz RL, Grannum PAT: Diagnosis and antepartum management of intrauterine growth retardation. J Reprod Med 1978;21:319.

38. Holmes GE, Miller HC, Hassanein K, et al: Postnatal somatic growth in infants with atypical fetal growth patterns. Am J Dis Child 1977;131:1078.

39. Ingardia CJ, Fischer JR: Pregnancy after jejunoileal bypass and the SGA infant. Obstet Gynecol 1978;52:215.

40. Jones KL, Chernoff GF: Drugs and chemicals associated with intrauterine growth retardation. J Reprod Med 1978;21:365.

41. Jones KL, Smith DW: Recognition of the fetal alcohol syndrome in early infancy. Lancet 1973;2:999.

42. Jones OW: Genetic factors in the determination of fetal size. J Reprod Med 1978;21:305.

43. Josimovitch JB, Kosor B, Bocella L, et al: Placental lactogen in maternal serum as an index of fetal health. Obstet Gynecol 1970;36:244.

44. Knox GE: Influence of infection on fetal growth and development. J Reprod Med 1978;21:352.

45. Koops BL: Neurologic sequelae in infants with intrauterine growth retardation. J Reprod Med 1978;21:343.

46. Krishna K. Tobacco chewing in pregnancy. Br J Obstet Gynaecol 1978;85:726.

47. Kruger H, Arias-Stella J: The placenta and the newborn infant at high altitudes. Am J Obstet Gynecol 1970;106:586.

48. Kurjak A, Latin V, Polak J: Ultrasonic recognition of two types of growth retardation by measurement of four fetal dimensions. J Perinat Med 1978;6:102.

49. Liggins GC, Howie RM: A controlled trial of antepartum glucocorticoid therapy for the prevention of respiratory distress syndrome in premature infants. Pediatrics 1972;50:515.

50. Low JA, Galbraith RS: Pregnancy characteristics of intrauterine growth retardation. Obstet Gynecol 1974;44:122.

51. Low JA, Galbraith RS, Muir D, et al: Intrauterine growth retardation: a preliminary report of long term morbidity. Am J Obstet Gynecol 1978;130:534.

52. Low JA, Pancham SR, Piercy WN, et al: Intrapartum fetal asphyxia: clinical characteristics, diagnosis and significance in relation to pattern of development. Am J Obstet Gynecol 1977;129:857.

53. Lubchenco LO, Bard H: Incidence of hypoglycemia in newborn infants classified by birth weight and gestational age. Pediatrics 1971;47:831.

54. Lubchenco LO, Hansman C, Dressler M, et al: Intrauterine growth as estimated from liveborn birth-weight data at 24 to 42 weeks of gestation. Pediatrics 1963;32:793.

55. Makowski EL, Battaglia FC, Meschia G, et al: Effect of maternal exposure to high altitude upon fetal oxygenation. Am J Obstet Gynecol 1968;100:852.

56. Molteni RA, Stys SJ, Battaglia FC: Relationship of fetal and placental weight in human beings. J Reprod Med 1978;21:327.

57. Naeye RL: Causes and consequences of placental growth retardation. JAMA 1978;239:1145.

58. Naeye RL, Dixon JB: Distortions in fetal growth standards. Pediatr Res 1978;12:987.

59. Niswander KR, et al: *The Women and Their Pregnancies: the Collaborative Perinatal Study of the National Institute of Neurological Diseases and Stroke*. Philadelphia, WB Saunders Co, 1972.

60. Nochimson DJ, Petrie RH: Glucocorticoid therapy for the induction of pulmonary maturity in severely hypertensive gravid women. Am J Obstet Gynecol 1979;133:449.

61. Odendall H: Fetal heart rate patterns in patients with intrauterine growth retardation. Obstet Gynecol 1976;48:187.

62. Oh W: Considerations in neonates with intrauterine growth retardation. Clin Obstet Gynecol 1977;20:99.

63. Ong HC, Sen DK: Clinical estimation of fetal weight. Am J Obstet Gynecol 1972;112:877.

64. Ounsted M, Ounsted E: Rate of intrauterine growth. Nature 1968;220:599.

65. Perry CP, Harris RE, Delemos RA, et al: Intrauterine growth retarded infants. Obstet Gynecol 1976;48:182.

66. Queenan JT, Kubarych SF, Cook LN, et al: Diagnostic ultrasound for detection of intrauterine growth retardation. Am J Obstet Gynecol 1976;124:865.

67. Resnik R: Maternal diseases associated with abnormal fetal growth. J Reprod Med 1978;21:315.

68. Rosso P, Winick M: Intrauterine growth retardation: a new systematic approach based on the clinical and biochemical characteristics of this condition. J Perinat Med 1974;2:147.

69. Stangstad LF: Birth weights in children with phenylketonuria and in their siblings. Lancet 1972;1:809.

70. Shanklin DR: The influence of placental lesions on the newborn infant. Pediatr Clin North Am 1970;17:25.

71. Shaul WL, Hall JG: Multiple congenital anomalies associated with oral anticoagulants. Am J Obstet Gynecol 1977;127:191.

72. Smith DW: Teratogenicity of anticonvulsive medications. Am J Dis Child 1977;131:1337.

73. Spellacy WN: Monitoring of high risk pregnancies with human placental lactogen, in Spellacy WN (ed): *Management of high risk pregnancy*. Baltimore, University Park Press, 1976, p. 107.

74. Stein H: Maternal protein depletion and small-for-gestational-age babies. Arch Dis Child 1975;50:146.

75. Stein ZA, Susser MW: The Dutch famine 1944-45 and the reproductive process: effects on six indices at birth. Pediatr Res 1975;9:70.

76. Stein, ZA, Susser, MW, Rush D: Prenatal nutrition and birth weight: experiments and quasi-experiments in the past decade. J Reprod Med 1978;21:287.

77. Stumpf DA, Frost M: Seizures, anticonvulsants, and pregnancy. Am J Dis Child 1978;132:746.

78. Tejani N, Mann LI: Diagnosis and management of the small-for-gestational-age fetus. Clin Obstet Gynecol 1977;20:943.

79. Tejani N, Mann LI, Weiss RR: Antenatal diagnosis and management of the small for gestational age fetus. Obstet Gynecol 1976;45:31.

80. Tulchinsky D: Endocrine evaluation in the diagnosis of intrauterine growth retardation. Clin Obstet Gynecol 1977;20:969.

81. Tulchinsky D, Osathanonoh R, Finn A: Dehydroepiandrosterone sulfate loading test in the diagnosis of complicated pregnancies. N Engl J Med 1976;294:517.

82. Turner G: Recognition of intrauterine growth retardation by considering comparative birth-weights. Lancet 1971;2:1123.

83. Usher RH: Clinical and therapeutic aspects of fetal malnutrition. Pediatr Clin North Am 1970;17:169.

84. Varma TR: Fetal growth and placental function in patients with placenta praevia. Br J Obstet Gynaecol 1973;80:311.

85. Vohr BR, Oh W, Rosenfield AG, et al: The preterm small-for-gestational age infant: a two-year follow-up study. Am J Obstet Gynecol 1979;133:425.

86. Warsof SL, Gohavi P, Berkowitz RL, et al: The estimation of fetal weight by computer-assisted analysis. Am J Obstet Gynecol 1977;128:881.

87. Westin B: Gravidogram and fetal growth. Acta Obstet Gynecol Scand 1977;56:273.

88. Wilson GS, Desmond MW, Verniaun WM: Early development of infants of heroin-addicted mothers. Am J Dis Child 1973;126:457.

89. Wood C, Ng KH, Hounslow D, et al: Time—an important variable in normal delivery. Br J Obstet Gynaecol 1973;80:295.

90. Zador G, Nilsson BA: Low dose intermittent epidural anesthesia in labor: influence on labor and fetal acid-base status. Acta Obstet Gynecol Scand 1974; 34(suppl):19.

91. Zelson C, Lee SJ: Casalino M: Neonatal narcotic addiction. N Engl J Med 1973;289:1216.

9

■ ■ ■

MANAGEMENT OF PROLONGED PREGNANCY

Fernando Arias

Until relatively a few years ago the existence of problems associated with prolonged gestation was a controversial matter. Today, there is general consensus that perinatal mortality and morbidity are increased severalfold when pregnancies become prolonged.[3,4,18] Controversy is now centered on the adequacy of different methods of fetal surveillance for detecting the fetus at risk of developing the problems associated with prolongation of pregnancy.

■ DEFINITION

A pregnancy becomes prolonged when it reaches or surpasses 42 weeks. In addition to *prolonged pregnancy*, other names commonly used for this situation are *postdatism* and *postterm pregnancy*. The terms *prolonged pregnancy*, *postdatism* and *postterm pregnancy*, are not interchangeable with *postmaturity*, another expression used commonly when referring to prolonged gestations. Postmaturity means intrauterine growth retardation associated with a prolonged gestation. Some authors use the term *dysmaturity* to refer to postmature infants. The difference between these terms is as follows:

prolonged pregnancy, postdatism, postterm pregnancy Pregnancy that reaches or surpasses 42 weeks of gestation.

postmaturity, dysmaturity Syndrome of intrauterine growth retardation occurring in a prolonged pregnancy.

■ INCIDENCE

According to Nägele's rule, human gestation lasts 40 weeks. There is some biologic variation; in fact, about 11% of all pregnancies end after 42 weeks of gestation (Table 9-1). The obstetrician, therefore, will be faced with the problems and dilemmas associated with the management of prolonged pregnancies in 1 of every 10 obstetric patients. Fortunately, only about 10% of

TABLE 9-1 ■ Time of spontaneous termination of pregnancy

Week	% of patients
37	0.6
38	3.6
39	6.9
40	20.9
41	31.0
42	26.0
43	8.5
44	2.5

Data from Park GL: The duration of pregnancy. Lancet 1968;2:1388.

173

those pregnancies that reach or surpass 42 weeks of gestation are associated with fetal complications. Thus only 1 of every 100 obstetric patients will develop problems associated with prolonged gestation.

■ PHYSIOLOGIC CHANGES ASSOCIATED WITH PROLONGED GESTATION

With prolongation of pregnancy a series of changes occur in the amniotic fluid, placenta, and fetus. Knowledge about these changes and their early detection allow the clinician to obtain evidence of the development of problems and are the basis for the management protocol to be described later.

Amniotic fluid changes

There are quantitative and qualitative changes in the amniotic fluid with prolongation of pregnancy. From a quantitative viewpoint the amniotic fluid volume reaches a peak of about 1000 ml at 38 weeks of gestation and decreases to about 800 ml at term. The reduction in volume becomes more marked after term, and the amount of fluid is approximately 480, 250, and 160 ml at 42, 43, and 44 weeks, respectively.[1,9,16] Thus in the absence of rupture of the fetal membranes, a marked decrease in amniotic fluid volume in a pregnancy at term is strong evidence that such a pregnancy has reached or exceeded 42 weeks. In general, an amniotic fluid volume under 400 ml indicates that the fetus is at risk of complications and that the pregnancy must be terminated.[12]

For the clinician the problem is how to evaluate amniotic fluid volume. Precise methods require the injection of radioactive tracers or dyes into the amniotic cavity to calculate the volume by dilution techniques. These methods require amniocentesis. A nonquantitative but extremely reliable method is ultrasound examination. Both real-time and static scanning instruments allow the expert to have a clear impression about the amount of fluid contained in the uterus. Some techniques indirectly measure the amount of fluid with ultrasound,[7] but for practical purposes a nonquantitative evaluation is adequate in the majority of cases.

In addition to changes in volume with prolonged gestation, there are changes in the composition of the amniotic fluid. The liquor becomes milky and cloudy because of the presence of abundant flakes of vernix caseosa coming out of the fetal skin and floating in the fluid. The presence of large amounts of vernix alters the phospholipid composition of the fluid, and the L/S ratio becomes very high (4:1 or more) when measured by the Gluck method[5] using reflectance spectrometry. Also, when the fetus has passed meconium, a situation that occurs frequently in prolonged pregnancies, the color of the fluid may have a green or yellow discoloration depending on how long meconium has been present.

Placental changes

There is an abundance of literature regarding the gross and microscopic changes occurring in the placenta after term: decrease in diameter and length of chorionic villae, fibrinoid necrosis, and accelerated atheromatosis of chorionic and decidual vessels are all changes occurring simultaneously or preceding the appearance of hemorrhagic infarcts, which are the foci for calcium deposition and formation of white infarcts. Infarcts are present in 10% to 25% of term and 60% to 80% of postterm placentas, and they are more common at the placental borders.[16] Similarly, postterm deposition of calcium in the placenta reaches up to 10 g/100 g of dry tissue weight, whereas it is only 2 to 3 g/100 g at term.

The morphologic changes that occur with placental senescence can be observed by ultrasound and have been described by Granum, Berkowitz, and Hobbins.[8] These changes are quite specific. During the first part of gestation the ultrasonic appearance of the placenta is homogeneous, without echogenic densities, and limited by a smooth chorionic plate (grade 0 placenta). With progression of pregnancy the chorionic plate begins to acquire subtle undulations, and echogenic densities appear randomly dispersed throughout the organ but sparing its basal layer (grade I placenta). Near term the indentations in the chorionic plate become more marked, echogenic densities appear in the basal layer, and commalike densities seem to extend from the chorionic plate into the substance of the placenta (grade II). Finally, when the pregnancy is at term or postterm the indentations in the chorionic plate become more marked, giving the appearance of cotyledons. This impression is reinforced by increased confluency of the commalike densities that become the intercotyledonary septa. Also, characteristically, the central

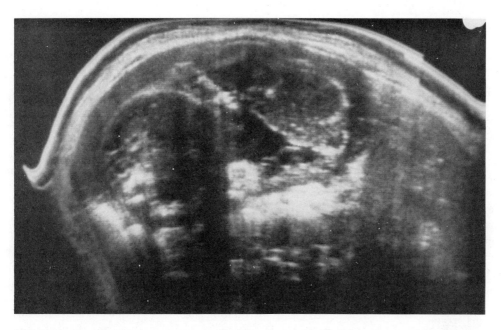

FIG. 9-1 ■ A grade III placenta seen with static ultrasound. The placenta is to the right, the circular fetal abdomen is to the left. Echo-free amniotic fluid is seen between the fetus and the placenta. The placenta has marked calcification and gives the appearance of being divided in cotyledons with central echo-free lakes.

portion of the cotyledons become echo-free (fall-out areas), and large irregular densities, capable of casting acoustic shadows, appear in the substance of the placenta (grade III placenta, Fig. 9-1).

The structural changes in the placenta may be reflected in changes affecting the biochemical tests used to evaluate the fetoplacental unit. Both human placental lactogen (HPL) and estriol concentration are affected, but these changes lack sensitivity and have a low positive predictive value. In other words, a normal serum estriol[6] or a normal estriol/creatinine ratio[10] is reassuring, but finding abnormally low levels does not necessarily indicate the presence of problems.

Fetal changes

With progression of a gestation beyond 42 weeks the fetus starts to lose the vernix caseosa. With this loss of the protective lipid layer the fetal skin directly contacts the aqueous environment and becomes wrinkled. Growth of the hair and fingernails continues, and in some cases wasting of the subcutaneous tissues is also apparent. If the fetus passes meconium, the skin will have a greenish or yellowish staining.

Unfortunately, the changes occurring in the fetus as a result of pregnancy prolongation cannot be assessed directly, and some can be observed only after birth. The loss of vernix caseosa and the presence or absence of meconium can be evaluated by amniotic fluid examination. Arrest in fetal growth and excessive fetal growth can be assessed by ultrasound examination. However, other fine details of the fetal postmaturity syndrome are still beyond the present capacities for antenatal evaluation of the fetus.

■ ANTEPARTUM MANAGEMENT OF THE PATIENT WITH PROLONGED GESTATION

Most protocols for the management of postterm pregnancies attempt to find solutions to this complex problem with the use of a single method of assessment (nonstress test [NST], contractions stress test [OCT], amniocentesis). Other protocols use simplistic solutions that ignore important aspects of the problem and may cause increased fetal and maternal morbidity, for example, induction of labor for every pregnancy that reaches 41 weeks. As in any other difficult clinical situation, adequate management of prolonged pregnancy must be based on known facts about the problem and must follow a rather rigorous sequence of steps. The first question to be answered when the obstetrician faces a patient suspected of a prolonged pregnancy is the following:

Are the patient's dates excellent?

It is important to notice that this question asks for the reliability of the patient's dates and not for the dates themselves. To answer the question requires going back to the original information that allowed the obstetrician to establish an estimated date of confinement (EDC) and submit them to critical analysis to find out whether or not that information is highly reliable. The reliability of the EDC is excellent if the following conditions are met:

1. The patient had at least three regular menstrual periods before the last menstrual period (LMP) in the absence of oral contraception, and the LMP was normal in duration and amount of flow.
2. At least one of the following pieces of corroborative information about the patient's dates is present:
   a. A positive pregnancy test 5 to 6 weeks after the LMP
   b. An ultrasonic crown-rump measurement before 12 weeks that is in agreement with the LMP
   c. A pelvic examination carried out by an obstetrician before 16 weeks of gestation with the finding of a uterine size in agreement with the LMP
   d. Uterine fundus at the umbilicus and fetal heart tones (FHT) heard with aural stethoscope 20 weeks after the LMP
   e. One or more ultrasound measurements of the fetal biparietal diameter (BPD) obtained between 16 and 30 weeks of gestation in agreement with the LMP

There are only two possible answers to the initial question. If the answer is yes, the dates are excellent, and the patient is, in fact, at 42 or more weeks of gestation. Then the next question is:

Is the patient's cervix ripe?

If the cervix is ripe (more than 6 points in the cervical evaluation score, Chapter 3), the patient with excellent dates must be admitted to the hospital and her labor induced with oxytocin under direct electronic monitoring. There is no good reason to prolong a pregnancy that by rigorous criteria has reached or surpassed 42 weeks, especially if the cervix is ripe, indicating a high probability of a successful induction.

If the patient's dates are not excellent or if the patient has excellent dates but an unripe cervix, the next step in our management protocol is an ultrasound examination. To obtain adequate information, the ultrasound laboratory must be informed of the nature of the problem. Patients with poor dates who are suspected of being postterm are frequently sent to the ultrasound laboratory with a request for the estimation of gestational age. This request ignores the large margin for error in the estimation of dates when single ultrasound measurements of the fetal BPD are taken at the end of pregnancy. The examination with ultrasound in patient's with prolonged gestation has as its first objective to answer the following question:

Is there any gross congenital malformation of the fetus?

This is an important question because some congenital defects, particularly neural tube defects, are relatively frequent in patients with prolonged gestations. An ultrasound examination rules out hydrocephaly and anencephaly, two defects often associated with prolongation of pregnancy. In anencephaly, a defect incompatible with life, concerns about fetal well-being disappear and with them the need for further testing. In hydrocephaly, careful evaluation is necessary, since extrauterine life with adequate neurologic and intellectual development is becoming possible for an increasing number of neonates afflicted with this problem (Chapter 2).

If no fetal abnormalities are detected, the second question to be answered in the ultrasound examination is:

What is the volume of amniotic fluid and the ultrasonic appearance of the placenta?

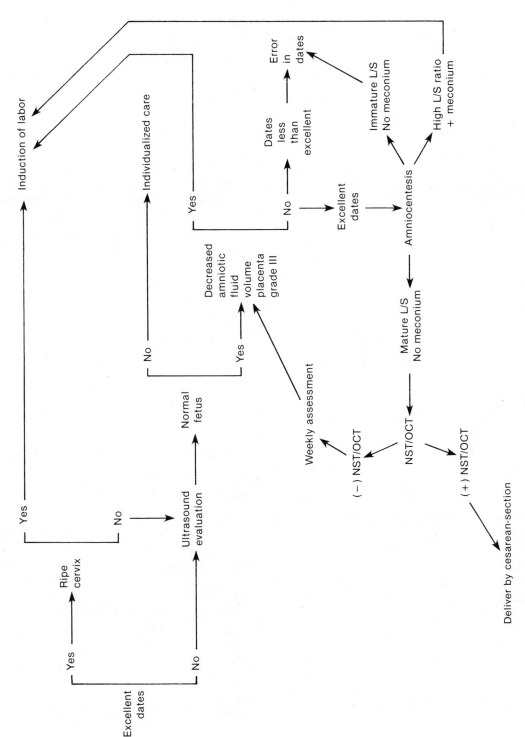

FIG. 9-2 ■ Antepartum management of patients suspected to have prolonged pregnancy.

A decreased amount of amniotic fluid or advanced placental aging (grade III placenta) are reliable signs indicating the need for pregnancy termination.[13,17] The patient must be admitted to the hospital for a trial of labor with intravenous oxytocin under careful fetal monitoring, ideally with fetal scalp electrode and intrauterine pressure catheter. If the induction fails, cesarean section must be chosen as the proper way of delivery.

If the amniotic fluid volume is normal and the placenta does not show signs of senescence, the chances that the pregnancy is postterm become small. Further evaluation will be necessary only for patients with excellent dates.

Those patients with less than excellent dates who have been analyzed up to this point in our protocol should be told that their pregnancy is not postterm and should be followed with weekly examinations of the cervix and ultrasound evaluations of the amniotic fluid volume.

Patients with excellent dates indicating postterm pregnancy, but with normal ultrasound findings with respect to fluid volume and placental appearance, should have amniocentesis as the next step to answer the following question:

> **What is the L/S ratio and the color of the amniotic fluid?**

An L/S ratio markedly elevated (4:1 or greater) when determined with the Gluck technique[5] is an early sign of postmaturity and an indication for pregnancy termination. Similarly, the presence of green or yellow meconium staining of the amniotic fluid in a patient with excellent dates indicating 42 or more weeks of gestation is a sign of postmaturity, and the pregnancy must be terminated. In cases of meconium staining detected antenatally and generally in all cases of postterm deliveries, the obstetrician and the pediatrician must be ready to institute measures to prevent meconium aspiration at the time of delivery.

If the L/S ratio is immature or mature but not markedly elevated and the fluid is clear, the patient's dates must be reviewed again in an attempt to discover any fault in the analysis that led to the classification of the patient's dates as excellent. The possibility of a condition causing delayed fetal lung maturation, such as maternal diabetes, must also be considered and ruled out.

If repeated analysis shows that, in fact, the dates are excellent, the patient must have an NST-OCT evaluation. The test is simple and may be useful in detecting a rare case of placental insufficiency not suspected with the previous tests. Obviously if the NST-OCT testing is abnormal, the pregnancy must be terminated. The NST-OCT testing will be abnormal only exceptionally in patients with prolonged pregnancy without signs of intrauterine growth retardation (IUGR), normal amount of amniotic fluid, placenta that does not show signs of senescence, clear amniotic fluid, and a L/S ratio that is not markedly elevated. If these tests are normal, the patient must have weekly evaluations, including pelvic and ultrasound examinations, amniocentesis, and NST-OCT testing, and the pregnancy is allowed to continue but checked weekly if negative results are obtained.

The most important point to remember with respect to NST-OCT testing in the evaluation of prolonged pregnancies is that they must not be the only tests used for assessing fetal well-being in this situation. The literature abounds in descriptions of antepartum and intrapartum fetal deaths within a few days of reassuring fetal evaluation with both NST and OCT in patients with prolonged gestation.[10,11]

A summary of the antepartum management protocol for patients suspected of prolonged pregnancies is shown in Fig. 9-2.

■ INTRAPARTUM MANAGEMENT OF THE PATIENT WITH PROLONGED GESTATION

Once it has been determined that a patient with prolonged gestation must be delivered (excellent dates and ripe cervix, oligohydramnios, placental aging, IUGR, fetal macrosomia, elevated L/S ratio, meconium-stained amniotic fluid, congenital malformations of the fetus), the obstetrician should be ready to face several potentially serious problems during the intrapartum period.

Intrapartum fetal hypoxia

It is not an uncommon event for signs of fetal hypoxia to appear during labor in patients with prolonged gestation. Decreased beat-to-beat variability and late decelerations are the most commonly observed indicators of fetal distress, and the presence of these signs is always significant in postterm pregnancies and must be followed by measurement of the fetal pH. If the cervix has not dilated enough to allow the performance of fetal scalp sampling, labor must be arrested with a tocolytic agent and the pregnancy terminated by cesarean section. If electronic monitoring is suggestive of fetal distress but the pH measurements show no evidence of fetal acidosis, labor may be allowed to continue.

A difficult situation occurs when scalp sampling is not possible and decreased variability is the only manifestation of the possibility of fetal hypoxia in patients with prolonged gestation and closed cervix. In these cases it is necessary to remember that if the variability appears to be decreased with the external monitoring, it will look worse with a direct lead and that the fetus at term and the healthy postterm fetus normally have *increased* variability. Also, in many cases of prolonged pregnancy, decreased beat-to-beat variability is the only monitoring sign preceding the sudden onset of fetal bradycardia frequently ending in intrapartum or neonatal death. Therefore termination of pregnancy by cesarean section may be necessary in this situation even if late decelerations are not present. Fetal tachycardia (190 to 200 beats/min) has also been reported preceding fetal death in postterm pregnancies.[14]

Fetal trauma

Labor in a patient with prolonged gestation must be preceded by an evaluation of the fetal size. If the clinic, ultrasonic, and radiologic examinations point to the existence of fetal macrosomia, close attention must be given to the development of abnormalities of labor and cesarean section used liberally if any arrest or protraction disorder occur. Unfortunately in some cases labor proceeds without detectable abnormalities until the moment when the fetal head is delivered and shoulder dystocia becomes apparent. The obstetrician must be aware of the possibility of shoulder dystocia in every postterm pregnancy with macrosomic fetus, even if labor is completely normal.

Meconium aspiration syndrome (MAS)

With the increased awareness of obstetricians about the complications associated with postterm pregnancies and with the increased use of biophysical and biochemical methods for antepartum and intrapartum fetal evaluation, the main complication associated with prolonged pregnancy is, at the present time, MAS. This extremely serious problem until recently had a mortality that in some series went up to 60% of the cases. Fortunately, with the use of nasopharyngeal aspiration before the first breath, followed by endotracheal aspiration immediately after birth,[2,15] both the mortality and morbidity associated with MAS have substantially decreased in the last few years.

In every delivery of a patient with prolonged pregnancy, and especially in those cases in which meconium has been detected antepartum or intrapartum, the obstetrician must be ready to prevent the occurrence of MAS. For this purpose a DeLee tube must be ready in the obstetrician's mouth at the time of delivery, and, as soon as the fetal head appears on the maternal perineum, or in the open uterus in the case of cesarean section, *and before the first fetal breathing effort*, the tube must be introduced through the nose and the nasopharynx aspirated completely. If there is abundant meconium, a second DeLee tube must be used. During this time, in the case of vaginal deliveries, the mother must be panting and avoiding expulsive efforts. Once the obstetrician feels certain that all or most of the meconium that existed in the oropharynx has been removed, the delivery is completed and the infant moved to an Ohio table where the obstetrician or the pediatrician, if present, must proceed to endotracheal aspiration in *every case* in which meconium has been removed from the upper airway. For this purpose another DeLee tube, or the largest endotracheal tube compatible with the baby's tracheal size, must be inserted in the infant's trachea and then removed slowly under continuous aspiration with the mouth or with a suction machine.

The literature shows excellent results (decreased neonatal mortality and morbidity) with the combined use of aspiration of the oropharynx before the first breath followed by endotracheal aspiration.[2,15] This technique must become routine in the delivery room management of the meconium-stained infant.

■ REFERENCES

1. Beischer NA, Evans JH, Townsend L: Studies in prolonged pregnancy. I. The incidence of prolonged pregnancy. Am J Obstet Gynecol 1969;103:476.
2. Carson BS, Losey RW, Bowes WA, et al: Combined obstetric and pediatric approach to prevent meconium aspiration syndrome. Am J Obstet Gynecol 1976;126:712.

3. Clifford SA: Postmaturity with placental dysfunction. J Pediatr 1954;44:1.
4. Field TM, Dabiri C, Hallock A, et al: Developmental effects of prolonged pregnancy and the postmaturity syndrome. J Pediatr 1977;90:836.
5. Gluck L, Kulovich MV, Borer RC, et al: The interpretation and significance of the lecithin/sphyngomyelin ratio in amniotic fluid. Am J Obstet Gynecol 1974; 120:142.
6. Goebelsmann U: The uses of estriol as a monitoring tool. Clin Obstet Gynecol 1979;6:223.
7. Gohari P, Berkowitz RL, Hobbins JC: In utero prediction of IUGR by determination of total intrauterine volume. Am J Obstet Gynecol 1977;127:255.
8. Granum PA, Berkowitz RL, Hobbins JC: The ultrasonic changes in the maturing placenta and their relation to fetal pulmonic maturity. Am J Obstet Gynecol 1979; 133:915.
9. Hytten FE, Thomson AM: Maternal physiological adjustments, in Assali NS (ed): *Biology of Gestation*. New York, Academic Press, Inc. 1968, vol. 1, pp. 449-479.
10. Khouzami VA, Johnson JWE, Hernandez E, et al: Urinary estrogens in postterm pregnancy. Am J Obstet Gynecol 1981;141:205.
11. Kiyazaki FS, Miyazaki BA: False reactive nonstress tests in postterm pregnancies. Am J Obstet Gynecol 1981; 140:209.
12. Morris ED: Placental insufficiency. Br Med Bull 1968; 24:76.
13. Rayburn W, Molley ME, Stempel L, et al: Antepartum prediction of the postmature infant, in *Proceedings of The Society of Perinatal Obstetricians*, second annual meeting, San Antonio, 1982, p. 41.
14. Ron M, Adoni A, Hchner-Celnikier D, et al: The significance of baseline tachycardia in the postterm fetus. Int J Gynaecol Obstet 1980;18:76.
15. Ting P, Brady JP: Tracheal suction in meconium aspiration. Am J Obstet Gynecol 1975;122:767.
16. Vorherr H: Placental insufficiency in relation to postterm pregnancy and fetal postmaturity. Am J Obstet Gynecol 1975;123:67.
17. Yeh S-Y, Petruch R, Platt LD: Possible role of ultrasonic placental grading in the management of post-term pregnancies, in *Proceedings of The Society of Perinatal Obstetricians*, second annual meeting, San Antonio, 1982, p. 139.
18. Zwerdling MA: Factors pertaining to prolonged pregnancy and its outcome. Pediatrics 1967;42:202.

10

■ ■ ■

CARDIAC DISEASE IN PREGNANCY

Carlton S. Pearse

The incidence of heart disease in pregnancy is probably about 1% with figures ranging from 0.2% to 3.7% in the literature.[9,14,23,45] In a recent large survey cardiac disease represented the most common (22%) nonobstetric cause of maternal mortality.[23] Pregnant patients with cardiac disease are of two types: (1) those who have a previously undiagnosed cardiac disease and (2) those who were diagnosed as having a cardiac disease before they became pregnant. In both cases it is of paramount importance for the obstetrician to know the cardiovascular physiology of normal pregnancy to recognize abnormalities in the diseased state. Therefore the initial part of this chapter deals with the hemodynamics of pregnancy and other normal physiologic changes that take place during pregnancy, labor, and the puerperium. The rest of the chapter covers general guidelines for managing the pregnant patient with cardiac disease and discusses specific cardiac conditions.

■ CARDIOVASCULAR CHANGES IN THE PREGNANT WOMAN WITH NO CARDIAC DISEASE
Hemodynamic changes

Pregnancy induces profound changes in the cardiovascular dynamics of all women. In women without cardiac disease these rather dramatic changes are tolerated with minimal or no symptomatology. However, in women with an altered cardiovascular system the ability to adapt to the stress of pregnancy, labor, and the puerperium may be limited, placing both fetus and mother at risk.

Before parturition. The major cardiovascular alterations seen during pregnancy are decreased peripheral vascular resistance, increased cardiac output, and increased blood volume.

Peripheral resistance decreases dramatically during pregnancy. The reasons for this decrease have not been completely worked out, but they are probably the result of a combination of (1) trophoblastic erosion of maternal endometrial vessels causing an effect similar to an arteriovenous fistula, (2) increased production of placental and ovarian steroid hormones that decrease vascular resistance, and (3) perhaps the effects of prolactin.[30,31,36,41] The result is a 20% to 30% fall in resistance at 21 to 24 weeks, which gradually returns to normal at term. As peripheral resistance decreases, so does systemic blood pressure that decreases near the end of the first trimester, continues to decrease through the second trimester, and then often begins to rise toward nonpregnant levels. The fall in diastolic pressure exceeds that of the systolic, resulting in a widened pulse pressure.

At least partially as a result of the fall in peripheral resistance, *cardiac output* rises during pregnancy reaching a maximum at about 20 weeks of gestation. This increase probably be-

181

gins as early as 10 weeks and persists until delivery. The maximal increase in output is approximately 30% to 50% and is achieved by an augmented stroke volume early in pregnancy and by an increase in heart rate as pregnancy advances.[30,31,44]

An important variable in the hemodynamics of pregnancy is maternal position. As length of gestation increases and the uterus grows, measurements made in the supine or seated positions reflect more the effects of the obstruction of the inferior vena cava by the pregnant uterus, which can decrease cardiac output by nearly 30% at term.[31] As vascular resistance drops and cardiac output increases, *blood volume* is also increasing by about 40% to 50%.[34,43] The volume expansion begins early in pregnancy and includes red cell and plasma volumes. Most authors have found that the increase in plasma outstrips that of red blood cells volume resulting in the physiologic anemia of pregnancy. However, recent work supports the contention that if adequate supplemental iron is given, no decline in hemoglobin concentration occurs.[31,45]

The demand on the heart in pregnancy is primarily to pump more blood, often with a lowered viscosity as a result of the drop in hemoglobin concentration against a lowered afterload. Resting oxygen consumption increases but proportionately less than cardiac output so that, especially in early pregnancy, the arteriovenous oxygen difference falls. There is some evidence that myocardial contractility increases during pregnancy and falls postpartum, and this has led some investigators to postulate that hormonal changes have a direct effect on myocardial contractility. In twin gestations the changes in heart rate and stroke volume are similar to those seen in singleton pregnancies, whereas the increase in blood volume and decrease in peripheral resistance are about 20% greater than in pregnancies with one fetus.

Exercise in the pregnant patient is a source of additional cardiac demand and may make a significant difference in management and outcome in the pregnant patient with cardiac disease.[47,48,49] In an effort to preserve the low arteriovenous oxygen difference normal to pregnancy, oxygen consumption and cardiac output increase more in the pregnant than in the nonpregnant patient if the same exercise is performed. As pregnancy progresses, this increase

in output results more and more from an increase in heart rate because the ability of the pregnant heart to increase stroke volume decreases during gestation, although stroke volume throughout pregnancy always exceeds that of a nonpregnant individual. Thus in pregnancy the heart is required to pay a much higher cost to keep the peripheral tissues (and the uterus) bathed in oxygen-rich blood during exercise. If the heart is unable to meet these demands, relative tissue hypoxia will be the inevitable result.

During labor, delivery, and the puerperium. Labor, delivery, and the early puerperium induce a whole new set of changes in the maternal cardiovascular system and often represent the period of peak risk for the patient with cardiac disease. During labor each contraction, by squeezing blood out of the uterus and back to the heart, increases cardiac output by 15% to 20% and thereby increases blood pressure and causes a reflex decrease in pulse rate. Between contractions the hemodynamic physiology is a function of anesthesia more than anything else. In patients suffering from pain and apprehension there is a progressive rise in cardiac output of about 40% above that of late pregnancy. Patients with continuous epidural anesthesia do not show an increased cardiac output between contractions. Cardiac output in labor, just as in late pregnancy, is a function of maternal position, since the pregnant uterus significantly interferes with venous return to the heart. All the hemodynamic changes of labor are less pronounced if the woman is permitted to labor in lateral recumbency. During the second stage of labor the Valsalva's maneuver, used to effect delivery, results in a transient but significant decrease in venous return as well as reflex bradycardia. Each of these changes contributes to a decrease in cardiac output that could be critical to the pregnant patient with cardiac disease.

Delivery, by virtue of the sudden decrease in blood demand of the uteroplacental tissues and the resolution of the inferior vena cava compression, results in a rapid increase in circulating blood volume that causes an increase in cardiac output and reflex bradycardia. These changes occur regardless of anesthesia (local or continuous caudal) but are transient with return to nonpregnant levels by 1 to 2 weeks postpartum.[46] A factor lessening the increase in blood volume and cardiac output at the time of delivery is the maternal blood loss occurring during parturition—about 600 ml within the first hour postpartum. A blood loss significantly larger than this amount causes additional alterations in maternal hemodynamics. Delivery by cesarean section produces maternal cardiovascular changes that at least in part are a function of the anesthetic agent or agents used.

Changes in the heart examination

Many of the cardiovascular changes occurring during normal pregnancy result in symptoms, signs, or physical findings that may mimic heart disease. It is essential that the clinician be able to distinguish between those findings that are normal for pregnancy and those indicative of heart disease. The most common complaints in normal pregnancy are *dyspnea*, a result of hyperventilation and increased work during breathing and *edema* caused by impairment to the return circulation by the pregnant uterus. Physical findings are many. As mentioned previously in discussing peripheral resistance, blood pressure is usually below nonpregnant levels with increased pulse pressure. Pulse and respiration rates are generally increased. The cardiac impulse may be more diffuse, the jugular veins may be distended, and the point of maximal impulse is usually laterally displaced as the elevated diaphragm gives the heart a more horizontal position. The heart sounds are often more pronounced, and the second heart sound is occasionally palpated at the pulmonic area.

Cutforth and McDonald[11] studied the cardiac examination of 50 normal pregnant women. They found that the auscultatory changes occur at about the twelfth week or shortly thereafter and disappear within 1 week postpartum. Eighty-eight percent of these normal pregnant women had a widely split S_1 caused by early closure of the mitral valve, 84% developed an S_3, and 16% an S_4. Ninety-two percent developed a systolic ejection murmur best heard at the left sternal border. As described by Harvey[22] this "innocent" murmur of pregnancy is usually short, occurs in the early or middle portion of systole, and is grade 1 to 3 over 6 in intensity. It may have a musical, vibratory, or buzzing quality and should not be confused with the holosystolic murmurs of mitral insufficiency, tricuspid insufficiency, and ventricular septal defect, or the harsh murmurs of pulmonic or aortic stenosis.

The latter two murmurs are often associated with early systolic ejection sounds, palpable thrills, or diastolic murmurs, any one of which is a clue to the significance of the auscultatory finding. The ejection murmur of normal pregnancy may be confused with that of an atrial septal defect (ASD) if care is not taken to listen for splitting of the second heart sounds. In a normal heart S_2 is single or narrowly split in expiration, but on inspiration an increased split is heard; whereas, in an ASD, S_2 is split and the degree of split is fixed through inspiration and expiration.

Diastolic murmurs are usually indicators of organic heart disease with the only exception being the occasional patient in whom aftervibrations of a prominent S_3 may mimic a murmur. The murmurs of preexisting aortic insufficiency or mitral regurgitation may disappear during pregnancy, most likely as a consequence of the profound decrease in peripheral vascular resistance. A continuous hum either from the jugular vein or breast is a consequence of the high cardiac output. A venous hum can be eliminated by compressing the jugular vein, whereas the mammary hum disappears with direct pressure over the arm in which it is localized. The pulmonary examination of a pregnant woman is remarkable for the finding of elevated diaphragms and often for the presence of scattered basilar rales caused by atelectasis, all resulting from the upward growth of the uterus.

Changes in radiographs, electrocardiograms, and echocardiograms

No consistent changes in chest radiographs have been noted during normal pregnancy although lordosis may lead to straightening of the left heart border and cause prominence of the main pulmonary artery segment. Also, collateral flow through the azygos vein may occasionally lead to prominence of that vein in a normal mother. In general, the same radiologic diagnostic criteria for cardiopulmonary disease used in nonpregnant patients apply to pregnant patients as well.

Electrocardiograms often reveal elevation and rotation of the heart. There is a leftward shift in the axis and often a Q wave and inverted T wave in lead 3. However, there should not be an accompanying Q wave in aV_F, and the changes in lead 3 should revert toward normal on deep inspiration. Disturbances in rhythm are relatively common in pregnancy, and atrial and ventricular extrasystoles are often seen. Even bigeminal rhythm and paroxysmal atrial tachycardia may occur in the absence of organic heart disease.[40] These arrhythmias are usually self-limiting and seldom require therapy. Transient ST and T wave changes similar to those seen with ischemia have been reported in the absence of disease. Atrioventricular conduction may also be prolonged, and a Wenckebach-type of heart block has been observed in normal pregnant patients.

A recent addition to the diagnostic tools at the disposal of the physician is echocardiography. This technique is noninvasive and can be helpful in diagnosing mitral valve disorders, idiopathic hypertrophic subaortic stenosis, septal defects, and pulmonic and aortic stenosis as well as tricuspid insufficiency. The most important change in the echocardiogram during normal pregnancy is the finding of pericardial effusions in close to 50% of all women. This finding is more common in the last trimester, and the accumulation of fluid is usually small.[20]

Cardiac catheterization is the ultimate diagnostic tool. However, it entails significant risk to mother and fetus and should be avoided in pregnancy unless absolutely necessary. Using the history, physical examination, and the various diagnostic tests mentioned before, the clinician should be able to identify those pregnant patients with organic heart disease, evaluate their risks, and manage them appropriately.

■ GENERAL GUIDELINES FOR MANAGING THE PREGNANT PATIENT WITH CARDIAC DISEASE

In discussing patients with heart disease a functional classification is useful, and in keeping with most authors, the classification of the New York Heart Association (NYHA) is used as follows:

Class I	Asymptomatic
Class II	Symptomatic with heavy exercise
Class III	Symptomatic with light exercise
Class IV	Symptomatic at rest

The main problem for the patient with cardiac disease during pregnancy is the possibility of cardiac decompensation with resulting congestive heart failure. Therefore if a successful outcome is to be achieved, those factors that contribute to the cardiac work load must be carefully controlled and monitored. Such factors include activity, emotional stress, anemia, salt and caloric overload, infection, hypertension, and significant arrhythmias.

Control of activity and stress

With the added demands of pregnancy, the patient with cardiac disease must observe rigorous limits on her physical activity in accordance with the severity of her disease. Those patients in NYHA Class III or IV often require strict bed rest throughout the entire pregnancy, and some may need to be admitted to the hospital for prolonged periods. Patients with cardiac disease must also avoid emotional strain as much as possible, since often this factor alone can lead to decompensation. Phenobarbital 15 to 30 mg every 6 hours may be used as needed to achieve this goal. Well-fitted support hosiery should be used throughout pregnancy to encourage venous return and discourage venous pooling that can lead to thrombophlebitis.

Correction of anemia

Anemia also increases cardiac work load and must be avoided. Supplemental iron in dosages providing 60 mg daily of elemental iron and 0.2 to 0.4 mg of folate per day are recommended to ensure adequate nutrition for the increase in blood volume of pregnancy.

Salt restriction and caloric intake

Salt restriction of about 2 grams of sodium daily is recommended by most authors in an effort to limit edema and prevent intravascular volume overload. If such a diet is adhered to, regular diuretic use should be limited to few patients. Obesity also places an additional burden on the heart and must be avoided. The inactive patient with cardiac disease needs significantly fewer calories, but the dietary protein should be about 80 to 100 g/day. One author[44] with considerable experience advises his patients with cardiac disease not to gain more than 15 pounds (6.8 kg) during pregnancy.

Prevention of infection

Infection poses two potential threats: (1) the fever produces increased cardiac work load and (2) in patients with valvular lesions, bacteremia poses the threat of endocarditis and its potentially devastating consequences. For these reasons pregnant patients with cardiac disease should avoid crowds and persons with known respiratory infections and should obtain influenza vaccines. Patients with artificial valves and severe valvular lesions should be on chronic antibiotic prophylaxis with oral penicillin or sulfadiazine or receive monthly injections of benzathine penicillin G. Erythromycin should be substituted for sulfa drugs in the third trimester to avoid untoward fetal effects. Patients should be advised to report any sign of infection with special emphasis on the respiratory and urinary tracts. At the first sign of infection, even an upper respiratory tract infection that is usually viral in etiology, caution should be taken and antibiotics begun. If the patient is already on chronic antibiotic therapy, an alternative regimen should be instituted. In patients with cardiac disease the risk of fulminant bacterial infection with its potentially devastating consequences far outweighs the risk of the prophylaxis. Obvious bacterial infections such as pneumonia and pyelonephritis demand immediate hospitalization and high dosages of intravenous antibiotics. If the diagnosis of bacterial endocarditis is entertained, prolonged high dosages of parenteral antibiotics are required as in nonpregnant patients. With a poor clinical response in an infected prosthetic valve, replacement may be necessary.

Hypertension

The subject of hypertension is dealt with in Chapter 6. Suffice it to say that poor control of either chronic or pregnancy-induced hypertension is a preventable cause of decompensation. In the noncompliant or brittle patient hospitalization may be warranted.

Arrhythmias

Arrhythmias may also cause decompensation, are usually supraventricular (ie, atrial tachycardia, fibrillation, and flutter) and are seen most commonly in the rheumatic heart. Second-degree heart blocks may also cause failure and require therapy. The risk of heart failure with *paroxysmal atrial tachycardia* (usually associated with mitral stenosis) is substantial because the rapid heart rate does not allow for adequate left ventricular filling. If the patient's condition is stable, this arrhythmia can often be termi-

nated by carotid sinus pressure or other vagal maneuvers, but this should be done only with continuous monitoring, since ventricular ectopy can be produced. If the patient is unstable (hypotension, chest pain, or dyspnea) or if these attempts are unsuccessful, cardioversion should be performed. This technique is safe in pregnancy and has no known deleterious fetal effects. Other modes of therapy include digitalization (0.25 to 0.50 mg digoxin IV, followed by 0.125 to 0.250 mg IV or orally every 4 to 6 hours for 24 hours as the loading dosage, followed by 0.125 to 0.250 mg orally, as daily maintenance dosages). Propranolol (1 to 3 mg IV or 10 to 40 mg orally) can be used acutely and also as prophylaxis if recurrent attacks are a problem. In a patient already on digitalis, paroxysmal atrial tachycardia may represent digitalis toxicity, especially if there is a coexisting block. In this circumstance cardioversion should be avoided, since it can potentiate digitalis toxicity, and phenytoin (Dilantin), 250 mg in normal saline solution given IV slowly over 10 minutes followed by 100 mg every 15 minutes as needed, should be used cautiously under constant cardiac monitoring. A total dose of 500 mg in 24 hours rarely should be exceeded.

Atrial fibrillation, often seen in rheumatic heart disease, carries an increased risk of both heart failure and thromboembolic complications.[40] The onset of this rhythm in a pregnant patient should be treated as an emergency. The patient should be admitted to the hospital and treated with digoxin to control the ventricular rate. Beta blocking agents may also be helpful in controlling ventricular rate. Pulmonary congestion or edema should be treated as outlined, and when the patient is stabilized, efforts to reestablish sinus rhythm should be made. Cardioversion is preferable to any type of medical therapy, and if the atrial fibrillation is not long-standing, there is a 90% chance of restoring and maintaining sinus rhythm.[39] Quinidine has also been used in pregnancy and has been found to be safe as long as toxic levels of the drug are avoided. Administration of quinidine often raises the digoxin level and necessitates lowering the daily digoxin dosage to avoid digitalis toxicity. If atrial fibrillation is chronic or refractory to therapy, anticoagulation is indicated on a long-term basis. No attempt at medical or electrical cardioversion should be attempted on a patient with long-standing fibrillation until she has been fully anticoagulated for at least 3 weeks. Anticoagulation therapy should be continued for 2 to 3 weeks thereafter.

Similar to atrial fibrillation, *atrial flutter* in pregnancy is treated with digoxin and if necessary cardioversion. *Ventricular tachycardia* is rare in pregnancy. If it occurs, intravenous lidocaine is the treatment of choice. If this fails and the rhythm is not caused by digitalis intoxication, cardioversion becomes the treatment of choice.

Wolff-Parkinson-White syndrome, the most common preexcitation syndrome, is occasionally seen in pregnancy. These patients are susceptible to recurrent episodes of supraventricular arrhythmias, most often paroxysmal atrial tachycardia. If the patient is hemodynamically compromised, cardioversion is the treatment of choice. If medical management is chosen, digitalis and propranolol are to be avoided because they may precipitate tachyarrhythmias by blocking conduction through the atrioventricular node, thus favoring impulse conduction over the aberrant pathways.

Cardiac decompensation

Since the most common manifestation of cardiac decompensation in pregnant patients is pulmonary edema, these individuals ought to be frequently monitored for pulmonary congestion by regular vital capacity measurements. This is a simple, fairly reproducible, and noninvasive method of measuring lung compliance. If the measures outlined previously, such as rest, avoidance of stress, and restriction of salt and calories, do not prevent pulmonary congestion as evidenced by rapid weight gain, dyspnea, tachycardia, or decreasing vital capacity, the patient should be admitted to the hospital. As in the nonpregnant patient, digitalis glycosides are the mainstay of therapy for congestive heart failure and can usually be given in standard dosages. Rapid digitalization should be reserved for emergency situations in which benefits outweigh the risks. Any patient on digitalis should have periodic serum digitalis and potassium level determinations to ensure safe and effective therapy. Diuretics, usually thought of as standard therapy for heart failure, should be used sparingly in pregnancy.[19] Thiazides have been linked to possible liver damage, thrombocyto-

penia, and neutropenia in the newborn, especially when used late in pregnancy. Patients with mild dyspnea or edema usually respond to bed rest, salt restriction, and digoxin. In severe pulmonary congestion or frank pulmonary edema, however, diuretic use is essential; furosemide with or without aminophylline is a reasonably safe choice. Other measures such as morphine sulfate, rotating tourniquets, or phlebotomy can be used in pregnancy when indicated. Most authors feel that prevention of such a dreaded complication as pulmonary edema warrants hospitalizing all patients at high risk for decompensation (severe mitral stenosis, etc) 2 to 4 weeks before the expected date of confinement so that continuous, controlled management is possible.

Anticoagulation

In certain patients with cardiac disease (ie, those with chronic atrial fibrillation or artificial valves) continuous full-dosage anticoagulation is necessary to prevent life-threatening thromboembolic complications. This poses a therapeutic dilemma, since no form of anticoagulation is 100% safe in pregnancy. In a recent review[21] it was concluded that regardless of whether a coumarin derivative or heparin was used, a normal outcome could be expected in only about two thirds of the cases.

Coumarin derivatives with molecular weights of about 1000 readily cross the placenta, whereas heparin with a molecular weight of 20,000 does not. When used during the first trimester (probably in weeks six to nine), coumarin derivatives have been associated with congenital malformations including nasal hypoplasia, stippling of bones, ophthalmologic abnormalities, intrauterine growth retardation, and developmental delay.[5,21,38] Other sequelae include death, scoliosis, blindness, congenital heart disease, and seizures.[48] When coumarin is taken in the second and third trimesters only, serious fetal or placental hemorrhage is possible but malformations are infrequent.[28] Labor and delivery are hazardous for the fetus anticoagulated through maternal coumarin administration.

Heparin, though it does not cause congenital anomalies, has problems of its own. The maternal complication rate may be higher, deaths in the literature from hemorrhage or treatment failure are more common with heparin than with coumarin drugs. The fetus is also at risk for prematurity or stillbirth, although these data may be a reflection of the mother's primary disease process more than the therapy.

Since there is not and probably never will be a controlled randomized study on the use of heparin versus coumarin drugs in pregnancy, the most commonly recommended regimen for anticoagulation in pregnancy is as follows: In those patients on chronic anticoagulation who are actively trying to conceive, early diagnosis of pregnancy is essential and warrants serial measurements of serum chorionic gonadotropin beta subunit beginning 1 or 2 days after a missed period. When pregnancy is diagnosed, the patient should be hospitalized and continuous infusion heparin anticoagulation substituted for oral coumarin derivatives. Heparin anticoagulation should continue for the duration of the first trimester or at least for 9 weeks, at which time oral drugs may again be used. Three to four weeks before the estimated date of birth the patient should again be hospitalized and given heparin so that an infant free of any coumarin anticoagulation may be delivered. With all the hospitalization and monitoring required, this is certainly a difficult and expensive regimen, but it probably gives the patient an adequate chance of a healthy, normal baby.

Since many of these infants are at increased risk for growth retardation and placental insufficiency, regular and frequent determinations of uterine fundal height are important. Also, serial ultrasound measurements must be used to assess fetal growth. After 32 weeks, nonstress or stress tests (weekly) are of value to detect a fetus at high risk for fetal distress or death in utero.

Management during labor, delivery, and puerperium

Management of labor uses many of the concepts already discussed. Elective induction of labor is discouraged, since a smooth and easy natural labor is more beneficial than a protracted and difficult induction. Most authors feel it is beneficial to admit Class III and IV patients to the hospital at least a few days before the expected date of confinement to optimize and stabilize cardiovascular dynamics before the onset of labor. Once labor has begun, the patient should be kept in the lateral recumbent position as much as possible to augment venous return. Oxygen therapy should be used liberally, es-

pecially in patients with cyanotic heart disease, to benefit both mother and infant. Continuous direct monitoring of the fetal heart tones and fetal scalp pH determinations as needed should be used as in all high-risk patients. Intravenous fluids should be used with caution, especially in patients prone to congestive heart failure.[1] Augmentation of labor with oxytocin is acceptable practice and may be of significant benefit to these patients, since protracted labor increases risk of untoward outcome. Cesarean section offers no advantage to mother or infant in the absence of fetal distress and should only be used if indicated for obstetric reasons.

Anesthesia with its potential for profound hemodynamic effects is an aspect of obstetric management that requires careful consideration in the patient.[33] There is agreement that relief of pain is advantageous in the patient with cardiac disease because it decreases the hemodynamic burden that occurs during labor and delivery.

Early in labor most authors recommend a combination of a narcotic plus a tranquilizer of the benzodiazepine or phenothiazine families. If used in combination and in relatively low dosages, they will have little or no effect on cardiovascular dynamics, and a tranquil, cooperative, and relatively comfortable patient should be the result. Barbiturates and scopolamine are of little if any benefit, may have adverse effects on the patient with cardiac disease, and should not be used. Inhalation agents have little to offer for analgesia when compared to other techniques. Paracervical block and pudendal block with local anesthetic in the hands of a physician skilled in its use are safe and effective forms of analgesia. In this high-risk situation, however, any of the potential untoward reactions to this type of anesthesia (systemic injection of anesthetic, fetal bradycardia) poses an additional hazard.

Spinal or saddle block anesthesia with its potential for profound hypotension ought not to be used in the presence of cardiac disease. However, epidural or caudal blocks, both of which allow for controlled, continuous amounts of anesthetic agent to be placed in the extradural space, have been used with good success in patients with cardiac disease. Although they are contraindicated in patients who are fully anticoagulated, they usually are the ideal anesthetic technique for patients with cardiac disease, including those requiring cesarean sections. The reason this technique is ideal is that cardiovascular dynamics remain stable during labor, parturition, and the critical period immediately following delivery if measures are taken to avoid hypotension. By pooling some blood in the lower extremities, the sudden and occasionally disastrous postpartum increase in venous return is avoided, and a more gradual transition to postpartum hemodynamics can be obtained.

Metcalfe and Ueland[30] studied the effects of various types of anesthesia on cardiovascular dynamics in *normal* pregnant patients at term. When epinephrine was mixed with the local anesthetic for spinal or epidural blocks, the blood pressure and cardiac output fell with the induction of anesthesia and rose 35% to 50% after delivery. Using anesthetics without epinephrine resulted in stable measurements; the average fall in cardiac output was less than 10% after induction, and the postdelivery rise in output averaged about 10% as well. With general anesthesia, marked (albeit transient) alterations in hemodynamics were noted during intubation, during extubation, and while awakening the patient. There was also a 40% increase in cardiac output after delivery in this group. Blood loss is an additional variable that influences postpartum hemodynamics, but all things being equal epidural analgesia is the technique advocated by most authors.

Other drugs commonly employed in the management of labor and delivery should be used with caution (if at all) in the patient with cardiac disease. Beta mimetic drugs like terbutaline or ritodrine often produce maternal tachycardia, and in the presence of heart disease (eg, mitral stenosis) their administration may result in high output congestive heart failure. Synthetic oxytocin, when given in intravenous bolus, may cause a transient but marked drop in blood pressure. Therefore oxytocics must be avoided unless the blood loss is excessive and when given must not be used in intravenous bolus fashion. Conversely, ergot compounds may cause significant hypertension and should be used with caution if at all.

Suggested antibiotic regimens for the prevention of bacterial endocarditis in patients with heart disease who have genitourinary and gastrointestinal instrumentation or surgery

ANTIBIOTIC DOSAGES*

Aqueous crystalline penicillin G (2 million units IM or IV) *or*
Ampicillin (1.0 gram IM or IV) *plus*
Gentamicin (1.5 mg/kg [not to exceed 80 mg] IM or IV *or*
Streptomycin (1.0 gram IM)
Give initial doses 30 minutes to 1 hour before the procedure. If gentamicin is used, give a similar dosage of gentamicin and penicillin (or ampicillin) every 8 hours for two additional dosages. If streptomycin is used, give a similar dosage of streptomycin and penicillin (or ampicillin) every 12 hours for two additional dosages.†

FOR THOSE PATIENTS WHO ARE ALLERGIC TO PENICILLIN*

Vancomycin (1.0 gram IV given over 30 minutes to 1 hour) *plus* streptomycin (1.0 gram IM). A single dose of these antibiotics given 30 minutes to 1 hour before the procedure is probably sufficient, but the same dose may be repeated in 12 hours.

---

*In patients with significantly compromised renal function it may be necessary to modify the dosage of antibiotics used. Some of these dosages may exceed the manufacturer's recommendations for a 24-hour period. However, since in most cases they are only recommended for a single 24-hour period, it is unlikely that toxicity will occur.
†During prolonged procedures or in the case of delayed healing, it may be necessary to provide additional dosages of antibiotics. For brief outpatient procedures such as uncomplicated catheterization of the bladder, one dose may be sufficient.

Those patients with cardiac lesions—congenital, acquired, or prosthetic—in whom delivery is anticipated require broad spectrum antibiotics. The 1977 American Heart Association's recommendations for genitourinary and gastrointestinal instrumentation or surgery are shown in the box on p. 188.

As soon as is safely possible, delivery should be accomplished with the aid of forceps. Valsalva maneuvers should be avoided in almost all patients with cardiac disease. The recommended position for delivery is lateral recumbency with legs outstretched. The legs should not be up in stirrups but held out laterally by assistants.

As mentioned before, there is a substantial increase in venous return immediately postpartum. This phenomenon in a patient with cardiac disease, especially one in Class III or IV, can result in fulminant congestive heart failure. If this possibility is anticipated, such measures as delivery in the seated position (legs down), epidural anesthesia (peripheral pooling of blood), rotating tourniquets, as well as other more standard methods (diuretics, morphine) may be used prophylactically.[29]

Termination of pregnancy

Termination of pregnancy is an important consideration in the cardiac patient. Abortion may be a needed if not essential treatment for certain patients, and it should be done as early as possible in pregnancy to minimize maternal risks. In some cases (Eisenmenger's syndrome) the maternal risk may be so high that termination is a life-saving procedure. Before 12 weeks of gestation the risk of an abortion is far less than that of continuing the pregnancy. However, after that point the risk rises appreciably. Prostaglandins with their significant side effects (vomiting, diarrhea) should be used only with great caution if at all in the debilitated patient with cardiac disease. Hysterotomy or a dilation and evacuation technique for second trimester abortions poses risks of anesthesia and blood loss, which can be substantial. In virtually every type of cardiac disease antibiotic prophylaxis should be employed preoperatively and for 72 hours after the procedure.

Contraception

The risks from oral contraceptives (ie, hypercoagulability, thromboembolic disease, hypertension, and hyperlipidemia) usually contraindicate use for patients with organic heart disease. Though it is yet to be proven that these risks exist in the so-called *mini* pills containing less than 50 mg of estrogen, most clinicians avoid using even low-dose pills in this high-risk population.

The intrauterine device (IUD) does not in itself have any effect on the cardiovascular system, but there are two risks involved. The first is the vagal syndrome of syncope, diaphoresis, hypotension, and bradycardia that can occur on insertion or removal of an IUD. In most women this is a transient and mild episode without sequelae, but in a severely debilitated patient with cardiac disease this could be a serious and even life-threatening side effect. The use of the smaller, less rigid, copper-containing IUD has diminished the incidence of this syndrome to less than 1%,[6] and for that reason this type is recommended in patients with cardiac disease. The other risk from the IUD is of infection that may result from the insertion through a nonsterile cervix and also from the presence of a foreign body in the uterine cavity. This risk is less in parous women with single sexual partners, the population for whom this method should be reserved. Studies have shown[6] that the endometrial cavity is usually sterile 24 hours after insertion and always sterile after 30 days. Prophylactic antibiotics are thus recommended for at least 72 hours at the time of insertion. A recommended protocol for the patient with cardiac disease is 1.2 million units of procaine penicillin and 0.5 gram of streptomycin IM given 1 hour before insertion followed by oral penicillin 250 mg every 6 hours for 3 days. Those patients with prosthetic heart valves should be kept on streptomycin every 12 hours for six dosages.

Conventional barrier forms of contraception (ie, diaphragm, condom, and foam) are safe in all patients; however, their low efficiency must be considered when recommending their use. In those patients in whom pregnancy poses an unwanted or life-threatening dilemma, sterilization should be strongly recommended.

■ SPECIFIC CARDIAC DISEASES DURING PREGNANCY AND THEIR MANAGEMENT

Cardiac diseases are of two types, congenital and acquired. The mortality figures resulting from both types of heart disease are shown in Table 10-1.

TABLE 10-1 ■ Fetal and maternal mortality in specific types of heart disease

Cardiovascular lesions	Fetal mortality (%)	Maternal mortality (%)	Reference number
Coarctation of aorta	13	9*†	2, 29
Marfan's syndrome	—	50	29
Tetralogy of Fallot	30	12	2, 29
Repaired tetralogy of Fallot	25	0	41
Eisenmenger's syndrome	—	27-66	31
Primary pulmonary hypertension	—	53	30
Mitral stenosis			
All patients	—	1	37
NYHA Class III, IV	—	4-5	7
Patients with atrial fibrillation	—	14-17	7
Pregnancy after closed valvulotomy	—	4-6*	41
Peripartum cardiomyopathy	—	15-60	43
Patent ductus, ventricular septal defect	—	5.5	1
Prosthetic heart valves (all)	28	2	40
Myocardial infarction	26	28	37

*Rate expressed as percent of patients, not pregnancies.
†Rate doubles for complicated coarctation.

Congenital heart disease

The incidence of various forms of congenital heart disease during pregnancy has been reported to be between 0.2% and 19% of patients with cardiac disease.[10] With a marked reduction in the incidence of rheumatic heart disease during the last 2 decades and improved cardiovascular surgical techniques, there is no question that congenital lesions now constitute a higher percentage of patients than they did 20 years ago. Also, as diagnosis and modes of therapy improve, more women with severe lesions are reaching the childbearing age after correction or improvement of their conditions by surgery.

Most patients with acyanotic heart disease tolerate pregnancy well, even multiple gestations, with no significant increase in maternal or fetal mortality. With careful monitoring these individuals most often can be managed as normal obstetric patients, as can those women with well-compensated surgically corrected lesions (see Table 10-1). Conversely, there is a population of patients with cyanotic heart disease or pulmonary hypertension who are at much higher risk of fetal mortality.[6]

Primary pulmonary hypertension. Primary pulmonary hypertension is characterized by high pulmonary vascular resistance and normal wedge pressure, indicating an obstruction to

pulmonary blood flow proximal to the pulmonary capillaries. This results in a low, probably fixed, cardiac output and in right ventricular hypertrophy. It should be obvious that this condition does not readily accommodate the demands of pregnancy (ie, increased blood volume, increased cardiac output, and diminished venous return). These patients frequently develop shortness of breath, chest pain, and syncope in pregnancy; in fact, maternal mortality of up to 53% can be found in the literature.[24] Death is more often the result of sudden circulatory collapse rather than right heart failure. Pulmonary arterial pressure gives an indication of the prognosis of an individual patient. Strict limitation of physical activity is mandatory in these patients because during pregnancy, as flow to the pulmonary system increases, so does pulmonary arterial pressure. The immediate postpartum period with its sudden increase in venous return is a critical time in the management of these patients. There is some evidence to suggest an increased risk of pulmonary thrombosis, and one author[45] suggests full-dose anticoagulation in the early puerperium.

In general, most authors feel that the risks of pregnancy in a patient with documented primary pulmonary hypertension are so high that such patients should be strongly advised against pregnancy. Patients in early pregnancy should be offered termination as a potentially life-saving procedure.

Eisenmenger's syndrome

Eisenmenger's syndrome is composed of a combination of right-to-left or bidirectional shunt with pulmonary hypertension and resultant central cyanosis. The shunt may be aortopulmonary, atrial, or ventricular, and the pulmonary vascular resistance often equals the systemis resistance. This syndrome constitutes about 3% of all congenital heart diseases and is a progressive condition. Complications in the nonpregnant patient include pulmonary infarction, heart failure, syncope, and arrhythmias, all of which often result in sudden death before age 40.

As in primary pulmonary hypertension, it is the degree of pulmonary hypertension and not the functional classification of the patient that determines the prognosis. Any patient with a significant septal defect or patent ductus arteriosus should have her pulmonary artery pressures measured, since even asymptomatic nonpregnant patients may be at high risk if pregnancy occurs.

The pertinent pathophysiology of this condition is that any increase in pulmonary pressure or decrease in systemic vascular resistance increases the right-to-left shunt, bypassing the lungs and lowering arterial oxygen saturation. In pregnancy the systemic vascular resistance falls; the pulmonary vascular resistance does not fall. As a result, there is a tendency to increase the right-to-left shunt. Labor, delivery, and puerperium, with the sudden and dramatic changes in hemodynamics and the potential for significant blood loss, are the most critical periods. Sudden fetal and maternal death is a real possibility in these patients, since their ability to adapt to hemodynamic changes is nonexistent.

In a review article on the topic, Gleicher et al[16] found in more than 40 reported cases in the literature that over half of all persons with Eisenmenger's syndrome who had ever experienced pregnancy died during or in connection with pregnancy. The majority of these patients died during parturition and in the first week after delivery. They also found that a patient who is successfully managed through one pregnancy has no less risk in subsequent pregnancies than her nulliparous counterparts. They feel that pregnancy is contraindicated in patients with Eisenmenger's syndrome, even in those who have survived one or more gestations.

Concerning fetal outcome, Gleicher et al found that 60% of all pregnant patients with Eisenmenger's syndrome had a live baby. Only 25% of pregnancies reached term, and about one third of infants born were growth retarded. The perinatal mortality, principally as a reflection of prematurity, was 28.3%.

Predisposing factors to pregnancy-associated sudden death in patients with Eisenmenger's syndrome include blood loss, thromboembolic phenomena, disseminated intravascular coagulation, and preeclampsia.[3,16,25,32] Some authors believe that a major factor in the pathogenesis of sudden death in these patients is the hypercoagulable state of pregnancy. This idea is supported by autopsy findings of disseminated microthrombi in the pulmonary vascular system causing increased right-to-left shunting. For this reason many authors recommend prophylactic anticoagulation, and some recommend anticoagulants in the second trimester as well as in the postpartum period.

An increased mortality has also been reported for patients undergoing cesarean sections, but the cases reported are limited in number and the statistics may be skewed by the fact that often the patient's condition was compromised before surgery was begun. There does seem to be good evidence, however, that patients with Eisenmenger's syndrome tolerate surgery poorly.

A course of clinical management for these patients begins with advising against pregnancy and urging permanent sterilization as a lifesaving procedure. Abortion should be used as a first-line management for early pregnancy, even in those patients with a successful obstetric history. Those patients who decline sterilization or termination of pregnancy should do so with the understanding that they run a 25% to 33% chance of death as a result of pregnancy.

In those patients opting for pregnancy, recommendations for therapy include the following:

1. Hospitalization, if not for the entire course of pregnancy, at least from 20 weeks of gestation until 2 weeks postpartum.
2. Anticoagulation from the second trimester until at least 48 hours postpartum.

3. Bed rest and oxygen supplementation as much as possible.
4. "Tuning up" the cardiovascular system with appropriate diet and drugs before delivery.
5. Vaginal delivery whenever possible, forceps delivery when safely possible.
6. Monitoring with Swan-Ganz catheter and frequent blood gas determinations during labor, delivery, and the early puerperium.
7. Epidural anesthesia to help stabilize hemodynamics during delivery, with great care taken to avoid sudden or pronounced systemic hypotension.

Perhaps with modern technology and a greater awareness of the pathophysiology of Eisenmenger's syndrome, an improvement can be made in the rather grim prognosis for these pregnant patients.

Patent ductus arteriosus and atrial and ventricular septal defects. Patent ductus arteriosus and atrial and ventricular septal defects are relatively common (14.5%, 17.5% and 17% respectively of all congenital heart diseases) and usually well-tolerated lesions. Often these lesions, if hemodynamically significant, are surgically repaired before the patient reaches the childbearing age. If this is the case and the patient is functional Class I, she stands a good chance of having an uncomplicated obstetric experience. These women need antibiotic prophylaxis and careful follow-up, but they should do well during pregnancy.

With normal pulmonary pressures most women with these lesions do well. In the uncorrected patient any history of cyanosis or elevated pulmonary artery pressure means she has Eisenmenger's syndrome, which places her at high risk. One potentially disastrous complication must be kept in mind with patients with uncorrected defects and that is a sudden reversal of flow through the defect resulting in right-to-left shunting and cyanosis. This most often occurs in early puerperium as a result of significant blood loss or after resolution of uncontrolled toxemic hypertension, either of which causes a sudden drop in systemic blood pressure. Pulmonary embolism with resultant pulmonary hypertension would also cause this life-threatening shunt. Careful obstetric management, including immediate availability of blood if needed, should prevent these complications in most patients.

Patients with uncorrected defects should receive antibiotic prophylaxis before and after delivery.

A few asymptomatic patients with these lesions develop congestive heart failure in pregnancy. If pulmonary hypertension is ruled out, those patients are often best managed by operative closure of their defect if medical therapy fails. Many reports of successful repair during pregnancy are found in the literature.

Tetralogy of Fallot. Tetralogy of Fallot, constituting about 14.5% of congenital heart lesions, consists of dextroposition of the aorta, pulmonary stenosis, ventricular septal defect, and right ventricular hypertrophy. Most patients with uncorrected tetralogy have severe pulmonary stenosis with increased right ventricular pressures and resulting right-to-left shunt. Cyanosis, clubbing, syncope, and even convulsions are seen in these patients. In the past, without corrective surgery, most of these patients died of heart failure, respiratory infections, infective endocarditis, or cerebral complications before they reached the childbearing age.

Although there are reports in the literature of pregnancies with successful outcome, perinatal and maternal mortality is high in patients with tetralogy of Fallot. The life-threatening complications in association with tetralogy of Fallot, such as heart failure and increased right-to-left shunting, are more common in pregnancy. As a result of the fixed pulmonary outflow, systemic vascular resistance decreases, right-to-left shunting increases, and this causes syncopal attacks, hematocrit levels greater than 60%, arterial oxygen saturation under 80%, and right ventricular pressure over 120 mm Hg. Once again the immediate postpartum period is a critical time, since a fall in systemic pressure as a result of blood loss increases the right-to-left shunt. These patients can benefit from the same type of high-risk obstetric management used in patients with Eisenmenger's syndrome, including prolonged hospitalization and Swan-Ganz catheterization for labor and delivery. There is no mention of anticoagulation in these patients in the literature, but since thromboembolic phenomena do occur, there may be good reason to give anticoagulants late in pregnancy and in the puerperal period. Antibiotic prophylaxis is mandatory.

At the present time palliative surgery is often performed on patients with tetralogy of Fallot, substantially improving the obstetric prognosis. Treatment includes the Blalock-Taussig operation in which there is the formation of an anastomosis between the subclavian or innominate artery and the pulmonary artery; the Potts-Smith-Gibson procedure in which an anastomosis between the aorta and pulmonary artery is made; the Brock's operation in which there is a pulmonary valvulotomy and an infundibular resection and in suitable cases a total correction. Successful pulmonary valvulotomy during pregnancy has been reported, but one of two patients miscarried after surgery.[37] There are eight reported pregnancies in patients with corrected tetralogy in which there was a 25% fetal loss and no maternal mortality. It has been recommended that at least 1 year should pass from the time of surgery until pregnancy is attempted. More data on these patients should become available as more women reach childbearing age after surgery.

Marfan's syndrome. Marfan's syndrome is an autosomal dominant syndrome thought to to be caused by a defect in elastic tissue synthesis. Though it is an inherited disease, more than 15% are said to be new cases, presumably the result of de novo genetic mutation.[42] It is characterized by hyperextensibility of joints, excessively long bones, arachnodactyly, and subluxation of the ocular lens. The most important clinical alteration, however, is the disruption of the normal elastin fibers in the media of the ascending aorta, sometimes referred to as cystic medial necrosis. This abnormality predisposes these patients to ascending aortic dilation with resultant severe aortic regurgitation and/or a dissecting aneurysm of the aorta.[26] Early death in these patients usually results from intractable congestive heart failure or rupture of a dissecting aneurysm.

The alteration in the ascending aorta is the problem that puts pregnant women with Marfan's syndrome at great risk because pregnancy causes additional structural changes in the media of the aorta that further weaken the vessel. This change in combination with the increased cardiac output and widened pulse pressure of pregnancy contributes to a high incidence of rupture of the aorta and maternal death during pregnancy. In a review of the literature Tricomi[42] found that in women under 40 years who had dissecting aneurysms, about half were in pregnant women, some of whom had Marfan's syndrome.

Though good data on the mortality of pregnant women with Marfan's syndrome are not available, it is estimated to be at least 50%, and of reported cases survivors seem to be the exception rather than the rule. In a review of 10 cases of death during pregnancy Tricomi[42] found that all the deaths resulted from dissecting aneurysms, most of which ruptured into the pericardial sac.

Because of the exceptionally high risk to the mother, pregnancy is contraindicated, and early abortion and sterilization should be performed to save the mother's life. In those patients who refuse abortion, management should be in accordance with the general guidelines given on p. 184. Hospitalization with strict bed rest must be enforced. Most authors also recommend propranolol therapy to diminish the increase in cardiac output and pulse pressure normally seen in pregnancy. In these cases the benefits of propranolol administration clearly outweigh the potential risks. Labor and delivery should be managed as described on p. 187, and since childbirth is a high-risk period, careful observation in the postpartum period is also essential. Antibiotic prophylaxis is recommended for the puerperium.

Coarctation of the aorta. This disease represents about 7% of all congenital heart diseases.[17] In patients with uncomplicated coarctation, pregnancy is said to be "relatively safe" for the mother, but fetal risks are increased.[12] In cases complicated by a significant associated cardiovascular defect, frequently a bicuspid aortic valve, the maternal risk is much greater. Maternal mortality of around 20% is quoted in the literature for these patients, a risk that some authors find excessive to the point of recommending abortion. Patients with bicuspid aortic valve and coarctation of the aorta have both obstruction of flow through the aorta during systole and regurgitation of flow through the incompetent valve in diastole. As cardiac output and pulse pressure increase in pregnancy, the left ventricle must work harder and harder in women with aortic coarctation. There is also some evidence that during pregnancy there are certain histochemical changes in the media that may cause dissection. The most common causes of maternal death in these women are aortic rupture, congestive heart failure, cerebral vascular accidents, and bacterial endocarditis. Management of these patients should include strict bed rest, prolonged hospitalization, and prophylactic antibiotics. These patients should also be informed that there is a fetal mortality of about 13% associated with this condition.

Medical management during pregnancy usually suffices, but occasionally emergency surgical repair may be necessary. Indications for repair during pregnancy include early signs of dissection or aneurysm or rarely systolic blood pressures of over 200 mm Hg. As with so many congenital lesions, more patients with aortic coarctation are reaching childbearing age after having corrective surgery, and if that is the case, pregnancy may be undertaken with minimal risk.

Ebstein's disease. Ebstein's anomaly, constituting less than 1% of all congenital heart diseases, is a serious lesion. It consists of displacement of the tricuspid valve into the right ventricle, resulting in an enlarged right atrium and a small right ventricle. This is often associated with an atrial septal defect and tricuspid regurgitation. With gross regurgitation, shunting can occur through the atrial septal defect resulting in a right-to-left shunt, cyanosis, and clubbing. There is a wide range of severity in this condition, but a mortality of over 50% by age 20 is reported in a large series of cases.[41] Death results from arrhythmias early in life or from congestive heart failure. Surgical replacement of the tricuspid valve and repair of the atrial septal defect can markedly improve the functional status of the patient, but the risk of fatal arrhythmias persists.

In pregnancy the abnormal right ventricle does not accommodate the increased demands, and often the result is increased tricuspid regurgitation and right-to-left shunting. Risks to these patients also include bacterial endocarditis and paradoxical cerebral embolization through the atrial septal defect. There are no good statistics for maternal or fetal mortality in this condition, but in the presence of maternal cyanosis fetal mortality is high and presumably the risk to the mother is substantial. In patients with surgical correction of their lesion there is a good chance of pregnancy without complications.

Congenital heart block. Congenital heart block is a rare condition of unknown etiology, but it may be associated with endomyocardial fibrosis. Most of these patients have adequate escape rhythm and tolerate pregnancy without complication. However, syncope, Stokes-Adams attacks, and heart failure have been reported in these patients. Prophylactic pacing seems unwarranted in the asymptomatic patient, but if complications occur, the implantation of an artificial pacing device should be undertaken. Women with pacing devices should experience no problem with labor and delivery.

Acquired heart disease

Rheumatic heart disease. The cardiac lesions associated with rheumatic heart disease result from a hypersensitivity reaction to the Lancefield group A beta hemolytic streptococcus. Streptococcal infections are common, but only a small proportion of the population is susceptible to acute rheumatic fever. Approximately 3% to 10% of group A infections are followed by rheumatic fever. A characteristic of rheumatic fever is its tendency to recur with the possibility of further cardiac damage with each attack.

The cardiac lesion begins with swelling and inflammation of the myocardium as well as the cusps of the mitral, aortic, and less commonly the tricuspid valve. Often vegetations consisting of necrotic collagen occur on the surface of the valves. As the inflammation subsides, fibrosis and resultant deformity of the valve leaflets and adjacent structures occur, causing significant functional impairment of the heart.

This disease, which formerly constituted the overwhelming majority of heart disease in pregnancy, has been steadily decreasing over the past 20 years, although it probably still represents the majority of pregnant patients with cardiac disease. The severity of the damage to heart valves in each case also seems to be on the decline, possibly because of changes in the virulence of the streptococcus or in the susceptibility of the host. These changes have resulted in a marked decrease in the number of pregnant patients with significant rheumatic carditis.

The diagnosis of acute rheumatic fever has traditionally been made on the basis of the Jones' clinical criteria. The major criteria are carditis, polyarthritis, chorea, subcutaneous nodules, and erythema marginatum. The minor criteria include fever, arthralgia, leukocytosis, and other clinical and laboratory findings. The presence of two major or one major and two minor criteria has been considered diagnostic of rheumatic fever. However, today with the diminution in the severity of the illness, rigid adherence to these criteria results in underdiagnosis. In as many as 40% of patients with rheumatic fever there is a history of only mild respiratory illness or none at all. Szekely and Snaith[41] feel that "an apical systolic murmur following a Group A hemolytic strep infection" indicates a high probability of rheumatic carditis, even in the absence of other clinical signs. Recurrences of this disease are seen in about 50% of patients, with approximately 80% occurring in the first 4 years after the initial attack. Patients who get rheumatic carditis generally do so on the first attack, and in these people recurrences pose the threat of further cardiac and valvular damage.

In patients with acute rheumatic carditis the mitral valve is most commonly affected, with the aortic valve affected in about half the cases. These patients (22%) show auscultatory signs of mitral regurgitation alone, 3% pure mitral stenosis, and 75% a combination of stenosis and regurgitation. However, as patients age, more begin to show signs of mitral stenosis, which is the most common rheumatic heart lesion found in patients of childbearing age. Aortic regurgitation resulting from an acute inflammatory episode can be completely resolved, but if the damage to the valve is serious, it may result in permanent regurgitation. Aortic stenosis generally takes years to develop and is uncommon in the childbearing years. Chronic rheumatic heart disease is a progressive deterioration in the myocardial or valvular condition that often occurs without other signs of an active rheumatic process. The sequelae of this chronic deterioration include congestive heart failure, atrial tachydysrhythmias, systemic embolization, and infective endocarditis.

Initial episodes of acute rheumatic fever are uncommon in pregnancy; it could be, however, that some of the signs and symptoms of the disease are masked by the pregnant state. Some data suggest that pregnancy may increase the tendency to recurrence of chorea, but it is a debated point. When chorea occurs in pregnancy, careful management is required because in severe cases spontaneous miscarriage, preterm labor, fetal death in utero, maternal hyperpyrexia, heart failure, and death have been reported.[7] The use of sedatives such as chlorpromazine or phenobarbital is recommended, and in cases of severe chorea (violent and un-

controllable movements, agitation, and psychiatric disturbances) termination of pregnancy has been recommended. Active carditis in pregnancy also requires careful attention, since it can lead to heart failure. Administration of steroids and salicylates in conjunction with eradication of any active streptococcal infection constitute the recommended medical management. Chronic continuous antistreptococcal antibiotic prophylaxis in patients with known prior acute rheumatic attacks reduces the incidence of recurrences, whereas streptococcal vaccinations may worsen the recurrence rate. There are data to suggest that parenteral benzathine penicillin is the optimal prophylactic agent, but oral penicillin or sulfadiazine is often more practical. Szekely and Snaith[41] quote the following recommendations for antibiotic prophylaxis in rheumatic patients:

> Those who had acute rheumatism but no cardiac involvement should have prophylaxis for five years following the attack or until the end of the school period whichever is the longer; those who had carditis but in whom the signs of cardiac involvement had disappeared should have prophylaxis for a longer period, and those with established valvular heart disease should have it throughout life.

For dental extractions and other potentially bacteremic events, patients on long-prophylaxis with cardiac lesions should have additional broad spectrum antibiotic coverage as treatment against penicillin-resistant bacterial endocarditis.

The most common and certainly the most significant rheumatic lesion seen in pregnancy is *mitral stenosis*. In a series published by Szekely and Snaith[41] of 761 pregnant patients with rheumatic heart disease, 90% had mitral stenosis. This lesion is said to be the principal nonobstetric cause of death during the childbearing years.

The pathophysiology of mitral stenosis involves obstruction of flow from the left atrium to the left ventricle causing increased left atrial pressure and in retrograde fashion increased pressure in the pulmonary veins and capillaries. This functional obstruction is worsened by the dramatic increase in blood volume seen in pregnancy. Also, since flow from the atrium to the ventricles occurs only in diastole, the potential for pulmonary congestion is increased during pregnancy because the increased basal heart rate causes a shortened relative ratio of diastole to systole. Anything that serves to increase cardiac output or heart rate would further aggravate this situation. As pulmonary capillary pressure increases to values above 25 mm Hg, it exceeds the opposing forces of colloid osmotic pressure and lung tissue tension. As a result, fluid begins to transudate into alveoli and alveolar walls, and this results in acute pulmonary edema. In this way an asymptomatic Class I nonpregnant patient with mitral stenosis can be pushed into florid pulmonary edema in pregnancy. In Szekely's and Snaith's series[41] 23% of pregnant patients with mitral stenosis experienced heart failure.

Successful management of these patients requires strict adherence to the principles outlined in the section of this chapter on general guidelines for managing the pregnant patient with cardiac disease. The increase in cardiac output must be minimized as much as possible. Digoxin is useful to help prevent tachycardia that can be life-threatening to these patients. Epidural anesthesia, shortening the second stage of labor as much as possible, and delivery in the Sims' position are important aspects of puerperal management.

Surgical intervention, though best reserved for the nonpregnant patient, may be a life-saving alternative if medical management fails. Recurrent pulmonary edema or hemoptysis resistant to medical management in a patient who refuses interruption of her pregnancy is grounds for surgical intervention. Although its effects may only be temporary and pulmonary congestion may occur in this or subsequent pregnancies, mitral valvulotomy has been successfully performed many times in pregnant patients with satisfactory results for mother and fetus.[37] Ideally, valvulotomy should be done as early in pregnancy as possible and is not advisable after the sixteenth week of gestation.[50] Szekely and Snaith[41] reported 29 patients who had closed mitral valvulotomy; of this number only one died, and there were only two neonatal deaths. Open heart surgery, however, with its attendant extracorporeal circulation is associated with a higher fetal loss. Of 22 patients treated this way only one woman died, but the fetal loss rate was 33%.

Isolated mitral regurgitation is a lesion that is associated with increased volume demands on both the left atrium and ventricle. In the absence of congestive heart failure, which usually develops after the childbearing years, there is no increase in pulmonary capillary pressure as the atrium dilates. Though these patients are at risk for endocarditis, supraventricular tachydysrhythmias, and pulmonary embolization, significant pulmonary congestion or edema is not seen as a rule. These patients for the most part have uncomplicated pregnancies.

Aortic regurgitation results in an increased volume load on the left ventricle and is also as a rule not associated with serious sequelae in pregnancy. Though the increase in blood volume serves to increase the work of the ventricle, the physiologic tachycardia and its associated shortened diastole allow less time for regurgitant flow. Again, congestive heart failure usually occurs in these patients when they are past the childbearing years, although it has been seen in pregnancy.

Aortic stenosis is a lesion that limits the flow from the left ventricle into the aorta. As the pregnant patient's blood volume and cardiac output increase, the result is an increase in left ventricular systolic pressure. Nonetheless, patients with aortic stenosis without associated mitral stenosis and even those with severe cases tolerate pregnancy well. Symptoms such as angina, syncope, and congestive failure usually occur late in the course of the disease.[4]

Tricuspid valve disease is not seen without associated mitral or aortic valve lesions, and the clinical picture is determined by the dominant left-sided valvular lesion.

Peripartum heart disease. *Peripartum heart disease* is defined by the following diagnostic criteria listed by Demakis and Rahimtoola[13]: "(1) development of heart failure in the last month of pregnancy or within the first five postpartum months, (2) absence of a determinable etiology for the cardiac failure, and (3) absence of demonstrable heart disease prior to the last month of pregnancy." Estimates of incidence range from 1 in 1300 to 1 in 4000 pregnancies.[18]

The etiology and pathogenesis of this disorder have not been clearly explained despite careful investigations. Nutritional and alcohol intake do not seem to play a conclusive etiologic role. Most patients in whom this diagnosis has been made are black and multiparous with a high percentage over 30 years of age. Toxemia and twin gestation are five and seven times more common respectively in these patients than in pregnant patients in general. More than 80% of the cases compiled by Demakis and Rahimtoola[13] occurred in the first 3 months postpartum, whereas only 7% occurred in the last month of gestation.

The signs and symptoms of peripartum heart disease are simply those of severe congestive heart failure with dyspnea, orthopnea, edema, hepatic enlargement, ventricular gallop, and cardiomegaly. In their initial episode of failure most of these patients respond to standard medical management. Subsequent prognosis is determined by how rapidly the patient's heart size returns to normal. Those patients whose heart size is normal 6 months after the initial attack do well and can withstand subsequent pregnancies with only temporary if any deterioration in their functional status. However, patients who have persistent cardiomegaly past 6 months have a poor prognosis. Most have recurrent episodes of congestive failure and often do not tolerate subsequent pregnancies without permanent functional deterioration. Of their 13 patients in this category, Demakis and Rahimtoola[13] reported 10 were dead within 8 years of their initial attack. Death in these patients usually results from congestive heart failure often associated with subsequent pregnancy, pulmonary emboli, or arrhythmias.

Peripartum cardiomyopathy must be a diagnosis of exclusion made only after all other possible etiologies have been ruled out. Heart failure as a result of hypertensive heart disease, toxemia, nutritional cardiomyopathy, pericardial disease, and thromboembolism should be considered as well as rarities such as cardiac tumor, silent mitral valve disease, precocious coronary artery disease, and obliterative pulmonary hypertension. Systemic illnesses like diabetes, thyrotoxicosis, hypothyroidism, hemochromatosis, scleroderma, or sarcoidosis may also masquerade as peripartum heart disease. Viral etiologies should be investigated by stool cultures and serologic studies. Specific viruses to look for include the echo strains 9 and 30, influenza A, and coxsackie B.

Once the diagnosis is made, therapy for peripartum heart disease begins with standard medical management of congestive heart failure. Since these people are at a high risk for pulmonary as well as systemic embolization, anti-coagulation is recommended for as long as cardiomegaly persists. Most authors recommend low dosage subcutaneous heparin unless patients have evidence of a previous or present thromboembolic process. Pregnant patients (as opposed to postpartum patients) merit a rather specialized regimen for anticoagulation. Since this syndrome occurs late in the third trimester when it occurs prepartum, induction of labor can usually be accomplished without compromising fetal outcome significantly. Labor, delivery, and the postpartum period should be managed as outlined previously (see management during labor, etc).

Cardiac valve prostheses in pregnancy. Patients with cardiac valve prosthesis usually have a single mitral aortic prosthesis, although it is possible to have two, and a successful obstetric outcome was reported in a patient with three valve prostheses.[2] In general, pregnancy subjects the mother to increased risk of thromboembolic phenomena. As discussed earlier, anticoagulation in pregnancy is difficult and increases morbidity and mortality risks to the fetus.

Patients with an aortic valve prosthesis tolerate the demands of pregnancy much better than patients with an artificial mitral valve or those with both. The reason is that the aortic valve allows for increased output required in pregnancy, whereas the mitral valve limits cardiac output and does not allow for increases of the magnitude required in pregnancy. Consequently, many authors feel abortion is the only safe method of managing pregnancy in patients with a mitral valve prosthesis.

Most authors[8,27,35] feel patients with these prostheses who elect to attempt pregnancy are best managed on full-dosage continuous anticoagulation despite the attendant difficulty and risk. Antibiotic prophylaxis is especially critical. The patient with a mitral valve prosthesis has a fixed cardiac output and should be managed like a patient with mitral stenosis to avoid cardiac overload.

Coronary artery disease. Arteriosclerotic coronary vascular disease is rare in women of childbearing age. The incidence of myocardial infarction in pregnancy is said to be approximately 1 in 10,000 deliveries.[15] Predisposing factors include diabetes, hypertension, family history, and hyperlipidemia.

Management of the pregnant patient with an acute myocardial infarction is no different from the nonpregnant patient. Since the value of anticoagulation in the nonpregnant patient with myocardial infarction is subject to some doubt, the additional risk this entails in the pregnant patient probably outweighs the potential benefit. After recovery from the acute event, management follows the guidelines given in the section on general guidelines.

The advisability of pregnancy subsequent on myocardial infarction was considered in a review by Szekely and Julian[39] who made the following comment:

> The safety of pregnancy subsequent to acute cardiac infarction depends on several factors. A time interval of at least one year between the acute attack and pregnancy, a younger age in the obstetric sense, not more than slight cardiac enlargement, the absence of angina and no history of recent use of contraceptive drugs can be regarded as favorable features.

They further recommend that a full diagnostic workup, including coronary arteriography, should be performed before these patients attempt pregnancy.

It has been shown that patients who have effort-induced angina during pregnancy do not have an increased risk of infarction in the nonpregnant state. Beta blocking agents may be useful in controlling symptoms in these patients, although there is some debate on their effect on the fetus and newborn. The prognosis for these patients is said to be good if appropriate medical management is observed.

■ REFERENCES

1. Adams JQ: Management of the pregnant cardiac patient. Clin Obstet Gynecol 1968;11:910.
2. Andrinopoulos G, Arias F: Triple heart valve prosthesis and pregnancy. Obstet Gynecol 1980;55:762.
3. Arias F: Maternal death in a patient with Eisenmenger's syndrome. Obstet Gynecol 1977;50:76s.
4. Arias F, Pineda J: Aortic stenosis and pregnancy. J Reprod Med 1978;20:229.
5. Bloomfield DK: Fetal deaths and malformations associated with the use of coumadin derivatives in pregnancy. Am J Obstet Gynecol 1970;107:883.
6. Brenner PF, Mishell DR Jr: Contraception for the woman with significant cardiac disease. Clin Obstet Gynecol 1975;18:155.
7. Bunim JJ, Appel SB: A principle for determining prognosis of pregnancy in rheumatic heart disease. JAMA 1950;152:90.
8. Buxbaum A, Aygen MM, Shabin W, et al: Pregnancy in patients with prosthetic heart valves. Chest 1971;59:639.
9. Conradsson T, Werko L: Management of heart disease in pregnancy. Prog Cardiovasc Dis 1974;16:407.
10. Copeland WE, Wooley CF, Ryan JM: Pregnancy and congenital heart disease. Am J Obstet Gynecol 1963;86:107.
11. Cutforth R, McDonald CB: Heart murmurs in pregnancy. Am Heart J 1966;71:741.
12. Deal K, Wooley CF: Coarctation of the aorta and pregnancy. Ann Intern Med 1973;78:706.
13. Demakis JG, Rahimtoola SH: Peripartum cardiomyopathy. Circulation 1971;44:964.
14. Enrenfeld EN, Brezizinski A, Braon K, et al: Heart disease in pregnancy. Obstet Gynecol 1974;23:363.
15. Ginz B: Myocardial infarction in pregnancy. Br J Obstet Gynaecol 1970;77:610.
16. Gleicher N, Midwall J, Hochberger D, et al: Eisenmenger's syndrome and pregnancy. Obstet Gynecol Surv 1979;34:721.
17. Goodwin JF: Pregnancy and coarctation of aorta. Clin Obstet Gynecol 1961;4:645.
18. Goodwin JF: Peripartal heart disease. Clin Obstet Gynecol 1975;18:125.
19. Gray MJ: Use and abuse of thiazides in pregnancy. Clin Obstet Gynecol 1968;11:568.
20. Haiat R, Halphen C: Occult pericardial effusion during pregnancy: a new entity. Am J Cardiol 1982;49:937.
21. Hall JG, Pauli RM, Wilson, KM: Maternal and fetal sequelae of anticoagulation during pregnancy. Am J Med 1980;68:122.
22. Harvey W: Alterations of the cardiac physical examination in normal pregnancy. Clin Obstet Gynecol 1975;18:51.
23. Hibbard LT: Maternal mortality due to cardiac disease. Clin Obstet Gynecol 1975;18:27.
24. Jewett JF: Pulmonary hypertension in pregnancy. Clin Obstet Gynecol 1961;4:630.
25. Jones AM, Howitt G: Eisenmenger syndrome in pregnancy. Br Med J 1965;1:1627.
26. Kitchen DH: Dissecting aneurysm of the aorta in pregnancy. Br J Obstet Gynaecol 1974;81:410.
27. MacDonald HN: Pregnancy following insertion of cardiac valve prostheses. Br J Obstet Gynaecol 1970;77:603.
28. Maharias GH, Weingold AB: Fetal hazard with anticoagulant therapy. Clin Obstet Gynecol 1963;85:234.
29. Mestman JH, Manning PR: Management of the postpartum period. Clin Obstet Gynecol 1975;18:169.
30. Metcalfe J, Ueland K: Maternal cardiovascular adjustments to pregnancy. Prog Cardiovasc Dis 1974;16:363.
31. Metcalfe J, Ueland K: The heart in pregnancy, in Hurst JW, Logue RB, Schlaut RC, et al (eds): *The Heart*. New York, McGraw-Hill Book Co., 1978, pp. 1721-1734.
32. Neilson G, Galea EG, Blunt A: Eisenmenger's syndrome and pregnancy. Med J Aust 1971;1:431.
33. Ostheimer GW, Alper MA: Intrapartum anesthetic management of the pregnant patient with heart disease. Clin Obstet Gynecol 1975;18:81.
34. Pritchard JA: Changes in the blood volume during pregnancy and delivery. Anesthesiology 1965;26:393.

35. Radnich RH, Jacobs M: Prosthetic heart valves. Tex Med 1970;66:58.
36. Rovinsky JJ, Jaffin H: Cardiovascular hemodynamics in pregnancy. III. Cardiac rate, stroke volume, total peripheral resistance and central blood volume in multiple pregnancy; synthesis of results. Am J Obstet Gynecol 1966;95:787.
37. Schenker JG, Polishuk WZ: Pregnancy following mitral valvotomy: a survey of 182 patients. Obstet Gynecol 1968;32:214.
38. Shanl WL, Hall JG: Multiple congenital anomalies associated with oral anticoagulants. Am J Obstet Gynecol 1977;127:191.
39. Szekely P, Julian D: Heart disease and pregnancy. Curr Probl Cardiol 1979;4:1.
40. Szekely P, Snaith L: Atrial fibrillation and pregnancy. Br Med J 1961;1:1407.
41. Szekely P, Snaith L: *Heart Disease and Pregnancy*. Edinburgh, Churchill Livingstone, 1974, pp. 21-79.
42. Tricomi V: The Marfan syndrome and pregnancy. Clin Obstet Gynecol 1965;8:334.
43. Ueland K: Maternal cardiovascular dynamics. VII. Intrapartum blood volume changes. Am J Obstet Gynecol 1976;126:671.
44. Ueland K: Pregnancy and cardiovascular disease. Med Clin North Am 1977;61:17.
45. Ueland K: Cardiovascular diseases complicating pregnancy. Clin Obstet Gynecol 1978;21:429.
46. Ueland K, Hansen J: Maternal cardiovascular dynamics. III. Labor and delivery under local and caudal analgesia. Am J Obstet Gynecol 1969;103:8.
47. Ueland K, Novy MJ, Peterson EN, et al: Maternal cardiovascular dynamics. IV. The influences of gestational age on the maternal cardiovascular response to posture and exercise. Am J Obstet Gynecol 1969;104:856.
48. Ueland K, Novy MJ, Metcalfe J: Hemodynamic responses of patients with heart disease to pregnancy and exercise. Am J Obstet Gynecol 1972;113:47.
49. Ueland K, Novy MJ, Metcalfe J: Cardiorespiratory responses to pregnancy and exercise in normal women and patients with heart disease. Am J Obstet Gynecol 1973;115:4.
50. Wallace WA, Harken DE, Ellis LB: Pregnancy following closed mitral valvuloplasty: a long-term study with remarks concerning the necessity for careful cardiac management. JAMA 1971;217:297.

11

■ ■ ■

INFECTION DURING PREGNANCY

Denise M. Main and Elliott K. Main

Infections during pregnancy contribute more than any other perinatal problem to maternal and infant morbidity and mortality. For example, the congenitally transmitted TORCH diseases—*t*oxoplasmosis, *o*ther diseases, *r*ubella, *c*ytomegalovirus, and *h*erpes—are the major cause of congenitally acquired mental retardation in the United States. Bacterial infections can also cause other severe problems for the fetus and the pregnant woman. It behooves the obstetrician to attempt to identify infections when they occur and to treat them promptly. Much remains to be learned about infections during pregnancy; this is a rapidly changing field that is challenging and often frustrating.

In this chapter we discuss the most important perinatal infections: the four viral TORCH diseases, congenital and maternal syphilis, and three bacterial infections—urinary tract infections, group B streptococcal infections, and chorioamnionitis.

■ CYTOMEGALOVIRUS INFECTION

A DNA virus and member of the herpes family of viruses, cytomegalovirus (CMV) possesses the ability to remain latent within the host for years, reactivating infection sporadically. Histologic evaluation of cells infected with CMV reveals large intranuclear inclusions, leading to the alternate name, cytomegalic inclusion disease.

Of all infants born in the United States, 0.5% to 2.0% are congenitally infected with CMV. The vast majority are clinically well at birth, but some develop severe neurologic and auditory or visual impairments. Approximately 10% of infants congenitally infected with CMV have clinically recognizable signs at birth, and these infants incur even more devastating sequelae. Since transmission occurs from mothers who have recently acquired the disease as well as from those with latent and recurrent infections, the solution of immunization is not always possible.

Transmission

Seroepidemiologic studies show that CMV is more commonly acquired in early infancy in some countries (eg, Japan) than in the United States. A second period of seroconversion occurs during adolescence. Inasmuch as CMV is excreted in semen, cervical secretions, and saliva, the virus is believed to be venereally transmitted.

Congenital transmission appears to occur transplacentally, with isolated cases reported in which the placenta has been involved but the fetus spared.[28] A primary maternal infection in any trimester has the potential for congenital transmission. One report concerns a woman who developed a CMV mononucleosis-like infection at 6 weeks' gestation and at 22 weeks' gestation had a therapeutic abortion that revealed an infected fetus.[10] Other studies by Monif et al[46] and Stern and Tucker[64] have also shown that maternal infections in any trimester can lead to fetal infection. Their study populations, however, are small. In the study by Monif et al more severely affected infants were born to mothers who developed infections during the second trimester than during the third trimester. Stern and Tucker found a transmission rate of 50% as determined by culturing neonatal urine and secretions.

Unlike the situation with rubella, women with latent CMV infections (already immune without change in titers) can transmit CMV to their offspring. Women have delivered consecutive siblings who have been infected, although in all cases reported only the first child was severely affected and the second was asymptomatic. In several cases the CMV of both children and the mother was of similar antigenic composition, suggesting transmission by reactivation of a latent virus rather than reinfection with a new strain of CMV.[30] In a prospective study of 239 seroimmune women in Alabama, 7 delivered infected infants (3.4%). All infants were clinically asymptomatic at birth.[62]

From 3% to 28% of women excrete CMV from the cervix at some point in gestation.[23] Like herpes, CMV infection can be acquired at the time of vaginal delivery.[55] A further common means of infection appears to be via breast-feeding. The virus is transmitted in the breast milk of 25.7% of women with serologic evidence of CMV infection.[63] Indeed breast-feeding may account for the high seroconversion during infancy in countries such as Japan.

Most CMV infections in pregnant women are asymptomatic, although occasional primary infections will show mononucleosis-like syndrome of malaise, lymphadenopathy, and hepatosplenomegaly. There is no clear evidence that CMV leads to spontaneous abortions.[23]

Overt congenital infection

Infants born with overt CMV disease often exhibit hepatosplenomegaly, thrombocytopenia with petechiae and purpura, hepatitis associated with icterus, pneumonitis, and chorioretinitis. Abnormalities that result from faulty neurologic development include microcephaly, optic atrophy, aplasia of various parts of the brain, and microphthalmia. There is only indirect evidence

that malformations outside the central nervous system (CNS) are secondary to CMV.[23] Unlike toxoplasmosis, the presence of intracranial calcifications is an indication that the infant will have at least moderate to severe retardation.[23]

Silent congenital infection

Follow-up studies of infants with congenital CMV infections that were "silent" at birth suggest that a significant number develop auditory difficulties and mild degrees of mental impairment. In one study, 44 of these infants were examined at 3½ and at 7 years of age.[24] The infected group's mean IQ was 102.5, whereas the matched control group's mean IQ was 117 ($p < .025$). Bilateral hearing loss was present in 5 out of 40 infected infants versus 1 in 44 in the control group. However, 3 of the antibody-positive children had profound deafness, an abnormality that occurs in approximately 1 out of 1000 children.

There have been no studies to date that differentiate between sequelae of infants infected from primary maternal infections versus those infected from seroimmune mothers. Also, there have been no reports of any children born to seroimmune women developing mental or auditory sequelae.

Follow-up studies of infants with neonatal-related or breastfed-related infections have only been reported to 1 year of age. No obvious sequelae were noted in these groups, but follow-up is still inadequate.[24]

Diagnosis

During acute infections the CMV virus may be recovered from the urine, throat, and blood. The most dependable source is a sample (5 ml) of the first urine voided in the morning. After the acute infection patients continue shedding the CMV virus in the urine for several weeks and even months. When blood samples are used for the diagnosis of acute infection, the yield is not as good as the urine culture. In the case of blood samples the leukocytes are separated and inoculated into human fibroblast cell cultures, which are examined a few days later for the presence of characteristic cytopathic effects. Serologic studies may also be useful in the diagnosis of acute infection. In fact, they are diagnostic if they show a fourfold increase in the antibody level between acute and convalescent phase sera, even if the urine or blood cultures are negative.

Prevention

Several field studies involving CMV vaccines have been initiated. Unfortunately, more information is needed about the effects of the vaccines and the sequelae of congenital infections in infants of seroimmune mothers before they can receive wide use.

■ RUBELLA

Rubella was considered an inconsequential disease until 1941 when the association between maternal rubella and fetal defects was discovered. The ensuing congenital rubella saga is not unlike the recent history of Rh isoimmunization. In a relatively short time the cause of the disease was identified, the pathogenesis explained, and a preventive measure created, with the result that public health measures have markedly reduced the incidence of the disease. But, like isoimmunization, congenital rubella still occurs at a higher than acceptable rate, and considerable work remains to be done.

Signs and symptoms

Rubella causes a usually mild exanthematous disease in children (fever, malaise, and lymphadenopathy) and a somewhat more severe form of the illness in young adults. Characteristic are a facial rash, postauricular adenopathy, flu-like symptoms, and arthralgia or arthritis. The symptoms of arthralgia and arthritis occur largely in women and more commonly involve the smaller joints. Rubella has a typical time relationship between clinical signs, virus shedding, and antibody development that is important in the evaluation of potential exposures. When a person first contracts rubella, the virus multiplies in the upper respiratory tract mucosa and associated lymph nodes. After 7 to 10 days the virus enters the bloodstream, and the viremia continues until antibodies appear—generally another 7 days. The viremia may occur as long as a week before the facial rash appears. The total incubation time (exposure to symptoms) is 14 to 21 days, most commonly 16 to 18 days.

Hemagglutination-inhibition (HI) antibodies begin to rise with the onset of symptoms and peak in 1 to 3 weeks. Complement-fixing (CF)

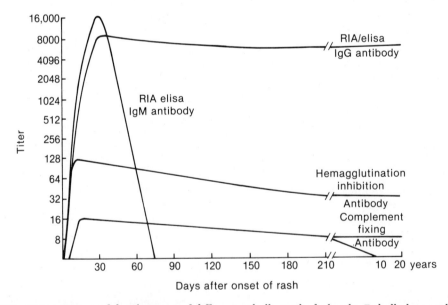

FIG. 11-1 ■ Pattern of development of different rubella antibody levels. Rubella hemagglutination-inhibition (HI) antibody develops rapidly after the onset of symptoms and remains relatively constant for several years. Complement-fixing (CF) antibody develops slower than HI and falls off after some years. IgM antibody appears shortly after the rash, peaks at about 30 days, and is undetectable by day 80 after the rash. The IgG antibody parallels the IgM but remains at high level indefinitely. Obviously the best marker of recent infection is the presence of specific IgM antibody. (From Sever JL: Clin Perinatol 1979;6:347.)

antibodies increase more slowly, reaching their maximum approximately 1 to 2 weeks after the peak of the HI antibodies (Fig. 11-1). The rubella-specific IgM antibody appears shortly before the onset of symptoms, peaks approximately 1 week later, and disappears approximately 1 month after the onset of the disease.[58]

Congenital rubella

The U.S. rubella pandemic of 1964-1965 made it possible to perform a tremendous amount of clinical, serologic, and virologic research on the congenital rubella syndrome. Some of the important lessons are as follows[13]:

1. Both clinically apparent and totally silent maternal infection can result in fetal infection.

2. Fetal consequences of first-trimester rubella may be no infection, inapparent infection with no clinical consequence, single-organ involvement (typically the ear), or multiple organ involvement with mild to severe damage. The most common abnormalities are cataracts, patent ductus arteriosus, and impaired hearing; they frequently are found together. The multiple abnormalities are as follows:

Common
  Growth retardation (intrauterine and postnatal)
  Deafness (sensorineural and/or central)*
  Cataracts, retinopathy

---

*Often detected only after 1 year of age.

Patent ductus arteriosus
Pulmonary artery hypoplasia (or valvular stenosis)
Hepatosplenomegaly
Less frequent
  Thrombocytopenic purpura
  Psychomotor retardation*
  Meningoencephalitis
  Radiolucency of the long bones
  Coarctation of the aorta
  Myocardial necrosis
Rare
  Microcephaly
  Brain calcifications
  Cardiac septal defects
  Glaucoma
  Hepatitis
Late-onset features (after 3 to 12 months)
  Interstitial pneumonitis
  Chronic rubella-like rash
  Recurrent infections
  Hypogammaglobulinemia
  Chronic diarrhea
  Diabetes mellitus
  Progressive CNS deterioration (onset in adolescence)

3. The risk of congenital disease is maximum at 4 to 8 weeks of gestation (as high as 50% to 60% affected in prospective studies), while the risk for the rest of the first trimester is about 25% to 35%. (These figures include late-onset deafness and retinopathy, which account for nearly half of the affected infants.) There is also some risk just before conception and as late as 20 weeks of gestation[69] (Fig. 11-2).

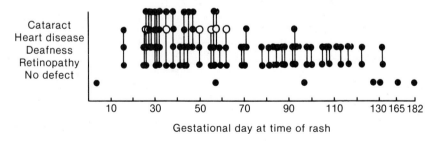

FIG. 11-2 ■ Clinical manifestations in 55 patients with congenital rubella in relation to the gestational age at the time of infection. The figure shows that deafness and retinopathy are the most common abnormalities of congenital rubella and that they appear when the infection occurs before 120 days of gestation. In contrast, cataracts and heart disease are almost completely limited to infections occurring before 60 days of gestation. The open circles in the line corresponding to heart disease indicate patients with patent ductus arterious. (From Ueda K, Nishida Y, Oshima K, et al: J Pediatr 1979;94:763.)

4. After 9 weeks of gestation, nearly all the cases of congenital disease result in hearing loss, retinopathy, and psychomotor retardation.
5. The fetus is at risk only during the primary infection. To date, there is no recorded evidence of a sibling of a child with congenital rubella being affected.
6. Infection in the first weeks of gestation is associated with a doubling of the spontaneous abortion rate.
7. Wild rubella virus is highly contagious, with only minimal contact necessary for transmission.

Serology

Every pregnant woman should have rubella immunity testing at her first prenatal visit. History of prior infection or immunization is often misleading or may not have resulted in adequate antibody response. The HI test is the most common screening test to assess immunity. A titer of $\geq 1:16$ (or $1:20$) is conclusive evidence of immunity. Titers of $1:8$ (or $1:10$) are more difficult to interpret.[25] In a recent study up to 17% of these patients lacked antibodies when tested with radioimmunoassay. These false positive results are probably the result of incomplete removal of nonspecific inhibitors present in all human sera.

To evaluate a person who is seen 7 days or less after potential exposure or exanthematous illness, a sample for the HI test is drawn or, if available, the results of the test performed at the first prenatal visit are referred to. The titer may be as high as $1:256$ in up to 15% of the normal immune population, and, if the test has been, in fact, obtained within 7 days after exposure, it does not indicate infection. If the patient is not immune ($<1:8$ or $<1:10$) or the titer is high ($\geq 1:256$), the HI test should be repeated 2 to 3 weeks later. If the second HI titer shows a similar value or an insignificant variation (less than two dilutions) in relation to the first sample, infection has not occurred. The repeat titer in 2 to 3 weeks will show at least a fourfold rise (two dilutions) if an infection has occurred.

When the patient is seen 1 to 5 weeks after exposure or up to 3 weeks after the onset of a rash, serum HI and CF antibody levels should

TABLE 11-1 ■ Examples of serologic interpretation of rubella titers*

History	Days after exposure or onset of illness	HI titer	Interpretation
Exposure to case; no clinical illness	1 14	$1:32$ ($1:40$) $1:64$ ($1:80$)	Mother immune and not at risk; twofold increase in titer not significant and within errors of test
Exposure to case; no clinical illness	2 18	$<1:8$ ($1:10$) $<1:8$ ($1:10$)	Patient susceptible but not infected
Exposure to case; no clinical illness	14 28	$1:16$ ($1:20$) $1:64$ ($1:80$)	Subclinical infection in a susceptible patient; first serum taken when antibody was beginning to appear
Fever rash; questionable case	2 16	$1:16$ ($1:20$) $1:16$ ($1:20$)	Patient immune as result of previous infection; illness not rubella
Fever, rash, lymphadenopathy compatible with rubella	4 18	$1:16$ ($1:20$) $1:128$ ($1:160$)	Clinical rubella confirmed in a susceptible patient

*Each example consists of a history (first column) and two consecutive HI titers (third column) carried out at different days after exposure or after the onset of illness (second column). The interpretation of the titers is given in the last (fourth) column.

be obtained immediately and 2 weeks later. A fourfold increase in either antibody will be evidence of acute infection. Absence of CF antibody in both specimens will rule out acute infection. Stable, elevated positive titers for both HI and CF antibodies will require testing to determine the presence of rubella-specific IgM in both specimens. In this case the patient should be informed about the possible risk of fetal abnormalities. It is important for the follow-up titers to be run simultaneously with sera saved from earlier samples to be certain of differences in titers.

Rubella-specific IgM antibody titers rise rapidly after a recent infection and disappear after 4 to 5 weeks, leaving only IgG as a residual antibody. A positive rubella-specific IgM is the most specific test indicating recent rubella infection and should be done in every case where infection is suspected and before abortion is performed. A negative rubella-specific IgM test is of little diagnostic value unless supported by other laboratory data. The rubella-specific IgM test is not commonly available, and specimens may need to be sent directly to the Centers for Disease Control (CDC) in Atlanta, Georgia. It is also important to remember that many "rubella exposures" are actually exposures to nonspecific viral exanthems. Therefore a medical history should be taken on the individual thought to be the *source* of exposure, and a physical examination and serologic tests should also be performed. For example, determination of prior immunization would make it very unlikely that the illness is rubella. Likewise, negative serologic titers in the source of exposure would rule out rubella. Table 11-1 gives examples of how serologic testing can aid in making a diagnosis.

Vaccination

In 1969 two vaccines were licensed in the United States—HPV77-DE5 and the Cedehill strain. HPV77 was the most commonly used vaccine until its replacement by RA27/3 in 1979. The vaccines produce seroconversions in 95% to 98% of susceptible individuals and cause symptoms resembling mild rubella in 10% to 15% of recipients. Transient arthralgias and arthritis are particularly common in adult women receiving the vaccine; in those over 20 years of age, up to 20% to 30% may experience joint involvement.

The major problem with the earlier vaccines was that they were not as immunogenic as the natural virus. Several recent studies have shown absent HI antibody titers in long-term follow-up in an alarming 10% to 25% of individuals vaccinated earlier, whereas the RA27/3 vaccine has had a serologic failure rate in 4 to 5 years of follow-up of only 3%.[5] However, there is some evidence that patients with absent titers after vaccination still have some protection against viremia. Their serologic response to reimmunization resembles a "booster" response more closely than a primary one.

After the 1964-1965 pandemic that resulted in approximately 20,000 cases of congenital rubella syndrome, live attenuated vaccines were quickly developed and field-tested. National immunization policy was based on the concept of herd immunity. Schoolchildren, who have a high incidence of acute rubella during epidemics, were vaccinated to prevent spread to susceptible pregnant women. In addition, follow-up vaccination of susceptible nonpregnant women was recommended. Since rubella epidemics occur in the United States in cycles about 6 to 9 years apart, the policy had a sense of urgency to it. The American program, which vaccinated boys and girls, while more costly than the British policy of only vaccinating pubertal girls was quicker in reducing the number of rubella victims and thus the number of birth defects.

The herd immunity concept worked reasonably well initially in the United States and has been responsible, in part, for the reduction of congenital rubella cases to an estimated 30 each year. However, several problems remain today with this policy. It has been difficult to maintain the size of the herd in these recent nonepidemic years. Public concern has fallen so that only 65% to 70% of children have been immunized. Consequently, there has been a dramatic shift in the age at which a person gets rubella. In 1977, 70% of the reported cases were in persons 15 years of age or older.[36]

The lack of immunity among medical and hospital personnel is a problem dramatized by several recent outbreaks of rubella in hospitals in New York and California. In the New York incident[43] a male obstetrics house officer exposed 170 persons to the disease, including susceptible pregnant patients. A similar report concerning a private obstetrician in Texas[41] again highlights the need for health personnel to be vaccinated.

Selective immunization of women of child-bearing age has been difficult and incomplete at best. Several studies have shown that, even when physicians obtain routine serologic tests of women, the results are rarely acted on.[7] Just as prenatal serologic testing has become commonplace in the United States, so should postnatal immunization of all susceptible patients. The newly vaccinated woman is not contagious to other pregnant women in the hospital, nor is her baby at risk even if she breast-feeds, although recently there have been several cases reported in which a breast-fed infant seroconverted without any evidence of the disease. There is some evidence that the serologic response rate may be slightly less when vaccination is performed in the postpartum period, but this is more than balanced by the decreased risk of pregnancy in the ensuing 2 to 3 months.

Rubella vaccine is absolutely contraindicated in pregnancy, as are the other live attenuated vaccines. Recent investigative work has shown, however, that the risk is not nearly as great as with the wild virus. In one study rubella virus was isolated from the products of conception (usually the placenta) in 21% (6 out of 28) of vaccinated women known to be susceptible. The timing of vaccination in the cases where the virus was isolated ranged from 7 weeks' preconception to 11 weeks' postconception. This 7-week case is the basis for the recommended waiting period of 3 months from vaccination to attempted pregnancy.[45]

The CDC have reviewed their data and estimated that the *maximum* risk of fetal infection after vaccination is between 3% and 5%, with the *real* risk probably less.[52] To date there has not been a reported live birth with the congenital rubella syndrome after immunization of the mother during pregnancy. Despite extensive testing, there is no documentation of spread of rubella vaccine virus from a vaccinated person to a susceptible contact. Therefore it is not necessary to vaccinate susceptible household members of a pregnant woman vaccinated after delivery.

The role of immune globulin for exposed first-trimester mothers remains controversial. Some investigators recommend its use by patients who will not accept therapeutic abortions. The CDC do not recommend its use, and it must be kept in mind that preparations of immune globulin vary greatly in their rubella antibody content and that, to be effective, the immune globulin needs to be given at the time of exposure (viremia occurs *before* the rash). Furthermore, only the studies carried out in the early 1960s demonstrated effective protection against infection. Later studies found either protection against some of the signs and symptoms of disease but not against infection, or no protection at all.[17] Apparently, immune globulin administration does not preclude serologic diagnosis (seroconversion indicates infection rather than acquisition of a passive antibody). Thus immune globulin is an uncertain option of controversial benefit that should be offered only to a small number of women in special circumstances.

■ HERPES

The herpes simplex virus (HSV) is of major obstetric interest because of the devastating, yet often preventable, effects that it can produce in the newborn. Since the major source of neonatal infection is the mother's birth canal, this fact has led to the use of cesarean section to minimize exposure of the infant.

Description of the virus

HSV types 1 and 2 belong to a large group of DNA viruses that includes at least three other human viruses—cytomegalovirus, varicella-zoster, and Epstein-Barr virus. These viruses have the ability to persist throughout the life of their hosts and to produce recurrent infections. They induce intranuclear inclusions in infected cells.

There are two main antigenic types of HSV, although antigenic variations can occur among strains of each of the two types. Several biologic and biochemical differences between HSV-1 and HSV-2 have been identified[49] and are summarized in Table 11-2.

Both types of HSV can affect the genital areas, and both can lead to neonatal infections of equal severity. Approximately three fourths of neonatal HSV infections are of type 2 and one fourth of type 1.[70]

Maternal infection

Genital HSV infections have been detected in 1% to 2% of low-income pregnant patients surveyed by cytologic or viral screening. The in-

TABLE 11-2 ■ Differences between HSV types 1 and 2

Characteristic	HSV-1	HSV-2
Clinical	Infects primarily nongenital sites	Infects primarily genital sites
Epidemiologic	Transmission primarily via nongenital route	Transmission primarily via genital route (venereal or mother to newborn)
Biochemical composition		
DNA guanine	67	69
Cytosine (moles%)	Around 50% homology in viral DNAs	
Biologic		
Chick embryo (chorioallantoic membrane)	Small pocks	Large pocks
Mice-genital or intramuscular inoculation	Less neurotropic	More neurotropic
Tissue culture cells	Differences exist between the two virus types in their ability to propagate and in their cytopathic characteristics in certain cell cultures	

Modified from Nahmias AJ, Visintine AM: Herpes simplex, in Remington JS, Kline JO (eds): Infectious diseases of the fetus and newborn infant. Philadelphia, WB Saunders Co, 1976, pp. 156-190.

cidence of positive studies at the time of delivery is lower, in the range of 1 case out of 250 to 364 as determined by viral cultures[61,65] and 1 out of 1000 as diagnosed by Papanicolaou smears.[48] Women of higher socioeconomic status and nonpregnant women have lower infection rates.[48,50]

In a study by Nahmias and Visintine[49] of a group of 140 pregnant women with HSV infection diagnosed by cytology, only 36% had vesicular or ulcerative lesions that could be characterized as herpetic. A number of women with characteristic lesions demonstrated nonspecific manifestations of genital infection, including cervical inflammation, dysuria, hematuria, leukorrhea, and pelvic pain. Such nonspecific findings were detected in the absence of typical lesions in 21% of women affected. However, 43% of the group was totally asymptomatic at the time of diagnosis. This asymptomatic rate is comparable to that found by other researchers.[50] The virus is shed between 1 week and 3 months after an infection, most commonly from 1 to 3 weeks. Shedding tends to be longer with primary infections.

Early pregnancy. Women with genital HSV infections during the first half of pregnancy have a significantly increased incidence of spontaneous abortions.[48,50] The risk of abortion seems to be higher in those with serologic evidence of

a primary infection. In a few instances HSV has been isolated from the abortus material, and in one case the placental membranes were noted to have intrauterine inclusion bodies.[2] However, there has been no histologic evidence, to date, of direct fetal involvement. Thus it remains unclear as to whether the increased abortion rate results from generalized maternal toxicity or whether it is related to a transplacentally acquired fetal infection. A handful of case reports have suggested a complex of congenital anomalies, including microcephaly, intracranial calcifications, microphthalmia, retinal dysplasia, and chorioretinitis that may result from early fetal infections with HSV.[71] However, none of these cases have been well documented. The occurrence of this sort of congenital syndrome appears to be very infrequent.

Late pregnancy. Maternal infection after 20 weeks of gestation is associated with an increased incidence of preterm delivery and direct transmission of HSV to the newborn. The risk of preterm delivery is most pronounced in women experiencing primary HSV infections. In the study of Nahamias et al,[48] 35% of a group of women experiencing primary infections after 20 weeks of gestation delivered prematurely, as compared to 14% of women of similar gestational age affected by recurrent infections.

TABLE 11-3 ■ Clinical course of infants with HSV infection

Clinical category	Number of infants	Fatalities (%)	Infants with sequelae (%)	Infants without apparent sequelae (%)
Disseminated				
With CNS involvement	104	72	15	13
Without CNS involvement	102	91	2	8
Localized				
CNS	63	37	51	12
Ocular	15	0	40	60
Cutaneous*	36	6	22	72
Oral	4	0	25	75
TOTAL	324	59	20	21

Adapted from Visintine AM, Nahamias AJ, Josey WE: Perinatal Care 1978;2:32.
*Infection in more than 20% of the infants with skin lesions and no other clinical manifestations eventually progressed to involvement of the CNS or eyes.

The most important source of infection to the neonate is the mother's genital tract at the time of delivery. Passage through virus-containing maternal secretions during the second stage of labor allows HSV to enter the infant via the eyes, upper respiratory tract, scalp (especially if internal fetal monitoring devices were used), and cord. Prolonged rupture of the membranes has also been associated with neonatal infections, suggesting an ascending spread of infection.

When an infant is delivered vaginally or by cesarean section at least 4 to 6 hours after rupture of the membranes of a HSV-infected mother, the reported risk of acquiring an HSV infection is 40% to 60%.[48] The risk is markedly decreased, however, if the infant is delivered by cesarean section before rupture of the membranes or within 4 hours of rupture of the membranes, although isolated cases of HSV infection have been reported even in these situations.[37,71] If the infant is delivered by cesarean section more than 4 hours after rupture of the membranes, it does not necessarily develop infection; Grossman et al[21] recently reported that of 58 pregnancies complicated by HSV infection, 6 infants were delivered by cesarean section more than 4 hours after rupture of the membranes and none of them became infected.

The risk of acquiring an HSV infection appears to be similar whether the infant is term or preterm and whether antibodies are present or absent.[48] Transplacentally acquired antibodies against HSV may protect the infant from dis-

seminated HSV infection but are not a protection against localized disease, which frequently is fatal.[1]

Visintine et al[70] reviewed the clinical course of 324 infants with HSV infections, and their data are summarized in Table 11-3. The disseminated form of HSV infection in the neonate involves primarily the liver and adrenal glands. Other organs also frequently involved include the larynx, trachea, lungs, esophagus, stomach, intestines, spleen, and heart. If the infant does not die early from visceral involvement, CNS disease is often manifest. Skin, oral, or ocular lesions are often also associated with disseminated disease. The incidence of asymptomatic infections appears very low, with no cases detected among 1600 infants screened by viral culture.[2,8]

Postpartum infection

There have been infrequent reports of infants acquiring HSV-1 and HSV-2 infections without apparent genital exposure.[57] Some of these infected infants were exposed to individuals with oral infections or to other HSV infants in the nursery. With the recent ability to "fingerprint" viral isolates on the basis of their DNA composition, it is possible to clarify the mode and frequency of nongenital HSV transmission to neonates.[38] One report cites postpartum acquisition of HSV-1 infection in a breast-fed newborn whose mother's milk culture was positive for HSV-1 while her genital and throat cultures were negative.[14]

Diagnosis

Cytologic techniques are a readily available, rapid means of identifying HSV infections. Cell scrapings are obtained from the base of lesions as well as from the cervix; they are smeared, fixed in alcohol, and then stained with Papanicolaou stain. The typical morphologic findings include intranuclear inclusions and multinucleated giant cells. In skilled hands, cytologic techniques will identify 60% to 80% of HSV infections.[70]

Viral isolation techniques are the most definitive means of establishing HSV infections. Specimens are obtained from any active lesions as well as from the cervix and vagina. If not tested within a few hours, the specimen should be frozen at −70° C or in dry ice or stored in a Leibowitz-Emory transport medium. A tentative diagnosis can usually be obtained by the viral laboratory in 1 to 3 days.

Serologic tests are of limited value because of the cross reactivity of HSV-1 and HSV-2. However, if an individual has had neither type of HSV infection, acute and convalescent titers can define a primary infection.

Management

Early pregnancy. A careful history of prior HSV infections, both genital and labial, and of exposure to the virus is useful during an initial evaluation. Any suspicious lesions should be cultured and smeared for cytologic evaluation. Each pregnant woman should have a routine Papanicolaou smear of the cervix, which can help detect asymptomatic infections.

If a woman has an active genital lesion suspected of being an HSV infection, every effort should be made to document it. If she has no history of prior genital or labial HSV infections, acute and convalescent serologic titers may be helpful. Because of the very low incidence of early congenital infections leading to affected infants and because of uncertain interpretation, additional diagnostic tests such as amniocentesis are probably not indicated. However, it should be remembered that there is a high incidence of spontaneous abortion, particularly with primary infections.

Late pregnancy. Women at high risk of acquiring HSV infections should be monitored at frequent intervals during the third trimester to detect any infection. Visintine et al[70] recom-

mend viral and/or cytologic screening at 28, 32, and 36 weeks of gestation and weekly thereafter for women with any of the following:

1. A documented genital HSV infection that has been detected earlier in pregnancy
2. A substantiated, preferably laboratory-confirmed, history of recurrent genital HSV infections
3. A sexual partner who has had a substantiated genital HSV infection

Frequent monitoring avoids operative delivery when genital HSV infection is present early in the third trimester but has been resolved before the onset of labor. In these cases a Papanicolaou smear or, if available, a double antibody immunofluorescence test for rapid diagnosis should be done when the patient goes into labor to detect any recurrence between the time of the last test and delivery. Cesarean section is indicated for women who have a laboratory-demonstrated virus or active genital lesions close to the time of delivery unless rupture of the membranes has already exceeded 6 hours. Recent data, however, suggest that in some cases cesarean sections may help even after 6 hours of rupture of the membranes.[21] HSV can be isolated from amniotic fluid in the absence of fetal infection,[80] so amniocentesis and fluid culture are not useful in determining route of delivery.

Postpartum. There is considerable controversy regarding an isolation policy for both mother and infant who may have an HSV infection. Isolation policies range from minimal, if any, isolation to removing mothers with HSV infections from obstetric floors and thus preventing maternal-infant contact. Also, there is no defined policy with respect to herpes labialis, which puts infants at greater risk, since it is almost impossible for mothers and nurses with "cold sores" to keep their hands from their face and the virus may be transferred to the hands and then to the baby. In general, as long as the mother maintains scrupulous handwashing after personal hygiene care, there is no increased risk of transmission of genital or labial HSV to other patients or to the baby.

Nosocomial transmission of HSV is extremely rare or nonexistent. With the ability to "fingerprint" HSV isolates, it will be possible to define nongenital transmission more accurately and recommendations will become more sensible. At present, because of the severity of neonatal

TABLE 11-4 ■ Recommendations for women with prior or concurrent HSV infection at the time of delivery

Genital herpetic lesions present at term	Group	Primary genital lesions	Recurrent genital lesions (or genital reinfection)	Status of membranes	Recommended route of delivery	Isolation of mother	Isolation of newborn
Yes	1	+	—	Intact or ruptured* <4 to 6 hours	Cesarean section	Yes	Yes
	2	+	—	Ruptured† >4 to 6 hours	Vaginal	Yes	Yes
	3	+	— or +	Baby delivered vaginally	—	Yes	Yes
	4	—	+	Intact or ruptured* <4 to 6 hours	Cesarean section	Yes	Yes
	5	—	+	Ruptured† >4 to 6 hours	Vaginal	Yes	Yes
No, but cervicovaginal culture or cytology positive for herpes	6	—	—	Intact or ruptured* <4 to 6 hours	Cesarean section	Yes	Yes
	7	—	—	Ruptured† >4 to 6 hours	Vaginal	Yes	Yes
No, but past history of genital herpes, presently inactive, or status unknown	8	—	—	Intact or ruptured	Vaginal	No	No
No, but nongenital herpes present at birth	9	—	—	Intact or ruptured	Vaginal	Yes	No, at birth; yes, after newborn goes to mother
No but past history of nongenital herpes	10	—	—	Intact or ruptured	Vaginal	No	No

*The shorter the interval between rupture of the membranes and cesarean section, the less the risk of fetal infection. The critical period appears to be 4 to 6 hr.
†Recent evidence suggests that cesarean section delivery may help even after more than 4 hours of ruptured membranes.

disease, a conservative approach appears indicated. A recent *JAMA* review article set forth some useful recommendations for the care of mothers with both genital and nongenital HSV infections;[33] these are summarized here:

Care of mother with proven or clinically suspected genital HSV infection

1. Mother should be in a private room.
2. All personnel having direct contact with the patient or with contaminated articles should wear gown and gloves.
3. Perineal pads and other genital dressings as well as bed linen should be handled as if infected (ie, double-bagged).
4. Mother may handle and feed her infant if:
   a. She is out of bed and has washed her hands carefully. (For mother-newborn contact, this is preferable to wearing gloves.)
   b. She puts on a clean gown before the baby is brought to her from the nursery.
5. Mother may leave room after washing hands and view baby through nursery windows.

Care of mother with active nongenital HSV infection

1. Mother should be in a private room.
2. All personnel having direct contact with patient or contaminated articles should wear gown and gloves.
3. Dressings covering lesions and bed linen should be handled as if infected (ie, double-bagged).
4. Attempts should be made to expedite crusting of lesions by applying drying agents such as providone iodine (Betadine), benzoin, or ethyl ether.
5. Once lesions are crusted (generally 2 to 3 days), mother may handle infant as described for mother with genital HSV infection, except she should wear a face mask.

In cases of both genital and nongenital infections, standard operating room technique and proper cleaning of labor and delivery rooms should be sufficient to prevent transmission of HSV infection in these areas. Table 11-4 is a summary of the recommended route of delivery and isolation procedures for HSV patients at the time of delivery.

■ TOXOPLASMOSIS

Approximately 3300 infants born every year in the United States are congenitally infected with toxoplasmosis.[54] Most of these infants are asymptomatic during the neonatal period, but many subsequently develop adverse sequelae. Early treatment—maternal or neonatal—may reduce the severity of the sequelae. The main challenge, then, lies in the early diagnosis of the usually asymptomatic infected gravidas and neonates.

Description of the parasite

The *Toxoplasma* parasite exists in three forms: the trophozoite, the tissue cyst, and the oocyst. The trophozoite requires an intracellular habitat to survive and multiply. Reproduction is endogenous (internal budding). During the acute phase of an infection the trophozoite invades virtually every type of cell. After invasion the organisms multiply until the cell cytoplasm is so filled that the cell is disrupted.

The second form of the parasite, the tissue cyst, is formed within the host cell as early as the eighth day of an acute infection and probably persists throughout the life of the host. The skeleton, heart muscles, and brain are the most common sites for latent infections.

The oocysts are produced in the small intestine of the cat. Once shed, the oocyst sporulates in 1 to 5 days and becomes infectious. Under appropriate conditions (warm moist soil), it may remain infectious for more than 1 year. The parasite, in addition to being transmitted by direct handling of contaminated soil and cat feces, can be transmitted to food via insect vectors (Fig. 11-3).[54]

All forms of the parasite are destroyed by adequate freezing and heating. Tissue cysts and oocysts are resistant to stomach and small bowel digestion and destruction.

Transmission of *Toxoplasma* to humans commonly occurs through the ingestion of undercooked meat (pork or lamb and occasionally beef) and through other foods contaminated with oocysts. Isolated cases have been transmitted by the transfusion of whole blood.

Acute maternal infection

Most maternal infections with *Toxoplasma* are mild or asymptomatic. The commonly recognized clinical signs are adenopathy and fatigue without fever. The groups of nodes most often involved are the cervical, suboccipital, supraclavicular, axillary, and inguinal nodes. The adenopathy may be localized in one node or diffused. Retroperitoneal and mesenteric nodes

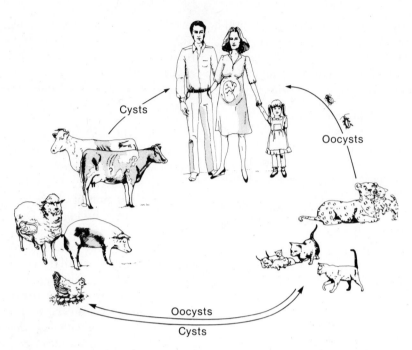

FIG. 11-3 ■ Life cycle of the *Toxoplasma* parasite. The cat seems to be the definite host. An enteroepithelial cycle occurs in the cat's intestine and results in the production of oocysts, which pass out with the feces. Ingestion of the oocysts by other animals or by humans initiates an extraintestinal cycle characterized by cell invasion by trophozoites followed by formation of tissue cysts. Humans and cats also may become infected by ingesting tissue cysts formed in other animals. (From Remington JS, Desmonts G: In Remington JS, Klein JO [eds]: Infectious diseases of the fetus and newborn infant. Philadelphia, WB Saunders Co, 1976, p. 199.)

may also be involved, as well as, at times, the spleen and liver. Occasionally there may be a fever or exanthem. Chorioretinitis rarely occurs in the acute infection, but several cases have been documented.[54]

Congenital transmission

Of major obstetric concern is the congenital transmission of the parasite. With very rare exceptions, congenital transmission occurs only during an acute infection acquired during pregnancy.[54] Most fetal transmission appears to be transplacental and usually occurs before labor as evidenced by cord antibody titers. *Toxoplasma* is rarely transmitted to the fetus when the acute infection occurs at conception or during the first 2 months of gestation. During this time the placenta appears to serve as a "barrier" to fetal infection more effectively than later in gestation and provides nearly 80% protection. Although the placenta is infected with *Toxoplasma*, there is evidence that, in some cases, transmission to

the infant does not occur until labor begins.[34] Occasionally women secrete *Toxoplasma* in their vaginal fluids, and exposure to the infant may be through vaginal delivery.[54]

The relative risk of acquiring toxoplasmosis during pregnancy is related in part to the overall incidence of the disease in each community. Studies of U.S. citizens reveal a wide variation of antibody positivity ranging from 13% to 67% and tending to increase with age. Studies of pregnant women with toxoplasmosis in the United States have been few. In one study in New York City of over 4000 pregnant women[34] the overall incidence of positive *Toxoplasma* antibodies was 31%. Women who were older, more affluent, and white had the highest incidence of prior infection. The higher income white patients also had the greatest risk of acquiring toxoplasmosis acutely during pregnancy; in this high-risk group 3 out of 189 women seroconverted during gestation.

Studies uniformly have shown that toxoplasmosis is transmitted to the fetus in less than 50% of the acute cases. Multiple prospective studies have been done in France where the incidence of toxoplasmosis is high and seroconversion during pregnancy frequent (6.3% in each pregnancy). In one group of 183 women who seroconverted during pregnancy, the results were an overall transmission rate of 33% to 39% and included 11 abortions, 7 stillborn or immediate newborn deaths, and 59 infants born with congenital toxoplasmosis.[11] Nine of the 59 infected infants were severely affected, 11 were mildly affected, and 39 had subclinical disease at birth. The severely infected infants all acquired their infections during the first two trimesters of pregnancy. Third trimester transmission resulted only in subclinical infection. None of the infants of 195 mothers with elevated antibody titers suggesting infection before gestation were infected.

Congenital infection

Infants with congenital toxoplasmosis may be stillborn, may be obviously affected at birth, may gradually develop symptoms in the first months of life or even later, or may remain asymptomatic. The "classic triad" of congenital toxoplasmosis includes hydrocephalus, chorioretinitis, and intracranial calcifications. Many affected infants have other symptoms, however, including hydrops fetalis or erythroblastosis, hepatosplenomegaly, and abnormal cerebrospinal fluid.

One prospective 5-year study of infants who had toxoplasmosis as neonates revealed that 85% of them were mentally retarded; 75% developed seizures, spasticity, or other major motor defects; 50% had severely impaired vision; and 15% had significant hearing impairment.[54] Even more worrisome are follow-up studies of infants detected by serologic screening who were completely asymptomatic at birth. A high percentage of these infants develop significant visual impairment, mental retardation, and other neurologic sequelae later in life. In one study[76] 20 of 23 asymptomatic infants developed significant visual impairment, with 6 becoming blind in both eyes and 5 more becoming blind in one eye. The mean IQ in this group was 89.4, with 5 children having IQs below 80. It is unclear whether early treatment of such infants reduces the incidence and severity of sequelae, although in preliminary studies treated infants appear to have done better than their untreated cohorts.[56]

Toxoplasma cysts can be isolated from the myometrium, endometrium, and vaginal secretions of chronically infected women who have stable low antibody titers. Likewise, the organism has been isolated from aborted products of conception, suggesting an association between toxoplasmosis and spontaneous abortion. Data indicate, however, that although chronic toxoplasmosis is associated with abortion, it is exceedingly uncommon.[54]

Diagnosis

A number of serologic tests have been developed for the diagnosis of toxoplasmosis. The two most helpful tests for the obstetrician are the Sabin-Feldman dye test and the IgM–indirect fluorescent antibody (IgM-IFA) test.

The Sabin-Feldman dye test rises relatively slowly following an acute infection, frequently taking 2 months to attain maximum levels, which are generally ≥300 IU/ml (≥1:1000) and may be as high as 3000 IU/ml (≥1:10,000) or more. High titers persist for months to years. Low titers almost always persist for life.

The IgM-IFA test becomes positive early in the course of an infection and may be the first serologic test to detect *Toxoplasma* antibodies. Titers in patients with an acute acquired infection vary widely, ranging from 1:10 to 1:1000. High titers persist for several months and then decrease steadily. In most cases the test becomes negative 3 to 4 months after infection (Table 11-5). Until proven otherwise, any pregnant woman with a dye test ≥300 IU/ml or 1:1000 and an IgM-IFA test ≥1:160 must be presumed to have active toxoplasmosis.[54]

Congenital infection may be diagnosed in several ways: (1) by isolating the protozoa from the placenta, a time-consuming and expensive method; (2) by lymphocyte transformation, a promising, more rapid method recently described[74]; and (3) by isolating toxoplasma from the amniotic fluid.[66] In the last method, failure to isolate *Toxoplasma* would not prove that the fetus is noninfected.

Management

Treatment during pregnancy attempts to decrease both the incidence and the severity of congenital infection. A combination of sulfonamides and pyrimethamine have been used, although because of possible teratogenic effects, pyrimethamine was not given during the first 12

TABLE 11-5 ■ Interpretation of *Toxoplasma* serologic studies in pregnancy

Time in gestation	Dye test	IgM-IFA test	Interpretation and follow-up
First trimester	Negative	Negative	No prior infection—mother susceptible to infection
	Positive	Negative	Prior infection months or years before pregnancy—regardless of dye test level, no risk to infant
	Positive	Positive	Recent infection—obtain follow-up IgM-IFA titers in 3 weeks—risk to infant low because so early in gestation but may have risk for spontaneous abortion
Midgestation	≥300 IU/ml	Positive	Recent maternal infection—significant risk to infant—look for adenopathy
	≤300 IU/ml	Positive	Probable infection—repeat serologic tests in 2 to 3 weeks
Immediately postpartum	≥300 IU/ml	Positive	Infection during pregnancy
	≥1000 IU/ml	Negative	Infection during pregnancy very likely
	300 to 1000 IU/ml	Negative	Infection early in gestation possible
	<300 IU/ml	Positive	Possible infection during late pregnancy—obtain follow-up titers
	<300 IU/ml	Negative	No infection during gestation

Adapted from Remington JS, Desmonts G: Toxoplasmosis, in Remington JS, Klein JO (eds): Infectious diseases of the fetus and newborn infant. Philadelphia, WB Saunders Co, 1976, pp. 191-332.

to 14 weeks of pregnancy.[54] With this treatment a definite reduction in the incidence of congenitally infected infants born to treated mothers was noticed (5% versus 16.6% for untreated mothers). In France women who seroconverted during pregnancy were treated with spiramycin (not available in the United States). The treated French women had significantly fewer infants who were congenitally infected (24% versus 45% of untreated mothers), although the incidence of clinically obvious infection was similar (11%) in both groups.[11] Thus treatment of mothers who seroconvert during pregnancy appears helpful. Data are insufficient to recommend therapy of women with chronic infections.

Prevention

Heating meat thoroughly to 66° C (150° F) or having meat smoked or cured eliminates tissue cysts. Pregnant women should thoroughly wash their hands after handling raw meats. If at all possible, seronegative pregnant women should avoid handling cat litter or soil contaminated with cat feces. Cat litter should be flushed away daily. To destroy viable oocysts, the empty

litter pan can be filled with nearly boiling water for 5 minutes daily.[54] Gloves should be worn when working in contaminated soil, and hands should be washed carefully.

Recommendations

Because of the relatively low incidence of acute toxoplasmosis during pregnancy in this country and the mixed reliability of serologic tests, routine serologic screening is generally not performed. However, experts are urging that regional screening programs be developed.[75] Patients at high risk for toxoplasmosis infections—women working in veterinary clinics, cat owners, raw and rare meat eaters—generally deserve screening with a dye test and, if possible, the IgM-IFA test. Similarly, any woman who develops adenopathy during pregnancy should be screened and have follow-up serologic testing.

Any woman who develops acute toxoplasmosis during pregnancy should be counseled about the possibility of legal abortion. Inasmuch as congenital toxoplasmosis is limited almost exclusively to women with acute infections, reassurances can be made regarding future pregnancies. The risk of fetal infection appears minimal if the mother's infection occurred during the first 2 months of gestation, but the risk is significant, although less than 50%, later in gestation.

Women with acute toxoplasmosis who do not elect to terminate their pregnancy or who are gestationally too far advanced for an abortion may benefit from treatment. In the United States one reasonable regimen includes pyrimethamine (1 mg/kg/day, maximum dosage 25 mg/day) and sulfadiazine or triple sulfonamides. (Before using these potentially toxic medications, see the report of Remington and Desmonts[54] on therapy.) When spiramycin is approved in this country, it should provide an easier, safer regimen. It is important to alert the pediatrician, so that, if indicated, evaluation of the infant and treatment are begun shortly after birth.

■ SYPHILIS

Congenital syphilis has served many generations of physicians as the model of fetal disease. With the spread of more complete prenatal care and the development of effective treponemicidal agents, the incidence of congenital syphilis has decreased markedly. This is fortunate because not only were these pregnancies marked by a very high rate of fetal death, but the affected infants bore a series of permanent sequelae that could not be erased even with neonatal treatment. However, the problem of congenital syphilis is far from dead; in fact, a minimum of 300 to 400 infants with congenital syphilis have been reported to the CDC each of the last 20 years. Furthermore, while penicillin is a highly effective treatment, the physician still has the problem of what to give to the pregnant woman who cannot take penicillin. The treatment of fetal syphilis serves today's physician as a paradigm for both the successes and the problems with intrauterine therapy.

Maternal syphilis

In the mother the manifestations of disease are unchanged by pregnancy. With exposure to *Treponema pallidum* there is a 50% chance of infection. After an average incubation period of 3 weeks a *primary* chancre appears (painless ulcer with an indurated base and local adenopathy). Disappearance of the ulcer in 2 to 6 weeks

heralds the beginning of secondary syphilis (rash, mucous patches, condyloma latum, generalized lymphadenopathy). These lesions also last from 2 to 6 weeks, at which point latent syphilis begins.

Congenital syphilis

Congenital syphilis is a multisystem disease that has a wide range in its severity and different forms in its presentation.[15] The manifestations resemble secondary syphilis (a fact that is not unexpected, since in congenital syphilis the treponemes obtain direct access to the fetal bloodstream), but unlike secondary syphilis quite often there is skeletal involvement such as osteomyelitis, osteochondritis, or periostitis. A list of common manifestations of congenital syphilis is presented on p. 216.

Examination of the placenta can often be helpful. On gross review, it is large, pale, and edematous. Microscopically, *Treponema pallidum* can often be identified with silver stain. The villae are often immature, enlarged, and with bullous projections, and the vessels have endovascular and perivascular proliferation.

A principle in congenital syphilis is that the more recent the maternal infection, the more severe the congenital disease. This is demonstrated in Table 11-6, which shows the differences in fetal outcome of *untreated* mothers with early, latent, and late syphilis.[15]

It has long been held that the placenta, via Langhans' cells, acts as a barrier for the first 16 to 18 weeks of pregnancy and protects the fetus from early infection. However, Harter and Benirschke[27] have clearly identified *Treponema pallidum* in first-trimester abortuses of women with recent syphilitic infections, and it seems more likely that the fetus has to develop an immune response for the treponemes to cause tissue injury.

Diagnosis

The diagnosis of syphilis is based on the type of lesions present. Serologic tests are less likely to be positive with primary lesions, so the test of choice is a darkfield examination of secretions from the chancre. In fact, this procedure (usually easily available from the venereal disease control branch of the local health department) is useful in any suspicious *moist* skin lesion (condyloma latum, mucous patches, or ulcers). Alternatives

Manifestations of congenital syphilis

Most infants look healthy at birth. A few have vesicular-bullous eruptions, usually in palm and soles.

From 4 days to 3 weeks of life, symptoms may begin and may be grouped as follows:
1. *Flu-like syndrome*
   a. Meningeal signs
   b. Lacrimation (iritis)
   c. Nasal discharge; mucous membranes red, swollen, eroded, loaded with *Treponema pallidum*
   d. Sore throat—pharynx with mucous patches
   e. Generalized arthralgia—splinting of arms and legs; osteochondritis on x-ray film; often periostitis, particularly of tibia (saber shin)
2. *Generalized lymphadenopathy*
   a. Cervical, epitrochlear, inguinal, axillary, popliteal
   b. Hepatosplenomegaly—if severe, probability of anemia, purpura, jaundice, edema, hypoalbuminemia
3. *Rash*
   a. Maculopapular, papular, and bullous eruptions may all appear together
   b. Occasionally papular lesions may coalesce to form condyloma latum

TABLE 11-6 ■ Outcome of normal pregnancy and pregnancy affected by untreated syphilis

Outcome of pregnancy	Status of mother			
	Without syphilis	Early syphilis (primary and secondary)	Latent syphilis	Late syphilis
Premature infants	9.0%	50.0%	20.0%	9.0%
Neonatal deaths	0.5%	—	4.0%	1.0%
Stillbirths	0.5%	—	16.0%	10.0%
Congenital syphilis (full term)	0.0%	50.0%	40.0%	10.0%
Normal infant (full term)	90.0%	0.0%	20.0%	70.0%

Adapted from Fiumara NJ: Clin Obstet Gynecol 1975;18:183.

in the absence of a positive darkfield examination are the serologic tests. The Venereal Disease Research Laboratories (VDRL) test and the rapid plasma reagin (RPR) test are quite similar and are the rapid screening nontreponemal antigen immunologic tests, while the fluorescent treponemal antibody-absorption (FTA-ABS) test and the newer and easier Treponema pallidum hemagglutination (TPHA) test are specifically used to verify a positive screening test. These tests are accurate in pregnancy. Their false positive and false negative rates appear to be no different in pregnancy[40] despite early suggestions that pregnancy itself may be the cause of false positive nontreponemal tests. Table 11-7 demonstrates the reactivity of the common tests in use today in each stage of syphilis.[53]

False positives in the screening tests are a significant problem. Their incidence is directly related to the prevalence of syphilis in the population; the lower the risk of syphilis, the higher the rate of false positives. The box on p. 217 lists the usual causes of false positive VDRL results. Women who have persistent unexplained

Biologic false positive reactions*

FALSE POSITIVE REACTIONS ARE TRANSIENT AFTER

Immunizations and vaccinations
Atypical pneumonia
Other bacterial and viral infections

FALSE POSITIVE REACTIONS ARE CHRONIC WITH

Systemic lupus erythematosus
Thyroiditis
Other autoimmune disorders
Narcotic addiction
Lymphoma
Leprosy
Elderly people

*Usually low titer range (1:1 to 1:4), usually positive VDRL, negative FTA-ABS.

TABLE 11-7 ■ Summary of reactivity of TPHA, FTA-ABS, and VDRL tests in syphilis*

Condition	Approximate % reactive†		
	TPHA	FTA-ABS	VDRL
Primary syphilis	75-80 (59-94)	85-88 (80-100)	50-70 (48-96)
Secondary syphilis	99 (90-99)	99-100	98-100
Late syphilis	96 (90-99)	97 (96-100)	98-100 (55-95)
Normal patients	0.9 (0-3.0)	0.5 (0-1.3)	1.0 (0.5-10.0)
Biologic false positive	1.5 (0-11)	1.5 (0-16)	‡

Adapted from Ravel R: Lab Med 1976;7(5):22.
*Tabulated from 10 independent studies.
†Numbers not in parentheses represent ranges most commonly reported. Numbers in parentheses refer to maximum ranges of values found in the literature.
‡From 20% to 40% of reactive VDRL results are reported to be false positive reactions.

false positive VDRL results are at high risk (>25% chance) for later development of connective tissue disease.

Latent (asymptomatic) and late syphilis need evaluation to rule out neurosyphilis and the need for longer treatment. Spinal puncture is an important step for all patients in this category.

A recent study demonstrates that 20% of pregnant patients with latent syphilis will have positive spinal fluid findings (ie, aysmptomatic neurosyphilis) and will need much closer follow-up to effect a cure.[31] Diagnostic and therapeutic recommendations are outlined in Tables 11-8 and 11-9.

TABLE 11-8 ■ Management of early (primary and secondary) syphilis in pregnancy

Clinical setting	Laboratory confirmation	Treatment	Follow-up
Moist lesion 1. Chancre or ulcer (genital, perioral, perianal) 2. Condyloma latum 3. Mucous patches	Positive darkfield examination (repeated in 24 hours if negative initially)	Benzathine penicillin G, 2.4 × 10⁶ units, IM, repeated in 1 week for a total of 4.8 million units	Monthly quantitative VDRL tests until delivery, then at 3, 6, 12, and 24 months
One of three suspicious lesions: 1. Maculopapular or papulosquamous rash 2. Patchy alopecia 3. Generalized lymphadenopathy History of sexual contact in last 3 months with partner with known or probable syphilis Documented positive VDRL result within last year	Positive VDRL and FTA-ABS results or equivalent (eg, TPHA)		

TABLE 11-9 ■ Management of latent syphilis and asymptomatic neurosyphilis in pregnancy

Clinical setting	Laboratory confirmation	Treatment	Follow-up
Positive VDRL and either of the following: 1. Asymptomatic with undetermined length of positive VDRL results 2. Suspicious history or examination compatible with a complication of syphilis	Positive quantitative VDRL and FTA-ABS results or equivalent (eg, TPHA) and spinal fluid quantitative VDRL test (all patients with latent syphilis in pregnancy should have lumbar puncture)	If VDRL test of cerebrospinal fluid is negative: Give Benzathine penicillin G 2.4 × 10⁶ units every week for 3 weeks	Monthly quantitative VDRL test until delivery, then at 3, 6, 12, and 24 months
		If VDRL test of cerebrospinal fluid is positive: Admit to hospital, give aqueous crystalline penicillin G, 2 to 4 million units every 4 hours for 8 to 10 days	Same as above plus quantitative cerebrospinal fluid test every 3 months

Management of the penicillin-sensitive patient

The penicillin-sensitive gravida poses a major dilemma in intrauterine therapeutics. Maternal and fetal toxicities, poor placental transmission, and low fetal tissue penetration cause many otherwise satisfactory treatment alternatives to be undesirable in pregnancy. At present there is *no* drug that can be recommended with experience.[68] As a result, skin testing is imperative to document serious allergy, and desensitization should also be considered. Table 11-10 discusses the possible options for a gravida with a documented allergy to penicillin. Any infant born to

TABLE 11-10 ■ Treatment alternatives for penicillin-sensitive patients during pregnancy*

There is *no satisfactory alternative* at this time. Every effort should be made to *document penicillin allergy* with *skin testing*, as more than 80% of persons who give a history of penicillin allergy can tolerate additional doses of the drug. Furthermore, desensitization should be considered in selected cases.

Medication	Comments
Erythromycin base (500 mg qid × 15 days)	The drug with the *most experience*. *Compliance* is a problem with this regimen. Lower maternal cure rate than with penicillin. Variable and often *quite low fetal levels* of the drug probably explain the many reports of *failure to cure fetal disease*. Erythromycin estolate should not be used, as it is associated with an estimated 10% incidence of *hepatotoxicity* in pregnancy. Overall, erythromycin is a *suboptimal choice*.
Deoxycycline (100 mg bid × 12 days)	Tetracyclines, in general, are quite effective at destroying treponemes and penetrate fetal tissue satisfactorily. The *risks* of deoxycycline in pregnancy are *much lower than those of tetracycline* (hepatotoxicity, drug absorption by fetal bones, and teeth with resultant defects). The drug has promise, but at present there is *minimal experience* in pregnancy.
Cephalosporins	Relatively *safe* drugs in the presence of penicillin allergy (provided no immediate sensitivity). In general, adequate fetal levels with *parenteral* administration, which would require a 2 week hospitalization. *Experience is quite limited*, and most of the published reports use cephaloridine, which is rarely used today because of its potential renal toxicity.
Cefoxitin/Cefamandole/third-generation cephalosporins	These new drugs may be useful agents in the future. Little data on their use in pregnancy are available, and there are *no reported data* on their use for syphilis during pregnancy.

*Before undertaking *any* of these treatment alternatives, it would be useful to contact the CDC in Atlanta, Georgia, to obtain their latest data and opinions on this very difficult choice.

Serologic response to antisyphilitic treatment

FTA-ABS TEST

Remains positive ≥2 years following treatment in 95% of patients with early syphilis

QUANTITATIVE VDRL TEST

Primary syphilis (seropositive)
Progressive decline in titer
Negative serologic results
in 3 to 12 months—75%
in ≥24 months—97%

Secondary syphilis
Progressive decline in titer
Negative serologic results
in 3 to 12 months—40%
in ≥24 months—75%

Latent syphilis
Expect progressive decline, but a high number of patients will maintain low titers

Fixed low titers
Do not need further evaluation (after following for 1 to 2 years).

Suspect treatment failure
Lack of two-dilution decline in titer 2 months after treatment
VDRL result fails to become negative or does not reach a fixed low titer in 1 year
Rise in titer (two dilutions)

TABLE 11-11 ■ Intrauterine infections

Disease	Maternal disease	Susceptibility	Infant findings	Prevention and/or treatment
Toxo-plasmosis (*Toxoplasma gondii*)	6 out of 1000 pregnancies; majority asymptomatic; occasionally mononucleosis-like illness	All trimesters; prognosis worst with first and second trimester infection	2 out of 1000 births; 70% asymptomatic at birth but later problems; 30% with chorioretinitis, seizures, microcephaly or hydrocephaly, systemic symptoms, growth retardation	Avoid cats, sandboxes and uncooked meats; perform broad maternal and/or neonatal serologic screening; give pyrimethamine (Daraprim) and triple sulfa drugs
Congenital rubella (virus)	1 to 2 out of 1000 pregnancies; one third asymptomatic; two thirds with malaise, adenopathy, arthralgia, conjunctivitis, rash	First trimester worst; can cause problems with infection up to sixth month	Sequelae in one third of maternal infections; congenital heart disease, cataracts, glaucoma, deafness, microcephaly, systemic symptoms	Immunize before pregnancy; recommend abortion in laboratory-documented cases; isolate infected newborns; give gamma globulin in selected cases
Cytomegalovirus disease (virus)	4% to 5% of pregnant women carry virus; majority asymptomatic; rarely, have mononucleosis-like illness	All trimesters	Virus can be cultured from 1% to 2% of all newborns; 90% will be asymptomatic at birth but may have later problems; 9% have only transient thrombocytopenia; 1% have severe symptoms with microcephaly or hydrocephaly, seizures, chorioretinitis, deafness, growth retardation, systemic symptoms	Perform broad maternal serologic screening and abortion in laboratory-documented infections; give cytosine-arabinoside(?), CMV vaccine(?)
Neonatal herpes (virus type 1 or 2)	1% pregnant women carry virus; 43% asymptomatic; 21% nonspecific vaginal discharge; 36% painful genital vesicles	First trimester—54% end in spontaneous abortion; at 32 to 40 weeks—10% of infants infected	One sixth develop vesicular rash only; five sixths develop disseminated disease with encephalitis, chorioretinitis, pneumonitis, systemic symptoms	Perform broad maternal Papanicolaou and culture screening; do cesarean section in selected cases; give cytosine-arabinoside(?), acyclovir(?)
Neonatal syphilis (*Treponema pallidum*)	Asymptomatic or chancre or rash	All trimesters, but virtually 100% cure if treated before 16 weeks	Usually none at birth; lacrimation, snuffles, osteochondritis at 2 to 4 weeks; late sequelae: saddle nose, Hutchinson's teeth, deafness, saber shins, Clutton's joints	Perform broad maternal serologic screening; give penicillin

a mother who receives one of these alternatives is suspect and should be treated with a full course of penicllin neonatally.

Serologic follow-up

Serologic follow-up of treatment is important to identify therapeutic success and reinfection. Most commonly, the FTA-ABS test result remains positive for the lifetime of the patient, while reaction to the VDRL test progressively declines and becomes negative. If the disease has already entered the latent phase before treatment, a large percentage of patients may never attain a completely negative VDRL result; these patients are called *sero-fast*. The box on p. 219 discusses the serologic responses to treatment.

Table 11-11 is a summary of important facts concerning the intrauterine infections of toxoplasmosis, rubella, cytomegalovirus disease, herpes, and syphilis.

■ URINARY TRACT INFECTIONS

In addition to the congenitally transmitted diseases, the obstetrician is concerned about bacterial infections during pregnancy. Of all bacterial infections, those of the kidney and lower urinary tract are most common.

Pyelonephritis is the most common serious antepartum infection encountered in obstetrics. Another infection, asymptomatic bacteriuria, can be detected and treated, and such treatment significantly reduces the incidence of pyelonephritis. Several factors predispose pregnant women to the development of kidney infections: hormonal action (presumably progesterone with its smooth muscle relaxant effects), decreased ureteral tone, decreased peristalsis, and pressure of the enlarging uterus on the ureters at the pelvic brim.

Asymptomatic bacteriuria

By definition, asymptomatic bacteriuria implies the presence of a significant number of virulent organisms in the urine of a patient with no symptoms of urinary tract infection. The number of colonies considered significant is 100,000 or more per milliliter of urine obtained by a clean-voiding technique.

The incidence of asymptomatic bacteriuria ranges from 2% to 3% in upper socioeconomic groups to 7% to 8% in the indigent clinic population. Roughly, only 1% to 2% of women without asymptomatic bacteriuria on initial screening develop a symptomatic urinary tract infection during pregnancy.[72] In contrast, other studies have shown that approximately 25% of all women with asymptomatic bacteriuria will develop an acute infection, often pyelonephritis, if not treated.[32] Treatment with antimicrobials in an attempt to eradicate asymptomatic infections decreases the rate of pyelonephritis to 1% to 3% in these high-risk patients.

The most common offending organism is *Escherichia coli*, isolated in one large study from Dallas[73] in 73% of cases. In this study 24% of the other organisms belonged to the *Klebsiella-Enterobacter* group, and the remaining 3% were *Proteus* species. Group A or B beta hemolytic streptococcus is an occasional urine pathogen in pregnancy, also. Whalley and Cunningham[73] have also shown that short-term antimicrobial therapy for asymptomatic bacteriuria is as effective as continuous antibiotic therapy. Follow-up cultures obviously need to be obtained.

Symptomatic infections

Cystitis, that is, inflammation of the bladder, generally involves dysuria, frequency, urgency, hesitancy, and sometimes incontinence. It may be accompanied by headache, low grade fever, and other signs of systemic infection. Urinalysis usually demonstrates white blood cells and bacteria and occasionally red blood cells.

Pyelonephritis implies involvement of the renal pelves, calyces, and parenchyma resulting from a bacterial infection. Symptoms usually include a prodromal history of lower urinary tract infection followed by fever, chills, and costovertebral angle pain. There may be accompanying anorexia, nausea, and vomiting. Urinalysis findings include white blood cells, frequently in clumps; white blood cell casts; and bacteria. An immunofluorescence test to evaluate the presence of antibody-coated bacteria can further substantiate renal involvement.[67] Although most patients respond readily to treatment, with 85% becoming afebrile within 48 hours of treatment,[9] others can develop septicemic shock and, in rare cases, may die.

Effects on fetal well-being

Many contradictory reports about the effects of maternal urinary tract infections on the fetus have been published during the past 20 years. Analysis by Naeye[47] of the 53,000 participants in the Collaborative Perinatal Project revealed that the incidence of premature delivery was significantly higher in bacteriuric women than in those without urinary tract infection. Furthermore, the combined perinatal mortality of eight common placental and fetal disorders was significantly higher in infected versus noninfected mothers. All deaths took place when the urinary tract infections occurred within 15 days of delivery. Death rates were highest when urinary tract infections coexisted with maternal hypertension and acetonuria. Only one disorder, placental growth retardation, was significantly increased in the bacteriuric gestations. Most of the increase in mortality resulted from disorders whose frequencies were not significantly increased. Thus the urinary tract infections seem to make already compromised infants more vulnerable.

Sever et al[59] analyzed data from the same collaborative study with respect to symptomatic urinary tract infections and pediatric findings. The associations with urinary tract infections included low birth weight, stillbirth, Rh incompatibility, eye infections, and poor motor performance at 8 months. A number of these are obviously not cause and effect related but represent coexistent disease in high-risk subgroups.

A number of studies have been carried out to determine if asymptomatic bacteriuria is associated with poor neonatal outcome or prematurity. The results from these studies are conflicting and almost equally divided between those showing association between urinary tract infections and prematurity and toxemia and those finding no significant association. One study[26] used fluorescent antibody techniques to evaluate 70 women with asymptomatic bacteriuria. Antibody-coated bacteria were found in 50% of these women, suggesting a renal source for the infection. The individuals with renal involvement had higher serum creatinine levels and lower creatinine clearances than the group without evidence of kidney infection. Furthermore, there was an increased incidence of intrauterine growth retardation among the offspring of the women with renal infections despite therapy. Another study[20] contradicts these findings.

Management
Asymptomatic bacteriuria and cystitis
1. All patients should be screened for bacteriuria on their first prenatal visit.
2. Treatment of initial infections includes a sulfonamide, ampicillin, cephalosporins, or nitrofurantoin. Therapy should be continued for 7 to 10 days. The sulfa drugs may cause worsening of neonatal hyperbilirubinemia in infants of mothers taking the drugs at the time of delivery. They do this by competing with the pigment binding to albumin and possibly by a direct effect on glucuronyl transferase. Since ampicillin is only slightly more expensive than sulfa drugs, it is an excellent choice for nonallergic patients. Cephalosporins reach high concentrations in the urinary tract and should be used when indicated by antibiotic sensitivity testing. Nitrofurantoin is also a good choice for initial therapy; however, it may precipitate hemolysis in G-6-PD–deficient patients. Tetracyclines, in general, should be avoided in pregnancy. They may cause discoloration of decidual teeth in the newborn. In addition, pregnant women with impaired renal function should not be given tetracycline, since hepatotoxic levels of the drug might be reached. Trimethoprim-sulfamethoxazole combination therapy is relatively contraindicated in pregnancy; this combination is teratogenic in rats (mainly causing cleft palate), although no effects have been noted in a limited study of humans during pregnancy.[77]
3. Following therapy, repeat cultures should be obtained to establish that treatment has been adequate. Thereafter follow-up cultures should be obtained at 6-week intervals to diagnose reinfections.

Acute pyelonephritis
1. Patients with acute pyelonephritis need to be admitted to the hospital for intravenous fluid and antibiotic therapy. Although uncommon, pregnant women are more susceptible to endotoxic shock than nonpregnant women. Attention is directed to blood pressure, pulse, temperature, and urine output. Serum creatinine level also must be monitored.
2. A urine culture—generally a clean-voided

specimen is adequate—is obtained before beginning antibiotic therapy. Blood cultures may be obtained depending on the clinical severity of the infection.

3. A large number of antimicrobial agents are available for treatment. Ampicillin is a useful starting drug in a dose of 1 to 2 grams intravenously at 4- to 6-hour intervals. Alternative treatments include aminoglycosides, cephalosporins, carbenicillin, and possibly chloramphenicol. If the condition of a patient already under therapy for acute pyelonephritis clinically worsens, a different medication should be used. If clinical response is not rapid, antimicrobial sensitivity tests available from the initial culture aid in the selection of the right drug.

4. Once the patient's fever subsides, medication by mouth can be used. Therapy should extend for at least 10 days.

5. As with lower urinary tract infections, repeat cultures are necessary to establish that treatment was adequate.

6. Many infectious disease specialists recommend continuous prophylaxis during pregnancy for all individuals who develop pyelonephritis. Prophylaxis may be maintained with nitrofurantoin or ampicillin.

■ GROUP B STREPTOCOCCAL INFECTIONS

Group B streptococcus is a major neonatal pathogen that is transmitted from mother to infant at the time of delivery. Conservative estimates suggest that 12,000 to 15,000 infants develop group B streptococcal sepsis each year.[4] Approximately 50% of these infants die, and of the survivors who had meningeal invasion up to 50% develop neurologic sequelae. Although safe and effective antimicrobial agents are available, they often are unable to arrest the fatal progression of neonatal disease, even when administered early in the course of the illness. Group B streptococcal sepsis, although relatively rare, has been estimated to be at least as frequent as the intrapartum deaths for which elaborate fetal monitoring techniques have been developed.

Description of the organism

Group B streptococcus is a gram-positive organism that most often is beta hemolytic on blood agar plates. Cell wall polysaccharides have been used to classify the organism into five serotypes: Ia, Ib, Ic, II, and III.

Maternal colonization and disease

Multiple studies of pregnant women have revealed vaginal colonization rates that range from 10% to 35%, with the higher rates reported in studies that used selective culture media and multiple culture sites. The frequency of group B streptococcal isolation significantly increases as one proceeds from the cervical os (lowest) to the introitus (highest).[4,42] Specimens from the urethra yield higher isolation rates than those from the rectum or throat.[42]

The distribution of serotypes of group B streptococci isolated from vaginal cultures reveals that approximately one third are types Ia, Ib, or Ic, one third type II, and one third type III. The prevalence of colonization does not appear to vary significantly from trimester to trimester.[3,4] Longitudinal studies show that roughly one third of patients with positive vaginal cultures are chronic carriers, one third are transient carriers, and one third are intermittent or indeterminant carriers.[3,78] Nearly 50% of the male sexual partners of colonized women have urethral colonizations by a similar serotype of group B streptococcus, a fact that suggests venereal transmission.[4]

Neonatal colonization and disease

Up to 65% of infants born to women with positive intrapartum cultures for group B streptococcus will have positive surface cultures for the same serotype.[3] It is estimated that 1 in 100 colonized infants will develop "early onset" invasive disease.[4] These infants develop symptoms within the first 5 days of life and often within the first 48 hours. This early onset disease is often associated with maternal obstetric complications, especially premature onset of labor and prolonged rupture of the membranes. Neonates with early onset disease are extremely ill, and more than 50% die. Although the majority of infants with early onset disease are preterm, term infants may also develop this fatal infection.

By screening with vaginal cultures all women with preterm (<34 weeks) labor or preterm rupture of the membranes and then by screening all infants of colonized women, Pasnick et al[51] were able to identify infants who had a 1 in 20 chance of developing early onset disease.

Nosocomial acquisition of group B streptococcus by infants with initially negative cultures has been reported in up to 40% of infants recultured after a 48-hour stay in the nursery.[4] The distributions of serotypes isolated from infants at birth, at 48 hours of age, and at 4 to 8 weeks of age are virtually identical, suggesting that all five serotypes persist on mucous membranes.[4]

In contrast to the early onset or septicemic type of disease, the late onset or meningitic type of infection occurs in infants after 1 week of life (generally 10 days to 4 months). Maternal obstetric complications are infrequently associated with the late onset disease. The infants are usually less severely ill at diagnosis, and the overall mortality is around 20%. However, up to 50% of the infants with meningeal disease develop neurologic sequelae.[29]

The overwhelming majority (>90%) of cases of late onset disease in infants can be attributed to type III organisms.[4] This is in contrast to the 35% to 40% incidence rate for type III streptococcus in asymptomatic mothers and infants. A factor of significance, at least with type III disease, is maternal antibody status. Mothers of infants with invasive type III disease were all antibody deficient, in contrast to a group of women colonized with type III organisms who delivered healthy infants.[22] Multiple preliminary studies are in process in an attempt to develop a vaccine to induce maternal immunity.

Management

Despite considerable research and clinical interest, the optimal approach to prevent group B streptococcal infection remains ill defined. Treatment of mothers and their sexual partners before term does not reduce colonization rates at the time of labor.[18,44] However, treatment of colonized mothers and their partners with oral penicillin beginning at 38 weeks of gestation and extending to delivery[79] or treatment of colonized women (documented by prior vaginal culture) with intravenous ampicillin during labor[79] will significantly decrease both maternal and infant colonization rates. Presumably, by decreasing infant colonization rates the incidence of invasive group B streptococcal disease will also decrease, although this has not been shown.

Although these maternal treatment regimens appear to effectively reduce colonization, rough-ly 200 women should be treated to prevent each case of early onset disease (assuming a transmission rate of 50% from mother to infant and a ratio of invasive disease to colonization of 1: 100 for term infants). Furthermore, since vaginal cultures are not usually obtained remote from term, the preterm infants who experience the highest mortality from the disease are not protected. Also, the long-term consequences of maternal treatment—for example, incidence of penicillin-resistant infection—have not been studied.

An alternative, still controversial, involves treating all newborns with a single intramuscular dose of aqueous penicillin G (50,000 units for infants $\geq$2.0 kg; 25,000 units for infants <2.0 kg) within 1 to 2 hours of birth. This therapy is effective prophylaxis for gonococcal ophthalmia and, as an added benefit, decreases the infant colonization rate of group B streptococcus. In a controlled trial of 18,738 newborns at Southwestern Medical School in Dallas,[60] the incidence of infant colonization was reduced from 50% in control infants born to colonized mothers to 12.2% in penicillin-treated infants. Furthermore, there was a significant decrease in the incidence of diseases caused by penicillin-susceptible organisms in the penicillin-treated group. However, the frequency of diseases caused by penicillin-resistant organisms was significantly increased in the penicillin-treated group in the first, but not the second, year of the study. We do not recommend routine administration of penicillin until the effect of treatment on the incidence of infection caused by penicillin-resistant organisms is further defined.

At present, what measures are reasonable to prevent group B streptococcus infection? Unfortunately, there are still more questions than answers. An area in which no data are available regards preterm labor and rupture of the membranes in a colonized mother, a situation in which 1 out of 20 infants will develop the invasive disease.[51] Should prophylactic drugs be given and delivery postponed? Or should intravenous antibiotic coverage be administered for delivery only? Will either of these regimens increase infections of penicillin-resistant organisms in either the mother or infant? For uncomplicated colonized women at term is it preferable to administer parenteral antibiotics to the mother or the infant, or should antibiotics be limited only to high-risk situations such as prematurity, prolonged rupture of the membranes, and perhaps very heavy maternal vaginal colonization? Some of our suggestions in the management of this problem are as follows:

1. Routine culturing of all women near term is probably not cost efficient.
2. Vaginal cultures in selective media should be obtained at 26 weeks of gestation from all women at high risk of preterm delivery and perhaps women who have had prior infants with neonatal sepsis.
3. All women admitted to the hospital for preterm labor or rupture of the membranes should have vaginal cultures for group B streptococcus as part of their admission evaluation.
4. Individual decisions regarding prophylactic treatment of colonized mothers can be undertaken in consultation with the pediatrician who will care for the preterm infant.

■ CHORIOAMNIONITIS
Diagnosis

Chorioamnionitis is a difficult diagnosis that usually is made by exclusion and confirmed days later by histology or microbiology. Estimates of the incidence of the problem vary tremendously from institution to institution according to the type of definition used. For example, leukocytic infiltration of the chorion and amnion on histologic examination, which is a commonly used criterion for the diagnosis of chorioamnionitis, can be demonstrated in 10% to 20% of all deliveries and is inversely proportional to gestational age, with more than 50% of membranes of infants under 32 weeks of gestation demonstrating inflammation.[12] Likewise, several authors have noted a rapidly rising proportion of histologically inflamed placentas with increases in the length of time of rupture of the membranes.[39] The problem is that, at most, about 1 in 10 of the histologically diagnosed cases will have clinical manifestations either in the mother or child. If a more rigorous criterion, positive amniotic fluid culture, is adopted, the difficulties persist. In fact, bacteria can be cultured from amniotic fluid in a high number of patients with preterm or prolonged rupture of the membranes who never become symptomatic.

The clinical diagnosis of chorioamnionitis is based on a coincidence of nonspecific signs—maternal fever, maternal or fetal tachycardia, uterine tenderness, preterm labor, or foul vaginal discharge. Peripheral leukocytosis is of little help unless the mother is not in labor or the count is above 20,000/mm^3 with a shift to the left. Even studies of the amniotic fluid are imperfect. Most authorities recommend examining a sample obtained by transabdominal amniocentesis or from an intrauterine pressure catheter (discarding the first 10 ml) if the patient is in labor. The presence of white blood cells in the amniotic fluid is a nearly universal finding in chorioamnionitis, but it is hardly diagnostic, since they are commonly present in early labor. The presence of bacteria is more specific, and their quantity is important. Bobitt and Ledger[6] have demonstrated that colony counts greater than 10^3/ml on quantitative amniotic fluid cultures are nearly universally associated with overt amnionitis. In a clinically suspicious situation the presence of white blood cells and bacteria on a centrifuged specimen of sterilely collected amniotic fluid can be considered as confirmation of infection. Absence of white blood cells and bacteria in such a situation suggests that the fever is from another source. Labor complicates the analysis, as both white blood cells and bacteria are frequently found in the amniotic fluid of gravidas in labor who never go on to develop clinical chorioamnionitis or endometritis. In the special situation of preterm rupture of the membranes without labor, where information concerning the presence of chorioamnionitis is critical in the management, the role of stained amniotic fluid specimens is yet to be adequately determined. Quantitative bacterial cultures and gas chromatography analysis appear to have more promise.

Any pregnant patient with fever without apparent cause is suspected to have chorioamnionitis. Membranes need not be ruptured nor labor commenced, although obviously the risks are much higher when these occur. After upper respiratory infection, otitis, urinary tract infection, pneumonia, and phlebitis are eliminated by history and physical examination, amniotic fluid should be examined (Gram's stain) and cultured in attempts to identify bacteria and make the diagnosis. It is important to be certain of the diagnosis, especially in preterm pregnancies, as the cornerstone of therapy is delivery. Although in recent years, with the advances in antimicrobial therapy, the serious sequelae of uncontrolled chorioamnionitis (septic shock, disseminated intravascular coagulation, severe endomyometritis with possible adverse effect on fertility or hysterectomy) are relatively rare, serious infectious morbidity still remains a clear threat to mother and fetus. The most common signs and symptoms of chorioamnionitis are as follows:

Maternal fever

Maternal tachycardia

Fetal tachycardia

Foul cervical discharge

Uterine tenderness

Preterm labor

Labor in a patient with preterm rupture of the membranes being treated with beta adrenergic tocolytic agents

Marked elevation of white blood cells (>5000) with a shift to the left

Multiple bacteria and white blood cells in amniotic fluid smear

Management

If the infant and the placenta are removed expeditiously, maternal morbidity is minimized. Obviously the infant is better off the sooner it is out of the hostile environment. However, the quickest route of intrauterine delivery—cesarean section—carries a very high rate of endometritis (30% to 60%). The two basic decisions the obstetrician must face in cases of chorioamnionitis are (1) how best to effect delivery and (2) when to start antibiotics.

Older literature (up to 5 years ago) recommended delivery as soon as possible. If vaginal delivery could not be obtained in 1 to 6 hours (depending on the study), cesarean section was indicated. Two recent studies[19,35] have reviewed experiences with large indigent populations, presumably those at highest risk for infectious complications. Both noted that maternal infectious morbidity was markedly increased with cesarean delivery, and it was hard to demonstrate any improvement in neonatal outcome with early cesarean section. In fact, 40% to 50% of the patients required abdominal delivery because of dysfunctional labor or fetal distress. Friedman[16] found abnormal labor patterns in 50% of his patients wtih clinical chorioamnionitis. In short, cesarean section should be performed for obstetric indications or if the cervix is very unfavorable in the face of serious maternal infection, but in other cases vaginal delivery is recommended. While it is difficult to demonstrate any critical interval from the time of diagnosis to the time of delivery, there are situations in which primary cesarean section without a trial of labor may be indicated. The patient with a long, closed posterior cervix, especially if she is a primipara, with a gestation several weeks from term, or with desultory responses to an oxytocin challenge may be a candidate for primary cesarean section.

The fetal distress (on the fetal monitor) so often diagnosed in chorioamnionitis may actually represent more fetal stress than hypoxia/acidosis. At Los Angeles County only 1 out of 25 infants whose mothers had chorioamnionitis and whose monitors demonstrated distress had an abnormal fetal scalp sampling (and that was a false positive!).[6] Clearly, close monitoring of the fetus is indicated, as are oxygen and intensive efforts to reduce maternal temperature when necessary.

If delivery is not anticipated in less than 2 hours, antibiotics are indicated. Unlike postpartum endometritis, chorioamnionitis is likely to be caused, at least initially, by a single agent (*Streptococcus*, *Peptostreptococcus*, *E. coli*). To maximize fetal and amniotic fluid levels, antibiotics that easily cross the placenta must be chosen. Ampicillin (1 to 2 grams every 6 hours intravenously via piggyback [IVPB]) is the choice for mild infections (temperature <38.5° C without severe symptoms), and a combination of ampicillin (2 grams every 4 to 6 hours IVPB) and gentamicin (80 mg every 8 hours IVPB) should be used for serious infections. If delivery is imminent (1 to 2 hours), antibiotics may be withheld until cord clamping, unless the mother is severely ill.

If the delivery is via cesarean section, a more complete coverage of anaerobic bacteria is indicated, and clindamycin (600 mg every 6 hours IVPB) may be given in place of or in addition to ampicillin. The extraperitoneal approach to cesarean section or a cesarean hysterectomy are probably not worth their added risks with the availability of modern antibiotics. However, if there is extensive uterine necrosis or invasion by gas-forming bacteria, a cesarean hysterectomy may still be necessary.

A summary of our approach to the treatment of chorioamnionitis is as follows:

1. *All cases*
   Close maternal and fetal monitoring
   Move toward delivery
2. *Mother mildly ill* (temperature <38.5° C)
   Induction of labor
   Cesarean section for obstetric indications, cover with antibiotics after cord is clamped
3. *Mother seriously ill* (temperature >38.5° C)
   Antibiotics if delivery expected in more than 2 hours:
   Ampicillin, 1 to 2 grams every 6 hours IVPB
   Gentamicin, 80 mg every 8 hours IVPB as needed
   Clindamycin, 600 mg every 6 hours IVPB as needed
   Induction of labor
   Cesarean section if delivery expected in more than 6 to 8 hours or for obstetric indications

With today's management, maternal mortality and serious morbidity secondary to chorioamnionitis have been nearly eliminated. Similarly, perinatal mortality has decreased by a factor of 10 (28% to 3%) in the last 15 to 20 years.

■ REFERENCES

1. Amstey MS, Monif GRG, Nahmias AJ, et al: Cesarean section and genital herpes virus infection. Obstet Gynecol 1979;53:641.
2. Andinan WA: Congenital herpes infections. Clin Perinatol 1979;6:331.
3. Anthony BF, Okada DM, Hobel CJ: Epidemiology of group B streptococcus: longitudinal observations during pregnancy. J Infect Dis 1978;137:524.
4. Baker CJ: Summary of the workshop on perinatal infections due to group B streptococcus. J Infect Dis 1977;136:137.
5. Balfour HH: Rubella reimmunization now. Am J Dis Child 1979;133:1231.
6. Bobitt JR, Ledger WJ: Amniotic fluid analysis: its role in maternal and neonatal infection. Obstet Gynecol 1978;51:56.
7. Cheldelin LV, Francis DP, Tilson H: Postpartum rubella vaccination: a survey of private physicians in Oregon. JAMA 1973;225:158.
8. Cherry JD, Soriano F, John CL: Search for perinatal viral infection. Am J Dis Child 1968;116:245.
9. Cunningham FG, Morris GB, Mickal A: Acute pyelonephritis of pregnancy: a clinical review. Obstet Gynecol 1973;42:112.
10. Davis LE, Tweed GV, Steward JA, et al: Cytomegalovirus mononucleosis in a first trimester pregnant female with transmission to the fetus. Pediatrics 1971;48:200.
11. Desmonts G, Couvreur J: Congenital toxoplasmosis: a prospective study of 378 pregnancies. N Engl J Med 1974;290:1110.
12. Driscoll SG: The placenta and membranes, in Charles D, Finland M (eds): *Obstetric and perinatal infections*. Philadelphia, Lea & Febiger, 1973, pp 529-540.
13. Dudgeon JA: Congenital rubella. J Pediatr 1975; 87:1078.
14. Dunkle LM, Schmidt RR, O'Connor DM: Neonatal herpes simplex infection possibly acquired via maternal breast milk. Pediatrics 1979;63:250.
15. Fiumara NJ: Syphilis in newborn children. Clin Obstet Gynecol 1975;18:183.
16. Friedman EA: Obstetric infection in labor, in Charles D, Finland M (eds): *Obstetrics and perinatal infections*. Philadelphia, Lea & Febiger, 1973, pp 501-518.
17. Fulginiti VA, Alexander ER: Rubella in pregnancy: a guide to rational counseling. JAMA 1981;245:1666.
18. Gardner SE, Yow MD, Leeds LJ, et al: Failure of penicillin to eradicate group B streptococcal colonization in the pregnant woman: a couple study. Am J Obstet Gynecol 1979;135:1062.
19. Gibbs RS, Castillo MS, Rodgers PJ: Management of acute chorioamnionitis. Am J Obstet Gynecol 1980; 136:709.
20. Gilstrap LC, Leveno KS, Cunningham FG, et al: Renal infection and pregnancy outcome. Am J Obstet Gynecol 1981;141:709.
21. Grossman JH, Wallen WC, Sever JL: Management of genital herpes simplex virus infection during pregnancy. Obstet Gynecol 1981;58:1.
22. Hall RT, Barnes W, Krishman L, et al: Antibiotic treatment of parturient women colonized with Group B streptococci. Am J Obstet Gynecol 1976;124:630.
23. Hanshaw JB: Cytomegalovirus, in Remington JS, Klein JO (eds): *Infectious diseases of the fetus and newborn infant*. Philadelphia, WB Saunders Co, 1976, pp. 107-155.
24. Hanshaw JB, Scheiner AP, Moxley AW, et al: School failure and deafness after "silent" congenital cytomegalovirus infection. N Engl J Med 1976;295:468.
25. Harris RE, Smith KO, Gehle WD, et al: Rubella immunity: comparison of hemagglutination inhibition and radio immunoassay antibody methods. Obstet Gynecol 1980;55:603.
26. Harris RE, Thomas VL, Shelokov A: Asymptomatic bacteriuria in pregnancy: antibody-coated bacteria, renal function and intrauterine growth retardation. Am J Obstet Gynecol 1975;126:20.
27. Harter CA, Benirschke K: Fetal syphilis in the first trimester. Am J Obstet Gynecol 1976;124:705.
28. Hayes K, Gibas H: Placental cytomegalovirus infection without fetal involvement following primary infection during pregnancy. J Pediatr 1971;79:401.
29. Horn KA, Zimmerman RA, Knostman JD, et al: Neurologic sequelae of group B streptococcal neonatal infections. Pediatrics 1975;53:501.
30. Huang ES, Alfort CA, Reynolds DW, et al: Molecular epidemiology of cytomegalovirus infections in women and their infants. N Engl J Med 1980;303:953.

31. Jones JE, Harris RE: Diagnostic evaluation of syphilis during pregnancy. Obstet Gynecol 1979;54:611.

32. Kaas EH: Bacteriuria and pyelonephritis of pregnancy. Arch Intern Med 1960;105:194.

33. Kibrick S: Herpes simplex infection at term: what to do with mother, newborn and nursery personnel. JAMA 1980;243:157.

34. Kimball AC, Kean BH, Fuchs F: Toxoplasmosis: risk variations in New York City obstetric patients. Am J Obstet Gynecol 1974;119:208.

35. Koh DS, Chan FH, Monfared AH, et al: The changing perinatal and maternal outcome in chorioamnionitis. Obstet Gynecol 1979;53:730.

36. Krugman S: Rubella immunization: progress, problems, and potential solutions, editorial. Am J Pub Health 1979;69:217.

37. Light IJ, Linnemann CC, Jr.: Neonatal herpes simplex infection following delivery by cesarean section. Obstet Gynecol 1974;44:496.

38. Linnemann CC, Jr., Buchman TG, Light IJ, et al: Transmission of herpes-simplex virus type 1 in a nursery for the newborn: identification of viral isolates by DNA "fingerprinting." Lancet 1978;1:964.

39. Mandsley RF, Brix GA, Hinton NA, et al: Placental inflammation and infection: a prospective bacteriologic and histologic study. Am J Obstet Gynecol 1966;95:648.

40. Manikowska-Lesinska W, Linda B, Zajac W: Specificity of the FTA-ABS and TPHA tests during pregnancy. Br J Vener Dis 1978;54:295.

41. McCubbin JH, Smith JS: Rubella in a practicing obstetrician: a preventable problem. Am J Obstet Gynecol 1980;136:1087.

42. McDonald SW, Manuel FR, Embil JA: Localization of group B beta-hemolytic streptococci in the female urogenital tract. Am J Obstet Gynecol 1979;133:57.

43. McLaughlin MC, Gold LH: The New York rubella incident: a case for changing hospital policy regarding rubella testing and immunization. Am J Public Health 1979;69:287.

44. Merenstein GB, Todd WA, Brown G, et al: Group B®-hemolytic streptococcus: randomized controlled treatment study at term. Obstet Gynecol 1980;55:315.

45. Modlin JF, Herrman K, Brandling AD, et al: Risk of congenital abnormality after inadvertent rubella vaccination of pregnant women. N Engl J Med 1976;294:972.

46. Monif GRG, Egan EA, Held B, et al: The correlation of maternal cytomegalovirus infection at varying stages in gestation with neonatal involvement. J Pediatr 1972;80:17.

47. Naeye RL: Causes of the excessive rates of perinatal mortality and prematurity in pregnancies complicated by maternal urinary tract infections. N Engl J Med 1979;300:319.

48. Nahamias AJ, Josey WE, Naib ZM, et al: Perinatal risk associated wtih maternal genital herpes simplex infection. Am J Obstet Gynecol 1971;110:825.

49. Nahamias AJ, Visintine AM: Herpes simplex, in Remington JS, Kline JO (eds): *Infectious diseases of the fetus and newborn infant*. Philadelphia, WB Saunders Co, 1976, pp. 156-190.

50. Ng ABP, Reagan JW, Yen SSC: Herpes genitalis. Obstet Gynecol 1970;36:645.

51. Pasnick M, Mead PB, Philip AGG: Selective maternal culturing to identify group B streptococcal infection. Am J Obstet Gynecol 1980;138:480.

52. Preblund SR, Stetler HC, Frand JA, et al: Fetal risk associated with rubella vaccine. JAMA 1981;246:1413.

53. Ravel R: Hemagglutination tests for syphilis (MHA) as alternative to the FTA-ABS. Lab Med 1976;7(5):22.

54. Remington JS, Desmonts G: Toxoplasmosis, in Remington JS, Klein JO (eds): *Infectious diseases of the fetus and newborn infant*. Philadelphia, WB Saunders Co, 1976, pp. 191-332.

55. Reynolds DW, Stagno S, Hosty TS, et al: Maternal cytomegalovirus excretion and perinatal infection. N Engl J Med 1973;289:1.

56. Saxon SA, Knight W, Reynolds DW, et al: Intellectual deficits in children born with subclinical congenital toxoplasmosis: a preliminary report. J Pediatr 1973;82:792.

57. Schreiner RL, Kleimar MB, Greshan EL: Maternal oral herpes: isolation policy. Pediatrics 1979;63:247.

58. Sever JL: Pattern of development of rubella antibody levels. Clin Perinatol 1979;6:347.

59. Sever JL, Ellenberg JH, Edmonds D: Urinary tract infections during pregnancy: maternal and pediatric findings, in Kass EH, Brumfitt W (eds): *Infections of the urinary tract*. Chicago, University of Chicago Press, 1979, pp. 19-21.

60. Siegel JD, McCracken GH, Threlkeld N, et al: Single-dose penicillin prophylaxis against neonatal Group B streptococcal infections. N Engl J Med 1980;303:769.

61. South MA, Rawls WE: Treatment of neonatal herpes virus infection. J Pediatr 1970;76:497.

62. Stagno S, Reynolds DW, Huang ES, et al: Congenital cytomegalovirus infection: occurrence in an immune population. N Engl J Med 1977;296:1254.

63. Stagno S, Reynolds DW, Pass RF, et al: Breast milk and the risk of cytomegalovirus infection. N Engl J Med 1980;302:1073.

64. Stern H, Tucker SM: Prospective study of cytomegalovirus infection in pregnancy. Br Med J 1973;2:268.

65. Tejani M, Klein SW, Kaplan M: Subclinical herpes simplex genitalis infections during the perinatal period. Am J Obstet Gynecol 1979;135:547.

66. Teutsh SM, Sulzer AJ, Ramsey JE, et al: *Toxoplasmosis gondii* isolated from amniotic fluid. Obstet Gynecol 1980;55:2S.

67. Thomas V, Harris RE, Gilstrap LC, et al: Antibody-coated bacteria in the urine of obstetrical patients with acute pyelonephritis. J Infect Dis 1975;131:S57.

68. Thompson SE: Treatment of syphilis in pregnancy. J Am Vener Dis Assoc 1976;3:159.

69. Ueda K, Nishida Y, Oshima K, et al: Congenital rubella syndrome: correlation of gestational age at time of maternal rubella with type of defect. J Pediatr 1979;94:763.

70. Visintine AM, Nahamias AJ, Josey WE: Genital herpes. Perinatal Care 1978;2:32.

71. Von Herzen JL, Benirschke K: Unexpected disseminated herpes simplex infection in a newborn. Obstet Gynecol 1977;50:728.

72. Whalley PJ: Bacteriuria of pregnancy. Am J Obstet Gynecol 1967;97:723.

73. Whalley PJ, Cunningham FG: Short-term versus continuous antimicrobial therapy for asymptomatic bacteriuria in pregnancy. Obstet Gynecol 1977;49:262.
74. Wilson CB, Desmonts G, Couvreur J, et al: Lymphocyte transformation in the diagnosis of congenital toxoplasma infection. N Engl J Med 1980;302:785.
75. Wilson CB, Remington JS: What can be done to prevent congenital toxoplasmosis? Am J Obstet Gynecol 1980;138:357.
76. Wilson CB, Stagno S, Remington JS: Follow-up of children with subclinical toxoplasmosis. Pediatr Res 1979;13:471.
77. Wormser GP, Keusch GT: Trimethoprim-sulfamethoxazole in the United States. Ann Intern Med 1979;91:420.
78. Yow MD, Leeds LJ, Thompson PK, et al: The natural history of group B streptococcal colonization in the pregnant woman and her offspring. I. Colonization studies. Am J Obstet Gynecol 1980;137:34.
79. Yow MD, Mason Ed, Leeds LJ, et al: Ampicillin prevents intrapartum transmission of group B streptococcus. JAMA 1979;241:1245.
80. Zervoudakis IA, Silverman F, Senterfit LB, et al: Herpes simplex in the amniotic fluid of an unaffected fetus. Obstet Gynecol 1980;55:16S.

12

. . .

HEMATOLOGIC PROBLEMS DURING PREGNANCY

Fernando Arias

Anemia is the most common hematologic abnormality diagnosed during pregnancy. It is most often caused by iron deficiency and occasionally by more complex situations involving deficient production or accelerated destruction of red cells. In the large majority of pregnant patients low hemoglobin or hematocrit values are not diagnostic of anemia; most of these patients are affected by a situation called *hemodilution of pregnancy*. In a demonstration of this phenomenon, Scott and Pritchard[32] measured the hemoglobin concentration of a large group of healthy young women with proven iron stores and normal folate status and found that they had a hemoglobin drop during pregnancy that was more marked during the second trimester. The drop in hemoglobin concentration is a consequence of the expansion of intravascular volume that starts at 8 weeks of gestation and is at its maximum during the second trimester. Since the increase in plasma volume is greater than the increase in red cell volume, the net result is a drop in hemoglobin/hematocrit (H/H) values in spite of the fact that the total number of red cells in circulation is increasing.

Unfortunately, in a large number of pregnant women the diagnosis of anemia is made on the basis of comparisons between H/H values obtained in midgestation and averages from non-pregnant women. This procedure ignores the changes just mentioned in red cell and plasma volumes that cause, as Pritchard[29] has demonstrated, an average drop in hematocrit values during the second trimester of five units for a singleton pregnancy and seven units for twin pregnancies.

Not every drop in H/H values is the result of hemodilution. Real anemia, considered by most authors a hemoglobin concentration below 10 g/dl or a hematocrit value under 30%, occurs frequently during pregnancy.

■ EFFECTS OF ANEMIA ON MOTHER AND FETUS

There is considerable evidence indicating that preeclampsia and eclampsia occur more frequently in patients with iron deficiency[31] and megaloblastic anemias[3,14] than in nonanemic-gravidas. However, the nature of the relation between anemia and preeclampsia-eclampsia has not been clarified. It is possible that preeclampsia interferes with the gastrointestinal absorption of blood-forming elements or causes hepatic or renal disfunction affecting the metabolism of folic acid or the production of erythropoietin.

Another maternal complication that seems to be associated with maternal anemia is abruptio

230

placenta. Studies in this respect, however, are contradictory. Some authors[17,35] have found a high correlation between folic acid and abruptio, whereas many others[15,39] deny that this association exists.

With respect to the fetus, studies have shown that anemia during pregnancy is associated with preterm births,[20] stillbirths, and neonatal deaths.[31] The high incidence of stillbirths and preterm births decreases significantly when iron is given to anemic mothers before they reach 30 weeks of gestation.[23] The mechanism behind the association between fetal problems and maternal anemia remains to be determined.

■ IRON-DEFICIENCY ANEMIA

Almost 80% of all anemias in pregnancy are caused by iron deficiency.[40] The reasons for the predominancy of this etiologic factor are (1) the inadequate iron content of the average American diet and (2) the lack of adequate iron stores in a majority of women during their reproductive years.

The daily iron requirement for an adult is about 2 mg of iron per day. Although the average diet in the United States provides between 5 and 15 mg of elemental iron per day, only about one tenth (0.5 to 1.5 mg) is absorbed in the gastrointestinal tract. This amount of dietary iron is probably enough to compensate for the daily losses plus the monthly menstrual loss of an average female, but it is not adequate for the formation of large iron stores. As a consequence, more than 20% of all women in the United States have no stored iron,[25] and probably twice that number have small stores that become exhausted quickly under the increased demands of pregnancy. The iron requirements of a normal pregnancy have been quantified by the Council on Foods and Nutrition[9] as follows:

To compensate for external iron losses	170 mg
To allow expansion of maternal red cell mass	450 mg
Fetal iron	270 mg
Iron in placenta and cord	90 mg
TOTAL	980 mg

The gastrointestinal absorption of iron increases during the last two trimesters of pregnancy to about 1.0 to 3.0 mg per day. Even if this increased absorption is taken into consideration, the iron content of an unsupplemented diet cannot provide more than one to two thirds of the normal requirements of pregnancy. A pregnant woman must have at least 500 mg of stored iron at the beginning of pregnancy to fulfill the requirements of gestation without the need for iron supplementation. Even if this deposit is present, it will be completely exhausted at the end of gestation. It is also important to notice that demands on maternal iron stores begin early in pregnancy, whereas increased gastrointestinal absorption of iron is only apparent after midgestation.[12]

Pathophysiology and diagnosis

In the body iron is complexed to transferrin (transport form), ferritin (storage form), or heme (such as in hemoglobin, myoglobin, or iron-containing enzymes). The iron necessary for the synthesis of hemoglobin is carried as transferrin. If the molecules of transferrin are less than 15% saturated with iron, production of red cells by the bone marrow will decrease, and the red cells produced under these conditions will be small (microcytosis) and will contain a reduced amount of pigment (hypochromic). Iron-deficiency anemia can be divided in three stages: (1) depletion of iron stores, (2) deficient erythropoiesis, and (3) frank iron-deficiency anemia.

Depletion of iron stores without overt signs of iron-deficiency anemia usually occurs during the first trimester of pregnancy. It can be detected by looking at the iron content of the bone marrow or by measuring the amount of plasma ferritin that is in equilibrium with the iron stored in the bone marrow. The first of these methods is invasive, and its routine use is unjustified. Conversely, determination of serum ferritin is becoming an increasingly popular means of evaluating the status of the iron stores in nonpregnant individuals. Each molecule of ferritin is a sphere of protein that may contain up to 4500 atoms of iron, although it usually contains less than the maximum. Serum ferritin is measured by radioimmunoassay, and the values reported by different laboratories tend to vary because ferritin from different sources is used to prepare the antibody used in the assay. The normal range of values of serum ferritin for females is 100 ± 60 ng/ml, and any value under 20 ng/ml is indicative of deficient iron stores. Routine evaluation of the iron stores in pregnant women using serum ferritin determinations is not recommended. In fact, the cost of iron supplementation for all pregnant women on the assumption that they have decreased iron stores is probably less than the cost of screening all of them with serum ferritin determinations.

The state of iron-deficient hematopoiesis without overt signs of iron-deficiency anemia can be diagnosed by measuring the serum transferrin iron-binding capacity and the serum iron concentration and calculating the percentage of transferrin that is saturated with iron. Another useful test for the same purpose is to measure the red blood cells' protoporphyrin concentration. The serum transferrin binding capacity (normal value 330 ± 30 μg/dl) increases progressively with the severity of the iron-deficiency state, whereas the serum iron concentration (normal value 115 ± 50 μg/dl) decreases. The result of these divergent changes is a decrease in transferrin saturation by iron (normally 35% to 50%) to under 15%. Simultaneously, since there is not enough iron to convert all the protoporphyrin to hemoglobin, the normal concentration of protoporphyrin (30 μg/100 ml of red cells) increases two to three times. All these changes precede the occurrence of gross morphologic changes in the red cells and happen before a significant drop in H/H values is apparent.

The final stage in the evolution of the process of iron deficiency is reached when clear signs of iron-deficiency anemia are present. At this stage the most important elements in the diagnosis are the blood smear and the red cell indexes: mean corpuscular volume (MCV), mean corpuscular hemoglobin (MCH), and mean corpuscular hemoglobin concentration (MCHC). Iron-deficiency anemia is characteristically microcytic and hypochromic. The blood smear in patients with iron-deficiency anemia shows abundant, small, well-rounded erythrocytes with characteristic pale centers. The MCV, MCH, and MCHC are below normal limits. Also, the serum transferrin iron-binding capacity, the serum iron concentration, and the red cell protoporphyrin concentration shows changes similar to those described before in relation to the stage of iron-deficiency hematopoiesis. However, most of these latter tests are unnecessary for the diagnosis of iron-deficiency anemia. Anemia is a late manifestation of iron deficiency, and when it is present, the situation

can be diagnosed easily without the need for complex and expensive laboratory determinations. Normal red cell values in the female are as follows:

Red blood cells	$4.8 \pm 0.6 \times 10^6$
Hemoglobin level	14.0 ± 2 g/dl
Hematocrit value	42.0 ± 5%
MCV	$90 \pm 9 \ \mu m^3$
MCH	29 ± 2 pg
MCHC	35 ± 2 g/100 ml
Reticulocyte count	0.5% to 1.5%

Prevention

Every pregnant woman needs iron supplementation during pregnancy. Iron supplements should be started as early as possible, usually when the patient is seen for her first prenatal visit. If the patient is affected by nausea and vomiting during the early part of her pregnancy, the administration of iron should be postponed until the gastrointestinal disturbances disappear in the second trimester. Multiple forms of iron, varying in their content of elemental iron, are available for supplementation during pregnancy. These different types of iron supplements include the following:

	Iron molecule content (mg)	Elemental iron content (mg)
Ferrous sulfate	300	60
Ferrous gluconate	320	36
Ferrous fumarate	200	67

A pregnant woman needs only one tablet of iron per day for prophylaxis of iron-deficiency anemia. In fact, one tablet of any of the different forms of iron shown in the material just listed provides enough iron to fulfill the needs of pregnancy as long as it is taken daily for at least the last two trimesters and, very important, provided that the patient is not already anemic. To give more than one tablet of iron per day for prophylaxis is a waste, since the excess iron is not absorbed and frequently causes gastrointestinal side effects.

Treatment

Oral iron therapy. If the patient is already anemic, the physician has a choice between oral and parenteral iron therapy. In most cases oral administration of one 300 mg tablet of iron sulfate three times daily after meals suffices. This dosage provides 180 mg per day of elemental iron of which 15 to 25 mg per day are absorbed. The patient's response to this dosage is fast, and a significant increase in reticulocyte count is observable 5 to 10 days after initiation of oral therapy. Hemoglobin rises from 0.3 to 1.0 gram per week, and this is reflected in a significant elevation in H/H values 2 to 3 weeks after initiation of treatment.

A prevalent problem associated with oral iron therapy is gastrointestinal intolerance that is experienced by about 10% of the patients undergoing treatment. The most common symptoms are nausea, vomiting, and diarrhea. Since the gastrointestinal side effects are dose-related, the treatment of choice is to reduce the doses to a tolerable level. Another useful maneuver is to give the iron pill with rather than after meals. Although this decreases the amount of iron that is absorbed and prolongs the time necessary to achieve normalization of the hematologic indexes, it is frequently the only way to continue the treatment. Gastrointestinal toxicity depends on how much ionic iron, the absorbable form of iron, gets in contact with the gastrointestinal mucosa. Thus iron preparations that produce fewer side effects deliver less iron available for absorption. It is cheaper to reduce the dose of the preparation that is causing gastrointestinal effects than to ask the patient to buy something else containing a lesser amount of an absorbable form of iron.

Parenteral iron therapy. Parenteral iron therapy is used with patients who (1) come to the obstetrician with severe iron-deficiency anemia (hemoglobin less than 8 g/dl) a few weeks before their expected date of delivery and require a rapid normalization of their hematologic indexes, (2) are noncompliant with oral therapy, and (3) develop marked gastrointestinal side effects with oral iron. Parenteral iron therapy is hazardous and expensive when compared with oral administration. Up to 2% of patients receiving parenteral iron may develop severe systemic reactions (hemolysis, hypotension, circulatory collapse, vomiting, muscle pain, and anaphylactic shock). Other patients suffer delayed reactions characterized by pyrexia, myalgias, and arthralgias. Parenteral iron may also cause dark staining of the skin and inflammation at the site of application. The frequency of side effects with parenteral iron therapy is such that the manufacturer recently recommended not to exceed 2 ml in a 24-hour period.

Before giving parenteral iron it is necessary to calculate the patient's iron deficit. Among the several formulas available for this purpose the following is useful:

Weight in pounds $\times$ 0.3 $\times$ 100 $-$ Hb% = Milligrams of iron needed

For this calculation 100% hemoglobin is equal to 14.2 g/dl. For example, the iron required by a pregnant woman with a hemoglobin concentration of 7.1 g/dl and a weight of 140 pounds (63 kg) is:

$$140 \times 0.3 \times 50 = 2100 \text{ mg}$$

Another formula, simpler and easier to remember, is to give 250 mg of elemental iron for each gram of hemoglobin below normal. In the hypothetical case just mentioned the calculation is:

$$250 \text{ mg} \times 7.1 \text{ g} = 1775 \text{ mg}$$

The iron dextrin for administration IV or IM comes as a solution containing 50 mg of elemental iron per milliliter. Since the maximal recommended dose of intramuscular iron is 2 ml per day, several injections may be necessary to correct the calculated deficiency.

Some authors[36] suggest diluting the iron dextrin in normal saline solution (1.5 g/1000 ml), administering initially at a rate of 1 ml/30 minutes, and if no side effects are apparent, continuing at a rate of 150 ml per hour. A syringe with epinephrine must be at hand as well as an ampule of a preparation of glucocorticoid suitable for administration IV. The incidence of phlebitis at the site of administration increases with the use of diluted iron solutions. Because of the multiple problems associated with parenteral iron administration, we do not recommend its use for the treatment of iron-deficiency anemia in pregnant patients.

■ MEGALOBLASTIC ANEMIA
Incidence and pathophysiology

Only 3 or 4 of every 100 women with anemia during pregnancy have megaloblastic anemia.[6,16] In the overwhelming majority of cases megaloblastic anemia is the result of a folic acid deficiency, and in only 1 out of every 8500 pregnant women anemia is caused by vitamin B_{12} deficiency.[22] The reason for the low incidence of megaloblastic anemia during pregnancy is the abundance of both folic acid and vitamin B_{12} in the American diet. Folate is present in fruits, green vegetables, and meats; vitamin B_{12} is found in meat, fish, poultry, and dairy products.

Folic acid deficiency may appear as a consequence of decreased ingestion, poor absorption, or increased use; examples of all three mechanisms may occur during pregnancy. The overwhelming reason is, however, inadequate ingestion. The reason is not a lack of available folate in the diet but the water-soluble characteristic of the vitamin that makes its content in the diet vulnerable to the cooking habits of the patient. In fact, prolonged cooking destroys the vitamin, and this habit combined with a lack of raw food in the diet are conditions that eventually lead to the production of megaloblastic anemia.

Poor absorption of folate in spite of adequate ingestion occurs rarely, usually in situations in which ingested folic acid polyglutamates cannot be degraded to absorbable monoglutamates because of the presence in the diet of an inhibitor of the enzyme responsible for this degradation (gluten-induced enteropathy) or because of the presence of an acid intestinal pH. Decreased use of folate is seen in about 60% of the patients with vitamin B_{12} deficiency.

Theoretically, vitamin B_{12} deficiency may occur like folic acid deficiency because of inadequate ingestion, poor absorption, or increased use. In practice, however, vitamin B_{12} deficiency means poor absorption, and perhaps the only situation in which inadequate ingestion may be suspected is in the case of strict vegetarians who do not ingest animal products of any kind.

Poor vitamin B_{12} absorption may occur because of a gastric defect resulting in inadequate secretion of intrinsic factor (pernicious anemia), an ileal defect causing poor absorption in the presence of adequate amounts of intrinsic factor, or finally, a pancreatic defect causing inadequate alkalinization of the intestinal content or inadequate removal of nonintrinsic factor binders. Until recently, almost all cases of megaloblastic anemia caused by vitamin B_{12} deficiency found during pregnancy were the consequence of inadequate secretion of intrinsic factor by the stomach. In the last few years, however, defects in ileal absorption have risen in frequency, mainly as a result of the popularization of gastrointestinal surgical procedures in the treatment of patients with morbid obesity.

Both folic acid and vitamin B_{12} deficiencies cause megaloblastic anemia through mechanisms affecting DNA replication. Folic acid is an essential cofactor for one-carbon metabolism, and its deficiency affects particularly the synthesis of thymidine. In the case of vitamin B_{12} deficiency, DNA replication is affected at the same step but by a mechanism that involves a deficiency in the conversion of circulating forms of folate to those involved in thymidine synthesis. As a consequence of the defect in DNA synthesis, more cells are in an unresting state trying to slowly complete the doubling of their DNA, and when examined microscopically, they show more than the normal amount of DNA despite their defect in DNA synthesis. Furthermore, since RNA and protein synthesis are not affected, these cells exhibit a large, mature cytoplasm. These nuclear and cytoplasmic changes are the basic element of megaloblastosis, and they affect not only the erythroid line but also the myelopoiesis with production of the neutrophils with hypersegmented nuclei that are characteristic of megaloblastic degeneration.

The similarities in mechanism of action and morphologic effects on the red and white cells caused by folate and vitamin B_{12} deficiencies and the fact that the anemia caused by the deficiency of one of them can be corrected by administering the other cannot obscure a fundamental difference between the two processes: vitamin B_{12} deficiency causes progressive demyelinization, whereas folate deficiency does not, and improper treatment of a B_{12} anemia with folate does not arrest the progression of the neurologic damage caused by the B_{12} deficiency. This is the reason the differential diagnosis between these two major causes of megaloblastic anemia is important and necessary.

Both folate and vitamin B_{12} deficiencies may mask an iron deficiency. In fact, red cell synthesis is inhibited during the vitamin deficiency, available iron is underused, and increased saturation of transferrin occurs. As soon as therapy with folate or B_{12} is initiated, red cell synthesis starts again, use of iron is maximal, and iron deficiency becomes apparent.

Diagnosis

Usually, the first indication of the presence of megaloblastic anemia in pregnancy is an elevated MCV found in the course of a routine prenatal evaluation of patients who may or may not be markedly anemic. In a few cases the elevated MCV is the result of maternal hypothyroidism, but in a majority of cases this finding is accompanied by the presence of hypersegmented neutrophils, and the diagnosis of megaloblastic anemia is obvious. As mentioned before, folate deficiency is generally the cause of the megaloblastic changes. The astute clinician, however, should obtain serum levels of both folate and vitamin B_{12} and evaluate the red cell folate concentration to avoid missing the rare case of vitamin B_{12} deficiency that someday will appear in his or her practice. Other tests that may be useful in the differential diagnosis between folate and vitamin B_{12} deficiency are the reticulocyte count that usually is normal in B_{12} and elevated in folate deficiencies and the amount of formiminoglutamic acid (FIGLU) eliminated in the urine, which will be high in cases of folate deficiency.

The serum vitamin B_{12} level may be low in cases of folic acid deficiency, and the serum folate may also be low in cases of B_{12} deficiency reflecting the intimal biochemical relation that exists between these two nutrients. A B_{12} serum level less than 100 pg/ml is diagnostic of B_{12} deficiency. A combination of a serum folate less than 3 ng/ml and a red cell folate less than 150 ng/ml is diagnostic of folate deficiency. Red cell folate reflects more appropriately than serum folate the tissue level, has fewer fluctuations in value, and is the test of choice for the diagnosis of folate deficiency.

Therapy. Treatment of folic acid deficiency requires no more than 1 mg per day of folic acid. Any amount in excess of 1 mg per day is unnecessary, since the daily requirements even in the presence of megaloblastic anemia probably do not exceed 100 to 200 μ per day.

Treatment of vitamin B_{12} deficiency requires about 250 μg of parenteral cyanocobalamin every month. The oral preparations of B_{12} have unreliable absorption properties and are inadequate for long-term therapy.

In severely anemic patients, especially if they are close to the date of confinement, exchange transfusion of packed red cells followed by parenteral therapy with folic acid (1 mg per day for 1 week) or cyanocobalamin (100 μg every day for 1 week), depending on the cause, may be necessary.

The reticulocyte count must show an appro-priate response to either folate or cyanocobalamin in 3 to 8 days. An underlying iron deficiency may be detected a few days after initiation of therapy for megaloblastic anemia if an appropriate follow-up is carried out.

■ HEMOLYTIC ANEMIAS

The life of a normal red cell is 120 days, but this life span is shortened in the case of hemolytic anemias because of the premature destruction of red cells. This premature destruction may occur extravascularly (ie, acquired immune hemolytic anemia) or intravascularly (ie, microangiopathic hemolytic anemia of preeclampsia). When hemoglobin is liberated intravascularly, the alpha chains bind to haptoglobin—an alpha 2 globulin—and the hemoglobin-haptoglobin complex is rapidly cleared in the liver. Thus a decrease in plasma haptoglobin is a reliable sign of hemolysis. After the haptoglobin becomes saturated with hemoglobin, free hemoglobin appears in the plasma, and when the amount of hemoglobin in the plasma exceeds the reabsorptive capacity of the tubular cells of the kidney, hemoglobinuria also occurs. The free hemoglobin in the plasma becomes oxidized to methemoglobin, and some of the heme groups of methemoglobin are bound to albumin molecules with formation of methemalbumin. As a compensatory mechanism to red cell destruction, bone marrow erythropoiesis increases markedly, and this is noticeable by an increase in reticulocyte count. Thus a decrease in or absence of haptoglobin; presence of free hemoglobin, methemoglobin, and methemalbumin; and presence of reticulocytosis are the diagnostic hallmarks of intravascular hemolytic anemia. Also, abnormalities in red cell morphology are frequent in this situation.

When red cells are destroyed extravascularly in the reticuloendothelial system, the hemoglobin liberated in the process is converted to bilirubin and an increase in indirect bilirubin is apparent in the patient's serum. The products of bilirubin metabolism (fecal and urinary urobilinogen) also increase. Erythropoiesis markedly increases, and an evident rise in reticulocytes is apparent. Thus elevated unconjugated bilirubin, increased urinary urobilinogen, and reticulocytosis are the hallmarks of extravascular hemolysis. Although classification of the hemolytic anemias with respect to the site of red cell destruction (intravascular or extravascular) is important for an adequate interpretation of the laboratory tests and for differential diagnosis purposes, in many hemolytic processes both sites of destruction are operative, and the laboratory tests reflect that fact.

It is apparent from the previous description of intravascular and extravascular hemolysis that in both cases there is a bone marrow response, characterized by marked erythroid hyperplasia and reticulocytosis. In some cases the erythropoiesis is so active that there is passage of immature red cells into the bloodstream. Also, in all cases of accelerated red cell destruction, plasma lactic dehydrogenase (LDH) increases as a consequence of the liberation of the red cell isoenzyme.

Microangiopathic hemolytic anemia

Microangiopathic hemolytic anemia occurs during pregnancy in some patients with severe forms of preeclampsia-eclampsia. It is also seen in the rare cases of thrombotic thrombocytopenic purpura that occur during gestation. Characteristically, the blood smear shows fragmented red cells, schistocytes, and helmet cells. Thrombocytopenia is always present. Immunofluorescent studies show marked and generalized fibrinogen deposition in the microvasculature, especially in the kidney, liver, and brain. The treatment of this condition is prompt termination of pregnancy. Delivery is followed by progressive improvement in the indicators of hemolysis. This subject is further discussed in Chapter 6.

Acquired immune hemolytic anemia

In cases of acquired immune hemolytic anemia the patient makes antibodies of the IgG type or warm antibodies against red cell antigens causing premature destruction of these cells. The abnormality may occur in association with several diseases (leukemia, lymphomas, viral infections) or as a consequence of an immune reaction to certain drugs (penicillin, sulfas, quinidine), but the most frequent cause of this situation in pregnant women is collagen vascular disease. On a few occasions no cause can be discovered, and the disorder is named *idiopathic acquired immune hemolytic anemia*.

In acquired immune hemolytic anemia IgG antibodies and complement coat the red cells' surface and attach to reticuloendothelial cells that contain receptors for both IgG and complement. When the red cells detach, some membrane fragments remain attached to the reticuloendothelial cells. As a consequence of this loss of membrane fragments, the red cells are transformed into spherocytes and easily destroyed in the spleen.

The diagnosis of acquired immune hemolytic anemia is made with the direct Coombs' test. In this test red cells of the patient are mixed with antihuman globulin antiserum, and since they are coated with IgG and complement, agglutination occurs immediately. Diagnosis of a connective tissue disorder, usually lupus erythematous causing the synthesis of antibodies against red cell antigens, is made with other laboratory tests such as ANA titers and determination of antiDNA antibodies. These tests are negative in the idiopathic variety of immune hemolytic anemia.

Treatment of acquired immune hemolytic anemia consists of drugs known to affect the body immune response. The first choice is glucocorticoids, used in doses equivalent to between 60 and 100 mg of prednisone per day. Glucocorticoids act preferentially by interfering with the recognition by the reticuloendothelial cells of the IgG and complement that cover the red cells' surface and, to a smaller extent, by interfering with the process of antibody synthesis.

In cases of acquired immune hemolytic anemia not responsive to glucocorticoids, the drug of choice is the immunosuppressant azathioprine. Also, in some cases splenectomy may be necessary to arrest the hemolytic process. However, not all patients with acquired immune hemolytic anemia respond to splenectomy, and it is important to determine the degree of splenic entrapment of radioactively tagged red cells before a surgical procedure is carried out.

Some patients with lupus-induced hemolytic anemia during pregnancy may exhibit hemoglobin concentrations under 5 g/dl. Transfusion therapy seems to be clearly indicated in these cases, but most patients quickly hemolyze the transfused red cells. The only hope of finding some compatible blood in these desperate situations is by in vivo crossmatching. For this purpose a small amount of red cells from the potential donor is tagged with ^{51}Cr and given to the patient. If the red cells are hemolyzed, radioactive chromium will be released from the cells and found in the plasma. If no hemolysis occurs, the radioactivity will remain contained in the red cells. In the majority of cases the best thing to do is to wait for the patient's response to glucocorticoids rather than transfusing red cells that quickly become hemolyzed. In some critical patients, however, cells that are quickly destroyed have to be transfused to keep the patient alive until the effect of the immunosuppressant drugs is apparent.

Hemolytic anemias associated with hemoglobinopathies

The abnormalities in hemoglobin synthesis most commonly found in pregnant patients in the United States are (1) sickle cell trait, (2) beta thalassemia minor, and (3) sickle cell disease (SCD).

Sickle cell trait. Sickle cell trait is present in about 10% of the black population of the United States. In spite of claims to the opposite, there is strong evidence[30] that these patients are not at greater risk of abnormal reproductive performance than individuals without the trait. The only problem with these patients is the transmission of the abnormal gene to their descendants. Patients with sickle cell trait should have preconceptional counseling, and the male should be examined to determine if he also carries the trait because in this case there is a 25% chance that an infant with homozygous SCD will be the result of pregnancy. As opposed to patients with SCD, patients with sickle cell trait require iron supplementation during pregnancy.

Beta thalassemia minor. Beta thalassemia minor is second in frequency to sickle cell trait among pregnant women with hemoglobinopathies. This disease is characterized by diminished synthesis of hemoglobin beta chains. These patients have a microcytic, hypochromic anemia with hemoglobin levels that fluctuate between 8 and 10 g/dl. The diagnosis of beta thalassemia minor is frequently missed, and the patients are repeatedly treated with large doses of oral and in some instances parenteral iron without therapeutic response. This is dangerous because they may develop hepatic and cardiac hemosiderosis as a consequence of excessive iron administration. To avoid this problem hemoglobin A_2 and serum iron determinations should be ordered in every pregnant patient with mycrocytic hypochromic anemia who does not respond

to oral iron with an elevation of her reticulocyte count or hemoglobin concentration. Patients with beta thalassemia minor characteristically show a hemoglobin A_2 concentration greater than 3.5% and normal or increased serum iron concentration.

Patients with beta thalassemia minor have a reproductive performance similar to patients with normal hemoglobin. They do not require iron supplementation during pregnancy unless there is laboratory evidence of iron deficiency. If it is necessary to raise their red cell concentration, the only way to do it is by blood transfusions.

Sickle cell disease (SCD). Although sickle cell trait and beta thalassemia minor are seen more often, the most important hemoglobinopathy encountered during pregnancy because of the frequency and severity of the problems exhibited by these patients is SCD. Pregnant patients with SCD are affected by the following problems:

1. *A significant maternal mortality.* Approximately 2% to 7% of women with SCD die during pregnancy. The causes of maternal deaths are multiple, but pulmonary infection, pulmonary infarcts, and pulmonary embolization are predominant.
2. *A high incidence of severe maternal morbidity.* Morbidity is frequent, severe, and prolonged in pregnant patients with SCD. Painful vasoocclusive episodes (sickle cell crisis), infections, cerebrovascular accidents, and preeclampsia-eclampsia are common in these patients.
3. *A high incidence of spontaneous abortion.* Early reproductive failure affects close to 20% of all patients with SCD who become pregnant.
4. *A high incidence of stillbirths and neonatal deaths.* Approximately 14.2% of all pregnancies in patients with SCD end with the delivery of stillborn infants. Neonatal mortality is also high, approximately 84.5 per 1000 live births.[24]
5. *A high incidence of low birth weight.* The incidence of infants with birthweight under 2500 grams in patients with SCD is 37.5%. A large number of these infants are born at term but growth retarded. Intrauterine growth retardation is also present in a large number of the stillborn babies delivered by patients with SCD.

The method generally employed in attempts to decrease the incidence and severity of pregnancy-related problems in patients with SCD is the use of blood transfusions. There are two approaches to the use of transfusion therapy for patients with SCD: in the first, transfusions are used prophylactically; in the second, transfusions are used only when specific indications (sickle cell crisis, infection, erythropoiesis arrest) appear.

The prophylactic administration of red cells containing hemoglobin A_1 has as its objective the prevention of fetal and maternal problems, and indeed there are uncontrolled observations suggesting that transfusions improve the pregnancy outcome. There are two protocols for prophylactic transfusions. In the first protocol[27] the pregnant patient with SCD has one partial exchange transfusion at 28 weeks of gestation with the purpose of obtaining a hematocrit value of 35% and a concentration of hemoglobin A_1 of at least 40%. The procedure is repeated if a crisis occurs, if the hematocrit value drops under 25%, if the hemoglobin A_1 drops under 20%, or when the patient reaches 36 to 38 weeks of gestation. In the second protocol[10] packed red cells are given by partial exchange transfusion or more commonly by simple infusion, starting as soon as the diagnosis of pregnancy is established and then intermittently throughout the rest of the pregnancy. The objective of the transfusions is to keep the hematocrit value above 25% and the circulating red cells that would sickle in sodium metabisulfite solution under 60%.

Proponents of the protocol in which prophylactic exchange transfusions begin at 28 weeks of gestation believe that most of the serious complications in patients with SCD appear in the last trimester of pregnancy, that these complications are prevented by this method, and that the number of transfusions and the total number of units of blood used are less than with the other method. Those who use the protocol with intermittent transfusions beginning early in pregnancy believe that there is nothing magic about 28 weeks of gestation and that it is better to correct the maternal oxygen carrying capacity as early as possible to avoid problems both in middle and late pregnancy.

There is no agreement about the therapeutic value of prophylactic transfusion for pregnant patients with SCD. In fact, the lack of knowledge about the relative importance of several variables with respect to the outcome of pregnancy makes it difficult to decide what variables must be modified to improve the result. In April 1979 the National Institutes of Health had a Consensus Development Conference on transfusion therapy in pregnant patients with SCD and concluded that the risks and benefits of prophylactic transfusions have not been established and that prophylactic transfusions are not ready for routine clinical use. Among the dangers associated with prophylactic transfusion protocols, the most important are (1) the development of hemosiderosis, (2) the development of alloantibodies making it difficult to carry out future transfusions, and (3) the possibility of transmitting infective agents (ie, virus of non-A or non-B hepatitis) with the transfusions.

The second approach to transfusions—to transfuse only when there is a specific indication—is at the present moment the best method to manage SCD in pregnancy. With this approach the hazards associated with prophylactic transfusions are decreased, and important information may be obtained about the natural history of this disease during pregnancy.

Partial exchange transfusions may be carried out by manual methods using phlebotomy followed by infusion, or as recently suggested by Morrison et al,[26] by using automated erythrocytopheresis with a cell separator. This technique allows a fast and rigorously controlled exchange that is valuable for the patient in crisis or congestive heart failure.

Patients with SCD do not require iron supplementation during pregnancy unless laboratory evidence of iron deficiency is obtained. In contrast, they need adequate folic acid supplementation to compensate for the increased consumption of this vitamin during the active process of cell replication that takes place in their bone marrow.

Patients with sickle cell hemoglobin C disease and sickle cell beta thalassemia disease have problems during pregnancy similar to patients with SCD, but the frequency and severity of these problems are substantially less. A similar relatively benign outcome occurs in patients with SCD who have an elevated (greater than 10%) concentration of fetal hemoglobin. In these patients the need for prophylactic transfusions is more questionable than in patients with SCD.

■ APLASTIC ANEMIA

Aplastic anemias occur rarely during pregnancy, and less than 50 cases have been reported in the literature. In most of these cases no association has been found between the anemia and exposure to chemicals, medications, or infections that may have affected the bone marrow. The disease has a serious prognosis, and the maternal mortality is about 30%.[21] However, recent advances in the treatment of aplastic anemias using bone marrow transplantation, androgen, and antithymocyte globulin may improve the maternal outcome.

■ BLEEDING DIATHESIS

Bleeding diathesis different from that occurring in some cases of abruptio placenta, severe preeclampsia, and prolonged fetal death in utero are extremely rare in obstetrics. Idiopathic thrombocytopenic purpura is the most common among these rare conditions, although the average obstetrician probably does not see more than one or two patients with this problem in the course of his or her professional career. Even more rare is to find a pregnant patient with von Willebrand's disease.

Idiopathic thrombocytopenic purpura (ITP)

ITP is a disorder rarely seen during pregnancy and is characterized by an antibody-mediated destruction of maternal platelets. The patients are usually asymptomatic, may complain of easy bruising or bleeding from their nose or mouth, and frequently have petechiae in different parts of their bodies. Laboratory evaluation reveals thrombocytopenia, enlarged platelets, and normal erythrocyte and leukocyte counts. The diagnosis of ITP is made by exclusion after finding no evidence that the thrombocytopenia is secondary to collagen vascular disease, is drug mediated, or is caused by isoantibodies.

When ITP appears during pregnancy, both the mother and the fetus are affected. Maternal problems result not only from the disease but also as a consequence of therapy. Maternal platelet count may reach low levels with the production of gastrointestinal, urinary, or intracranial bleeding. Also, splenectomy, corticosteroid, and immunosuppressant therapy have side effects that may be serious in the mother with ITP. The greatest concern in these cases, however, is with the fetal effects of ITP: perinatal mortality is

close to 20%, and the majority of infant deaths are caused by intracranial bleeding resulting from fetal or neonatal thrombocytopenia. Fetal and neonatal thrombocytopenia in turn are the result of transplacental passage of maternal antiplatelet antibodies that bind to antigenic sites on the surface of the infant's platelets and facilitate their destruction in the spleen. Since the antigenic composition of the infant's platelets is not identical to that of the mother, it is impossible to predict before labor if the baby's platelets have reacted with the maternal antibodies and if fetal thrombocytopenia is present.

A traditional index to predict the fetal platelet count has been the maternal platelet count. The literature shows that if the maternal platelet count in nonsplenectomized mothers is greater than 150,000/mm^3, the possibilities of neonatal thrombocytopenia are almost nil.[5] This makes sense because if the antibodies are incapable of causing significant maternal thrombocytopenia, they should not be producing significant fetal problems. Unfortunately, maternal platelet counts are frequently under 150,000/mm^3, and in these cases the neonatal prognosis cannot be established antepartum. Therefore it is necessary to measure the fetal platelet count in labor when the cervix reaches 2 to 3 cm of dilation. If the fetal platelet count is greater than 50,000/mm^3, the possibilities of neonatal thrombocytopenia and intracranial bleeding are small,[33] and vaginal delivery is permissible. If the fetal platelet count is less than 50,000/mm^3, cesarean-section delivery is indicated.

Measurement of the fetal platelet count requires the collection of a scalp blood sample similar to the procedure used to measure fetal pH. The blood must be collected in a special pipette (Unopette test system 5855 from Becton-Dickison). The procedure must be performed early in labor to avoid the error introduced when a caput has formed and to minimize fetal trauma during labor if the fetus has thrombocytopenia.

The patient with ITP who has had a splenectomy is an exception to the statement that if the maternal platelet count is greater than 150,000/mm^3, the possibilities of neonatal thrombocytopenia are small. Splenectomy does not change the ability of the mother to make antiplatelet antibodies; it removes the place where platelets are destroyed and consequently prolongs platelet life and improves the platelet count. Therefore a splenectomized pregnant woman with a normal platelet count may have abundant antibodies that cross the placenta causing fetal and neonatal thrombocytopenia. The only way to evaluate the fetal situation in the splenectomized patient is by measuring the fetal platelet count early in labor.

Measurements of maternal circulating[11] or platelet bound[7] antibodies are unreliable to predict fetal or neonatal platelet count. As mentioned before, the antigenic composition of the surface of the baby's platelets is different from the mother, and the concentration of maternal antibodies is irrelevant if those antibodies do not react with the infant's platelets.

When the nonsplenectomized patient with ITP is seen early in gestation, the therapy of choice is glucocorticoid treatment. Prednisone 60 to 100 mg per day must be given until the platelet count is above 150,000/mm³. Then the dose should be tapered until the minimum required to keep the platelet count at the 150,000/mm³ level is reached. In these cases it is also important to measure the fetal platelet count early in labor to avoid missing the rare occurrence of a thrombocytopenic baby in a mother with a platelet count greater than 150,000/mm³.

Corticosteroids have also been used shortly before delivery. In the only controlled study about this approach to the problem,[19] infants from women with ITP treated with glucocorticoids had platelet counts high enough to prevent intracranial bleeding during labor and delivery. In seven pregnancies without glucocorticoid therapy, four infants had purpura at the time of delivery, and one of the four had abdominal wall hemorrhage around the umbilicus. The neonatal platelet count was significantly lower in untreated cases than in those treated. However, the number of cases in this study was small, and 6 of the 12 treated pregnancies resulted in babies with platelet counts under 50,000/mm³. In our opinion, more studies are necessary if maternal corticosteroid administration before delivery is to be adopted as a mode of therapy in pregnant patients with ITP.

von Willebrand's disease

von Willebrand's disease is a blood coagulation disorder resulting·from a quantitative or qualitative deficiency in von Willebrand's factor. This coagulopathy is rarely found during pregnancy, and only a few well-studied cases have been reported in the literature.[28,38] The bleeding disorder is inherited autosomally, but because of the marked clinical variability of the disease, the recessive or dominant mode of its inheritance has not been clearly determined. Characteristically, these patients have a prolonged bleeding time and moderate to marked decrease in von Willebrand's factor activity. The von Willebrand factor is a high molecular weight glycoprotein that is part of the factor VIII complex. In some cases of von Willebrand's disease the factor VIII procoagulant activity—the other component of the factor VIII complex that is reduced in cases of hemophilia A—is also decreased, and the activated partial thromboplastin time (PTT) is increased. von Willebrand's factor can be measured indirectly by observing the capacity of the patient's plasma to agglutinate washed platelets in the presence of ristocetin (von Willebrand's factor activity), or the factor can be measured directly by means of radioimmunoassay (factor VIII-related antigen).

The diagnosis of von Willebrand's disease must be suspected in any pregnant patient with normal platelet count, prolonged bleeding time, and prolonged PTT. A definite diagnosis can be made by measuring the von Willebrand's factor activity and factor VIII-related antigen.

The course of pregnancy in the majority of patients with von Willebrand's disease is benign. The most frequent complication is bleeding during labor and delivery or during the postpartum period. However, pregnancy causes an increase in von Willebrand's factor, and the possibility of bleeding is inversely related to the magnitude of such an increase. In general, if von Willebrand's factor rises to about 50% of the normal concentration, the possibilities of intrapartum or postpartum bleeding are almost nil. If the concentration of von Willebrand's factor by the end of pregnancy is less than 30%, the patient must be treated with cryoprecipitate to prevent the occurrence of abnormal bleeding.

■ THROMBOEMBOLIC DISEASES

The thromboembolic diseases occurring more frequently during pregnancy are (1) the intravascular deposition of fibrinogen-like material that occurs in the course of severe preeclampsia and eclampsia, (2) deep vein thrombosis (DVT) of the lower extremities, and (3) pulmonary embolization. The first of these problems has been analyzed in Chapter 6. In this chapter the discussion is limited to the last two problems.

Deep vein thrombosis of the legs (DVT)

The incidence of thrombophlebitis of the legs in the antepartum period is 2.0 per 1000 pregnancies (about the same for nonpregnant women). The large majority of cases of antepartum thrombophlebitis are superficial (1.7 per 1000 pregnancies), and DVT is a rare event (3.6 of each 10,000 pregnancies).

The incidence of superficial thrombophlebitis increases seven times (12 per 1000 pregnancies), and the incidence of DVT increases four to five times (15 per 10,000 pregnancies) during the postpartum period.[1] It is paradoxical that the postpartum period is the time of significant risk for thromboembolic complications, since this is when a rapid rise occurs in plasma and whole blood fibrinolytic activity.[2]

The overwhelming majority of patients who develop superficial and deep thrombophlebitis during pregnancy belong to a high-risk population characterized by the presence of one or several of the following problems: (1) cesarean-section delivery, (2) obesity, (3) use of estrogen to suppress lactation, (4) obstetric complications (such as prolonged labor, multiple labor inductions, and difficult deliveries) making prolonged bed rest necessary, and (5) age greater than 30 years and high parity.

The clinical diagnosis of leg DVT is in error 50% of the time. Therefore in any situation in which this diagnosis is being considered, the clinical impression must be confirmed with laboratory tests. The first test that must be carried out is impedance phlethysmography (IPG) using the occlusive cuff technique. This method measures changes in electrical impedance between two electrodes applied to the calf. When the venous return is impaired with a cuff applied to the thigh, there is a local increase in blood volume as well as a decrease when the cuff pressure is released. These changes in volume are reflected in changes in electric impedance that are altered when DVT is present. The test is highly specific (less than 5% false positives) and very sensitive (less than 5% false negative) for the diagnosis of popliteal and suprapopliteal DVT, and there is at least one report of its use in pregnant patients as a screening test for DVT.[8]

If the IPG test is negative, no further studies are necessary. If the IPG test is positive, a venogram must be ordered to confirm the diagnosis and to evaluate the characteristics of the clot.

Once the diagnosis of DVT has been established, treatment with intravenous heparin is mandatory. If untreated, 19% of pregnant patients with DVT develop pulmonary embolization, and 29% of those with pulmonary embolism die.[37] Our protocol is to give 5000 units of heparin via intravenous push as soon as the diagnosis is established, followed by continuous intravenous administration of 30,000 units of heparin per day (1250 units per hour) using a Harvard pump. The treatment is monitored by daily measurements of the PTT, and the goal is to maintain the PTT at one and one half to two times the normal rate (approximately 60 to 80 seconds). The amount of heparin administered daily is increased or decreased as necessary to reach this goal. Treatment with intravenous heparin is continued for a minimum of 7 days or until the pain has subsided completely. If the IPG remains positive at the end of the heparin treatment and the patient has already delivered, she is switched to oral anticoagulants, and full anticoagulation is continued until the IPG, venogram, or both are negative. If the patient has not delivered and the IPG remains positive at the end of 7 days of intravenous heparin treatment, continuous intravenous infusion of heparin should continue until normalization of the IPG. Once the IPG becomes normal, the patient should be maintained in prophylactic heparinization (5000 units subcutaneously every 12 hours) for the duration of pregnancy and during the postpartum period to avoid a recurrence with its potential risk of pulmonary embolization. In fact, 20% to 35% of those patients who have an episode of DVT during pregnancy and receive no treatment experience a recurrence.[37] Traditionally, patients have been kept fully anticoagulated for the duration of pregnancy after an episode of DVT. However, the need for this practice is open to question, and if the experience with prevention of thromboembolization in nonpregnant patients may be extrapolated to pregnancy, prophylactic heparinization will be all that is needed to prevent recurrences.

If it is decided to keep the patient with DVT fully anticoagulated during pregnancy, heparin is the drug of choice. Coumadin has been used

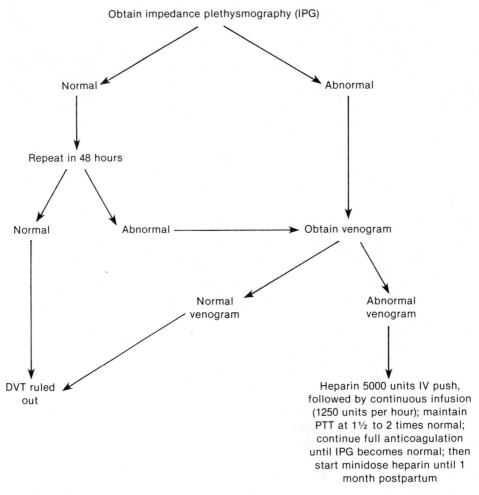

Obtain impedance plethysmography (IPG)

Normal

Abnormal

Repeat in 48 hours

Normal   Abnormal ──────────▶ Obtain venogram

Normal
venogram

Abnormal
venogram

DVT ruled
out

Heparin 5000 units IV push,
followed by continuous infusion
(1250 units per hour); maintain
PTT at 1½ to 2 times normal;
continue full anticoagulation
until IPG becomes normal; then
start minidose heparin until 1
month postpartum

FIG. 12-1 ■ Management of the patient suspected of having leg deep vein thrombosis (DVT) during pregnancy.

and continues to be used for this purpose (see protocol for the use of Coumadin during pregnancy in Chapter 10), but the occurrence of fetal congenital abnormalities[34] and the frequent occurrence of spontaneous intracranial bleeding with fetal death in uterus[37] in patients treated with Coumadin during the second and third trimester of pregnancy are powerful reasons to avoid this drug during pregnancy.

Once the patient is discharged from the hospital, full anticoagulation with heparin is difficult because of the need for parenteral administration of the drug. The following three modes of treatment are available:

1. Repeated subcutaneous injections of heparin by the patient herself every 4 to 6 hours in amounts that vary from 4000 to 6000 units, with the treatment monitored by PTT measurements carried out 1 hour before an injection. This method causes wide fluctuations in blood clotting with increased risk of bleeding complications and produces multiple small, painful, darkly stained hematomas at the injection sites.

2. Repeated intravenous injections of heparin administered by the patient herself via a heparin lock placed and secured in a peripheral vein of the arm. This method also causes wide swings in blood coagulation and requires an intelligent patient capable of adequately handling the heparin lock.

3. Continuous subcutaneous or intravenous injection of heparin using a micropump. With the development of sophisticated and

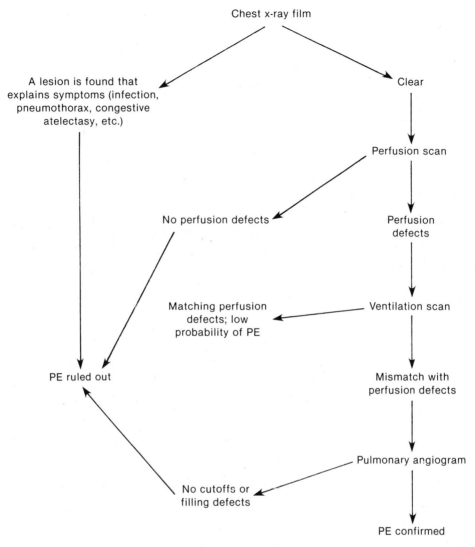

FIG. 12-2 ■ Diagnostic steps in patients suspected of pulmonary embolization (PE).

very small programmable pumps for continuous intravenous or subcutaneous infusion, it is possible to inject continuous small volumes of highly concentrated solutions of heparin and secure a steadier level of hypocoagulation. However, these pumps are expensive and may fail, producing bleeding or inadequate coagulation levels.

Once evidence has been obtained (by IPG or venogram), indicating that full anticoagulation with heparin is no longer necessary, our preference is to maintain the patient with minidose heparin (5000 units subcutaneously every 12 hours) for the duration of pregnancy and the

postpartum period. There is no evidence that minidose heparin prevents recurrences of DVT or pulmonary embolization in pregnant patients. However, the evidence accumulated in randomized trials of thousands of nonobstetric patients[18] is so strong that it seems logical to extrapolate these results to the obstetric situation and avoid the multiple inconveniences associated with full-scale prophylactic anticoagulation.

A summary of our approach to pregnant patients suspected of DVT is shown in Fig. 12-1.

Pulmonary embolism

Pulmonary embolism (PE) occurs rarely during pregnancy. Friend and Kakkar[13] reported an incidence of 2.7 per 1000, but almost certainly this is a high estimate caused by overdiagnosis. In about 95% of the cases PE is secondary to DVT of the thigh, and in the majority of cases it occurs in the immediate postpartum period.

All the clinical signs and symptoms of PE are inconsistent and unreliable, and only a pulmonary angiogram provides absolute evidence of the presence of this condition. In fact, approximately 80% of all patients with signs and symptoms of PE, including those with arterial hypoxemia and positive perfusion scans, do *not* have PE when examined with a pulmonary angiogram.[4] Since the diagnosis of PE has important therapeutic and prognostic implications, pulmonary angiograms must be obtained in every pregnant patient in whom this diagnosis is suspected. Fig. 12-2 shows the sequence of steps that must be followed in the evaluation of patients suspected of PE. If the clinical presentation is strongly suggestive of PE, the diagnostic studies must be initiated after giving the patient an intravenous injection of 10,000 units of heparin, and the treatment with heparin may be continued or discontinued later depending on the results of the diagnostic workup. It is also important to look for leg DVT in all cases in which PE is suspected, since DVT is present in about 95% of all cases of PE.

With respect to the diagnostic protocol (Fig. 12-2), the following are the most important points to remember:

1. Most patients with PE have a clear chest x-ray film.
2. A positive perfusion scan is sine qua non evidence of PE. If the perfusion scan is *negative,* the patient does not have PE, and no further testing is necessary.
3. A ventilation-perfusion mismatch is not diagnostic of PE, since there are other causes of pulmonary vascular obstruction (ie, inflammation). However, the probability of PE is high.
4. Pulmonary angiography is the only procedure to definitely establish the diagnosis of PE.

The duration of anticoagulation therapy for patients with PE is a matter of discussion. Traditionally, patients have been managed with continuous heparin infusion for 10 to 15 days followed by oral anticoagulation for several months. Nowadays, however, heparinization is

discontinued after 10 days provided that (1) the ventilation-perfusion scan is negative, (2) the leg IPG is negative, and (3) the patient is not at high risk for a recurrence. If the first and second conditions are fulfilled but the patient is at high risk for recurrence (ie, pregnant), treatment should continue with minidose heparin. If either the first or second condition is not fulfilled, continuous intravenous heparin infusion should be continued.

■ REFERENCES

1. Aaro LA, Johnson MR, Juergens JL: Acute deep vein thrombosis associated with pregnancy. Obstet Gynecol 1966;28:553.
2. Arias R, Andrinopoulos G, Zamora J: Whole blood fibrinolytic activity in normal and hypertensive pregnancies and its relation to the placental concentration of urokinase inhibitor. Am J Obstet Gynecol 1979;133:624.
3. Banedoch J, Callender S, Evans JR, et al: Megaloblastic anemia of pregnancy and the puerperium. Br Med J 1955;1:1245.
4. Bell WR, Simon TL: A comparative analysis of pulmonary perfusion scans with pulmonary angiogram. From a national cooperative study. Am Heart J 1976;92:700.
5. Carloss HW, McMillan R, Crosby WH: Management of pregnancy in women with immune thrombocytopenic purpura. JAMA 1980;244:2756.
6. Charain I, Rothman D, Perry J, et al: Folate status and requirements in pregnancy. Br Med J 1968;2:390.
7. Cines DB, Dusak B, Tomaski A, et al: Immune thrombocytopenic purpura and pregnancy. N Engl J Med 1982;306:826.
8. Clarke-Pearson DL, Creasman WT: Diagnosis of deep vein thrombosis in obstetrics and gynecology by impedance phlebography. Obstet Gynecol 1981;58:52.
9. Committee on Iron Deficiency: Iron deficiency in the United States. JAMA 1968;203:407.
10. Cunningham FG, Pritchard JA, Mason R, et al: Prophylactic transfusion of normal red blood cells during pregnancies complicated by sickle cell hemoglobinopathies. Am J Obstet Gynecol 1979;135:994.
11. Dixon R, Rosse W, Ebbert L: Quantitative determination of antibody in idiopathic thrombocytopenia purpura. N Engl J Med 1975;292:230.
12. Fenton V, Vavill L, Fisher J: Iron stores in pregnancy. Br J Haematol 1977;37:145.
13. Friend JR, Kakkar VV: Deep vein thrombosis in obstetrics and gynecological patients, in Kakkar VV, Joular AJ (eds): *Thromboembolism: Diagnosis and treatment.* London. Churchill Livingstone, 1972, pp. 131-138.
14. Getanby PPB, Lillie EW: Clinical analysis of 100 cases of severe megaloblastic anemia of pregnancy. Br Med J 1960;2:1111.
15. Giles C: An account of 335 cases of megaloblastic anemia of pregnancy and the puerperium. J Clin Pathol 1966;19:1.
16. Hibbard BM: The role of folic acid in pregnancy with particular reference to anemia, abruption and abortion. Br J Obstet Gynaecol 1964;71:529.

17. Hibbard BM, Jeffcoate TNA: Abruption placentae. Obstet Gynecol 1966;27:155.

18. Kakkar VV, Corrigan TP, Fossard DP, et al: Prevention of fatal postoperative pulmonary embolism by low doses of heparin. Lancet 1975;2:45.

19. Karpatkin M, Porges RF, Karpatkin S: Platelet counts in infants of women with autoimmune thrombocytopenia. N Engl J Med 1981;305:936.

20. Klein L: Premature birth and maternal prenatal anemia. Am J Obstet Gynecol 1962;83:588.

21. Knispel JW, Lynch VA, Viele BD: Aplastic anemia in pregnancy: a case report, review of the literature, and a re-evaluation of management. Obstet Gynecol Surv 1976;31:523.

22. Layrisse M, Aguero O, Blumenfeld N, et al: Megaloblastic anemia of pregnancy: characteristics of pure megaloblastic anemia and megaloblastic anemia associated with iron deficiency. Blood 1960;15:724.

23. McGregor MW: Maternal anemia as a factor in prematurity and perinatal mortality. Scott Med J 1963; 8:134.

24. Milner PF, Jones BR, Dobler J: Outcome of pregnancy in sickle cell anemia and sickle cell-hemoglobin C disease. Am J Obstet Gynecol 1980;138:239.

25. Monsen ER, Kuhn IN, Finch CA: Iron status of menstruating women. Amer J Clin Nutr 1967;20:842.

26. Morrison JC, Douvas SG, Martin JN: Methods of exchange transfusion in pregnant patients with sickle hemoglobinopathies. Read before the 30th annual meeting of American College of Obstetricians and Gynecologists, April 26, 1982.

27. Morrison JC, Schneider JM, Whybrew WD, et al: Prophylactic transfusions in pregnant patients with sickle hemoglobinopathies: benefit vs. risks. Obstet Gynecol 1980;56:274.

28. Noller KL, Bowie EJW, Kempers RD, et al: Von Willebrand's disease in pregnancy. Obstet Gynecol 1973;41:865.

29. Pritchard JA: changes in blood volume during pregnancy and delivery. Anesthesiology 1965;26:393.

30. Pritchard JA, Scott DE, Whalley PJ, et al: The effect of maternal sickle cell hemoglobinopathies and sickle cell trait on reproductive performance. Am J Obstet Gynecol 1973;1117:662.

31. Roszowski I, Wojeicka J, Zaeska K: Serum iron deficiency during the third trimester of pregnancy: maternal complications and fate of the neonate. Obstet Gynecol 1966;28:820.

32. Scott DE, Pritchard JA: Iron deficiency in healthy young college women. JAMA 1967;199:147.

33. Scott JR, Cruikshank DP, Kochenour NK, et al: Fetal platelet counts in the obstetric management of immunologic thrombocytopenic purpura. Am J Obstet Gynecol 1980;136:495.

34. Shaul WL, Hall JG: Multiple congenital anomalies associated with oral anticoagulants. Am J Obstet Gynecol 1977;127:191.

35. Streiff RR, Little B; Folic acid deficiency as a cause of uterine hemorrhage. J Clin Invest 1965;44:1102.

36. Van Nagell J, Koepke J, Dilts PV: Preventable anemia and pregnancy. Obstet Gynecol Surv 1971;26:551.

37. Villa Santa U: Thromboembolic disease in pregnancy. Am J Obstet Gynecol 1965;63:142.

38. Walker EH, Dormandy KM: The management of pregnancy in Von Willebrand's disease. Br J Obstet Gynaecol 1968;75:459.

39. Whalley PJ, Scott DE, Pritchard JA: Maternal folate deficiency and pregnancy. Am J Obstet Gynecol 1969;105:670.

40. Zuspan F: Anemia in pregnancy. J Reprod Med 1971;6:73.

13

■ ■ ■

RENAL DISEASE AND PREGNANCY

Fernando Arias

The situations that obstetricians commonly encounter in the case of renal disease and pregnancy are basically two: (1) the onset of signs and symptoms of renal disease in a pregnant patient with no history of kidney problems before pregnancy and (2) the development, usually unexpected, of pregnancy in a patient with known renal disease. The problems posed by each of these situations are different and require separate analysis.

■ RENAL DISEASE IN PREVIOUSLY HEALTHY PREGNANT PATIENTS
Acute renal failure

Before the legalization of abortion in the United States acute obstetric renal failure was a serious problem with an incidence that varied from 1 out of every 2000 to 1 out of every 5000 pregnancies.[14] At the present time with the availability of voluntary early pregnancy termination, acute renal failure secondary to septic abortion has almost completely disappeared. Thus for practical purposes acute renal failure of obstetric origin occurs mainly as a complication of severe preeclampsia or eclampsia or following hemorrhagic shock secondary to placenta previa or abruptio placentae.

The term *acute renal failure* describes a functional abnormality of the kidney characterized by a urine output of less than 400 ml/24 hours or less than 20 ml/hour.

The diagnosis of acute renal failure is easy as long as some attention is given to the patient's urine production. Unfortunately, occasionally the physician's attention is preferentially directed to the monitoring of some other aspects of the underlying disease (abruptio placentae, placenta previa, etc.), and oliguria and anuria remain undetected for several hours. In many cases this delay in the diagnosis of acute renal failure represents the difference between complete functional recovery of the kidney and chronic renal failure. In fact, all the available information suggests that variations in the *severity* and *duration* of an acute renal insult produce several clinical pictures with different prognoses. For example, an obstetric patient with oliguria or anuria following hemorrhagic shock may be suffering from a severe but immediately reversible impairment of kidney function. However, if this situation is not diagnosed and treated rapidly, it may reach a stage not susceptible to immediate return to normal function, or it may reach a stage of irreparable renal damage in the form of acute bilateral cortical necrosis. The role of the obstetrician is to detect the onset of the problem as early as possible to avoid the progression of the renal lesion to a point of irreversibility.

Etiology. Acute oliguria late in pregnancy is usually the result of an acute deficit in blood flow to the renal cortical region. Preeclampsia-eclampsia is the primary disease in about 60% of the cases of acute renal failure of obstetric origin.[24] Renal hypoperfusion in these patients is the consequence of decreased intravascular volume, spasm of afferent arterioles, and deposits of fibrinogen in the subendothelial region of the glomerular capillaries. In about 30% of the cases of acute renal failure of obstetric origin the disease is placenta previa or abruptio placentae. In these situations a massive blood loss causes acute intravascular volume depletion and severe reactive vasospasm, both responsible for the renal hypoperfusion. When abruptio placentae occurs, the presence of acute disseminated intravascular coagulation with formation of microvascular thrombi in the renal vasculature is a contributory factor to the defect in renal perfusion. In another 5% of the cases of acute renal failure of obstetric origin the primary disease (severe nephrotic syndrome, congestive heart failure, malignant hypertension, postpartum nephrosclerosis) acts on the kidney through mechanisms such as lack of effective blood volume or microvascular occlusion. Finally, in a small number of cases acute oliguria in pregnancy is the consequence of ureteral obstruction by an overdistended uterus or the result of an acute renal inflammatory process such as lupus nephritis.

In summary, in most cases the basic problem behind acute renal failure in obstetric patients is a defect in renal perfusion. The existence of a common pathogenic mechanism in spite of variations in the etiology of the problem allows a certain degree of uniformity in the diagnostic steps and the treatment of these patients.

Pathophysiology. Renal blood flow and glomerular filtration rate increase markedly during pregnancy; it has been calculated that about 25% of the increased cardiac output of the pregnant woman is destined to adequately maintain the increase in renal perfusion.[4] This may be why the kidneys of pregnant women are more easily damaged by an ischemic insult than those of nonpregnant women. The situation has some analogy with the frequent occurrence of panhypopituitarism (Sheehan's syndrome) after hypovolemic shock in obstetric patients and the rarity of this complication when hypovolemia occurs in the nonpregnant person.

Studies using radioactive tracers have shown differences in the rate of blood flow and the reactivity of the vasculature between the cortical and the medullar areas of the kidney. In fact, following profound hypovolemia, blood flow to the cortex decreases and almost disappears, whereas the perfusion to the medullar area is preserved.[12] This preferential cortical ischemia results in marked decrease in glomerular filtration rate, concentrating ability, and urinary volume. If cortical hypoperfusion persists, the initial functional changes will be replaced by anatomically recognizable damage that may progress to cortical necrosis. In some instances renal hypoperfusion may occur in the presence of an adequate intravascular volume if there is a low perfusion pressure (heart failure) or a lack of effective filtration pressure caused by a decrease in plasma colloid osmotic pressure (nephrotic syndrome).

The initial response of the kidney to hypoperfusion is to preserve the intravascular volume, and this results in the production of a concentrated urine (urine to plasma [U/P] osmolality ratio greater than 1.2) with a low sodium concentration (urinary sodium less than 20 mEq/L). If the situation remains uncorrected, the kidney will lose its ability to concentrate the urine and save sodium, and this will be reflected in a U/P osmolality ratio close to 1.0 and a urinary sodium concentration greater than 20 mEq/L, frequently in the 50 to 70 mEq/L range (Table 13-1). Further persistence of the insult may affect the kidneys to a point at which there is no production of urine (anuria), but this is uncommon and usually indicates the need to look for a urinary flow obstruction (postrenal azotemia).

The important role of the sympathetic-parasympathetic system in the renal circulation

TABLE 13-1 ■ Laboratory studies in the differential diagnosis of acute renal failure

	Prerenal failure	*Acute tubular necrosis or bilateral cortical necrosis*
U/P osmolality ratio	>1.2	<1.2
Urinary sodium	<20	>40
U/P creatinine ratio	>40	<20
Fe_{Na}	<1	>3

changes during hypovolemic states is demonstrated by experiments in which administration of alpha blockers prevent the redistribution of renal blood flow in animals in hypovolemic shock. This means that renal hypoperfusion secondary to a deficit in intravascular volume is further aggravated by arterial vasoconstriction. In cases of abruptio placentae and preeclampsia, capillary flow obstruction resulting from endothelial swelling and formation of microthrombi is also a contributory factor to the pathogenesis of the renal damage.

Diagnosis. For practical purposes the obstetric patient with acute renal failure usually falls into one of two groups. In the first group the patient arrives at the hospital several hours after the onset of a severe obstetric emergency (eclampsia, abruptio placentae, or placenta previa), and catheterization of the bladder yields only a few milliliters of dark or bloody urine. The patient is in renal failure, and the questions concern the degree of renal damage and the potential reversibility of the problem. The second group is made up of patients with complications of pregnancy (usually severe preeclampsia) who become oliguric while at the hospital, and the question is how to avoid the progression of the functional renal problem to a state of acute tubular necrosis (ATN) or bilateral cortical necrosis (BCN). In either case there are measures that should be carried out immediately.

Insertion of a central venous pressure (CVP) line or a Swan-Ganz catheter. Insertion of a CVP line or Swan-Ganz catheter is an important maneuver for both diagnosis and monitoring of therapy. An elevated CVP or pulmonary wedge pressure (PWP) in the presence of oliguria or anuria indicates fluid overload and suggests ATN or BCN rather than prerenal azotemia. In contrast, if the CVP or PWP is low, the presumptive diagnosis should be intravascular volume depletion, and intravenous fluids should be administered without fear of overload as long as the CVP or PWP remains within normal limits. The position of a CVP line should always be confirmed by a chest x-ray film. Details concerning the insertion of CVP or Swan-Ganz lines are described in Chapter 15.

Examination of the urine. Complete anuria is rare and usually indicates obstructive uropathy or profound kidney damage. In the majority of cases of acute renal failure in obstetric patients

it is possible to obtain a few milliliters of urine that must be sent to the laboratory for sodium, creatinine, and osmolality determinations. Simultaneously, a sample of serum should be sent to the laboratory to determine the same variables. In our opinion, the most valuable diagnostic test is the U/P osmolality ratio. In fact, the finding of a U/P osmolality ratio larger than 1.2 indicates that the oliguria or anuria is prerenal in origin. Usually a U/P osmolality ratio larger than 1.2 is accompanied by a low or negative CVP, a low urinary sodium concentration, and a high U/P creatinine ratio. In cases of ATN or BCN the U/P osmolality ratio is 1.0 or close to that, indicating the lack of capacity of the kidneys to concentrate the urine; the urinary sodium concentration is high, reflecting the lack of ability of the kidneys to reabsorb sodium; the CVP may be elevated, especially if the patient has been submitted to vigorous efforts to achieve intravascular volume expansion; and the U/P creatinine ratio is low, reflecting the lack of ability of the kidneys to eliminate nitrogen-retention products.

Another useful test to differentiate prerenal azotemia from ATN is the analysis of the fractional excretion of sodium or Fe_{Na} test.[7] The test is based on the fact that tubular handling of sodium is different in prerenal failure (when the tubes avidly reabsorb filtered sodium) from ATN (when sodium reabsorption is impaired because of the tubular damage). The Fe_{Na} is calculated using the following equation:

$$Fe_{Na} = \frac{U/P \text{ sodium}}{U/P \text{ creatinine}} \times 100$$

An Fe_{Na} less than 1.0 indicates prerenal azotemia, and a value larger than 3.0 indicates ATN.

Smelling the urine may be valuable in the differential diagnosis between prerenal failure and ATN, especially when there are difficulties in obtaining the necessary laboratory tests just mentioned. The urine of a patient in ATN does not have any particular smell (it smells like water), whereas the urine of patients in prerenal azotemia has a clearly distinguishable odor of urine. Examination of the urine sediment is also valuable in the diagnosis of the situation. In fact, the urine sediment of patients in ATN is characteristic and contains numerous renal tubular cells, renal tubular cell casts, and muddy-brown pigment casts. Many nephrologists accept the presence of pigment casts as a pathognomonic sign of ATN.

Blood chemistry. In addition to determining serum sodium, creatinine, and osmolality, it is important to obtain other baseline laboratory information that is useful in monitoring the evolution of the renal status and the effects of therapy. BUN and uric acid serum concentrations are, together with the serum creatinine, indexes for evaluating the ability or lack of ability of the kidneys to excrete nitrogen products. K^+ should be measured frequently, since elevations of this ion are common in the course of acute renal failure and may reach a point at which hemodialysis becomes mandatory. Changes in serum sodium concentration are also common, especially in obstetric patients who may have received large amounts of diuretics and isotonic solutions as part of their treatment.

Other blood tests may be important depending on the nature of the underlying disease. In patients with severe preeclampsia or eclampsia SGOT, lactic dehydrogenase (LDH), and bilirubin concentrations are important to follow the evolution of the liver lesion; a platelet count is important to assess the impact if any of the disease on platelet concentration. Patients who have had severe bleeding (abruptio placentae or placenta previa) require continuous monitoring or hemoglobin/hematocrit values to assess the adequacy of therapy. Finally, a useful laboratory determination in the obstetric patient is the measurement of plasma colloid osmotic pressure or in its absence serum albumin concentration. There are situations in which all tests show the presence of prerenal azotemia, but an adequately placed CVP line indicates a normal right atrial filling pressure suggesting adequate expansion of the intravascular volume. In this situation the effective intravascular volume may be inadequate because of a low serum albumin concentration. In these patients the urine output increases dramatically with intravenous administration of albumin followed or not by furosemide.

Prerenal failure

The large majority of obstetric patients in acute renal failure are in prerenal azotemia, and their kidney function impairment is immediately reversible with adequate management. Once the diagnosis of prerenal failure is established and the patient has a CVP line and Foley catheter in place, there are certain steps that should be taken to reestablish the urine flow.

Intravascular volume expansion. Whole blood, packed red cells, fresh frozen plasma, salt-poor albumin, low molecular weight dextran, cryoprecipitate, and isotonic and hypertonic crystalloid solutions may be used in the treatment of real or effective intravascular volume deficits, depending on the nature of the primary problem and the presence or absence of associated complications. For example, in cases of abruptio placentae the agent of choice for intravascular volume replacement is fresh whole blood. If fresh blood is not available, packed red cells, cryoprecipitate, and fresh frozen plasma are the agents of choice. In a patient with preeclampsia with low serum albumin concentration the agent of choice for volume expansion is salt-poor albumin. With patients in profound shock the administration of strong hypertonic solutions (7.5% NaCl) may be lifesaving.[5]

In all cases therapeutic expansion of intravascular volume should be monitored by frequent measurements of the CVP. *The CVP is not a measurement of the intravascular volume.* The CVP reflects right atrial filling pressure and indicates the capacity of the right heart to accept a given fluid load. To give large amounts of volume expanders without evaluating the capacity of the heart to accept that load is extremely dangerous and may lead to pulmonary edema. The CVP should remain between 10 and 15 cm H_2O during treatment, and any elevation above 15 cm H_2O should be answered with a decrease in the rate of intravenous fluid administration.

In cases of prerenal azotemia in which administration of blood or blood products is not necessary, intravascular volume expansion may be achieved by intravenous administration of 500 to 1000 ml of normal saline solution over 30 to 60 minutes. This maneuver should cause a modest elevation of CVP and result in an increase in urine production. Others prefer to use a "synthetic extracellular fluid" solution (750 ml of 0.9% NaCl, 225 ml of 5% dextrose in water, and 25 ml of a solution of HCO_3^- containing 3.75 g/50 ml) for the intravenous fluid challenge. In either case after the initial intravenous fluid challenge, administration of isotonic NaCl should be continued at a rate (125 ml to 200 ml/hour) compatible with a normal CVP and urinary output above 30 ml/hour. However, frequently the urinary volume response is transient, and soon the patient is requiring 200 or 300 ml/hour to maintain a marginal urinary output. The tendency in these cases is to push further the rate of administration of intravenous fluids, a decision that frequently results in the production of pulmonary edema. What is happening is that the patient (usually a mother with severe preeclampsia) is generating a large "third space" because of capillary leakage, and the majority of the intravenous fluids are being deposited in the interstitial space and have no influence on the renal perfusion pressure.

There are two main reasons for the formation of a third space in the obstetric patient in prerenal failure. The first is a low serum albumin concentration. This causes a drop in plasma colloid osmotic pressure and allows fluids to move toward and remain in the interstitial rather than the intravascular space. When the difference between plasma colloid osmotic pressure (usually 21 to 25 mm Hg) and PWP (usually 6 to 10 mm Hg) is reduced to less than 3 mm Hg, pulmonary edema usually occurs.[20] The solution to this problem is to increase the plasma colloid osmotic pressure by administering salt-poor albumin or low molecular weight dextran.

Another reason for the formation of a third space in patients with preeclampsia is capillary damage caused by tissue hypoxia. This happens in patients with severe forms of preeclampsia and is also common in those who have sustained large blood losses with inadequate replacement. If capillary hypoxic damage is the main reason for the third spacing, therapy should be directed toward mobilization of fluids from the third space into the intravenous space with the use of furosemide. Intravascular fluids should be maintained at a moderate rate (100 to 150 ml/hour) and diuresis forced with intravenous pushes of 20 mg of furosemide. This treatment depletes the plasma volume initially, but the losses from the intravascular space are compensated by mobilization of fluids contained in the third space.

Frequently patients with severe preeclampsia or eclampsia develop a third space as a result of both hypoalbuminemia and capillary hypoxia. In these cases therapy with intravenous albumin (50 to 100 grams) should precede the administration of furosemide.

Obstetricians are reluctant to use potent diuretics in pregnant patients before delivery. The concepts of expansion of intravascular volume → adequate placental perfusion → fetal well-being and decreased intravascular volume → decreased placental perfusion → fetal distress are so deeply engraved in the obstetrician's mind that frequently patients are overloaded with intravenous fluids in an attempt to obtain a diuresis that could be easily obtained with an injection of furosemide. Fetal well-being is an important consideration in the management of obstetric patients with oliguria-anuria, but it cannot be forgotten that this is a serious maternal emergency, and in these cases the benefits of furosemide administration (prevention of maternal renal damage) outweigh the fetal risks of the procedure.

Pregnancy termination. The development of oliguria-anuria in an obstetric patient is in the majority of cases an indication for pregnancy termination. Delivery is not only beneficial for the infant, who is removed from a progressively hostile environment, but also offers distinct maternal advantages. In fact, patients who have oliguria or even anuria for several hours before delivery often begin to produce copious amounts of urine once the fetus is removed from the uterus. This raises a question about the possibility of an obstructive factor (compression of the ureter by the pregnant uterus) being present. However, in a majority of cases the diuresis that follows delivery in the obstetric patient with prerenal azotemia is a consequence of the improvement in renal perfusion caused by the redistribution of blood volume and cardiac output that follows cessation of the placental circulation. In fact, approximately 25% of the cardiac output and a large part of the intravenous volume of a pregnant patient are destined to fulfill the needs of the placental circulation.[1] This need disappears abruptly after placental separation, and there is a redistribution of the cardiac output and an increase in the blood flow to the kidneys.

Another advantage of pregnancy termination is that after delivery it is possible to use large doses of diuretics and other medications and to perform diagnostic procedures using radioactive isotopes without fear of doing harm to the fetus. However, it is important to caution against the overenthusiastic use of pregnancy termination in obstetric patients with oliguria. In fact, patients with mild or moderate preeclampsia are frequently submitted to primary cesarean-section delivery because of a "drop in urinary output." A rigorous analysis of these cases generally leads to the conclusion that the oliguria was not adequately evaluated, medical treatment of the situation was not attempted, and often the diagnosis of the oliguria can be seriously questioned. As mentioned earlier, acute renal failure is the production of less than 400 ml of urine in 24 hours or less than 20 ml/hour. There is a clear indication to terminate the pregnancy by cesarean section *only* when the urinary output has dropped to less than 20 ml/hour and has remained at that level for 2 or more hours despite adequate treatment with volume expanders and furosemide and *only* if vaginal delivery is not in sight within an additional 2 hours. To proceed to surgical intervention because of a low urinary output without any effort to understand and treat the mechanism of the problem is not adequate.

Diuretics. Two groups of pregnant patients in acute renal failure should be given diuretics: (1) patients in prerenal failure (U/P osmolality ratio greater than 1.2, low CVP) who respond *inadequately* or fail to respond to an intravenous fluid challenge with crystalloids and colloids because of third space formation and (2) patients in early stages of ATN (U/P osmolality ratio between 1.05 and 1.20, CVP around 15 cm H_2O).

Patients in the first category have already been discussed in the section on intravascular volume expansion. As far as patients in the second group are concerned, there is a controversy in the literature about the possibility of reversing ATN with the use of high doses of furosemide.[6,11] It is possible that patients who respond to furosemide are not in real ATN but in a situation in which the physiological renal response to the primary insult is highly exaggerated. The obstetric patient in severe oliguria unresponsive to intravascular volume expansion and with laboratory indicators pointing to the presence of ATN should have a trial of high doses of furosemide because this is the last chance to obtain an immediate reestablishment of normal renal function. Also, there are some indications that furosemide treatment may produce a milder course for patients in acute renal failure who develop ATN. If the patient has not received furosemide before, we prefer to start with 20 mg injected IV. If there is no response in 30 minutes, the dose is increased to 100 mg. If there

is no diuresis, dosages of 200 and 500 mg are administered at 30-minute intervals. If the 500 mg dosage does not induce brisk diuresis, the patient is considered to be in established ATN and managed accordingly.

Acute tubular necrosis and bilateral cortical necrosis

In the past it was adequate to manage conservatively (without dialysis) patients who developed ATN as the result of obstetric complications. Dialysis was indicated in patients who developed (1) cardiovascular overload because of unsuccessful fluid restriction during the oliguric phase of ATN, (2) hyperkalemia that could not be controlled with the use of potassium exchange resins, and (3) pericarditis, uremic encephalopathy, electrolyte imbalances, or metabolic acidosis. In modern times patients with ATN are dialyzed earlier with the result being the ease and convenience of the management of their fluid and dietary intakes. Thus once the diagnosis of ATN has been clearly established (U/P osmolality ratio equals 1.0, urinary sodium more than 40 mEq/L, elevated CVP, lack of response to furosemide), the role of the obstetrician is threefold—to terminate the pregnancy if this has not been done previously, to restrict the fluid intake to an amount equivalent to the urinary output plus the insensible losses, and to refer the patient to a place with adequate facilities for hemodialysis.

Rigorous fluid restriction of the obstetric patient with ATN is mandatory as soon as the diagnosis is established. In fact, the most common indication for emergency dialysis in obstetric patients in renal failure is fluid overload. However, a severe fluid restriction makes it difficult to maintain an adequate caloric intake, and the result is increased protein degradation for energy generation purposes and accumulation of nitrogen products in the blood. One of the advantages of dialysis is that it allows a more liberal fluid intake and makes it easier to adjust the diet to an optimal caloric and protein intake.

The overwhelming majority of obstetric patients with ATN recover without sequelae. Most are able to leave the hospital 2 to 3 weeks after the onset of ATN, and most of them exhibit normal creatinine clearance and blood chemistries 6 to 12 months after the acute episode. Prognosis is different for those patients who develop BCN.

Often they have to remain in hemodialysis for the rest of their lives, and most of them never recover adequate renal function.

Postrenal failure

There are few cases of obstructive uropathy during pregnancy reported in the literature. This is usually the result of ureteral compression at the level of the pelvic brim by an overdistended uterus.[19] This situation is more likely to occur in twin pregnancies and in cases of severe polyhydramnios. Although in both prerenal and renal azotemia urine production rarely ceases completely, in obstructive uropathy complete anuria is frequently present. If complete anuria develops in a patient with an overdistended uterus, the possibility of obstructive uropathy should be strongly considered. In these cases termination of pregnancy is followed by profuse diuresis.

Nephrotic syndrome

A nephrotic syndrome is characterized by the presence of proteinuria greater than 3 grams per day, hypoalbuminemia of less than 3 g/dl, edema, and hypercholesterolemia. This constellation of signs and symptoms of renal disease appears infrequently during gestation, approximately once every 1500 pregnancies.[27]

Etiology and diagnosis. The etiology of nephrotic syndrome is varied, but the most common causes found in the pregnant patient include the following:

1. Preeclampsia and eclampsia
2. Lupus nephritis
3. Acute glomerulonephritis (GN)

The key element in the differential diagnosis among these possibilities is the presence or absence of hypertension. All the diseases causing nephrotic syndrome may produce elevation of blood pressure, but since this is a cardinal sign of preeclampsia, the most common cause for the nephrotic syndrome during pregnancy, the presence of hypertension automatically classifies the patient with nephrotic syndrome as having preeclampsia, and the burden of proof is on the person who proposes a different diagnosis. If the patient is not hypertensive, preeclampsia may be ruled out and a careful search for other diseases should be initiated.

The second most valuable element in the differential diagnosis of the cause of nephrotic syndrome during pregnancy is examination of the urinary sediment.[23] The presence of red cells and red cell casts is diagnostic of acute GN. A benign sediment with occasional large coarse granular casts is the usual finding in preeclampsia. The presence of lipid droplets, cellular casts, and birefringent lipids points to chronic renal disease.

Other laboratory tests useful in the differential diagnosis of the cause of nephrotic syndrome are the ANA titer, the complement battery, and the urinary protein electrophoresis. A positive ANA titer is strongly suggestive of systemic lupus erythematosus, which may be confirmed by the finding of a significantly elevated titer of antinative DNA antibodies in the patient's serum. The finding of an alteration in the complement battery (C_3, C_4, and CH_{50}) may also be useful for diagnostic purposes.[28]

The four renal conditions that cause a decrease in serum complement levels are (1) poststreptococcal GN, (2) membranous-proliferative GN, (3) the nephritis of patients with chronic bacteremia, and (4) lupus nephritis. Poststreptococcal GN is rare during pregnancy, and when it causes nephrotic syndrome, it is usually transient. Normal antistreptolysin (ASO) and antihyaluronidase titers are useful to rule out this disease. Membranous-proliferative GN, especially the variety called *dense deposit disease* or MPGN type II, characteristically depresses C_3, whereas C_4 remains normal. This is a disease of children and is extremely rare during pregnancy. Patients with chronic infectious processes who develop nephrotic syndrome are unusual in obstetrics. Thus for all practical purposes a decrease in complement levels in a pregnant patient with nephrotic syndrome means the presence of lupus nephritis.

In the majority of cases the diagnosis of lupus nephritis causing nephrotic syndrome during pregnancy is not difficult. Hypertension is usually not present, and this allows ruling out preeclampsia. The urine sediment is not inflammatory (no red cell casts), the ANA titer is positive, and the total complement activity and the C_3 and C_4 values are below normal limits. Also, frequently, there are signs of extrarenal disease such as hemolytic anemia, thrombocytopenia, or cutaneous alterations. Most cases of severe nephrotic syndrome with acute onset correspond to membranous lupus nephritis, although any of the five different histologic types may be present.

Urinary protein electrophoresis is another important test in the analysis of pregnant patients with nephrotic syndrome.[3] With this method it is possible to evaluate the predominant molecular size of the proteins appearing in the urine, which in turn is an index of the degree of glomerular permeability damage (size of the glomerular "hole"). There are methods such as the comparison of the clearance of IgG (molecular weight 160,000) to the clearance of transferrin (molecular weight 88,000) that allow a precise measurement of the "selectivity" of the proteinuria, but for routine evaluation the ratio of gamma globulin (formed mainly by immunoglobulins with molecular weight greater than 150,000) to albumin (molecular weight 69,000) as measured by urinary electrophoresis is adequate. A gamma globulin/albumin ratio of 0.1 or less indicates a selective proteinuria. If the proteinuria is not selective, the ratio will be more than 0.1, since a relatively larger proportion of IgG is lost in the urine. Studying the selectivity of the proteinuria in a patient with nephrotic syndrome is valuable because high selectivity (small glomerular hole) characterizes certain renal diseases, and this finding suggests a high probability that the patient will benefit from glucocorticoid therapy.

High selectivity (preferential excretion of small molecular weight protein molecules) is characteristic of minimal change disease, although it also may occur in a few cases of membranous GN and in rare cases of focal sclerotic and mesangial proliferative GN. The proteinuria that occurs in cases of excessive protein production (multiple myeloma, acute leukemia) or when there is a defect in tubular reabsorption of proteins (Fanconi's syndrome) is also highly selective but rarely is large enough to fulfill the definition of nephrotic syndrome. Thus for practical purposes the finding of high selectivity proteinuria in a pregnant patient with nephrotic syndrome is strongly suggestive of the presence of minimal change disease. Although minimal change disease is the most common cause (95%) of nephrotic syndrome in children, its prevalence quickly decreases during adulthood, and it is responsible for only 10% of the cases of nephrotic syndrome observed after age 40. In contrast, membranous GN is unusual in children

but is the underlying problem in about 50% of the cases of nephrotic syndrome occurring outside of pregnancy after 30 years of age.

Fig. 13-1 is a summary of the diagnostic steps to be followed in the study of patients with nephrotic syndrome during pregnancy. From a practical viewpoint the differential diagnosis is limited to the following four possibilities:

1. *Preeclampsia:* elevated blood pressure, negative ANA titer, normal complement, proteinuria not selective, urinary sediment benign.
2. *Lupus nephritis:* positive ANA titer, positive DNA antibodies, low complement, nephritic sediment.
3. *Minimal change disease:* high selectivity of proteinuria, normal complement, negative ANA, responsive to steroids.
4. *Acute GN:* extremely rare, nephritic or inflammatory urinary sediment (red cell casts).

Other causes of nephrotic syndrome are rare during pregnancy, and in some of them (diabetes, amyloidosis) the diagnosis is usually known before pregnancy or early in pregnancy, and the development of the renal complication is anticipated.

Renal biopsy is difficult to perform during pregnancy. In cases of idiopathic nephrotic syndrome, biopsy and histologic examination of the renal tissue should be postponed until 6 weeks postpartum.

Management of nephrotic syndrome. In the majority of cases (80%) the cause of nephrotic syndrome during pregnancy is preeclampsia, and the most important part of the treatment is termination of pregnancy. Quick recovery is the rule following delivery. If the diagnosis is lupus nephritis or minimal change disease, the treatment is administration of glucocorticoids (prednisone, 60 to 100 mg per day). If the etiology of the nephrotic syndrome is unknown, treatment should be symptomatic and follow certain measures.

Diet. The pregnant patient with nephrotic syndrome needs a diet rich in high quality protein and poor in cholesterol and saturated fats. The sodium intake does not need to be restricted unless edema is massive and poorly responsive to diuretics.

Anticoagulation. Patients with nephrotic syndrome have a marked tendency to develop deep

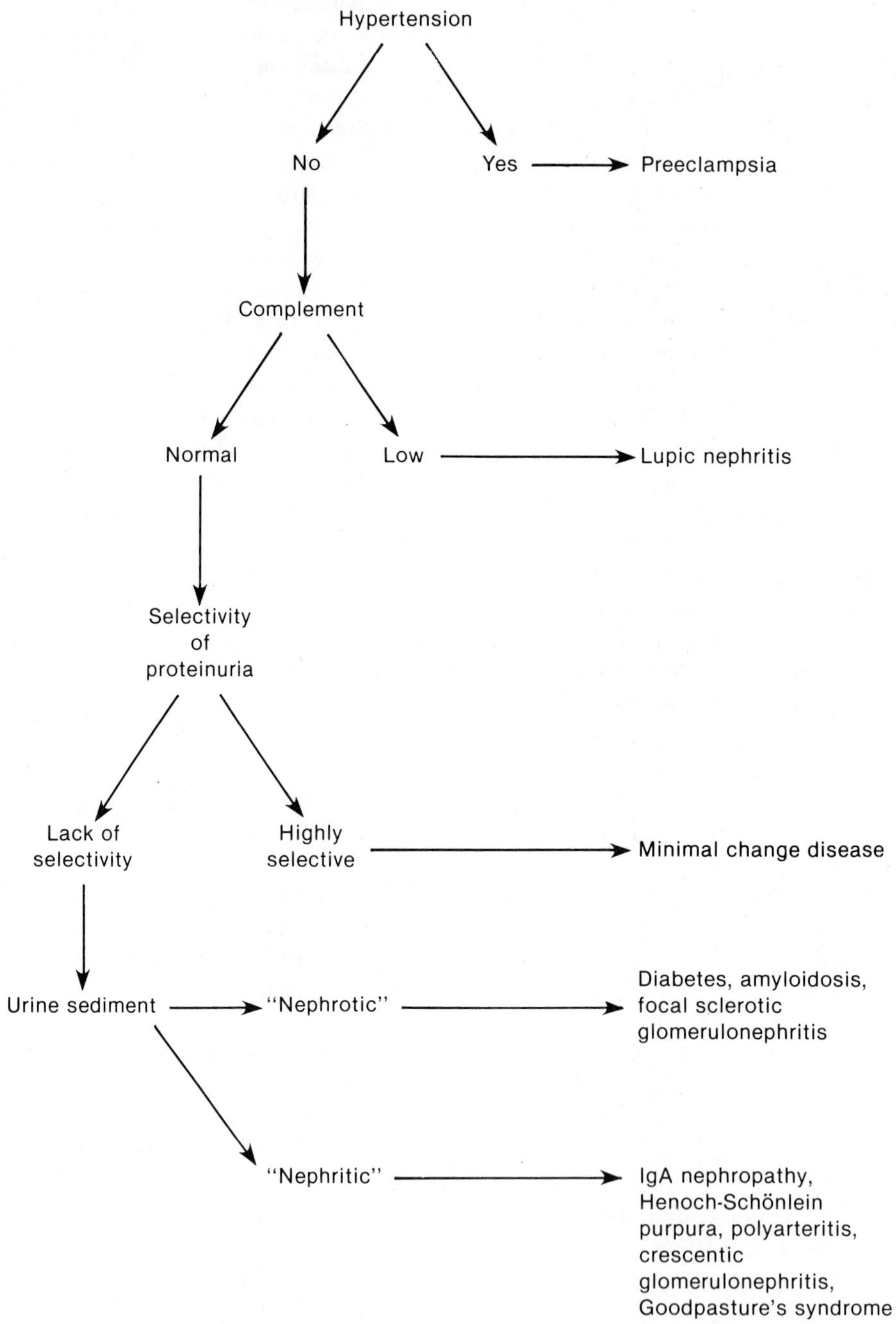

FIG. 13-1 ■ Differential diagnosis of the cause of nephrotic syndrome during pregnancy.

vein thrombosis, especially renal vein thrombosis,[16] and pregnancy may aggravate this tendency. Since severe hypoalbuminemia is associated with a high risk for venous thrombosis, there is justification for the prophylactic use of heparin (5000 units subcutaneously every 12 hours) in pregnant patients with nephrotic syndrome and a serum albumin concentration under 2 g/dl. Prophylactic heparinization is important during the last trimester and should be continued during the intrapartum and postpartum periods.

Diuretics. In some cases of nephrotic syndrome during pregnancy it is possible to avoid the use of diuretics. Patients usually become edematous early in the course of their disease, but they should not be treated with diuretics unless they become uncomfortable with the accumulation of interstitial fluid. Decreased physical activity and periods of rest in the lateral supine position are usually effective in promoting diuresis and curtailing the development of more edema. If a diuretic is required, furosemide is the agent of choice.

Albumin. If edema progresses to a state of anasarca, the plasma albumin concentration is low, and the hematocrit value shows progressive elevation, expansion of the intravascular volume with salt-poor albumin is indicated. Most physicians are reluctant to administer albumin because of possible lack of efficiency in view of the continuous urinary loss. However, intravenous albumin administration is indicated in obstetric patients with nephrotic syndrome showing constriction of the intravascular volume because if this situation persists, it will cause decreased placental blood flow and impairment of the fetal nutrition.

Glucocorticoids. There is no place for glucocorticoids in the treatment of nephrotic syndrome unless a corticoid responsive lesion (lupus erythematous, minimal change disease) is the etiology of the problem.

Prophylactic antibiotics. Pregnant patients with nephrotic syndrome are at high risk for the development of infections, especially urinary tract infections. For this reason they should receive prophylactic antibiotic treatment. Preferred regimens are ampicillin 500 mg, cephalosporin 500 mg, or nitrofurantoin 200 mg taken before bedtime every night.

Maternal monitoring. An important complication that pregnant patients with nephrotic syndrome may develop is elevation of blood pressure. They should have their blood pressure monitored at least weekly, and ideally they should obtain their own sphygmomanometer for daily checks at home. If hypertension develops, they should be admitted to the hospital, and the majority will require termination of pregnancy. For evaluation of the degree of fluid accumulation the best index is serial body weights. The renal function should be monitored periodically by measuring BUN, creatinine, and uric acid concentration. Because of urinary losses of transferrin, pregnant patients with nephrotic syndrome often develop anemia that does not respond to iron therapy. The diagnosis of anemia in these patients is complicated by the fact that in the initial phase of their disease they expand their plasma volume and dilute their hemoglobin/hematocrit values. Patients should have a transfusion if the hematocrit value drops under 30% and there is no response to iron therapy.

Fetal monitoring. The fetus of the pregnant patient with nephrotic syndrome is at risk of growth retardation, preterm delivery, and antepartum fetal distress, complications that usually occur if the condition of the mother worsens. As a general rule, if the mother remains stable, the risk of fetal complications is small. The best available methods for assessing the fetal status in the patient with nephrotic syndrome are (1) serial ultrasound examinations to follow the fetal biparietal diameter growth and (2) weekly nonstress tests after 32 weeks of gestation. The complication having the largest impact on the fetal outcome is the development of maternal hypertension; if this happens, the patient should be managed as an individual with preeclampsia with different alternatives, depending on the severity of the hypertension (see Chapter 6).

Acute glomerulonephritis

The diagnosis of acute GN is rarely made during pregnancy partly because of its low incidence in obstetric patients and also because the diagnosis is often confused with preeclampsia or idiopathic nephrotic syndrome. In fact, if a pregnant patient develops acute GN with hypertension and proteinuria, the diagnosis should be preeclampsia, and the treatment should be one for preeclampsia. The poor fetal and maternal prognosis associated with conservative therapy of severe preeclampsia, the frequent occurrence of preeclampsia versus the rarity of acute GN, and the difficulties in making a differential diagnosis between these two diseases make it necessary to discard the possibility of GN and to treat all these patients as having preeclampsia. For practical purposes the most common situation in which the possibility of GN is considered is in the differential diagnosis of patients who develop proteinuria without hypertension and have an inflammatory urinary sediment containing red cell casts. The latter point is important because if red cell casts are absent from the urinary sediment, an acute glomerular lesion is unlikely.

In those rare cases in which it is possible to establish the diagnosis of acute GN during pregnancy, and especially if the proteinuria is highly selective, the patient deserves a trial of glucocorticoids. Prednisone (60 to 100 mg per day) should be given for 3 or 4 weeks, and its effect on urinary protein and the level of nitrogen products in the blood should be assessed quantitatively on a weekly basis. Only exceptionally is the use of glucocorticoids justified in pregnant patients with nonselective acute GN. Glucocorticoids may confuse the clinical picture by causing sodium and water retention, volume expansion, and secondary hypertension development.

Acute nephrolithiasis

Acute nephrolithiasis is a rather unusual complication of pregnancy that occurs once in every 1500 deliveries,[15] usually during the third trimester. The main symptoms are flank and lower quadrant pain and microscopic hematuria. Pregnant patients with these symptoms should be approached similarly to nonpregnant patients suspected of kidney stones with the following two exceptions:

1. The use of x-ray examinations should be avoided or kept to a minimum.
2. In cases requiring surgical intervention palliative measures are the first choice, and definitive procedures should be postponed until the postpartum period.

If a pregnant patient develops symptoms suggesting the presence of stones in the urinary tract, the following should be ordered (Table 13-2):

1. All urines should be strained to assess the passage of gravel or stones.
2. The urine should be cultured. The finding of a *Proteus mirabilis* infection in patients with a history of chronic recurrent urinary tract infections is strongly suggestive of the presence of magnesium ammonium phosphate (struvite) stones.
3. A 24-hour urine collection for quantitative determination of calcium and uric acid should be obtained. Hypercalciuria (greater than 250 mg per day) suggests the presence of calcium oxalate stones, whereas hyperuricemia (greater than 800 mg per day) suggests uric acid stones. However, a diagnostic error can easily be made during pregnancy because hypercalciuria may be found in normal patients who are taking a large amount of calcium.
4. A careful family history should be elicited. If stone disease exists in several members of the family, cystinuria or hyperoxaluria may be present. In these cases a 24-hour urine collection should be sent to the laboratory for cystine and oxalic acid determination.
5. The urine pH should be determined several times a day for several days to determine the predominant pH of the urine. If the pH is persistently acid, this suggests uric acid stones; a persistently alkaline urine suggests magnesium ammonium phosphate stones.
6. Serum calcium, uric acid, and electrolyte concentrations should be measured. If hypercalcemia is present, it will be necessary to determine parathormone concentration to rule out the possibility of hyperparathyroidism, a situation frequently associated with calcium oxalate stones. Hyperchloremia suggests renal tubular acidosis and calcium phosphate stones. Hyperuricemia suggests uric acid stones.
7. A renal ultrasound examination must be ordered. It is useful for the detection of stones in the upper urinary tract and for the diagnosis of upper urinary obstruction.

If the diagnosis of nephrolithiasis or ureterolithiasis cannot be established with certainty by the previously mentioned laboratory tests and the patient is symptomatic enough to justify fur-

TABLE 13-2 ■ Laboratory studies in patients with renal stones

Test	Finding	Diagnostic possibility
Urine culture	Proteus mirabilis	Struvite stones
24-hour urine collection for calcium	Hypercalciuria (>250 mg/day)	Calcium oxalate stones
24-hour urine collection for uric acid	Hyperuricosuria (>800 mg/day)	Uric acid stones
Urine pH (several days)	Acid	Uric acid stones
	Alkaline	Struvite stones
Serum calcium	Hypercalcemia	Hyperparathyroidism
Serum uric acid	Hyperuricemia	Uric acid stones
Plasma chloride	Hyperchloremia	Renal tubular acidosis

ther diagnostic procedures, a flat plate of the abdomen and a modified intravenous pyelogram (IVP) should be carried out. Approximately 80% of the stones are seen in the flat plate. The modified IVP consists of a single exposure minutes after injection of contrast medium. The objective is to keep the amount of direct radiation to the fetus to a minimum. The modified IVP is useful only if a positive diagnosis is reached; a negative IVP does not necessarily mean that stones are absent.

Treatment of patients with nephrolithiasis of acute onset during pregnancy varies with the severity and duration of the symptoms and the presence of absence of obstruction to the urinary flow. In situations in which acute hydropyonephrosis develops as a consequence of obstruction, removal of the stone should be attempted using cystoscopy and retrograde ureteral catheterization. If this fails, a pyelostomy or nephrostomy should be carried out to avoid further damage to the renal parenchyma. Definitive removal of ureteral stones in patients in the late second and third trimesters is difficult because of the excessive vascularization and mechanical problems generated by the pregnant uterus. Such surgery should be postponed until after delivery.

More than 50% of the patients admitted to the hospital with symptoms of renal lithiasis pass their stone spontaneously and become asymptomatic.[15] This is why treatment with analgesics and increased dietary and intravenous fluids to keep the urine to about 2 liters per day is all that is necessary for the management of most of these patients. As long as there is no evidence of obstruction and the patient remains calm, spontaneous passage of the stones should be ex-

pected and intervention deferred. If the situation does not improve after a reasonable waiting period, attempts to remove the stone by cystoscopy and retrograde catheterization are justified.

Once the acute crisis is over, further treatment depends on the etiology of the nephrolithiasis. For example, a low calcium diet and thiazide diuretics are beneficial for patients with idiopathy hypercalciuria; patients with uricosuria and uric acid stones benefit from a low purine diet; patients affected by hyperparathyroidism stop producing stones once the underlying problem is corrected; patients with magnesium ammonium phosphate stones require intensive and prolonged treatment of their chronic urinary infection.

Postpartum malignant nephrosclerosis

Postpartum malignant nephrosclerosis is a condition characterized by the sudden onset and rapid progression of hemolytic anemia, thrombocytopenia, and renal failure in the postpartum period.[21] The onset of symptoms is usually preceded by a flu-like syndrome, and in a majority of the cases hypertension is also present. The disease may occur at any time from 1 day to 10 weeks after delivery.

There is confusion in the literature about the pathogenesis of this rare problem. Some investigators[22] believe that there are significant differences between the renal histology of pediatric patients with hemolytic uremic syndrome and that of adult patients who develop the disease in the puerperium or while taking oral contraceptives. The name *postpartum malignant nephrosclerosis* was proposed for the disease associated with pregnancy. This name reflects the anatomic pathology found in the kidneys of these patients and is more appropriate than postpartum renal failure, which is a generic denomination for a situation that may be caused by multiple etiologic agents. Other investigators[13] believe that postpartum hemolytic uremic syndrome, like nephrotic syndrome, is an entity that may be caused by different etiologic agents (virus, gram negative bacilli, oral contraceptives, pregnancy, malignancy) causing similar symptoms and histologic findings.

The essential anatomic feature in postpartum nephrosclerosis is the damage to the glomerular capillaries and renal arterioles by subendothelial deposits of fibrin. These deposits reduce the vascular lumen and cause ischemic changes that eventually result in renal cortical necrosis. Formation of microthrombi, especially in the afferent arterioles, is another feature of this disease that contributes to tissue ischemia. Erythrocytes and platelets are fragmented during their passage through the affected vessels, and this is the reason for the hemolysis and the thrombocytopenia that are part of the disease (microangiopathic hemolytic anemia).

The diagnosis of postpartum nephrosclerosis must be differentiated from severe preeclampsia with hematologic abnormalities, and the best way to avoid this confusion is by strict adherence to the following criteria:

1. Patients with postpartum nephrosclerosis should *not* have any signs or symptoms of preeclampsia before delivery, at the time of delivery, or in the immediate postpartum period.
2. The diagnosis of postpartum nephrosclerosis is more likely if there is a symptom-free period of several days after delivery.

The differentiation between preeclampsia and postpartum nephrosclerosis is important from a prognostic viewpoint, since recuperation is the rule in preeclampsia, and death or chronic renal insufficiency is the usual course for patients with postpartum nephrosclerosis. The differential diagnosis is also important from the therapeutic viewpoint, since heparin is probably indicated in postpartum nephrosclerosis but is not recommended for preeclampsia.

There is no evidence favoring a specific medication or mode of treatment in the management of patients with postpartum nephrosclerosis. However, all survivors reported in the literature have been treated with heparin, and this drug may be beneficial. Hemodialysis, antihypertensive drugs, anticonvulsants, antiplatelet medications, and dietary management are also important elements in the management of this almost uniformly fatal disease.

■ PREGNANCY IN PATIENTS WITH KNOWN RENAL DISEASE

When a pregnant patient known to have renal disease arrives in the obstetrician's office, three main questions arise.

1. What are the fetal and maternal prognoses for the pregnancy?
2. What are the possible complications and risks for the pregnancy?
3. What are the basic rules to be followed in the patient's management?

Although it is true that the correct answers to these questions depend to a large extent on the nature and severity of the underlying renal problem, it is also true that some general answers are valid for most of these patients. For instance, the maternal and fetal prognoses when pregnancy occurs in a patient with chronic renal disease are directly related to the presence or absence of hypertension and to the severity of the renal functional impairment; this general concept applies irrespective of the type of renal disease affecting the individual patient. It is also generally accepted that the main maternal and fetal complications for pregnant patients with underlying renal disease are development or aggravation of hypertension, progression of renal damage, fetal growth retardation, and preterm birth. Also, the basic elements in the management of these patients, irrespective of their particular type of renal lesion, are bed rest, antihypertensive drugs, and diuretics.

Maternal and fetal prognosis

One important concern for the pregnant woman with renal disease is whether or not pregnancy will accelerate the progress of her kidney lesion. A majority of investigators[18,25] believe that the answer is no and that pregnancy does not significantly increase the anatomic or functional renal damage as long as hypertension is under control. However, an important work[8] contains morphologic evidence suggesting that there is a definite progression in kidney damage with pregnancy in patients with nephrotic syndrome. The answer probably lies midway between these opposite views. The majority of pregnant patients with renal disease have only mild to moderate degrees of functional and anatomic impairment of their kidneys and are capable of tolerating pregnancy without further demonstrable impairment. A minority of patients (with severe functional and anatomic kidney damage) tolerate pregnancy poorly and develop hypertension resistant to conventional treatment, severe proteinuria, and progressive deterioration of their kidney function.

Therefore the answer to what the prognosis is for pregnancy should be chosen on an individual basis. Prognosis will be poor and complications will occur frequently if the pregnant patient with renal disease shows hypertension, large proteinuria, or elevated serum creatinine concentration. Of all these signs, the most reliable prognostic indicator is the presence or absence of hypertension; it is exceptional for a renal patient with significant hypertension (diastolic 100 mm Hg or more in spite of treatment with antihypertensive drugs) to go through pregnancy without developing severe complications.[9] Patients who are normotensive because of antihypertensive treatment have a better prognosis than those who are poorly controlled with treatment. Also, many patients with marked restriction of their kidney function (creatinine clearance between 20 and 30 ml/minute, serum creatinine between 2.5 and 3.5 mg/dl) are able to carry a pregnancy to term as long as hypertension is not a part of their disease.

Second to hypertension, the most valuable prognostic index for pregnant patients with chronic renal disease is the degree of functional impairment of their kidneys. Patients with creatinine clearances under 30 ml/minute and especially under 20 ml/minute have a much worse prognosis than those with better clearances, and the prognosis should be optimistic if the creatinine clearance is between 50 and 70 ml/minute. Patients have a relatively benign prognosis if the serum creatinine concentration is 1.5 mg/dl or less, but the prognosis becomes guarded for patients with values above that level.[2]

Finally, another important prognostic sign is the presence or absence of proteinuria. As a general rule, if the renal patient has significant proteinuria (2+ or more in qualitative tests, 3 grams or more in 24-hour urine collections) at the be-

ginning of pregnancy, the tendency will be toward increased urinary protein losses and development of a full-blown nephrotic syndrome. Patients without proteinuria at the beginning of gestation have a better prognosis.

In summary, renal patients without hypertension, without proteinuria, and with creatinine clearances of 50 to 70 ml/minute have an excellent prognosis for pregnancy and should be encouraged to get pregnant and have children before these indexes deteriorate. Fortunately, the majority of patients seen by obstetricians belong to this category, since patients with more severe kidney damage have serious difficulties in getting pregnant. However, these latter patients occasionally become pregnant, and if seen early enough in the course of gestation, they should be presented with detailed information about possible complications; the alternatives of abortion and sterilization should be openly discussed.

Complications

Hypertension. The development of hypertension, frequently severe (diastolic blood pressure 110 mm Hg or higher), often occurring early in pregnancy (before 28 weeks of gestation), and frequently resistant to conventional treatment (methyldopa, hydralazine, propranolol, and diuretics), is the most common and serious complication for patients with renal disease during pregnancy. Hypertension is the most important reason behind the elevated perinatal mortality (25% to 35%) and the high incidence of preterm delivery (37%) associated with renal disease during pregnancy.[10] In many cases hypertension is accompanied by proteinuria and edema, and the diagnosis is "superimposed preeclampsia" or "pregnancy-aggravated hypertension."

The pregnant patient with renal disease who develops hypertension or whose hypertension becomes worse during pregnancy is in serious danger. Maternal mortality may occur because of intracranial bleeding, abruptio placentae, or renal shutdown, and fetal mortality may also happen because of decreased placental blood flow, abruptio placentae, or intrapartum hypoxia.

Aggravation of the renal lesion. In some pregnant patients with renal disease progression of pregnancy is parallel with increases in proteinuria, a decrease in glomerular filtration rate, accumulation of nitrogen products in blood, and considerable water and sodium retention. In these patients pregnancy causes a worsening of the renal status. In many instances preeclampsia develops, causing additional deterioration of renal function. In a few cases, however, worsening of kidney function occurs in the absence of hypertension, and the clinical picture is that of a nephrotic syndrome with massive proteinuria, hypoalbuminemia, and hypercholesterolemia.

Fetal growth retardation. Infants born to patients with renal disease often exhibit anthropomorphic features (weight, length, head circumference) that are well below average for their gestational age. This inadequate somatic development occurs more often and is more marked in patients with high blood pressure, suggesting that decreased uteroplacental blood flow is the explanation for the abnormal fetal growth. Intrauterine growth retardation may also occur in normotensive patients with renal disease, although in these cases it rarely reaches the extreme deviation from normality seen in patients with hypertension.

Fetal growth retardation occurs in about 10% of normotensive patients with renal disease and about 35% of hypertensive pregnant patients with chronic renal illness. In most cases the abnormality is suggested by slow or static uterine fundal growth and is strongly indicated by the occurrence of a late flattening pattern of the biparietal diameter in serial ultrasound examinations. The diagnosis is almost certain when, in addition to the clinical picture and the abnormal biparietal diameter growth, the ultrasound examination shows an abnormal fetal head/abdomen circumference ratio (see Chapter 8).

Preterm birth. There are two main reasons for the high frequency (37%) of preterm births in patients with renal disease. In about half of the cases preterm birth is the result of medical intervention because of the development of maternal or fetal problems. In the other half of the cases preterm birth is the consequence of spontaneous preterm labor. In both cases the result is a high perinatal mortality and morbidity.

Antepartum and intrapartum fetal distress. Antepartum and intrapartum fetal distress occurs mainly in pregnancies complicated by intrauterine growth retardation. However, occasionally a fetus with adequate clinical and ultrasonic growth cannot tolerate the repetitive

hypoxic stress of labor, compensatory mechanisms are exceeded, and the result is fetal acidosis. All patients with renal disease should be monitored during labor, preferably using a fetal scalp electrode. Also, any abnormality in the monitoring trace in these patients should be taken seriously.

Management

General measures. Interruption of work is not necessary unless complications develop or the patient is symptomatic from the beginning of pregnancy. However, physical activity should be moderate, and prolonged periods of bed rest in the lateral supine position are beneficial and help to mobilize fluid that causes edema. The diet should be rich in high quality protein, especially if there is a considerable urinary loss of protein. Sodium intake may require adjustments if the patient is hypertensive and does not respond adequately to therapy or if there is excessive accumulation of sodium and water.

Hypertension. If the patient is hypertensive at the beginning of pregnancy, a serious effort should be carried out to reduce her blood pressure to a normal range with medications. Maximal doses of propranolol, methyldopa, and hydralazine should be used with diuretics added if necessary. If the blood pressure cannot be maintained within normal range with these drugs, the prognosis for the pregnancy outcome is poor and the chances of complications are high.

Hypertensive patients should be advised to obtain their own sphygmomanometer and measure their blood pressure daily at home. Highly motivated and intelligent patients should also be allowed to modify their therapeutic regimen by increasing or decreasing some of their medications in response to their blood pressure measurements.

If a previously normotensive patient with renal disease develops hypertension late in the second or third trimester of pregnancy, the diagnosis is preeclampsia, and pregnancy should be terminated if the hypertension becomes severe (greater than 120 mm Hg diastolic). All kinds of catastrophic events may occur when conservative therapy is adopted in cases of severe pregnancy-aggravated hypertension. These catastrophies usually happen when a diagnosis different from severe preeclampsia is entertained or when there is a predominant concern about the fate of the preterm infant.

Monitoring of renal function. The functional status of the kidneys should be monitored by determinations of serum creatinine every 4 to 6 weeks and by daily or every-other-day qualitative determinations for protein in the urine. At the beginning of the prenatal care a creatinine clearance determination is of value, but for subsequent checkups measurements of serum creatinine are adequate. In the majority of patients the initial serum creatinine concentration remains unaltered during pregnancy. Any significant elevation of serum creatinine (more than 0.2 mg/dl) requires repetition of the test, and if the elevation persists, evaluation with a creatinine clearance is indicated. It is unnecessary to order periodic 24-hour urine collections for quantitative protein determinations unless there is significant proteinuria as shown with Albustix strips. The patient should be instructed to check for albuminuria in the first urine voided every morning and to call the obstetrician if significant changes are apparent.

Excessive retention of sodium and water with marked peripheral edema is a frequent problem in the pregnant patient with renal disease. In these cases the first thing to do is to decrease working time, avoid prolonged periods of standing up or sitting, and increase the number of hours of daily rest in the lateral supine position. If these measures are not successful and the patient becomes uncomfortable with the accumulation of fluid that causes edema, diuretics may be used, but the degree of intravascular volume constriction caused by the diuretic should be monitored with serial hematocrit values to avoid a marked depletion and impairment of the placental blood flow.

If the patient has nephrotic syndrome, she should be managed as described earlier in that section. These patients often need intravenous albumin to partially compensate for their urinary losses, mobilize fluid out of the interstitial space, and maintain the integrity of their intravenous volume.

Fetal evaluation. The most reliable method for following fetal growth in pregnant patients with renal disease is by serial ultrasound determinations of the fetal biparietal diameter. The first ultrasound examination should be carried out between 20 and 22 weeks of gestation with

follow-up examination every 4 weeks thereafter. Any deviation from normal in these patients is significant and requires further investigation with measurements of the head/abdomen circumference ratio and initiation or continuation of nonstress testing to evaluate fetal well-being.

The renal patient who remains stable during pregnancy should be allowed to go to term and develop spontaneous labor. If the patient is unstable or symptomatic, delivery should be as soon as fetal pulmonary maturity is reached. A word of caution is necessary, however, about the use of tests for evaluating fetal lung maturation. If the mother becomes severely ill, there is no place for amniocentesis and lecithin/sphingomyelin (L/S) ratio determination, and immediate delivery is indicated. Frequently, amniocentesis and L/S ratio are carried out in these sick patients, and delivery is postponed at the expense of considerable maternal and fetal risks.

Specific problems

Chronic pyelonephritis. In pregnant patients with chronic pyelonephritis it is important to detect urinary tract infections and when they occur, to treat them vigorously. These patients often have chronic bacterial infections of the renal parenchyma that may flare up during pregnancy causing acute pyelonephritis, septic shock, and poor pregnancy outcome. Therefore they should have urine cultures every 4 to 6 weeks, and the finding of any pathogen should be followed by antibiotic treatment according to in vitro sensitivity testing. If there is a recurrence of the infection, the patient should receive urinary antibiotic prophylaxis (ampicillin 500 mg, nitrofurantoin 200 mg, or cephalosporin 500 mg) every night for the duration of pregnancy.

Hyponatremia may occur in pregnant patients with chronic pyelonephritis when they receive diruetics because these agents may intensify their sodium-losing tendency. In these cases they may exhibit a clinical syndrome similar to severe preeclampsia that improves with administration of sodium.

Renal transplants. Most patients with renal transplants tolerate pregnancy well if their kidney function is adequate and if hypertension is not present.[17] In most cases they are taking azathioprine and prednisone when they become pregnant, and they should continue taking these immunosuppressant agents during gestation. So far, no congenital malformations have been reported in these patients as a consequence of the use of these medications.

The most common problems with these patients are preterm labor and preterm delivery. Fortunately, this usually happens at a stage of pregnancy when the chances for fetal survival are excellent. In the management of patients with renal transplants delivery should be accomplished without delay if they develop preterm rupture of the membranes because of the risk of overwhelming infection.

Chronic hemodialysis. Few pregnant patients in chronic hemodialysis have been able to carry the pregnancy far enough to make fetal survival possible.[26] The large majority develop polyhydramnios and preterm labor and deliver immature infants who fail to survive. In most cases the frequency of dialysis has to be increased, and this is one reason for the high incidence of preterm labor, since often they develop regular contractions during dialysis.

One of the most difficult and frustrating experiences is to try to adjust the intravascular volume of the patient on dialysis to the level of expansion that occurs during normal pregnancy. It is probably better not to make special efforts to manipulate volume status.

■ REFERENCES

1. Assali NS, Brinkman CR: Disorders of maternal circulatory and respiratory adjustments, in Assali NS (ed): *Pathophysiology of Gestation*, New York, Academic Press, 1972, vol 1, pp. 270-347.
2. Bear RA: Pregnancy in patients with renal disease. Obstet Gynecol 1976;48:13.
3. Boyer M: Selectivity of proteinuria. Major Probl Clin Pediatr 1974;11:432.
4. Chesley LC: Disorders of kidney, fluids and electrolytes, in Assali NS (ed): *Pathophysiology of Gestation*, New York, Academic Press, 1972, vol. 1, pp. 355-478.
5. DeFelipe J, Timoner J, Velasco IT, et al: Treatment of refractory hypovolemic shock by 7.5% sodium chloride injections. Lancet 1980;2:1002.
6. Epstein M, Schneider NS, Befeler B: Effect of intrarenal furosemide on renal function and intrarenal hemodynamics in acute renal failure. Am J Med 1975;58:510.
7. Espinel CH: The FE$_{Na}$ test. JAMA 1976;236:579.
8. Fairley KF, Withworth JA, Kincaid-Smith P: Glomerulonephritis and pregnancy, in Kincaid-Smith P, Becker M (eds): *Perspectives in Nephrology and Hypertension*, New York, John Wiley & Sons, Inc, 1972, pp. 997-1011.
9. Felding CF: Obstetrics aspects in women with histories of renal disease. Acta Obstet Gynecol Scand 1969;48 (suppl 2):1.
10. Felding CF: The obstetric prognosis in chronic renal disease. Acta Obstet Gynecol Scand 1968;47:168.
11. Fries D, Pozet D, Dubois N, et al: The use of large doses of furosemide in acute renal failure. Postgrad Med J 1971;47(suppl):18.
12. Hollenberger NK, Epstein M, Rosen SM, et al: Acute oliguric renal failure in man: evidence of preferential renal cortical ischemia. Medicine 1968;47:455.
13. Kaplan BS, Drummond KN: The hemolytic-uremic syndrome is a syndrome. N Engl J Med 1978;298:904.
14. Knapp RC, Hellman LM: Acute renal failure in pregnancy. Am J Obstet Gynecol 1959;78:570.
15. LaHanzi DR, Cook WA: Urinary calculi in pregnancy. Obstet Gynecol 1980;56:462.
16. Llach F, Koffler A, Finck E, et al: On the incidence of renal vein thrombosis in the nephrotic syndrome. Arch Intern Med 1977;137:333.
17. Makowski EL, Penn I: Parenthood following renal transplantation, in de Alvarez RR (ed): *The Kidney in Pregnancy*, New York, John Wiley & Sons, Inc, 1976, pp. 215-227.
18. Oken DE: Chronic renal diseases and pregnancy: a review. Am J Obstet Gynecol 1966;94:1023.
19. O'Shaughnessy R, Wepsin SA, Zuspan FP: Obstructive renal failure by an overdistended uterus. Obstet Gynecol 1980;55:247.
20. Robin ED, Cross CE, Zelis R: Pulmonary edema. N Engl J Med 1973;288:239.
21. Robson JS, Martin AM, Rucley VA, et al: Irreversible postpartum renal failure. Q J Med 1968;37:423.
22. Schoolwerth AC, Sandler RC, Klahr S, et al: Nephrosclerosis postpartum and in women taking oral contraceptives. Arch Intern Med 1976;136:178.
23. Scully RE, Galdabini JJ, McNelly BI: Case records of the Massachusetts General Hospital. N Engl J Med 1978;299:136.
24. Smith K, Brown J, Shackman R, et al: Acute renal failure of obstetric origin: an analysis of 70 patients. Lancet 1965;2:351.
25. Strauch BS, Haylett JP: Kidney disease and pregnancy. Br Med J 1974;4:578.
26. Trebbin WM: Hemodialysis and pregnancy. JAMA 1979;241:1811.
27. Weisman SA, Simon NM, Herdon PB: Nephrotic syndrome in pregnancy. Am J Obstet Gynecol 1973;117:867.
28. West CD, McAdams AJ, McConvile JM, et al: Hypocomplementemic and normo-complementemic glomerulonephritis: clinical and pathological characteristics. J Pediatr 1965;67:1089.

14

■ ■ ■

MULTIPLE GESTATION

Fernando Arias

Few topics in obstetrics have stimulated more interest and generated more literature than the subject of multiple gestation. Communications on twins are not only abundant but extremely diverse reflecting the multidisciplinary approach to the study of this biologic phenomenon. Therefore it is not surprising that serious efforts have been made to unify all kinds of contributions on twins into a new branch of science named *gemellology*. In this chapter the emphasis is on the management of problems associated with twin gestations and the reasons behind the management, and only a small part is devoted to the study of gestations with higher fetal numbers. In fact, most of the different problems associated with twin gestations may be applied to triplet, quadruplet, and higher fetal number gestations. Also, the incidence of pregnancies with more than two infants is so low that there is no reason for a generous treatment of that subject in this book.

■ CLASSIFICATION

There are two types of twins: (1) monozygotic, identical, uniovular, or single-egg twins and (2) dizygotic, fraternal, biovular, nonidentical, or two-egg twins. Monozygotic twins have identical genotype and therefore are of the same sex. The similarity of their genetic composition is the result of their origin in the early division of an ovum singly fertilized by one sperm cell into two cell masses containing identical genetic information. In contrast, dizygotic twins are the result of the fertilization of two ova by different spermatozoids resulting in separate maternal and paternal genetic contributions to each infant.

The method most frequently used to determine the zygosity of twins is the examination of the placenta at birth.[4] This technique has significant possibilities for error and does not always permit an adequate classification. To minimize errors, the findings on gross examination should be confirmed by microscopic examination of a piece of the septum dividing the two fetal cavities. From a pathologic viewpoint placentae in twin gestation may be any of the following (Fig. 14-1):

1. Dichorionic-diamniotic
   a. Separated
   b. Fused
2. Monochorionic
   a. Monochorionic-monoamniotic
   b. Monochorionic-diamniotic

The finding of a monochorionic placenta is unequivocal proof of monozygosity. However, it is difficult in some cases to decide if a single placenta is monochorionic-diamniotic or a fused dichorionic-diamniotic. Also, the presence of a dichorionic-diamniotic placenta does not necessarily imply the existence of a dizygotic state, as it may represent separate implantations of

DICHORIONIC DIAMNIOTIC

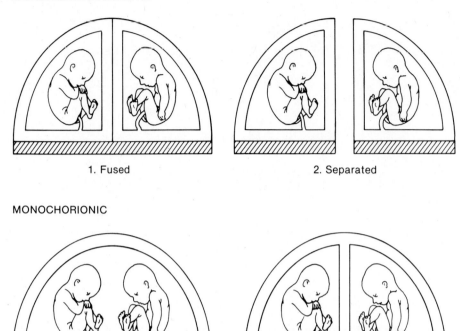

1. Fused   2. Separated

MONOCHORIONIC

3. Monoamniotic   4. Diamniotic

FIG. 14-1 ■ Placental morphology in twin pregnancy.

monozygotic twins. Approximately 80% of twin placentas are dichorionic, and 20% are monochorionic. In dichorionic-diamniotic placentae there is chorionic tissue present between the two amnions when the septum separating the two fetal sacs is examined. In monochorionic-diamniotic placentae the septum consists of two amnion layers without interposing chorion. Several other methods have been used with varied success to determine twin zygosity. Among them the study of blood groups and types (ABO, MNSs, Rh, Kell, Duffy, Kidd, etc) seems to be the most accurate.[39] Fingerprinting and histocompatibility studies may also be valuable.

■ INCIDENCE

The frequency of twinning is highest among the pure black race and consistently lowest among Orientals. The white race is between these two extremes. For example, in China there are 3 twins per each 1000 live births; in Scotland 12.3 per 1000; and in Nigeria 57.2 per 1000. These differences in frequency are the re-

sult of variations in double-ovum twinning because the rate of monozygotic twins is apparently constant (3.5 per 1000) throughout the world.

Factors influencing the frequency of dizygotic twinning are maternal age, parity, and conception soon after cessation of oral contraceptives. In fact, it has been reported that the incidence of twin gestation increases with maternal age (up to 35 to 39 years) and with parity. Also, studies show that if oral contraceptives have been used for more than 6 months and conception occurs within 1 month after discontinuation, the chances of a twin gestation doubles.

With the development of ultrasonic techniques for the evaluation of pregnancy it has become apparent that the incidence of multiple gestation in the human may be more common than indicated by the figures just given. In fact, the incidence of multiple gestation in a white population may be as high as 20 per 1000 pregnancies. The reason about half of these pregnancies fail to be recognized as twin gestations is that a high number of patients spontaneously

TABLE 14-1 ■ Causes of perinatal death in twins and singleton pregnancies in the United States

Cause	Perinatal deaths per 1000 births		
	Twins	Singleton	p
Amniotic fluid infection with intact membranes	22.6	5.9	<0.001
Premature rupture of membranes	15.9	3.5	<0.001
Fetal hypoxia of unknown cause	15.1	2.6	<0.001
Twin transfusion syndrome	11.7	—	
Congenital anomalies	10.1	3.2	<0.04
Large placental infarcts	10.9	2.1	<0.001
Hydramnios	8.3	0.1	<0.001
Overall perinatal mortality	138.7	33.4	<0.001

Data from the Collaborative Perinatal Project, in Naeye RL, et al: Am J Obstet Gynecol 1978;131:267.

abort early in pregnancy and another high number have spontaneous reabsorption of one of the gestational sacs. For example, in a recent study[36] 30 multiple pregnancies were found by first trimester ultrasonic examination among 1500 pregnant patients (incidence of 20 per 1000). Only 14 of these patients, however, produced live multiple-birth infants (13 twins and one set of triplets). In 7 of the 30 patients (23.3%) one of the sacs developed normally, and the other became smaller and showed no heart movements: two of them aborted, and the remaining five delivered single babies. The other nine patients (30%) of the original 30 aborted, eight early in pregnancy and one at 24 weeks of gestation. This and other studies[15] strongly suggest that the presence of a blighted ovum or the reabsorption of a gestational sac does not have any adverse effect on a coexisting normal pregnancy.

■ COMPLICATIONS

The mortality and morbidity of mother and infant are increased three to seven times in multiple gestations. The main causes of maternal mortality and morbidity are increased incidence of hypertension during pregnancy (14% to 20% in twins versus 6% to 8% in singleton pregnancies), sepsis associated with premature rupture of the fetal membranes (three times more frequent in twins than in singleton pregnancies), and excessive postpartum bleeding (about 20% of all twin pregnancies). The main problems affecting the fetal and neonatal outcome are preterm labor, premature rupture of the membranes, congenital abnormalities, umbilical cord

problems, abruptio placentae, placental transfusion syndrome, malpresentations, and other intrapartum complications. Table 14-1 compares the most frequent causes of perinatal mortality in twins and singleton pregnancies as found in the Collaborative Perinatal Project of the National Institute of Neurological and Communicative Disorders and Stroke.[23]

Hypertension

Most reviews of twin pregnancies agree on the existence of an increased frequency of preeclampsia and eclampsia in multiple versus singleton gestations. It is possible, however, that a considerable number of patients with twins develop hypertension and edema because of an excessive expansion of intravascular volume and are erroneously classified as having toxemia or preeclampsia. In these cases the glomerular filtration rate is increased, proteinuria is minimal or absent, and serial hematocrit determinations show expansion of plasma volume. These patients improve markedly with bed rest at home or at the hospital. However, it is important to recognize that the patient with multiple gestation may also develop vasoconstrictive preeclampsia that occasionally may be extremely severe. In these cases proteinuria is marked, and there is clinical and laboratory evidence of vasoconstriction and decreased intravascular volume.

Anemia

Maternal anemia is frequently quoted as a common complication of twin pregnancy. It has been demonstrated[30] that the largest degree of intravascular volume expansion in pregnancy occurs during twin gestation. Since the predominant element in the expansion is the plasma volume, the net result is a drop in hematocrit and hemoglobin levels, especially during the second trimester. In reality, these patients have an active hematopoiesis, and their total red cell volume is larger than at the beginning of pregnancy. This large increase in red cell synthesis during a twin pregnancy may exhaust limited iron storages in some women and become the trigger of an iron-deficiency anemia. The best way to differentiate between physiologic hemodilution and iron-deficiency anemia in patients with twin gestation is to examine their blood smear. The presence of red cells with adequate hemoglobin content shown by their homogenous staining rules out iron-deficiency anemia. In contrast, the presence of a dimorphic red cell population in which a large number of erythrocytes exhibit a pale central core is diagnostic of iron-deficiency anemia. A similar assessment may also be obtained (at a larger cost) by measuring the serum iron and the serum iron binding capacity and calculating the percentage of saturation of the iron transport protein, which is more than 15% under normal circumstances.

Postpartum bleeding

In most cases severe postpartum bleeding following the delivery of twins is a consequence of uterine atony that in turn is directly related to the enlargement reached by the uterus during gestation. Postpartum hemorrhage is more common in twin pregnancies delivered near term when the uterine muscle fibers have been stretched to their maximum. This complication may be prevented by aggressive use of oxytocic agents immediately after delivery of the placenta. If excessive bleeding occurs in spite of adequate use of oxytocin, the intramyometrial administration of prostaglandin $F_{2\alpha}$ may be life-saving.[12] Additional information about the management of postpartum hemorrhage may be found in Chapter 19.

Preterm birth

The single largest factor associated with fetal and neonatal mortality and morbidity in twin gestation is low birth weight. A review of 26

large series of twin pregnancies[25] shows that 55.85% of twins have a birth weight under 2500 grams. Since low birth weight overshadows any other risk factor in twin gestation, investigators have tried to find the etiology of this problem with the goal of attacking it at its roots. In the large majority of cases low birth weight in twins results from preterm birth. Thus the crux of the problem is to find out if preterm birth in twins is a natural consequence of crowding and constriction of the intrauterine environment or if it is the result of a high prevalence of certain pathologic problems specific to this type of gestation.

The first hypothesis—that is, preterm birth as a natural consequence of twinning—blames overstretching of the uterine muscle and decreased uteroplacental blood flow as the main reasons for the onset of preterm labor. There is limited experimental support for these ideas in contrast to the large popularity they enjoy in textbooks and review articles. In fact, the hypothesis that uterine distensibility is the factor limiting length of gestation in twins comes from comparative observations of length of gestation versus litter number and size in humans[20] and in other species. The data show an inverse correlation between uterine stretching and initiation of parturition but are not adequate to demonstrate a cause-effect relationship.

The evidence for the existence of decreased uteroplacental blood flow in twin gestation comes from experiments in which the clearance of $^{24}NaCl$ injected into the placenta was taken as an expression of the blood flow through the organ.[21] The difference between normal and twin pregnancies found in this experiment was small, and its significance was not calculated. Also, this work is hampered by large possibilities of error and has not been validated using more precise techniques. However, the prolongation of twin gestations with beta mimetics and bed rest may be taken as indirect evidence that decreased uteroplacental blood flow is a determinant of the onset of parturition in these patients.

The second hypothesis about the cause of preterm birth in twins is rather recent and comes mainly from the Collaborative Perinatal Project.[23] In this study autopsies were carried out on 171 twin and 1264 single-born infants, and the causes of death were analyzed and compared. Amniotic fluid infection with intact membranes or with preterm rupture of the fetal membranes was the single leading cause of perinatal mortality in twins. It seems that the excessive growth of the uterus in twin gestation results in an early opening of the cervix and a larger degree of exposure of the fetal membranes to the bacterial flora of the vagina, leading to amnionitis with intact membranes and in more severe cases to amnionitis with ruptured membranes. Variations in the virulence of the vaginal pathogens would account for differences in the severity and natural history of the process. This evidence implying that infection may be the most important cause of preterm birth in twin gestation needs validation. If further evidence suggesting that infection is the major cause of preterm birth in twins is collected, it may change completely our present approach to the antenatal management of multiple pregnancies.

Twin transfusion syndrome

Twin transfusion syndrome is a complication affecting 4% of all twin pregnancies and is unique to monochorionic twins. The problem is created by the existence of vascular communications between the infants causing a circulatory imbalance that results in anemia for one of them and polycythemia for the other. Since there is wide variation in the number and size of the vascular anastomosis, the degree of hematologic imbalance between the twins may also vary greatly. The existence of this syndrome is considered certain if there is a difference in hemoglobin concentration greater than 5 g/dl. This difference may be large, more than 15 g/dl.

The twin transfusion syndrome carries a perinatal mortality as high as 66%.[27] In fact, the effects of the parabiotic circulation are often severe for both the donor and the recipient. The recipient, as a consequence of the maximally increased intravascular volume, often develops cardiomegaly and congestive heart failure. Recipients frequently die in uterus and when born alive, may develop respiratory distress and congestive heart failure in the first 1 or 2 hours of life. They also frequently develop hyperbilirubinemia. Because of anemia the donor has retarded somatic growth and if the lack of red cells is severe, the donor develops hydrops fetalis and high output heart failure.

In monochorionic-diamniotic placentations polyhydramnios occurs frequently in the sac of the polycythemic twin and oligohydramnios in the donor twin. Thus the diagnosis of twin transfusion syndrome is strongly suggested by the development of polyhydramnios in discordant twins (see the following discussion), especially if the excessive amount of amniotic fluid is located in the amniotic sac of the larger twin. As previously mentioned, a positive diagnosis can only be made at birth by finding a significant difference in hemoglobin concentration between the infants.

If this complication is suspected in the antenatal period, the obstetrician should terminate the pregnancy as soon as evidence of fetal lung maturation of both infants is obtained. The smaller, anemic twin usually achieves lung maturation earlier than the other, and glucocorticoids should be used to accelerate lung surfactant production in the recipient twin. Once the infants are delivered, their respective hemoglobin/hematocrit values should be determined, and bleeding with or without blood for plasma exchange of the plethoric twin and transfusion of the anemic twin should be carried out as soon as possible after birth.

Congenital abnormalities

Congenital malformations occur more often in twins than in singleton pregnancies. This fact has been constant in all studies on perinatal mortality and morbidity in twins, but there is some variation in the figures reported by different investigators. Hendricks[9] in his review of 438 multiple pregnancies found an incidence of congenital abnormalities of 10.6% for twins versus 3.3% for all births. Guttmacher and Schuyler[6] in their analysis of 1327 twin deliveries found 6.86% of twins and 3.98% of singletons had congenital abnormalities. In the material collected for the Collaborative Perinatal Project[23] the malformation rate was 17.4% and 17.2% in monochorionic and dichorionic twins, respectively. However, malformations among monochorionic twins were multiple or lethal, whereas those occurring on dichorionic infants were mostly minor. The congenital abnormalities affecting twin pregnancies are mostly multifactorial. The most common are harelip, cleft palate, central nervous system defects, and heart defects.

Conjoined twins

An interesting anomaly that is unique to multiple pregnancy is the presence of conjoined twins. This is a rare complication affecting 1 of every 900 twin pregnancies and one out of every 50,000 deliveries. Conjoined twins are monovular and have the same sex and karyotype. The phenomenon occurs predominantly in females (female to male ratio of 3:1), and its cause is unknown. As the best explanation for the occurrence of this problem, most investigators favor an incomplete fission of the embryonic inner cell mass rather than a partial fusion of two separate centers of growth. In any case the phenomenon happens early in gestation, most probably before the second week after fertilization.

Conjoined twins are classified according to the site of union of their bodies. The different types include the following[14]:

Thoracopagus, (40%), joined at the chest

Omphalopagus or xylopagus (35%), joined at the anterior abdominal wall

Pygopagus (18%), joined at the buttocks

Ischiopagus (6%), joined at the ischium

Craniopagus (2%), joined at the head

The antepartum diagnosis of conjoined twins is possible if an effort is made to rule out the presence of this condition in all cases of twin gestation. As is discussed later in the section on diagnosis, if a twin pregnancy is suspected on clinical grounds, a sonographic evaluation should be obtained to confirm the diagnosis. If twins are discovered by ultrasound, the examination should include a careful inspection of the thorax and abdomen of the infants, especially if they are in the same position (vertex-vertex or breech-breech) or if it is difficult to separate the sonographic images of the two fetuses. If the ultrasound examination is suggestive of conjoined twins, a fetogram should be obtained and careful attention paid to the presence or absence of the following criteria formulated by Gray[5] for the diagnosis of this situation:

1. The twins face each other.
2. The heads are at the same level and plane.
3. The thoracic cages are in unusual proximity.
4. Both fetal heads are hyperextended.
5. There is no change in the relative position of the fetuses with movement, manipulation, or in repeat film obtained hours or days later.

If the sonogram and fetogram are suggestive of conjoined twins, the diagnosis should be confirmed by introducing 15 ml of Lipiodol (fat-soluble radiopaque material) and 40 ml of Conray-75 (water-soluble radiopaque material) into the amniotic cavity. This technique (amniography) makes it possible to demonstrate the existence and location of the union between the fetuses. Repeated ultrasound examinations and computed tomography (CT) scanning may be useful to determine antenatally the presence or absence of cardiac connections between the twins.[7]

Once the diagnosis of conjoined twins is made, plans should be formulated to terminate the pregnancy by the abdominal route unless there are special circumstances indicating the possibility of a safe vaginal delivery. If allowed to labor, the overwhelming majority of conjoined twin gestations will show abnormal patterns of cervical dilation and descent. In many cases reported in the literature abnormal labor is the first clinical sign in the chain of events leading to the diagnosis of conjoined twins.

The first successful surgical separation of conjoined twins was achieved in 1953. Because of recent advances in organ imaging (ultrasound, angiography, CT scanning), it is possible to obtain at the present time a more accurate assessment of the characteristics of the union between conjoined twins and the feasibility of separation than it was 20 years ago. The absence of malformations, the lack of bone unions, and the existence of separate hearts are the most important indicators of the possibility of a successful surgical outcome.

Fetal malpresentations during labor

There is a high incidence of fetal malpresentations at the time of delivery in twin gestations. In the review by Farooqui et al[2] the relative frequency of different fetal presentations was as follows:

Vertex-vertex	39.6%
Vertex-breech	27.7%
Vertex-transverse	7.2%
Breech-breech	9.0%
Breech-vertex	6.9%
Breech-transverse	3.6%
Other combinations	6.9%

A rare malpresentation occurring with the same frequency as conjoined twins (one case per every 1000 twins and per every 50,000 births) is the *interlocking of twins*. The perinatal mortality of this complication is high (62% to 84%)

probably because most cases are recognized late in the expulsive phase of labor. A typical case is a primipara who has generous pelvic measurements and twins in a breech-vertex presentation and who is allowed to deliver vaginally. Everything proceeds smoothly until the moment when twin A is partially delivered and the obstetrician finds an unusual amount of difficulty in delivering the infant head that remains high in the pelvis. Manual examination at this time reveals the head of twin B interposed between the body and the head of twin A. In most cases attempts to move up twin B's head using combined pelvic and abdominal maneuvers fail, and it is necessary to proceed to an emergency cesarean section. Death for twin A is an almost certain outcome.

To avoid a disastrous sequence of events such as that just described, it is necessary to rule out interlocking twins in every case of breech-vertex presentation that is going to be allowed to be delivered vaginally. Interlocking may also happen in the course of vertex-vertex, vertex-transverse, and breech-breech presentations, but the overwhelming majority of cases are breech-vertex. Perhaps the first indicator that the condition is present is the development of an abnormal labor pattern, usually an arrest disorder. In these cases it is necessary to obtain anteroposterior and lateral x-ray films of the twins and to repeat the films after 2 hours of active labor.[3] If the head of twin B is descending below the level of the head of twin A suggesting collision of the twins, cesarean-section delivery will be the most adequate method of delivery.

■ DIAGNOSIS

One of the most important contributions of the obstetrician to the successful outcome of a twin pregnancy is early diagnosis. In fact, studies demonstrate that perinatal losses are significantly larger when the diagnosis of twin gestation is made after 28 weeks as compared with cases diagnosed earlier in pregnancy. The reason for the improved outcome is that early diagnosis allows early implementation of measures that may be important in the prevention of prematurity. Early diagnosis is also important in allowing a planned approach to the delivery of the twins, thus avoiding the improvisation and mistakes that usually happen when the diagnosis is made in the delivery room. Unfortunately, as

many as 50% of twin pregnancies remain undiagnosed until the time of delivery,[2] although there has been a considerable improvement since the advent of real-time ultrasound.

The optimal method for the early diagnosis of twins is examination with real-time ultrasound.[17] Before the development of this technique x-ray examination and static B-scan ultrasound were the most reliable methods. Roentgenography should be avoided if possible during pregnancy and may be difficult to interpret if the examination is carried out before there is significant calcification of the bone structure of the fetuses. Static B-scan ultrasound may give as high as 10% false negative results mainly because the continuous changes in the position of the fetus in early pregnancy generate a major problem for static imaging. Also, static B-scan requires a good amount of technician time and expertise. Conversely, real-time ultrasound is not affected in its accuracy by the presence of fetal movement that may be visualized and used as a diagnostic index. Also, the chorioamniotic membrane separating the twins is more easily visualized with real-time than with static B-scan ultrasound. Once the diagnosis of twin gestation is established early in pregnancy, further examinations may be carried out using static B-scan ultrasound.

Even though modern echography permits an early diagnosis of multiple pregnancy in almost 100% of the cases, an important problem remains—the adequate selection of patients at risk for twin gestation who should be screened with real-time ultrasound. An easy solution would be the scanning of the entire obstetric population, but this would be extremely costly and unrealistic for such a large group. The selection of a "high risk for twins" group using serum determination of human placental lactogen[32] or alpha fetoprotein[38] in the overall obstetric population is also costly and lacks the accuracy of screening with real-time ultrasound. Under these circumstances the selection of patients at risk for twin pregnancy should be made by clinical means. If that is the case, the cardinal rule for the obstetrician is the following:

> **The presence of a uterine size that is larger than expected for the patient's dates requires examination with real-time ultrasound to rule out a multiple gestation.**

In addition to a discrepancy between the uterine size and the patient's dates, other useful clinical criteria for suspecting the existence of a twin pregnancy include pregnancy achieved through the use of fertility agents, family history of twins, auscultation of two fetal hearts, and abdominal palpation of three fetal poles. There is no substitute, however, for early initiation of prenatal care followed by careful, meticulous evaluation of the growth of the uterus as the basic elements for recognizing the presence of a multiple pregnancy.

■ ANTEPARTUM MANAGEMENT

Once the diagnosis of twin gestation is made, the efforts of the obstetrician must be directed toward prevention of preterm birth, evaluation of fetal growth, and determination of the best mode of delivery.

The most commonly used measures for the prevention of preterm birth and low birth weight in twins are bed rest and administration of beta mimetic agents. Also, in view of the findings of the Collaborative Perinatal Study, it is possible that eradication of bacterial pathogens present in the urogenital tract of the mother may be of benefit in preventing amnionitis with or without rupture of the fetal membranes. Another modality of treatment, the surgical cerclage of the uterine cervix, should be mentioned only to indicate that this therapy has not been rigorously evaluated.

Bed rest

Bed rest is widely used for the prevention of preterm labor in twin pregnancies. The rationale behind its use is that bed rest in the lateral position reduces pressure on the cervix and causes an increase in uteroplacental blood flow. The increase in blood flow in turn has a quiescent effect on myometrial contractility.

There are several reports, mainly from European literature, showing the positive effect of bed rest on prolongation of pregnancy and infant birth weight in twin pregnancies. Unfortunately, none of the studies have been carried out following adequate methodology or have been rigorously designed to avoid patient selection bias. Other equally poorly designed studies have concluded that bed rest in twin pregnancies has a questionable therapeutic value and adds a significant cost to the patient's care. A solution to the controversy about the role of bed rest in twin pregnancy is of extreme importance; this is an area in which a controlled trial is necessary.

Even if it is accepted that bed rest improves the outcome of twin pregnancies, there is no clear definition as to when bed rest should be started and when it should be stopped. As to when to begin, the retrospective study of Jeffrey et al[13] at the University of Colorado shows that if deliveries of twins occurring before 30 weeks of gestation are excluded from consideration, bed rest does not significantly change perinatal mortality or length of gestation. It is clear that the worst morbidity and mortality caused by preterm labor in twins occur before 30 weeks of gestation; consequently, bed rest probably should be started as early as possible after the diagnosis is made. Another retrospective study by Powers and Miller,[26] in agreement with the Colorado data, shows that twins are most vulnerable if born between 27 and 34 weeks. The tentative conclusion is that bed rest should begin before the initiation of that critical period (before 27 weeks) and finish after 34 weeks when the chances of the infants' survival are almost 100%. Some obstetricians prefer to stop bed rest after obtaining evidence of fetal lung maturation by amniotic fluid analysis rather than after an arbitrary period of weeks of gestation.

Beta mimetics

Several papers in the literature indicate a role for beta mimetic drugs in twin pregnancy. In one of them[34] 42 patients with twin pregnancies were treated with Salbutamol from the time of diagnosis, and their outcome was compared with an equal number of matched twin pregnancies who were treated with bed rest alone. The treated patients received an amount of Salbutamol that kept the maternal pulse above 100 beats per minute during weekly checks. The authors found a significant increase in the length of gestation and in the birth weight in the Salbutamol-treated group. Only four of the Salbutamol-treated babies weighed less than 2000 grams, and only one infant weighed less than 1500 grams. It is not clear in this study, however, if there was a significant difference at the time of initiation of therapy between the gestational age of the infants in the bed rest group and those who received Salbutamol or if there were significant differences in the duration of treatment for each group.

As in the case of bed rest, the administration

of beta mimetics to a pregnant woman causes an increase in uteroplacental blood flow. Beta mimetic drugs are powerful tocolytic agents not only through the increase in blood flow but also through a process that involves synthesis of myometrial cyclic adenosine monophosphate (AMP) (see Chapter 3). It is possible that beta mimetics not only prevent premature uterine activity but also may be useful in promoting fetal growth and development.

Infection surveillance and control

As mentioned previously, the data from the Collaborative Perinatal Project[23] indicate that infection of the amniotic membranes, which may or may not cause a premature rupture, is the most common pathologic finding underlying prematurity in twin gestations. This information should be incorporated into the management of twin pregnancies, and infections of the urinary tract, the cervix, and the vagina in the patient carrying twins must be aggressively treated to avoid propagation into the amnion. Urine, cervical, and vaginal cultures should be part of the care of the patient with twins, and adequate antibiotic treatment should follow the identification of pathogens in any of those organs.

Monitoring of fetal growth

Alterations in fetal growth that happen frequently in twin gestations are the initial indicator of the possibility of fetal and neonatal distress and death. Thus monitoring of fetal growth has become an essential component of the antenatal management of twin pregnancies, with serial measurements of the fetal biparietal diameter (BPD) being the most commonly used method of following fetal growth.

There are conflicting results among different studies on BPD growth in twin gestations. The data of Leveno et al[16] and Schneider et al[29] indicate that the growth of normal twin fetuses is different from the growth of singletons. According to these authors, the BPD of a twin is consistently smaller throughout gestation than the BPD of a singleton, with the difference averaging 3.5 mm between 16 and 40 weeks of gestation. This difference may be difficult to detect, since the error inherent in BPD measurements is about 2 mm, but it is of extreme importance because it may cause underevaluation of the gestational age of twin babies. The data of Leveno et al,[16] showing that twins are consistently small-

er than singletons from term as far back as week 16 of gestation, are in contradiction with data from Naeye et al[22] who found that twin weight was similar to singleton weight until 33 weeks of gestation and smaller thereafter. Naeye's findings suggest a relative lack of ability of the uteroplacental circulation near term to adequately supply nutrients for the full development of multiple pregnancies.

The data of Crane et al[1] are also in contradiction with the conclusions of Leveno et al.[16] These investigators have shown that BPD standards derived from observations of singleton pregnancies can be applied to twins even in the third trimester. They also have shown that BPD discordance alone cannot be taken as absolute evidence of markedly different twin size; they recommend that when the BPD difference between twins is 5 mm or more, the head circumference of the infants should be measured. Only if there is a difference greater than 5% in the head circumferences should the diagnosis of discordancy be accepted. The same group of investigators[1] also demonstrated that BPD discordancy has a more serious prognosis when it occurs early in gestation because it is suggestive of twin to twin transfusion syndrome.

The main problem that the obstetrician attempts to detect through ultrasound monitoring of a twin pregnancy is the presence of discordant fetal growth. In fact, if a significant difference in the BPD of twins is detected, the possibility of catastrophic events becomes distinctly clear. According to Houlton,[10] when the BPD difference before delivery was between 2 and 6 mm, the incidence of growth retardation at birth was 40%; when the difference was 6 mm or more, the incidence of small-for-gestational age infants at birth was 71%. In the work of Haney et al[8] 6.8 mm was the mean value for the BPD difference in a group of twin pregnancies in which intrauterine fetal death or severe intrauterine growth retardation happened after the initial scan.

In summary, every twin pregnancy should be followed with serial BPD measurements. If discordant BPDs are detected, there is a possibility that intervention and preterm delivery will be necessary. When the BPD difference between twins exceeds 5 mm, the head circumference should be measured, and if they differ more than 5%, the diagnosis of discordancy is almost certain.

Amniocentesis and lung maturation

Since evaluation of fetal lung maturation is often required in the management of twin pregnancies, especially in cases of discordant fetal growth, the question arises about the need for amniotic fluid studies of each separate sac. The evidence collected so far[31,33,37] indicates that lung maturation in normal twins happens at the same time, and therefore the information obtained through the biochemical analysis of the content of one amniotic sac may be applied to the other. However, this general rule does not apply to twins with discordant growth. In these cases the problem usually is the status of lung maturation in the larger twin. In fact, the growth-retarded twin has a more advanced degree of lung maturity than the other. A serious error may occur if a premature delivery is carried out on the basis of mature biochemical indexes in the amniotic liquor of the growth-retarded twin because the outcome of the case may be the death of both infants: the normally grown twin may die because of severe hyaline membrane disease, and the growth-retarded twin could die as a consequence of intrauterine malnutrition and hypoxia. Therefore in cases of discordant twins requiring premature delivery, the timing of delivery should be based on the biochemical analysis of the amniotic fluid surrounding the larger twin.

Summary of antenatal management

In summary, once twins are diagnosed, the following rules should be observed:

1. The patient should be scheduled for office visits every 2 weeks. Attention should be paid during those visits to the presence of abnormalities in blood pressure, urine composition, uterine fundal growth, and fetal movements.
2. The patient should be scheduled for ultrasonic measurements of the fetal BPD every 4 weeks to detect discordant fetal growth.
3. Cultures should be obtained from urine, cervix, and vagina. If pathogen bacteria (*Escherichia coli*, group B streptococci, *Neisseria gonorrhoeae*, *Haemophilus influenzae*, etc) are detected, they should be treated with an adequate antibiotic.
4. The patient should be counseled to stop working and to rest in the lateral position for a minimum of 2 hours each morning and afternoon and sleep at least 10 hours each night. More rest may become necessary if pelvic examinations show evidence of progressive cervical effacement and dilation.
5. Vaginal examination should be a part of every office visit beginning between 20 and 24 weeks of gestation with the purpose of detecting as early as possible the occurrence of cervical changes indicating a high possibility of preterm labor. In the course of the examination the obstetrician should avoid the introduction of the fingers through the cervix. This manuever causes prostaglandin release with production of contractions and places a rather large inoculum of vaginal bacteria in close contact with the amniotic membranes. At least initially, what should be observed with the vaginal examination is the development of the lower uterine segment and the length of the cervix. The finding of a bulging low segment and a short (less than 0.5 cm) cervix is indicative of a high risk for preterm delivery. In these cases administration of beta mimetics (terbutaline sulfate 2.5 to 5.0 mg orally four times a day) and progesterone (Delalutin 250 mg IM every week) should be initiated at 20 weeks of gestation and continued until 36 weeks with the objective of preventing the onset of preterm labor.
6. Administration of glucocorticoids (dexamethasone or betamethasone 12 mg IM per day during 2 consecutive days at 28 weeks of gestation, followed by 12 mg pulses every week as long as the patient remains undelivered and until 34 weeks of gestation) to accelerate fetal lung maturation should be part of the management of every twin gestation for which premature birth is a strong possibility, such as patients showing a discordant growth pattern in serial ultrasound, patients showing cervical changes indicative of a high probability of preterm delivery, and patients showing poor compliance with bed rest and medications.
7. If discordant fetal growth is observed in serial ultrasound examinations, weekly fetal reactivity testing of the slow growing twin should be instituted when the head

circumference difference is greater than 5%. The probability that the small twin is growth retarded is large, and early delivery may become necessary to avoid intrauterine fetal death. Evaluation of lung maturation and the use of glucocorticoids in the unaffected twin is pertinent if the lecithin/sphingomyelin ratio or the Foam Stability Index test shows lack of maturity. As mentioned previously, it should be assumed that the lung maturity of the small twin is better than that of the large twin. Estriol and human placental lactogen determinations are useless as a means of evaluating the state of the small twin in cases of discordant fetal growth.

■ MANAGEMENT OF LABOR AND DELIVERY

One of the most important decisions in the intrapartum management of a twin gestation is to choose between vaginal or cesarean-section delivery. Ideally, this decision should be made when the patient is in the early stages of labor. In fact, in a large proportion of cases of twin pregnancies with poor outcomes, fetal mortality and morbidity can be assigned to intrapartum problems that could have been prevented if the overall situation had been carefully analyzed at the beginning of labor.

The most important elements in the decision between vaginal versus cesarean-section delivery are the assessment of the gestational age of the twins and their presentation at the time of labor. Ideally, the gestational age should be known exactly, but in reality a large number of patients with twins have uncertain dates or confusing prenatal information derived from the large size of the uterus in relation to their dates. In the latter cases the obstetrician must use all the available elements such as dates and ultrasound and fetogram to assess the gestational age of the twins.

To determine the presentation of the twins a fetogram should be obtained from every twin gestation patient in labor. The fetogram should be obtained, even if the patient had a recent ultrasound examination, to avoid mistakes caused by variability of the fetal position and errors in ultrasonic evaluation because of intrauterine crowding. A fetogram at the time of labor avoids the surprise and frustration of finding

twins in vertex-vertex presentation during a cesarean section, when an ultrasound examination obtained a few days before the surgery had shown a vertex-breech or vertex-transverse presentation. The fetogram also provides information about some congenital abnormalities not detected during ultrasound scanning.

If the twins are under 34 weeks of gestation and delivery is imminent, unavoidable, or indicated, they must be delivered by cesarean section unless both are in vertex presentation. The objective of this policy is to avoid the fetal trauma and the hypoxic insult frequently associated with the vaginal delivery of preterm infants in presentations other than vertex.

Another situation requiring cesarean-section delivery in twin pregnancies is the presence of a single amniotic sac for both infants. The fetal mortality in these rare monoamniotic gestations is greater than 50%, and the overwhelming cause is cord accidents such as cord prolapse or entanglement of the cords. Therefore if a membrane separating the twins is not visualized by real-time ultrasound, it must be assumed that a single sac is present, and the pregnancy must be terminated by cesarean section.

If the pregnancy is at term and the first twin is in transverse lie or in a breech presentation, cesarean section is the adequate way of delivery. In fact, to allow vaginal delivery a first twin in breech presentation has to fulfill all the conditions required for vaginal delivery of a singleton breech (see Chapter 17). Therefore if the fetal head is hyperextended, cesarean section must be carried out to avoid transection of the fetal spinal cord. Another factor that makes the vaginal delivery of a first twin in breech presentation riskier than in a singleton breech is the possibility of interlocking of the twins. Admittedly, this is an infrequent complication, but when it happens, it is usually discovered at a moment in labor when it is too late to save the life of the infant. Early detection of interlocking requires taking anteroposterior and lateral x-ray films of all patients with fetuses in breech-vertex presentation who are allowed to deliver vaginally to evaluate the pattern of descent of both fetal heads.

The main problem making breech presentation of a second twin unusually dangerous as compared with singletons is the high chance of cord prolapse. In fact, singleton babies in frank

---

Indications for cesarean-section delivery in twin pregnancy

Monoamniotic twins
Premature twins $\longrightarrow$ All cases

First twin $\longrightarrow$ $\begin{cases} \text{Breech presentation} \\ \text{Transverse lie} \end{cases}$

Second twin $\longrightarrow$ $\begin{cases} \text{Any breech with hyperextended head} \\ \text{Transverse lie that remains unchanged after delivery} \\ \quad \text{of the first twin} \end{cases}$

---

breech presentation fill the low uterine segment and the vagina with their buttocks preventing the occurrence of cord prolapse, but second twin breech infants are high within a uterus that remains large and flaccid after the birth of the first twin. They do not occlude the birth canal, and if the membranes rupture spontaneously or artificially or if there is only one amniotic sac (monoamniotic twins), the probability of a cord prolapse is high (overall incidence of 4.2% in twins). Another problem is the frequent use of manual and instrumental maneuvering by the obstetrician when a second twin is in breech presentation. This is a consequence of the desire to keep the time between delivery of the infants as short as possible. These obstetric manuevers, however, carry an unacceptably high fetal mortality and morbidity.

The complications just mentioned (cord prolapse, trauma) associated with the vaginal delivery of second twins in breech presentation do not constitute absolute contraindications to labor and vaginal delivery. In fact, the indications for operative intervention based on the presentation of the second twin are more limited than for the first twin (see box above), and only breeches with hyperextension of the head are legitimate indications for cesarean section. Second twins in other presentations (breech presentation with normally flexed head and transverse lies) should be allowed to labor unless there is an operative indication based on the presentation of the first twin.

The reason a transverse lie in the first twin is an indication for cesarean section though it is not in the second twin has to do with the stability of the presentation. It is exceptional that a first twin in transverse lie changes position during labor. In contrast, a transverse lie in a second

twin is unstable and easily changes to vertex or to breech after delivery of the first infant. Only a few of these infants remain in transverse lie after the delivery of the first twin, and they require delivery by cesarean section.

Vaginal delivery

If a patient with twins is allowed to labor and vaginal delivery is anticipated, oxytocin may be used if necessary in the course of labor.

Analgesia should be kept to a minimum, and ideally only paracervical and pudendal blocks are to be used to relieve marked maternal discomfort. Electronic monitoring should include both twins; this can be done by using a simple technique[28] for the coupling of the intrauterine pressure transducer to two fetal heart tone monitoring instruments. In *all* cases once the first twin is delivered, electronic monitoring of the second twin is mandatory to detect signs of fetal hypoxia that may result from a partial placental separation following the birth of the first twin, but this occurs rarely. Twins must be delivered in a delivery room prepared for the performance of an emergency cesarean section because of fetal distress in the second twin, and the necessary personnel (nurses, anesthesiologist, etc) must be on standby until the second twin is delivered.

In the past it was thought that the interval between delivery of the first and second twin was important for the fetal outcome. Little and Friedman[18] found a perinatal mortality of 22.2% when the interval was less than 5 minutes, 7.3% when the interval was between 5 and 15 minutes, and 29.3% when the interval exceeded 15 minutes. Thus came the recommendation of an ideal interval of 5 to 15 minutes between the delivery of twin A and twin B. In the more recent series of Farooqui et al[2] 54.6% of second twins were delivered after an interval of less than 5 minutes, and the corrected neonatal mortality was 1.1%; an additional 84 infants (25.2%) were delivered from 6 to 10 minutes after twin A, and the mortality was 1.2%. These data invalidate the need for a minimal interval of 5 minutes between births. The greatest danger with a prolonged interval between twin deliveries is unrecognized placental separation causing fetal hypoxia and fetal bleeding. This does not happen frequently. In contrast, there are reports in the literature of intervals of several weeks between the deliveries of healthy twin infants.[35]

As stated before, electronic monitoring of twin B should be started or continued after the delivery of the first infant. If the monitoring trace is normal and uterine contractions have not resumed in 10 minutes, augmentation with intravenous oxytocin should be started. The bag of waters of the second twin must *not* be ruptured until the presenting part of the second infant is firmly engaged in the pelvis. To do otherwise is to risk the occurrence of cord prolapse. Once the presenting part is engaged, the membranes are ruptured and a scalp electrode for direct fetal heart rate monitoring is applied. As long as the monitoring trace remains normal, there is no reason to speed the delivery. If a sinusoidal rhythm (indicative of fetal anemia) or a pattern of late decelerations with loss of beat-to-beat variability (indicative of fetal distress) is detected, the pregnancy should be terminated immediately by cesarean section or forceps.

When the second twin is in transverse lie, the real-time ultrasound equipment should be available in the delivery room to monitor a possible change in lie. The obstetrician influences that change by applying pressure with the ultrasound transducer and external palpation of the uterus. No *intrauterine* maneuvers are carried out to influence or determine a change in presentation. If the infant converts to a breech or a vertex spontaneously or with the help of external manipulation of the uterus, the possibilities of a safe vaginal delivery are excellent. If the infant remains in a transverse lie, pregnancy should be terminated by cesarean section. Some obstetricians perform total breech extractions in cases of transverse lie or breech presentations. The expertise of the obstetrician in intrauterine manipulation is the most important factor in this decision. If that expertise does not exist, the safe

management is a cesarean section. It is not acceptable obstetric practice to perform internal version and total breech extraction for the delivery of a second twin in vertex presentation. This is a maneuver that has no place in modern obstetrics because of its lethal and morbid consequences on the fetus.

After delivery of the second twin and placenta, the attention of the obstetrician should be directed to the prevention of postpartum hemorrhage. Intravenous oxytocin (30 units in 1000 ml of 5% dextrose in lactated Ringer's solution) should be administered, and ergonovine and prostaglandin $F_{2\alpha}$ should be available if the uterus is unresponsive to oxytocin administration.

Cesarean-section delivery

The ideal anesthesia for the cesarean-section delivery of twins is epidural anesthesia because it allows a systematic and unhurried approach to the delivery of the infants without fetal hypoxia or depression caused by the transplacental passage of general anesthetics. Ideally, epidural anesthesia should be administered by an obstetric anesthesiologist who is aware of the peculiarities of twin pregnancy and is ready to prevent and treat the hemodynamic changes caused by the anesthetic blockade.

The best abdominal wall incision for the delivery of twins is a vertical incision. It can be made quickly, the blood loss is smaller than in transverse incisions, it gives a great deal of room for manipulation of abnormal presentations, and it allows a better exploration of the abdominal cavity. Also, it is easier to close and does not offer unusual difficulties when reintervention (repeated cesarean section) is necessary. The disadvantages are a higher chance of dehiscence and a less acceptable esthetic result than with transverse incision.

The best incision on the uterine wall is a transverse incision. Any vertical uterine incision condemns the patient to the threat of spontaneous uterine rupture and to termination of future pregnancies by repeated cesarean section. In contrast, the patient who receives a low transverse uterine incision should be allowed to labor in a subsequent normal pregnancy and has a high chance of a normal vaginal delivery. In spite of the strength of these arguments, the practice of vertical or classical incisions on the uterine wall to deliver twins in breech or transverse presentations continues. Vertical incisions on the uterine wall are rarely if ever needed if the twins are near term, if the exact position of their heads and buttocks is known before the operation, and if the incision on the abdominal wall is vertical. This allows room for the first assistant to introduce his or her hands around the uterus and in coordinate movements with the hand of the surgeon inside the uterus, to rotate the infant, thus making delivery by breech or vertex possible.[24]

■ MANAGEMENT OF GESTATIONS WITH HIGH FETAL NUMBER

Everything that has been said about twin pregnancies applies to gestations with higher fetal numbers. They are a rare event (triplets once in every 8000 to 9000 deliveries in the United States, quintuplets once in every 41 million births), although in recent years they are becoming more frequent as a result of the use of ovulation-inducing drugs in the management of infertility. In patients treated with gonadotropins the occurrence of multiple pregnancies is 20% of which 75% are twins and 25% are triplets or gestations of higher number. In infertility patients treated with clomiphene the occurrence of multiple pregnancy is 10%.

As in the case of twins, prematurity is the most important hazard for patients with high fetal numbers. The fetal mortality and morbidity is high and closely related to fetal weight, order of birth, and fetal position. Small babies, babies born last or close to last, and babies in breech or transverse presentations have the worst outcomes.[11,19] The complexity of the antepartum, intrapartum, and neonatal care of multiple pregnancies of high fetal number necessitates their referral to third-level perinatal centers adequately staffed and equipped to manage this type of problem.

■ REFERENCES

1. Crane JP, Tomich PL, Kopta M: Ultrasonic growth patterns in normal and discordant twins. Obstet Gynecol 1980;55:678.
2. Farooqui MO, Grossman JH, Shannon RA: A review of twin pregnancy and perinatal mortality. Obstet Gynecol Surv 1973;28:144.
3. Fox RL, Nathanson HG, Tejani N, et al: Interlocking twins. Obstet Gynecol 1975;46:53.
4. Fujikura T, Froehlich LA: Twin placentation and zygosity. Obstet Gynecol 1971;37:34.
5. Gray CM, Nix HG, Wallace AJ: Thoracopagus twins: prenatal diagnosis. Radiology 1950;54:398.
6. Guttmacher AF, Schuyler GK: The fetus of multiple gestations. Obstet Gynecol 1958;12:528.
7. Halwa S, Wojtowica J, Gradzki J, et al: Computed tomography in preoperative diagnosis of conjoined twins. J Comput Assist Tomogr 1979;3:411.
8. Haney AF, Crenshaw MD, Dempsey PJ: Significance of biparietal diameter differences between twins. Obstet Gynecol 1978;51:609.
9. Hendricks CH: Twinning in relation to birth weight, mortality and congenital abnormalities. Obstet Gynecol 1966;27:47.
10. Houlton MCC: Divergent biparietal diameter growth rates in twin pregnancies. Obstet Gynecol 1977;49:542.
11. Itzkowic D: A survey of 59 triplet pregnancies. Br J Obstet Gynaecol 1979;86:23.
12. Jacobs MM, Arias F: Intramyometrial prostaglandin F$_{2\alpha}$ in the treatment of severe postpartum hemorrhage. Obstet Gynecol 1980;55:665.
13. Jeffrey RL, Bower WA, Delaney JS: Role of bed rest in twin gestations. Obstet Gynecol 1974;43:822.
14. Kling S, Johnston RJ, Michalyschyn B, et al: Successful separation of xyphopagus-conjoined twins. J Pediatr Surg 1975;10:267.
15. Kurjak A, Latin V: Ultrasound diagnosis of fetal abnormalities in multiple pregnancy. Acta Obstet Gynecol Scand 1979;58:153.
16. Leveno KJ, Santos-Ramos R, Duenhoelter JH, et al: Sonar cephalometry in twins: a table of biparietal diameters for normal twin fetuses and a comparison with singletons. Am J Obstet Gynecol 1979;135:727.
17. Levine SC, Filly RA: Rapid B-scan (real-time) ultrasonography in the identification and evaluation of twin pregnancies. Obstet Gynecol 1978;51:170.
18. Little WA, Friedman EA: The twin delivery: factors influencing second twin mortality. Obstet Gynecol Surv 1958;13:611.
19. McFee JG, Lord EL, Jeffrey RL, et al: Multiple gestations of high fetal numbers. Obstet Gynecol 1974;44:99.
20. McKeown T, Record RG: Observations on fetal growth in multiple pregnancy in man. J Endocrinol 1952;5:387.
21. Morris N, Osborn SB, Wright HP: Effective circulation of the uterine wall in late pregnancy measured with ^{24}NaCl. Lancet 1955;1:323.
22. Naeye RL, Benirschke K, Hagstrom JW, et al: Intrauterine growth of twins as estimated from live born birthweight data. Pediatrics 1977;37:542.
23. Naeye RL, Tafari N, Judge D, et al: Twins: causes of perinatal death in 12 United States cities and one African city. Am J Obstet Gynecol 1978;131:267.
24. Pelosi MA, Apuzzio J, Fricchione D, et al: The "intraabdominal version technique" for delivery of transverse lie by low segment cesarean section. Am J Obstet Gynecol 1979;135:1009.
25. Powers WF: Twin pregnancy: complications and treatment. Obstet Gynecol 1973;42:795.
26. Powers WF, Miller TC: Bed rest in twin pregnancy: identification of a critical period and its cost implications. Am J Obstet Gynecol 1979;134:23.
27. Rausen AR, Seki M, Strauss L: Twin transfusion syndrome. J Pediatr 1965;66:613.

28. Read JA, Miller FC: Technique of simultaneous direct intrauterine pressure recording for electronic monitoring of twin gestation. Am J Obstet Gynecol 1977; 129:228.

29. Schneider L, Bessis R, Tabaste JL, et al: Ecographic survey of twin fetal growth: a plea for specific charts for twins. Prog Clin Biol Res 1978;24:123.

30. Scott DE: Anemia in pregnancy. Obstet Gynecol Annu 1972;1:219.

31. Sims CD, Cowan DB, Parkinson CE: The lecithin/sphyngomyelin ratio in twin pregnancies. Br J Obstet Gynaecol 1976;83:447.

32. Spellacy WM, Buhi WC, Birk SA: Human placental lactogen levels in multiple pregnancies. Obstet Gynecol 1978;52:210.

33. Spellacy WN, Cruz AC, Buhi WC, et al: Amniotic fluid L/S ratio in twin gestation. Obstet Gynecol 1977;50:68.

34. TambyRaja RL, Atputharajah V, Salmon Y: Prevention of prematurity in twins. Aust NZ Obstet Gynaecol 1979;18:179.

35. Thomsen RJ: Delayed interval delivery of a twin pregnancy. Obstet Gynecol 1978;52:375.

36. Varma TR: Ultrasound evidence of early pregnancy failure in patients with multiple conceptions. Br J Obstet Gynaecol 1979;86:290.

37. Verduzco R, Rosario R, Rigatto H: Hyaline membrane disease in twins. Am J Obstet Gynecol 1976;125:668.

38. Wald N, Barker S, Peto R, et al: Maternal serum alpha-fetoprotein levels in multiple pregnancy. Br Med J 1975;1:651.

39. Wilson RS: Blood typing and twin zygosity. Hum Hered 1970;20:30.

15

■ ■ ■

THIRD TRIMESTER BLEEDING

Alfred B. Knight and Fernando Arias

Although vaginal bleeding during any stage of pregnancy constitutes a significant concern to the patient and her doctor, discussions of third trimester bleeding are predominant in the obstetric literature and in educational programs. This emphasis is appropriate because in the third trimester *both* patients, the mother and fetus, are at risk for long-term morbidity and loss of life. Massive maternal hemorrhage may occur before 28 weeks of gestation, but it is rare, and when it happens the mother's management is not markedly influenced by considerations for fetal survival. Once the third trimester is reached, maternal vaginal bleeding is more frequently life threatening, and fetal survival is at least a significant possibility. Indeed, in many university centers an uncompromised neonate at 28 weeks of gestation may have a greater than 75% chance of survival.

The etiologies of third trimester bleeding most often emphasized are placenta previa and abruptio placentae. Modern obstetrics has markedly reduced the maternal mortality resulting from these conditions, and fetal outcome has also shown constant improvement, perhaps as much from more sophisticated neonatal care as from obstetric therapeutics. Yet perinatal mortality of 30% to 50% for abruptio placentae and 7% to 25% for placenta previa leaves little room for complacence. In addition, vaginal bleeding from other causes, most of which remain "unclassi-

fied," constitutes a real threat to the fetus and leads to mortality of 7% to 15%.[28,32] These vaginal bleeding episodes for which no etiology can be assigned may constitute 50% of all vaginal bleeding beyond the first trimester.

Most patients have less than massive hemorrhage and allow a careful and thoughtful evaluation. Unfortunately, even with the most sophisticated approach to diagnosis, the etiology for the bleeding can be assigned in only half of these pregnancies and then often *after* delivery of the fetus. Therefore the clinician is usually in the position of managing a high-risk condition without a clear diagnosis—certainly an uncomfortable situation. This chapter reviews the literature for the classic etiologies for third trimester vaginal bleeding and proposes a general plan for management of these conditions.

■ PLACENTA PREVIA

The high maternal (approaching 10%) and neonatal (ranging from 30% to 70%) mortality associated with placenta previa before 1925 changed dramatically with the advent of blood transfusion, liberal cesarean section, and later with a "conservative approach" to management. From 1945, when the conservative approach began, to the 1970s, however, little change has been noted in perinatal mortality (10% to 25%), although maternal death is now a very rare occurrence.

Definition and incidence

The diagnosis of placenta previa can only be confirmed at the time of vaginal examination or at the time of operative delivery when it is found that the placenta covers some portion of the potential space at the level of the internal cervical os. According to the latest edition of *Williams Obstetrics* there are four types or degrees of placenta previa:

1. *Total placenta previa,* when the internal os is completely covered by the placenta
2. *Partial placenta previa,* when the internal os is partially covered by the placenta
3. *Marginal placenta previa,* when the edge of the placenta is at the margin of the internal os
4. *Low-lying placenta,* when the placental edge may be palpated by the examining finger when introduced through the cervix

Most authors in the older literature based their clinical management plans on these types of placenta previa. There is very little agreement in the literature, however, as to the exact definition of some of the subdivisions, specifically marginal and low-lying placenta previa. Also, if one includes cervical dilation in the definition of placenta previa, a single patient during the course of normal labor may change from total to partial to marginal previa, although, by convention, the definition is based on the findings at the initial vaginal examination or at the time of cesarean section. In our opinion an unacceptable high fetal and maternal risk is present with every type of placenta previa, and the management should depend on careful fetal and maternal evaluation rather than on highly variable anatomic definitions.

The incidence of placenta previa varies greatly from one series to another, ranging from 1 out of 167[5] to 1 out of 327[21] in pregnancies beyond 24 weeks of gestation. The incidences of the different types also vary but they are, roughly, the following:

Total	23% to 31.3%
Partial	20.6% to 33%
Marginal	37% to 54.9%

Etiology

No specific etiology can be found for most cases of low placental implantations. Much teleologic discussion about the relatively avascular lower uterine segment and the resulting necessity for hypertrophy of the placenta over a larger area to maintain adequate diffusion capacity has been offered with little clinical or experimental research support. Associations are many and include increasing maternal age, increasing parity, multiple gestations, previous abortions, cesarean sections and uterine incisions, anemia, abnormal presentation, closely spaced pregnancies, tumors distorting the contour of the uterus, and endometritis. It is often difficult to separate out independent variables in these patients. Brenner et al[5] have also suggested a sex predilection with male fetuses predominant. The frequency of recurrence of placenta previa is 12 times the expected incidence.

Clinical presentation

Overwhelmingly, the most common symptom with placenta previa is vaginal bleeding. The bleeding may occur as early as the second trimester or even continue through from the first trimester. However, according to Crenshaw et al,[6] most patients (65%) have their first bleeding episode after 30 weeks of gestation. The data of Crenshaw et al also reveal that roughly a third of these patients initially bleed under 30 weeks, a third from 30 to 35 weeks, and a third after 36 or more weeks of gestation. No maternal fatality has been associated with the initial bleeding episode, barring inappropriate vaginal examination, which may precipitate massive hemorrhage and maternal shock.

Abnormal fetal presentations and congenital malformations are strongly associated with placenta previa. Breech, shoulder, and compound presentations may be found in up to 30% of the cases. Also, Hibbard[11] has shown that the incidence of placenta previa is 50 times greater in patients with a fetus in transverse lie at term than in patients with the fetus in vertex position. In addition, patients with placenta previa and fetus in vertex presentation are in persistent occiput posterior or transverse positions in as many as 15% of the cases. The complementary data are also most revealing: 60% of transverse lies and 24% of breech or compound presentations are associated with placenta previa.

Diagnosis

As mentioned before, the diagnosis of placenta previa can only be confirmed by vaginal examination or by direct visual observation at the time of operative delivery. With respect to vaginal examinations, *there is no justification for vaginal digital examination in patients with last trimester bleeding unless it is carried out under the conditions of a double setup*. The prohibition of vaginal examinations in these patients without appropriate operative preparation may appear, particularly to the young intern or resident, to be a holdover from less sophisticated days. Hibbard[11] reiterates the dangers: "Even with the knowledge that it is prudent to be both cautious and gentle, one out of every 16 examinations produced a major hemorrhage and one out of every 25 examinations resulted in hypovolemic shock." The only indication for this examination would be to attempt diagnosis; however, Hibbard points out that in known cases of placenta previa, if the examination is confined to the fornices, the disorder is identified in only 43% of cases, and even if the cervix is explored with the fingers, the accuracy is only 69%. A gentle speculum examination in the same series was not associated with any increased risks. Brenner et al[5] do not feel that even a speculum examination is worth the risk because the local causes of significant third trimester bleeding are so rare as to eliminate the necessity of the examination. We do not agree, since no data have ever shown a risk associated with this diagnostic maneuver.

Attempts to diagnose this clinical condition without the inherent risks of a direct physical examination have included many other techniques, such as listening for the placental souffle, soft tissue x-ray films, ^{125}I-labeled albumin scans, and technetium scans. Placental scanning techniques have approached 85% accuracy, but they have the inconvenience of fetal and maternal irradiation. Placental localization with ultrasound has superseded all previous techniques, since to date, it is associated with no known risks or dangerous sequelae and is painless, efficient, and relatively simple. Its accuracy approaches 98% for localizing the placenta within the uterine cavity.

A thorough understanding of the evolution of uterine anatomy throughout pregnancy is necessary for an appropriate ultrasonic diagnosis of placenta previa. Early in pregnancy the placenta appears to cover the cervical os *most* of the time. As the uterus enlarges and the lower uterine segment develops, the placenta appears to move cephalad away from the cervical os. This movement is referred to as *migration*. Before 24 weeks of gestation only a cautionary significance should be attributed to the relative cervical-placental apposition, particularly in asymptomatic patients. In the large majority of these cases (63 out of 67 in Kurjak and Barsic's series[16]) the placenta is free of the cervical os by term. Therefore *all diagnoses of placenta previa based on ultrasonic evaluation must be confirmed well into the third trimester*. In our experience, if the placenta extends both anteriorly and posteriorly over the cervix (that is, the bulk of the placenta is centered over the internal os of the cervix) *after* 24 weeks of gestation, it is much less likely to be away from the cervix at term.

In a small percentage of cases ultrasound cannot unequivocally diagnose placenta previa in symptomatic patients. Most often this situation occurs beyond 32 weeks of gestation, when elevation of the presenting part is essential for obtaining adequate resolution of the area of the cervix. In these cases a double setup is necessary for confirmation. Other areas of potential confusion include the presence of a blood clot at the level of the internal os, which can mimic placental tissue, the presence of a succenturiate lobe, and the existence of a thick "decidual reaction," which can appear like a very thin placenta. These problems are indeed unusual. Gray-scale ultrasound can provide a definitive diagnosis of placenta previa better than 95% of the time. The other 5% will require a double setup to confirm the diagnosis.

Outcome

A placenta previa is destined to bleed unless the pregnancy is interrupted by abdominal delivery. Patients with early bleeding are more likely to have total placenta previa but, clinically more important, the earlier the bleeding the less chance of carrying the fetus near term. The first bleeding episode has never been associated with a maternal death, a fact that provides the basis for the management of these patients. As we will see later, less than 35% of pregnancies complicated by placenta previa are terminated because of active bleeding.

The amount of blood loss does correlate with the degree of previa. With total, partial, and marginal placenta previa the number of 500 ml units of blood replaced per patient were, respectively, 4.7, 3.6, and 2.5 in Crenshaw et al's series.[6] However, the *number* of bleeding episodes did not correlate with total amount of blood loss or perinatal mortality. The origin of the vaginal blood is presumed to be maternal. However, a fetal component could be significant if some disruption of the villi occurs. Certainly, if a portion of the vaginal blood is fetal, the gestation would be at much higher risk for intrauterine (and possible neonatal) mortality. We have used the Fetaldex test to detect hemoglobin in blood collected from the vagina in patients with third trimester bleeding, but there are wide variations and technical difficulties. The following, simple test of Ogita et al* to determine the presence of fetal hemoglobin in patients with third trimester bleeding may be useful to assess the occurrence of fetal bleeding in this situation.

Reagents

A. 0.1 N KOH
B. 400 ml of 50% saturated $(NH_4)_2SO_4$ with 1 ml of 10 N HCl.

Procedure

1. Mix in a small test tube 5 drops of reagent A with 1 drop of vaginal blood. Shake vigorously for at least 2 minutes.
2. Add 10 drops of reagent B. Shake well.
3. Using a hematocrit capillary tube, apply a few drops of the mixture in the center of a filter paper. The liquid will diffuse to the periphery of the filter paper from the point of application. Stop the application when the liquid has diffused enough to form a circle 2 cm in diameter.

Results

Denatured hemoglobin and cell debris will remain as a dark spot at the point of application (origin). The alkali-resistant fetal hemoglobin will move away from the origin, forming a colored ring at the outer limit of the application circle. The dark brown color of the fetal hemoglobin peripheral ring will become darker with increasing concentration of fetal hemoglobin in the blood sample. The technique detects concentrations of fetal hemoglobin as low as 3%.

---

*From Ogita, S., et al: Obstet. Gynecol. 1976; 48:237.

Fig. 15-1, based on the data of Crenshaw et al,[6] shows the high perinatal mortality when the first bleeding episode occurs at less than 28 weeks of gestation and a progressive decline in mortality with advance in gestational age until a new elevation occurs after 36 weeks of gestation. Overwhelmingly, the main etiology for the perinatal mortality is preterm birth. When Crenshaw et al's data are broken down into gestational age groups and fetal weight, the predominance of preterm fetuses is evident. Most authors suggest that if preterm delivery could be avoided the perinatal mortality problem would disappear. However, Brenner et al's data[5] suggest that other factors in addition to preterm birth exist and compromise the infants of mothers with placenta previa. In fact, for babies born after 28 weeks of gestation there is a greater neonatal mortality associated with placenta previa. This is also evident if the data are broken down by fetal weights. For fetal weights above 1000 grams and under 3000 grams there is a greater neonatal mortality associated with placenta previa. Fetal and neonatal hypovolemic shock or fetal asphyxia are the logical culprits. In the past, delivery could also have contributed to the high mortality, since total breech extractions, internal versions, and fetal tamponade were used rather freely, but these procedures are rare now. In *none* of the more than 50 papers on placenta previa and other bleeding disorders we have recently reviewed were neonatal hematocrits or blood pressures routinely recorded. All babies from these series were born *before* 1970 and there has been no significant review of placenta previa material since that time. Brenner et al[5] did record Apgar scores and showed a higher frequency of low scores, but the means for patients with and without placenta previa were not significantly different. The long-term prognosis for these infants remains optimistic. In a 4-year follow-up of children at risk for intrauterine hypoxia, Niswander et al[22] could find no statistical differences between the risk and control groups in IQ scores and gross and fine motor skills.

Increased perinatal mortality is associated with earlier bleeding, greater amount of bleeding, and greater extent of placenta previa. However, all degrees of placenta previa, whatever the gestational age at the first bleeding episode

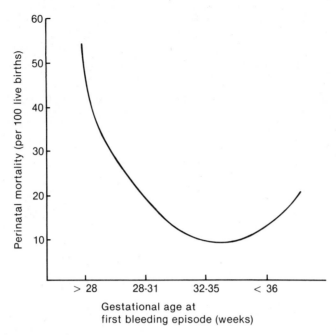

FIG. 15-1 ■ Perinatal mortality and gestational age at the time of the first bleeding episode in patients with placenta previa.

or the amount of bleeding, are associated with a very high perinatal mortality. This perinatal mortality will occur until therapeutic approaches to prolong the gestation or decrease the complications of preterm delivery are developed. If the mother is in hypovolemic shock at the time of delivery, perinatal mortality approaches 70%.

Beyond hemorrhage, the single most common cause for termination of pregnancy in patients with placenta previa is preterm labor, occurring in as many as 30% of these patients. Very likely, many patients who had increased bleeding also had spontaneous uterine activity that was inadequately recorded. Other indications for pregnancy termination are preterm rupture of the membranes (even with total previa), physician anxiety, and "term gestation."

A persistent finding in the offspring of mothers with placenta previa is a two to four times increased risk of congenital malformations. It is a sobering experience to aggressively manage a patient and maintain her pregnancy only to deliver an infant with no capacity for extrauterine life. No specific abnormalities are seen, and only a few, such as neural tube defects, omphalocele, and renal agenesis, can be identified antenatally by ultrasound or fetogram.

Management

Three fundamental areas of concern must be evaluated quickly and efficiently when dealing with a patient bleeding as a consequence of placenta previa: (1) the mother's condition as primarily evidenced by the degree of obstetric hemorrhage; (2) the fetal condition, including most particularly gestational age estimation; and (3) the ability of the neonatal unit to handle an infant of that gestational age. A massive hemorrhage threatening maternal life must be terminated without regard to the maturity of the fetus. A mild to moderate bleeding episode in a patient at term may be approached by preparation for delivery, but if she is preterm, a more conservative evaluation of mother and fetus is appropriate. No single issue is as important in obstetrics as gestational dating. All management problems require a balance of the risk of fetal demise in utero and the risk of neonatal morbidity and mortality. A 2-week discrepancy between clinical dates and gestational age can significantly alter the timing of delivery and certainly can alter neonatal outcome. Finally, the ability of pediatricians to handle preterm infants must also be strongly considered. Intervention on behalf of a fetus at 28 weeks of gestation is inappropriate when a neonate at 32 weeks of gestation has a great deal of difficulty surviving in the same hospital. Even the immediate transport after birth of these high-risk preterm infants to a neonatal center does not produce the same good outcome found when the infant is delivered at a tertiary hospital. If neonatal facilities are limited, the mother should be transported to a perinatal center where obstetric intervention on behalf of a 28-week fetus is relatively common and is producing increasingly normal outcomes.

For the purpose of discussion of the management of these patients, gestations will be called *previable* if between 16 to 26 weeks, *preterm* if between 27 to 36 weeks, and *term* if beyond 36 weeks of gestation. Within the preterm group, high-risk infants will be those classified between 27 and 32 weeks of gestation and lower risk those between 33 and 36 weeks. This latter subdivision is particularly important in evaluating risks of in utero or neonatal morbidity and mortality.

Evaluation of obstetric hemorrhage. To make an adequate evaluation of the severity of a bleeding episode in the third trimester of pregnancy is difficult. Visual inspection of the patient and her blood-stained clothes is notoriously inaccurate. Blood pressure and pulse may remain within normal range despite considerable blood loss because of the unusual tolerance to bleeding of the hypervolemic pregnant woman. Hematocrit and hemoglobin determinations during or shortly after a bleeding episode may be within normal range because of compensatory vasoconstriction. Measurements of blood volume are usually inaccurate during bleeding and, indeed, may be normal in spite of significant blood loss. Finally, the absolute amount of bleeding may be less important than the premorbid clinical status in a given case: an anemic patient may lose 1 unit of blood and show signs of profound hypovolemia, whereas a normal patient may handle this loss without any significant change in vital signs.

We use the following clinical criteria to classify the severity of a bleeding episode:

mild bleeding No change in vital signs. No postural hypotension. No peripheral evidence of circulatory volume deficit. Normal urinary output. In a mild bleeding episode the patient has lost less than 10% of her intravascular volume.

moderate bleeding Postural changes in pulse rate (increase of 10 to 20 beats/min when changing from the supine to the upright position) and in diastolic blood pressure (drop of 10 mm Hg or more). Evidence of inadequate circulatory volume (dyspnea, thirst, pallor, tachycardia, clammy extremities). Mental status changes may be present (apathy or agitation). A patient with moderate bleeding has lost between 10% and 25% of her intravascular volume.

severe bleeding Patient in shock with decreased or unrecordable blood pressure. Persistent loss of fresh blood from the vagina. The fetus may be dead or showing signs of distress. Oliguria or anuria. A patient with severe acute hemorrhage has lost more than 25% of her blood volume.

Severe bleeding. Little emphasis should be placed on finding the etiology of the hemorrhage in patients with severe acute third trimester bleeding. It should be assumed that a catastrophic event (placenta previa or abruptio placentae) is present. These patients could exsanguinate in a matter of minutes, and an efficient management plan including life-support measures as well as immediate operative intervention may be their only hope. Management includes constant observation and monitoring, administration of intravenous fluids, taking of blood samples, assessment of renal function and intravascular status, assessing of the fetus, and preparing for pregnancy termination.

Intensive observation and monitoring. These patients should never be left alone. Frequent monitoring of vital signs, fluid management, recording the amount of vaginal bleeding, and keeping complete records of what has transpired are essential for a positive outcome. Retrospective reconstruction of what went on in an emergency is, at best, inadequate. One health professional must be in charge of directly executing the physician's orders without leaving the room to get intravenous fluids, carry blood samples, answer telephones, etc.

Intravenous fluids. A large-bore cannula, at least 18 gauge, should be inserted for the administration of a balanced electrolyte solution such as lactated Ringer's solution. If the patient is in shock, two lines should be started. If shock becomes more profound, the second line, which may be lifesaving, is exceedingly more difficult to initiate than it is earlier.

The blood bank needs to be kept informed about the progress of this patient. Initially, type O Rh-negative packed red blood cells should be available. These should be used only when time is not available for crossmatch. The next level of crossmatch is type specific, which takes roughly 15 to 30 minutes. Both of these types of units need a physician's release and are an indication of the extreme emergency of the situation. The risk of incompatibility reaction is significant with these transfusions. A complete crossmatch usually requires 45 to 60 minutes if no major antibodies are found. As blood is used for these patients, more units need to be crossmatched to *constantly* have 4 units available. With massive transfusions, a dilution of clotting factors occurs that can increase the hemorrhage. Fresh whole blood, cryoprecipitate, and platelet packs may all be necessary. Close contact with the source of these products (blood bank) is very important.

Blood samples. Samples should be obtained for the following tests: complete blood count (CBC), type and cross (at least 4 units), electrolytes (Na, K, Cl, CO_2), glucose, creatinine (or blood urea nitrogen [BUN]), and disseminated intravascular coagulation (DIC) profile. Although the hemoglobin and hematocrit have been the basis for evaluation of blood loss for decades, acute and dramatic changes can often remain hidden in a constant blood cell level, only to be fully revealed a few days later after complete vascular equilibration. On the other hand, rapid fluid infusion can expand the intravascular space and produce a decrease in blood cell level that a few days later will also reequilibrate, only at a higher value. During the acute phase of hemorrhage other parameters (such as pulse, blood pressure, urine output, and estimated blood loss) may provide a better measure of the intravascular status. The electrolyte, glucose, and creatinine levels are baseline, primarily in preparation for anesthesia, and a "crude" screen for major problems. Repetitive values are valuable in continuously monitoring patients.

The DIC or coagulopathy profile is essential to identify the rare patient who needs even more sohpisticated management. The DIC profile includes determination of prothrombin time (PT), partial prothromplastin time (PTT), platelet count, fibrinogen, and fibrinogen degradation products (FDP). A simple screening test for a *clinically significant* coagulopathy is to observe a clot tube. Five milliliters of fresh whole blood are placed in a glass test tube. A clot should occur in 5 minutes; if no clot forms, a coagulopathy exists. If a clot forms, observation of the quality of the clot over the next 60 minutes will reveal evidence of clinically excessive fibrinolysis. This will identify a patient who may clinically be in trouble before the specific and sophisticated tests are back. A more complete discussion of DIC in obstetrics is found at the end of this chapter.

Renal function. Most long-term complications from severe hemorrhage are related to shock. Particularly, acute tubular and cortical necrosis are associated with anuria or oliguria resulting from hypovolemic shock. Thus urine output observation is critical for appropriate management. These patients need a Foley catheter and aggressive therapy for decreased urine output. Their initial treatment should consist of expansion of the intravascular volume—*not diuretics*. Maintenance of a urine output of 30 ml/hr should protect the kidney from permanent damage. Furosemide in an intravenous dosage of 20 to 60 mg bolus is usually sufficient to reestablish urinary output once adequate hydration and blood replacement have been obtained.

Central venous pressure. A patient in critical condition needs an accurate monitoring of her intravascular status. Hemoglobin, pulse, and blood pressure can all be misleading, particularly in the presence of a decreased urine output. A peripherally inserted central venous pressure line (particularly if there is coagulopathy) or a more centrally inserted line (subclavian, internal jugular, etc.) will provide the necessary information for safe and rapid expansion of the intravascular space. A more precise evaluation is obtained by placement of a Swan-Ganz catheter and measurements of the pulmonary wedge pressure. Unfortunately, this may not be available in all clinical settings.

Fetus. During the first critical minutes when preparations are being made to terminate the pregnancy, no time is usually available for obtaining a lecithin/sphingomyelin (L/S) ratio, using ultrasound for rough dating, or even making a fetogram to rule out gross malformation. Often a quick clinical assessment is all that can be expected.

Vaginal examination. In the acutely bleeding patient, there is no indication for a vaginal examination, even a speculum examination, until preparations are complete for operative delivery. At the time of a double setup, visual inspection will reveal the very rare local causes of hemorrhage. The decision whether to rupture the membranes in anticipation of a vaginal delivery is made at this time.

Other medical problems. Systemic maternal disease must be quickly evaluated in preparation for surgery. A history of hypertension, diabetes, renal disease, etc, will alter management and certainly choice of anesthesia. Diabetic patients should receive less glucose, those with hypertension fewer electrolytes, and patients with renal disease strict electrolyte and fluid management.

Pregnancy termination. The method of delivery, whether abdominal or vaginal, was a controversial issue in most of the older literature.[11,28] In our opinion, with the exception of some clearly previable infants, *all types of pregnancies with placenta previa should be terminated by abdominal delivery.*

The type of anesthesia to be used depends on the expertise of the anesthetist/anesthesiologist, the clinical setting, and the desire of the patient. It would be better to treat the patient who is hemorrhaging or who may hemorrhage (ie, as a result of a double setup) with general anesthesia and endotracheal intubation after induction with sodium pentothal and succinylcholine, to be followed after delivery by the choice of the administrator of the anesthesia (eg, narcotics, halothane).

Once the method of delivery is determined, a decision as to the type of uterine incision must be made. Overwhelmingly, it has been the custom to elect a low transverse incision regardless of placental location or fetal lie. Delivery of the placenta first with rapid clamping of cord or even delivery through the placenta has rarely been associated with fetal exsanguination. However, effective delivery of a transverse lie or a preterm infant through the lower uterine segment may be difficult. The low transverse incision is appropriate if the presenting part is easily accessible and the lower uterine segment is adequately developed to allow a generous incision. Otherwise, a low vertical incision provides greater flexibility in the approach to delivery and perhaps somewhat less trauma to the fetus.

Moderate bleeding. Only rarely should the pregnancy in a patient with placenta previa be continued if adequate fetal lung maturation is obtained or if the fetal gestational age is more than 36 weeks. Therefore in a patient with moderate bleeding, immediate evaluation of fetal maturity is essential as soon as the acute bleeding episode subsides and the patient's condition is stabilized. With a positive shake test result or a mature L/S ratio, immediate delivery of the fetus should occur.

If the fetal lungs are immature, the patient with placenta previa and moderate bleeding should remain under intensive care (usually in the labor and delivery unit) for a period of 24 to 48 hours. A hemoglobin level of roughly 11 g/dl should be maintained by transfusion. The uterus should be kept quiescent with the *prophylactic* use of beta mimetics. Steroids to induce lung maturation should be administered. If the patient's condition remains unstable, with steady blood loss in moderate amounts, or if she requires more than 2 units of blood in 24 hours to compensate for losses, she should be delivered in spite of the early gestational age or lack of fetal lung maturation. The pediatrician should be alerted to the imminent delivery of a baby at risk for developing respiratory distress syndrome (RDS). Should this patient's condition rapidly become stable and remain stable for 24 to 48 hours, she becomes a candidate for chronic care, as described later.

Most patients with placenta previa and moderate bleeding stop bleeding and return to a stable condition shortly after admission, thereby becoming candidates for chronic care or expectant management. However, in some cases rare complicating factors such as premature rupture of the membranes, other maternal medical conditions, or fetal distress may make continuation of the pregnancy inappropriate. Attempts have been made to identify patients at high risk for life-threatening hemorrhage so as to preclude their being included in an expectant management protocol. For example, if the initial bleeding episode results in hemorrhage of more than 600 ml or "more than moderate" or if the pla-

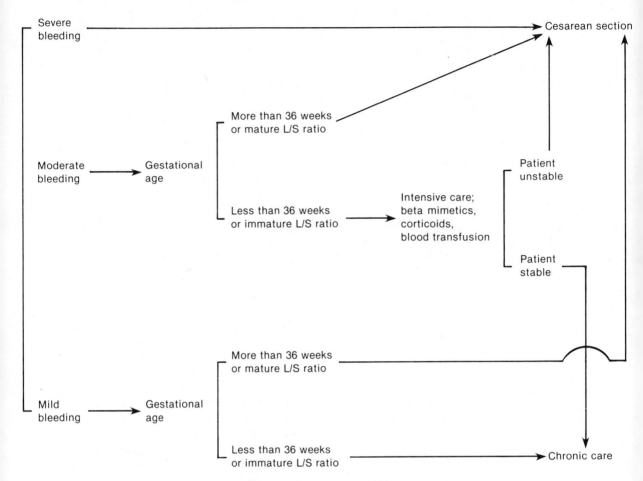

FIG. 15-2 ■ Management of placenta previa.

centa previa is total, some authors would recommend immediate termination of pregnancy. Objective evaluation of published series on placenta previa does not substantiate these caveats. Indeed, even a few days of delay in delivery may radically improve the neonatal outcome, as discussed later.

Mild bleeding. As with moderate bleeding, fetal maturity dictates management of patients with mild bleeding. Immediate delivery of mature fetuses is the appropriate course, regardless of the minor degree of bleeding. Each published series on placenta previa recounts term infants dying while awaiting cesarean section. If the fetal lungs are immature or gestational age is less than 36 weeks, the patient with mild bleeding and placenta previa becomes a candidate for chronic care, as described later.

A flow chart for management of patients with placenta previa is shown in Fig. 15-2.

Chronic care. The "conservative" or "expectant" management of placenta previa is an attempt to reduce the high fetal mortality associated with early delivery. Around 1920, before the capability for transfusion and decreased risk of abdominal delivery, maternal mortality was as high as 10% and fetal mortality as high as 70%. When more aggressive management became safe and practical, a uniform decision for immediate delivery, regardless of gestation, was made. Roughly 25 years later, in 1945, a reevaluation of this approach suggested that maintenance of the pregnancy under close supervision might decrease perinatal mortality. This clinical approach, as founded by MacAfee, Tomlinson, Williams, and Semmens, cannot be shown in any studies, however, to have unquestionably resulted in decreased perinatal mortality. In individual cases one must balance the risk of maintenance of the pregnancy in terms of the chances that massive hemorrhage will result in fetal demise against the chance of complications of preterm delivery. In most studies only 40% to 60% of the patients are eligible for inclusion in a chronic care protocol. The other patients are at term, are bleeding too much, have ruptured membranes, etc. Other authors have suggested that if gestation is maintained for only 1 to 2 weeks, expectant management will not be successful. In modern obstetrics, however, a delay of delivery for even a few days may be highly significant in neonatal outcome.

The following discussion outlines some characteristics of our expectant management regimen.

Patient selection. The importance of proper selection of patients cannot be overemphasized. Only patients with proven fetal pulmonary immaturity or less than 36 weeks of gestation should be admitted to chronic care. Patients with unstable vital signs or bleeding in moderate amounts should remain in intensive care until bleeding stops and vital signs become stable.

Hospitalization. Although the financial implications are appreciated, continued hospitalization is the best management plan that can be offered to these patients. Because of the potential financial burden, attempts have been made to isolate a "safe" group of patients who could be managed at home with constant supervision. However, no data can predict which patients will have recurrent hemorrhage and fetal demise.

Prevention of labor. Up to 30% of all patients with placenta previa have their pregnancies terminated because of preterm labor. Whether the lower implantation of the placenta predisposes to early labor or whether these pregnancies were destined for preterm delivery is a moot question. In the past there has been no consistent therapeutic approach to preterm labor in patients with placenta previa. Once the patient's condition is stabilized, the use of terbutaline (Chapter 3) is strongly recommended. Because of terbutaline's cardiovascular side effect (tachycardia), the patient should not be actively bleeding and her vital signs should be in the normal range. The patient should continue this medication until termination of the pregnancy is elected. In 1975 Johnson[12a] showed the usefulness of Delalutin in prophylaxis of premature labor, but he did not specifically discuss placenta

previa. Patients with placenta previa may benefit from Delalutin treatment not only because of the effect of progesterone in decreasing myometrial contractility, but also because the ability of progesterone to regenerate beta mimetic receptor sites may increase the therapeutic effect of terbutaline.

Fetal lung maturation. With massive hemorrhage the question is simply whether or not the fetus is viable. With less than massive bleeding, if the fetus is term, delivery is appropriate. For the preterm fetus an attempt to determine fetal lung maturation should be made except when there is a strong suspicion of placental abruption, discussed more fully later. Appropriate tests include ultrasound dating, realizing its limitations when done after 30 weeks of gestation, and amniocentesis for the shake test and for determination of the L/S ratio.

Multiple studies have shown about a 50% reduction in the incidence of hyaline membrane disease (HMD) in preterm infants born after the mother received glucocorticoids. The time course necessary for this effect can be as little as 24 hours or as much as 72 hours. In the clinical situation of placenta previa and preterm gestation, glucocorticoids may be lifesaving for the baby. Under 32 weeks of gestation it should be assumed that the fetal lungs are immature, and the medication should be given empirically without first evaluating the amniotic fluid L/S ratio. Between 32 and 36 weeks of gestation, however, a mature L/S ratio and a positive shake test result are more likely to occur and amniocentesis is recommended. If immediate access to an amniotic fluid test is not available, steroid treatment should be given without hesitation. The known risks of HMD far outweigh the unknown risks of brief fetal exposure to steroids.

After the diethylstilbestrol (DES) experience of the last decade, there remains an appropriate reluctance to intervene pharmacologically on behalf of the fetus. Steroids, however, have been used extensively for other diseases in pregnancy without significant fetal side effects. Also, Howie and Liggins[12] have preliminarily reported a 7-year follow-up on their initial group of glucocorticoid-treated and control infants with no significant differences found.

It is important that the significant reduction in HMD found by Liggins and Howie[17] was restricted to preterm babies delivered 1 to 7 days after maternal glucocorticoid treatment. After 7 days they found no difference between glucocorticoid and placebo groups, and there was a rebound effect in the treated group that was not statistically significant. Thus it is possible that if pulmonary maturation is obtained with glucocorticoids at an early gestation, it may not persist if more than 1 week intervenes before delivery. For this reason, we give a pulse of glucocorticoids (12 mg dexamethasone) every week as long as the patient remains undelivered or until 36 weeks of gestation is reached.

Vaginal and rectal rest. Although the clinician is acutely aware of the danger of vaginal manipulation, the patient may not appreciate the significance of the problem. Naturally, intercourse, douching, and vaginal suppositories are contraindicated. In addition, straining at defecation and urination should be avoided. Stool softeners are appropriate.

Bed rest is strongly recommended. Limited bathroom privileges are usually allowed after the patient has been asymptomatic for a number of days.

When to deliver. Controversy exists concerning when to deliver the fetus if lung maturation is obtained at a very early gestational age. That is, are the non-RDS-related neonatal complications frequent and severe enough at 32 weeks of gestation, for example, to warrant continuation of intrauterine life at an unknown risk? No clear answers are available at this time. In our opinion, in patients with placenta previa the termination of pregnancy is to be carried out before 36 weeks of gestation mainly for maternal reasons. After reaching this gestational age, the pregnancy should be terminated (even if there are no maternal indications) once the fetal lungs are mature. Therefore in pregnancies very remote from term (30 weeks, for example), we give an initial course of glucocorticoids at the time the patient is admitted to the hospital, prescribe beta mimetics and bed rest, and continue giving a pulse of glucocorticoids every week as long as the patient remains undelivered. If there is no maternal indication for delivery, weekly amniocentesis for L/S ratio is initiated at 36 weeks and the patient is delivered as soon as a mature L/S ratio is obtained.

• • •

Following is a summary of the main points in the chronic care of patients with placenta previa:

1. *Selection criteria:* Only patients whose conditions are stable and whose pregnancies are far from term should be in chronic care. Patients actively bleeding or with unstable vital signs should remain under intensive care conditions. Patients with pregnancies near term should be delivered.
2. *Duration of hospitalization:* The patient should stay in the hospital for the duration of her pregnancy.
3. *Medications:*
   a. Terbutaline, 2.5 to 5 mg orally every 4 to 6 hours.
   b. Delalutin, 250 mg IM every week.
   c. Dexamethasone, 12 mg IM every 24 hours for two doses initially, followed by 12 mg IM every week thereafter.
   d. FeSO$_4$, 325 mg orally three times a day.
   e. Stool softeners, high residue diet.
4. *Laboratory tests:*
   a. Hemoglobin concentration every week. Maintain hemoglobin level above 11 g/dl using blood transfusion if necessary.
   b. L/S ratio after pregnancy reaches 36 weeks.
5. *Criteria to deliver:*
   a. Before 36 weeks of gestation, most indications for delivery are maternal (continuous or recurrent bleeding, etc).
   b. After 36 weeks of gestation, if no maternal indication for delivery, pregnancy should be terminated as soon as a mature L/S ratio is obtained.

In conclusion, there is a modern approach to placenta previa. If we can stop labor and allow further intrauterine growth, intervene pharmacologically to treat the fetus's immature surfactant system, and deliver abdominally under controlled conditions, thereby giving the neonatologists the best possible baby for their sophisticated care, the perinatal mortality from placenta previa can be significantly reduced.

Complications

Major long-term complications of placenta previa are related to hemorrhagic shock and hypotension. Irreversible renal damage (renal cortical necrosis) is the most common terminal event. Naturally, all complications inherent in cesarean section and emergency surgery pertain. However, a few specific complications are unique to placenta previa.

DIC. DIC occurs in connection with placenta previa quite infrequently. It most likely is secondary to hemorrhagic shock or abruptio placentae and less likely a characteristic of placenta previa alone. Treatment is not unique to the placenta previa situation.

Placenta accreta. The combination of placenta previa and accreta, although certainly a rare event, must be actively considered. In retrospective studies[4,8] 17.5% to 34% of placenta accreta was associated with placenta previa. Since placenta accreta is said to be related to lack of or decreased amount of decidua formation, thereby allowing invasion of the myometrium by the trophoblast, implantation of the placenta in the lower uterine segment would logically predispose to this complication. If extensive accreta is found at the time of cesarean section, primary hysterectomy is the treatment of choice. Lesser degrees of invasion may be treated with local curettage and figure-of-eight hemostatic sutures.

Postpartum uterine atony. In every series of patients who had diagnosed placenta previa a small percentage had postpartum hysterectomy for "hemorrhage." The older literature suggests that many of these cases were the result of uterine atony. More recent series, however, do not confirm this association. Bleeding from the placenta implantation site was said to be more commonly seen with placenta previa (usually treated with figure-of-eight sutures), but subsequent series were not conclusive.

Abruptio placentae. The incidence of abruptio placentae in association with placenta previa is certainly greater than in the general population. Whether it is a true abruption—the etiology of which is rarely identified—or whether it is secondary to dilation of the cervix and disruption of the placenta off the lower uterine segment will most likely never be truly known. If the clinical situation is such that abruption is suspected with placenta previa, a situation requiring clinical acumen of the highest degree, delivery should be effected immediately.

Couvelaire uterus. The extravasation of blood into the myometrium is rarely associated with placenta previa, although Kalstone[13] has reported one case. Treatment should be conservative unless the hemorrhage cannot be controlled.

Rh-negative patients. Special care should be taken to assure that an appropriate amount of RhoGAM is given to Rh-negative mothers delivering Rh-positive infants. A positive Coombs' test on the third day postpartum provides assurance of adequate treatment.

■ ABRUPTIO PLACENTAE

Obstetricians have been in a quandary about the management of abruptio placentae since it was first described. The evolution of ideas through the years has little altered a high perinatal morbidity and mortality, and a rare maternal mortality still is a hazard associated with this diagnosis.

Definition and incidence

Abruptio placentae is best described as the premature separation of the normally implanted placenta. Different classes of abruption are often defined by the size of the retroplacental blood clot present at delivery or by the clinical setting (discussed more fully under the section on management).

The pathology associated with abruption is hemorrhage into the decidua basalis, which then separates or splits. The hematoma thus formed causes the acute withdrawal of the adjacent placental tissue from maternal life support. Naeye et al,[19] in a large prospective study of abruption with fetal demise, have described an increased frequency of thrombosed arteries and necrosis of the decidua basalis, suggesting that in some abruptions a vascular component may play an etiologic role.

Knab[15] reviewed a large number of articles and found the overall incidence for abruption to be 1 out of 120 deliveries, with a range of 0.52% to 1.29% of all deliveries. This wide range most likely represents different definitions and variations in the completeness of review of the clinical material. The incidence certainly varies with different populations and within one population as the socioeconomic status changes. The incidence of abruption increases as term approaches. More than 90% of infants involved weigh more than 1500 grams at the time of abruption.[3]

Marginal sinus rupture in the older literature represents a distinct pathological entity. Pritchard[27a] feels that it is an abruption limited to the margin of the placenta. Since it is a postpartum diagnosis with no way to distinguish it from antepartum bleeding of unknown etiology, it will not be discussed further. It may, however, be associated with a significant perinatal mortality.[7]

Etiology

Multiple etiologies have been associated with abruptions as outlined by Pritchard et al.[27] Few data support short umbilical cord, uterine anomaly, inferior vena cava occlusion, or maternal folate deficiency as significant etiologies. External trauma, if acute, and decompression of polyhydramnios can lead to abruption but are rare. Maternal hypertensive and/or vascular disease as a significant etiology remains controversial. Pritchard et al[27] unquestionably showed an association in their large study of abruption severe enough to cause fetal demise in which 45% of the patients had elevated blood pressure. However, these were intrapartum blood pressures. Naeye et al[19] confirmed this association with *intrapartum* hypertension but could not correlate an increased risk with preabruption hypertension. Both of these series deal with severe abruption. The data for lesser degrees of abruption do not confirm the anticipated association with chronic hypertension. Hypertension intrapartum *as a result* of the abruption (not as the etiology for it) has been suggested to explain the high association, with little pathophysiologic or experimental basis.

In multiple studies high parity increases the risk of abruption. For example, a woman with a parity of seven has a risk of abruption six times greater than a primipara and three times greater than a woman with a parity of three. Age as a separate factor does not appear to be significant. Rapid successive deliveries, however, are associated with an increased frequency of abruption, which may simply represent high parity. The strongest association with abruption is a previous history of abruption. Hibbard and Jeffcoate[10] showed that the recurrent risk of abruption is roughly 17% with one previous abruption and as high as 25% with more than one previous abruption. Concern is expressed that subsequent abruptions are often more severe than the previous one.

Grieve,[9] in a poorly controlled study, proposed that a high protein diet could eliminate abruption. Naeye[20] confirmed a strong association of abruption and poor weight gain, sug-

gesting that nutrition does play a significant role. He also demonstrated that maternal smoking (particularly in association with anemia) may be a significant contributory factor to the development of placental infarction and thereby abruption. Placentas from these patients showed an increased incidence of necrosis of the decidua basalis, which supports the hypothesis that relative or intermittent hypoxia may predispose to abruption.

Clinical presentation

The classic clinical presentation of abruptio placentae—vaginal bleeding, hypertonic tender uterus, no fetal heart tones, varying degrees of hypovolemia, and coagulopathy—represents the *unusual* patient. Most patients will have at least one of these, but occasionally none of these clinical symptoms will be manifest.

Less than one third of all cases of third trimester bleeding are diagnosed as placental abruption, and a good deal of these are retrospective diagnoses after delivery and examination of the placenta. Although dark (old) bleeding throughout the cervical os is classically associated with abruption, any type and amount of bleeding can occur. Indeed, no bleeding may be observed in concealed abruption (35% of all cases), which clinically may be the most severe type. The presence of a hypertonic tender uterus may be apparent in about half of the cases of abruption, with the incidence increasing as the severity of the process increases. If an intrauterine catheter is placed, baseline hypertonus (increased resting pressure) may be present, as well as demonstrable superimposed frequent contractions. Generalized or localized tenderness is a far less persistent clinical finding. Fetal demise happens before admission to the hospital in 25% to 35% of patients, representing the most severe, complicated cases. An additional number of fetuses will be lost before delivery and after admission to the hospital. Clinically significant bleeding disorders are usually limited to those abruptions associated with fetal demise and, even then, to less than 50% of these cases.[25]

Diagnosis

Little beyond clinical acumen may be offered in the diagnosis of abruptio placenta. Certainly placenta previa must be excluded, as discussed previously. A few reports suggest that ultrasound might be useful in the diagnosis of retroplacental clots, but our experience has not confirmed its usefulness. Serial DIC profiles (discussed later) might suggest abruption in the patient with bleeding of unknown cause. However, not many cases have been reported showing changing DIC profiles as the only objective finding.

Fetal and neonatal outcome

Naturally, little can be done to alter the outcome in the 20% of patients with abruptio placentae where fetal death is diagnosed at admission. Counseling and appropriate preparation for the next pregnancy are certainly worthwhile, however. The perinatal mortality remains high for those patients with infants alive at admission, with fetal and neonatal demise figures varying from 22.2%[31] to 40.2%.[3] The analysis of perinatal deaths is, however, most difficult, since in most series acute intervention was not attempted for fetuses weighing less than 2000 grams even when distress was detected. The neonatal deaths, as with all types of antepartum hemorrhage, are overwhelmingly associated with preterm birth, although a rare neonatal coagulopathy has been reported. Little can be done to alter the incidence of preterm birth in these situations, but delivery of a baby in better condition might significantly alter neonatal morbidity and mortality.

Hibbard and Jeffcoate[10] confirmed the impression that these infants are more likely small for gestational age (SGA). In their study 81% of babies born secondary to severe abruption before 36 weeks of gestation had low birth weight for age, suggesting a long-standing pathologic process. Others have supported these findings, although with less impressive correlations. Consistent with other types of antepartum hemorrhage, the incidence of congenital malformations is increased in this condition by two to five times. Again, no specific syndromes predominate.

Each series concerning abruptio placentae recounts patients in whom fetal heart tones could not be heard, particularly with the aural stethoscope, but who later delivered viable infants. Whether the taut uterine wall or the interposition of a retroplacental blood clot interfered with auscultation of the fetal heart recording is not known. A Doptone stethoscope or, preferably, real-time ultrasound must be used to confirm fetal demise.

The natural history of placental abruption remains controversial. The frequency of extension of abruption after the initial insult cannot be clearly documented. In addition, whether the extension will be preceded by classic monitoring signs of fetal distress, which would allow acute intervention on behalf of the fetus before it becomes severely compromised, has yet to be completely determined.

Classification

Sher,[31] in a review of clinical material from the Groote Schur Hospital in Cape Town, South Africa, proposed a *clinical* grading system for placental abruption:

Grade I incorporates those cases in which the causes of antepartum hemorrhage are uncertain and the diagnosis of abruptio placentae is made retrospectively. Most of these patients had a retroplacental clot volume of 150 ml, and none were more than 500 ml. Sher's results demonstrate that these fetuses are usually not at risk and that a favorable perinatal outcome may be achieved through delivery as soon as fetal lung maturation is obtained.

Grade II incorporates those cases in which antepartum hemorrhage is accompanied by the classic features of abruptio placentae (tenderness and tenseness of the uterus in abdominal palpation) and the fetus is alive. The retroplacental clot in these patients was usually 150 to 500 ml, with roughly 27% having a clot larger than 500 ml. Of the 26 patients in this category, 24 (92%) had an abnormal fetal heart pattern. Sher's definition of abnormal fetal heart pattern was any variation of heart rate above 160 or below 120 beats/min or "abnormal variation with contraction" as monitored by a monaural stethoscope. Seventeen of the 24 patients so identified were delivered by cesarean section, with one stillbirth. Of the remaining 7 who delivered vaginally there were four stillbirths. In contrast, only 2 patients admitted with a live fetus and tense uterus (8%) *did not* show an abnormal tracing. It appears that the *palpably* tense uterus represented a significant high-risk situation for the fetus in this small series. Sher specifies a *palpably tense uterus*, which should be distinguished from the hypertonic labor usually found at the time of placement of intrauterine catheters. The palpably tense uterus may represent the more severely hypertonic labors, although no data were presented to confirm this hypothesis. An important characteristic of Sher's patients was the identification of abnormal fetal heart patterns, although not defined by continuous heart tracing methods.

Grade III incorporates the features of grade II but fetal demise is confirmed. It is further subdivided based on the presence (A) or absence (B) of coagulopathy. Virtually all maternal mortalities in association with abruptio placentae occur in grade III patients. Meticulous attention to the cardiovascular and renal status of these patients is necessary to ensure a good maternal outcome.

Management

The rational basis for management of placental abruption has usually centered on decreasing maternal morbidity and mortality by advocacy of immediate delivery. Studies based on postpartum measurement of a retroplacental clot and its association with perinatal mortality rarely can be used to manage patients prospectively, that is, in the acute clinical situation. In our opinion immediate evaluation of the condition of the fetus and mother provides the keys to the successful management of this potential obstetric catastrophe.

The question of fetal viability in abruptio placentae is particularly important, as it alone provides an index for evaluating the severity of the disease, measuring the size of the retroplacental clot, and judging the probability of existence of a coagulopathy. Assessment of fetal death in abruptio placentae has become much more precise with the availability of ultrasonic Doppler devices to hear the fetal heart and with real-time ultrasound that permits visualization of the heart movements. Before these technologic developments, errors happened frequently, since the rigidity of the uterine wall and, in many instances, the presence of large retroplacental hematomas located in the anterior aspect of the uterus made auscultation with the fetoscope quite difficult and imprecise.

Today, as soon as the patient is admitted into the labor and delivery intensive care area with signs and symptoms strongly suggestive of abruptio placentae, a diagnosis of fetal life or death should be established using the Doppler or real-time scanner.

Fetal demise. Fetal life is perhaps the best available clinical index for the evaluation of the extension of the placental detachment (usually greater than 50% with loss of fetal life). Therefore every incidence of abruptio placentae with fetal death in utero should be classified as severe. Management of this situation includes steps discussed here.

Evaluation and replacement of blood loss.

Pritchard[25] and Pritchard and Brekken[26] have demonstrated that if abruptio placentae is severe enough to kill the fetus, the average intrapartum blood loss (most of it retroplacental) is about 2500 ml. Therefore the patient with abruptio placentae this severe has had a significant blood loss and requires aggressive measures to avoid a progressive impairment in the perfusion of vital organs. Immediate transfusion of at least 2 units of blood *regardless* of the initial vital signs is appropriate. The obstetrician should never be satisfied with a "normal" blood pressure. A previously hypertensive patient with a "normal" blood pressure may be close to shock. The pulse rate in these patients may also be "normal" until appropriate hydration produces a tachycardia. Particularly in concealed hemorrhage, a vast underestimation of blood loss frequently occurs, and when the vital signs deteriorate it may be difficult or impossible to catch up. Similar caution should be expressed in relation to the interpretation of hemoglobin and hematocrit values in patients with severe abruptio placentae. Very frequently the hemoglobin and hematocrit are within the normal range as a consequence of intense reactive vasoconstriction. The patient with abruptio placentae severe enough to kill the fetus should be transfused without consideration of the presence of normal hematocrit/hemoglobin values or normal vital signs.

Fresh whole blood is the ideal replacement, although it is rarely available. Packed red blood cells and lactated Ringer's solution are the best alternatives. After every fourth unit, evaluation of clotting status must occur, since hemodilution can create a coagulopathy itself. A unit of fresh blood or clotting factors may have to be introduced at this point. It may take up to 60 minutes to prepare these components for use, and all involved personnel should be kept aware of the clinical condition of the patient.

Intravenous fluids and central venous pressure. In cases of severe abruptio placentae the administration of large amounts of intravenous fluids should be anticipated and a central venous pressure line should be inserted through a peripheral vein to monitor the administration of these fluids. If the patient is in shock, an arterial line may be necessary to monitor the blood pressure. Our preference is to insert the line through the femoral artery. The procedure to be followed for internal jugular vein catheterization and placement of a central venous pressure line is as follows:

1. Position the patient in Trendelenburg's position and turn her head away from the side chosen for catheterization. The catheter will be inserted at the apex of the triangle where the sternal and clavicular heads of the sternocleidomastoid muscle meet. Prepare the area (from the lower mandible to below the clavicle) with povidone-iodine (Betadine), cover with drapes, and perform a skin wheal in the site of insertion using 1% mepivacaine (Carbocaine).
2. Insert an 18-gauge catheter-needle assembly at an angle of 45 degrees to the skin and aspirate while advancing the needle, which is aimed toward the ipsilateral nipple. Free flow of venous blood indicates that the needle is in the internal jugular vein.
3. Holding the needle in place, advance the catheter in the vein 4 to 5 inches. Then, holding catheter in place, withdraw the needle and connect the catheter to the intravenous line and central venous pressure manometer.
4. Apply povidone-iodine gel at the point of insertion of the catheter. Attach the catheter to the skin using two "mesentery" tapes and cover the whole thing with sterile 4 × 4 gauze.
5. Check the position of the tip of the catheter with a chest x-ray film.

The procedure to be followed for central arterial catheterization for the monitoring of central arterial pressure is as follows:

Site

The first choice is the femoral artery. It is remote from the other sites of manipulation and is easier to catheterize than other arteries. The incidence of complications is lower than with the use of other arteries.

Technique

The use of aseptic technique during the procedure is mandatory. Use a 16- or 18-gauge Intracut catheter and advance the needle into the artery until a spontaneous, pulsatile backflow of arterial blood is obtained. Then advance the catheter several inches into the vessel while the needle is simultaneously withdrawn. Cover the site of penetration of the catheter into the skin with povidone-iodine ointment and immobilize

the catheter with a mesentery tape. Apply pressure to this site for at least 5 minutes. Cover with dry gauze and nonallergic tape. Mark the time and date of insertion and the type of device inserted in the covering tape. Attach a three-way disposable stopcock to the arterial catheter. Connect the port of the stopcock opposite the catheter to the pressure transducer and the right-angle port to an intravenous fluid infusion source containing 5 units of heparin per milliliter.

The guidelines for administration of red blood cells and intravenous fluids have been established by Pritchard.[25]: *to maintain adequate organ perfusion in the patient with severe abruptio placentae, it is necessary to give blood and crystalloid solutions in amounts large enough to have at all times a hematocrit of at least 30% and a urinary output of at least 30 ml/hr.* To this may be added a third criterion—maintain a normal central venous pressure. Pritchard's two criteria are of fundamental importance; by keeping the hematocrit at 30% or more the adequacy of the patient's oxygen-carrying capacity is sustained, and by maintaining the urinary output at 30 ml/hr or more it is possible to be relatively certain that the kidneys will not succumb to acute tubular necrosis or bilateral cortical necrosis, the most common causes of death for patients with abruptio placentae. In fact, the large majority of patients with abruption die because of renal failure secondary to hypovolemia. Evaluation of the urine output is one of the most important and frequently neglected variables in the evaluation and monitoring of the patient with severe abruptio placentae. The presence of oliguria below 30 ml/hr for 2 hours in a patient with abruption constitutes a true medical emergency requiring the most urgent and aggressive corrective therapy (to be described under complications).

Coagulopathy (DIC). According to Pritchard and Brekken,[26] 38% of patients with abruptio placentae severe enough to kill the fetus have plasma fibrinogen concentrations below 150 mg/dl, and in 28% the fibrinogen level is below 100 mg/dl. Acute DIC is responsible for this alteration in fibrinogen concentration as well as for changes in other coagulation tests. In fact, simultaneously with the drop in fibrinogen, patients with abruptio placentae and DIC may also show prolonged thrombin time (TT), prolonged PT, increased FDP, positive protamine sulfate precipitation test (PSP), and low platelet count.

DIC is a syndrome that may complicate illnesses with very different etiologies, such as sepsis, giant hemangiomas, and malignancies. The syndrome occurs rather frequently in obstetric conditions such as abruptio placentae,[26] amniotic fluid embolization,[24] and prolonged fetal death in utero.[2] In the case of abruptio placentae, DIC seems to be the consequence of a massive release of placental thromboplastin within the circulation causing intravascular formation of fibrin, consumption of coagulation factors, and compensatory activation of the fibrinolytic system.

For the evaluation of the hemostatic system in patients with abruptio placentae we use a *DIC profile*. This is a battery of laboratory tests, including PT, PTT, TT, FDP, PSP, quantitative fibrinogen determination, platelet count, and euglobulin lysis time. Normal values for the DIC profile are shown in Table 15-1. The DIC profile has completely replaced old and unreliable systems for evaluating the ability of the patient to make clots. One of those tests is the whole blood clot time, which is prolonged whenever there is a severe deficiency of any coagulation factor except thrombocytopenia and deficiency of factors VII and XIII. This is a most insensitive test and is altered only in obvious severe deficiencies. A coagulation factor may be as low as 5% of normal without affecting the whole blood clotting time.

TABLE 15-1 ■ DIC profile

Test	Normal results
Fibrinogen	150 to 600 mg/dl
Prothrombin time (PT)	100% of control (control should be 11 to 16 seconds)
Partial thromboplastin time (PTT)	22 to 37 seconds
Thrombin time (TT)	Within 5 seconds of control
Platelet count	150,000 to 350,000/mm³
Fibrinogen degradation products (FDP)	Positive at less than 1:8 dilution or less than 4 µg/ml
Protamine sulfate precipitation (PSP) tests	Negative
Euglobulin lysis time	More than 120 minutes

Other tests used in the past for the evaluation of hemostasis in patients with abruptio placentae were the observation of the clot retraction and the whole blood clot lysis test. Clot retraction depends on adequate functioning of intact platelets and the presence of divalent cations. The degree of retraction does not correlate well with the platelet count, and the test may give normal results with platelet counts as low as 20,000/mm³. The clot lysis test is a gross way of observing the fibrinolytic system. The increased amount of plasmin in patients with DIC should result in dissolution of a clot, while a normal clot should remain intact for at least 48 hours. If the clot dissolves within 24 hours, fibrinolysis is increased. If fibrinolysis is very active, the clot may be dissolved within 1 hour. This test provides information usually obtained with more precise measurements, and it can be misleading, since clot lysis must be differentiated from clot retraction, and fragmentation of a friable clot may be mistaken for lysis.

The DIC profile is useful for evaluating and following the patient's coagulopathy, but abnormal results are not necessarily an indication for therapy, that is, without *clinical* evidence of excessive bleeding no therapy is warranted. Vaginal delivery can be managed in the presence of extremely low clotting components if unusual trauma is avoided. Even a cesarean section can be initiated before replacing coagulation factors, and the degree of bleeding during the operation can be used to monitor the amount of factor replacement. After delivery of the fetus and placenta the coagulopathy will resolve within hours with appropriate blood replacement and intravascular pressure maintenance. The uterus is rarely a source of excessive bleeding, as the contraction mechanism inherent in the myometrium will allow hemostasis independent of clotting factors. Sher[30] has proposed that high levels of FDP inhibit myometrial contractility and that treatment with the protease inhibitor aprotinin (Trasylol; not available in the United States) may decrease the FDP and allow the return of normal uterine activity. We have already expressed our concern that by inhibiting the degradation of fibrin, clots may persist throughout the vascular tree with consequent potential for decreasing organ perfusion and inducing greater morbidity. Also, as will be seen in the discussion of complications, there are other extremely effective measures to combat postpartum uterine atony in these patients.

It has been unfortunate that the prognostic importance and the management implications of DIC in patients with abruptio placentae have been magnified out of proportion. This has generated problems such as the use of heparin for the treatment of DIC complicating abruption. This therapeutic modality frequently recommended by internal medicine and hematology consultants should be strongly condemned. DIC in the patient with abruption has its origin in the premature separation of the placenta. The use of heparin in these cases often magnifies hypovolemia by causing additional blood loss, thereby increasing the need for additional transfusions. Another unfounded caveat is that the presence of DIC in a patient with abruptio placentae is an indication for immediate cesarean section. In reality, in the context of a generalized hemostatic defect, *any type of operative intervention should be avoided if at all possible*. An additional management error is the unnecessary replacement of coagulation factors with blood bank preparations when replacement is only necessary under specific circumstances. Finally, as mentioned earlier, the attempt to treat DIC in patients with abruptio placentae by means of fibrinolysis inhibitors lacks theoretic and experimental justification. Increased fibrinolysis in abruption represents a compensatory effort to get rid of intravascular fibrin deposits. The inhibition of this response will not affect the primary process causing DIC and may cause further impairment in organ perfusion.

Fetal presentation and size. The basic obstetric evaluation of fetal position and size is frequently forgotten when dealing with this extreme emergency. Because of the rigidity of the uterine wall and the presence of a closed, uneffaced cervix, it is often difficult to evaluate clinically the fetal presentation and size. Therefore a fetogram or sonogram should be obtained in every case of abruptio placentae where there is the slightest doubt about the fetal presentation. If a malpresentation is detected, pregnancy should be terminated by cesarean section, with the exception of very small infants (less than 800 grams) that may be delivered vaginally even if they are in transverse lie. As for patients with placenta previa, the anesthesia and uterine incision at the time of the cesarean section need

to be carefully considered. A failure in properly evaluating the fetal presentation in patients with abruptio placentae may result in a catastrophic uterine rupture when oxytocin stimulation of the uterus is carried out in the presence of an undetected dystocic presentation.

Delivery. Without a malpresentation, every effort should be made to deliver the patient with abruptio placentae and fetal death in utero vaginally. Amniotomy should be carried out as soon as practicable, followed by the insertion of an intrauterine pressure catheter. Oxytocin infusion for induction or augmentation of labor should be used irrespective of maternal age and parity unless there is clear evidence of active spontaneous labor. The rigidity of the uterus or the presence of a high intrauterine resting pressure should not deter the use of oxytocin. In many instances it will be necessary to use rather large amounts (50 to 100 mU/min) of oxytocin to obtain progressive cervical dilation and effacement. However, total intrauterine pressure at the peak of contractions should not exceed 100 mm Hg.

The clinical pattern and the monitoring characteristics of spontaneous or induced labor in patients with severe abruptio placentae are different from those observed in normal pregnancies at term. In fact, in these patients the uterus remains rigid at all times. There is constant pain that is superimposed on the cyclic and intermittent pain of labor. With the use of an intrauterine pressure catheter, the resting pressure is very high (usually around 40 mm Hg) and contractions are seen as small waves on top of the resting pressure recording. Despite the lack of clinical and monitoring signs of cyclic uterine activity, the cervix starts to change, and after complete effacement dilation is usually fast.

Pritchard[25] has demonstrated that there is no arbitrary limit of time for obtaining a vaginal delivery in patients with abruptio placentae and fetal death in utero. In the past there was a dictum that these patients should be delivered in 4 to 6 hours, thus possibly introducing morbidity by aggressive and excessive uterine stimulation and operative delivery. Today we know that with appropriate maintenance of the maternal status the time period to obtain vaginal delivery may be extended safely up to 24 hours. Urine output of 30 to 60 ml/hr in the absence of diuretic administration and maintenance of a hematocrit above 30% can go a long way to assure a good maternal outcome. If there is an abnormal fetal presentation, if the patient had a previous cesarean section, or if cephalopelvic disproportion is suspected, the patient with abruptio placentae and fetal death in utero should be delivered by cesarean section. In these cases, fortunately a minority, evaluation of hemostasis with a DIC profile before surgery is mandatory. Patients with fibrinogen concentration less than 100 mg/dl will benefit from the administration of 10 to 20 units of cryoprecipitate immediately before and during the operation. This amount of cryoprecipitate contains enough fibrinogen to secure adequate hemostasis during surgery and prevent the loss of additional blood volume. Very rarely is a platelet transfusion necessary; the criteria for platelet transfusion are abnormal bleeding with a count below 20,000/mm^3.

Following is a summary of measures to be taken in the initial management of the patient with severe abruptio placentae:

1. Initiate transfusion of whole blood (ideally *fresh* whole blood) regardless of the initial vital signs and the initial hemoglobin and hematocrit concentrations. *Confirm fetal demise with real-time ultrasound*.
2. Insert a Foley catheter and evaluate the urine output every hour.
3. Give blood and crystalloid solutions in amounts large enough to maintain at all times a hematocrit of at least 30% and a urinary output of at least 30 ml/hr.
4. Obtain a sonogram. If there is no fetal malpresentation, start an intravenous infusion of oxytocin. Remember that high doses of oxytocin may be required, that monitoring of uterine activity is unreliable, and that the best index of progress in labor is the cervical changes.
5. Obtain a DIC profile. Patients with consumption coagulopathy *may* require the administration of fresh frozen plasma or cryoprecipitate if cesarean section or episiotomy is carried out.

Following are some indications of what *not* to do in patients with abruptio placentae and DIC:

1. *Do not give heparin*. There is no place for heparin in the management of obstetric bleeding. Heparin use in abruptio placentae is dangerous and contraindicated.

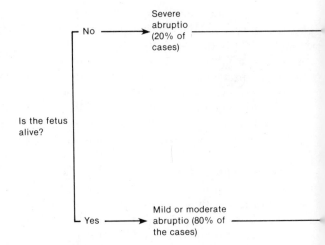

FIG. 15-3 ■ Management of abruptio placentae.

2. *Do not intervene by performing a cesarean section unless there is a clear indication for the procedure*. Remember that DIC by itself *is not* an indication for cesarean section but rather a strong contraindication. Surgical procedures should be avoided if at all possible in the presence of existing or impending generalized hemostatic defect. The presence of a long, hard cervix *is not* an indication for cesarean section. The cervix very quickly will efface and dilate after oxytocin induction.
3. *Do not administer fibrinolysis inhibitors*. Increased fibrinolysis in patients with abruptio placentae is a homeostatic compensatory mechanism, and its inhibition will not affect the primary process causing the coagulopathy.

A live fetus. If the fetus is alive, complexity of management of the patient with abruptio placentae increases.[18] Mother and fetus are at risk for loss of life. No condition requires more sophisticated obstetric care. There are two main subgroups of patients: those with a palpably hypertonic uterus and those with a palpably soft uterus.

Patients with palpably hypertonic uterus. If the infant is alive and the uterus is rigid at all times, the abruption is probably large but under 50% (moderate abruptio placentae) and the

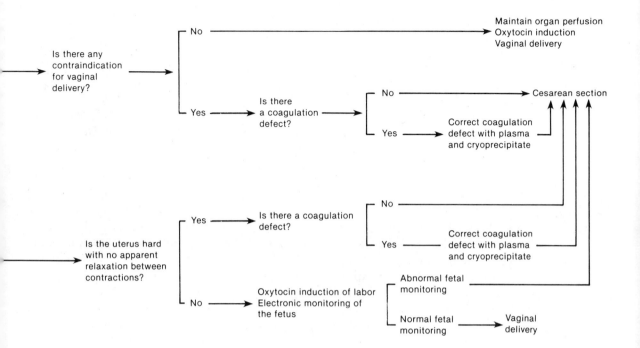

chances of fetal distress being present or happening later are more than 90%.[31] The patient should be prepared for a cesarean section unless there are very special circumstances that preclude surgical intervention (eg, maternal shock, previable fetus). The preparations for cesarean section should include evaluation of the patient's hemostasis profile and availability of at least 4 units of blood for potential use during surgery. The occurrence of overt coagulopathy when the abruption has not been large enough to kill the fetus is extremely rare. However, coagulopathy, bleeding, and maternal death may occur as a result of precipitous surgical intervention without appropriate preparation. As with most fetal indications, there is a strong inclination to rapidly intervene by cesarean section. This decision must be carefully balanced against the possibility of increased maternal morbidity and mortality resulting from operating on a subject whose condition may be severely compromised.

Some concern has been expressed that, with an aggressive policy of abdominal delivery of patients with moderate abruptio placentae, intrapartum fetal death is simply converted to neonatal death or to survival of a neurologically impaired infant. The older data dealing with gestational age and morbidity unfortunately cannot be compared to neonatal survival since 1970. The clear impression is that small babies born

early as a result of abruptio placentae do a great deal better now than before 1970. Niswander et al[22] was not able to document any neurologic deficit in his 4-year follow-up study of infants born with intrapartum complications such as placenta previa, abruptio placentae, and cord prolapse when compared with matched controls. The most significant correlation of neurologic deficit was with gestational age at the time of birth.

Patients with palpably soft uterus. If the uterus is soft but the clinical history strongly suggests abruptio placentae, the pregnancy should be terminated by induction of labor using amniotomy and intravenous oxytocin. If an abruption is present, it probably will not be greater than 25%. The chance of significant coagulopathy is extremely low, and the prospects for a vaginal delivery with good fetal and maternal outcome are excellent. Should the uterus become hypertonic during labor or should signs of fetal distress appear, it must be assumed that an extension of the abruption has happened and the pregnancy should be terminated by cesarean section. In the absence of uterine rigidity, fetal distress, or obstetric contraindication for vaginal delivery, the large majority of patients should have an uneventful course.

Fig. 15-3 summarizes the overall plan of management for patients with abruptio placentae.

Complications

The overwhelming majority of complications in abruptio placentae are the consequence of hypovolemia and its inadequate treatment. The situation is such that the older literature is rich in references to "obstetrical shock" defined as "shock out of proportion to the blood loss" thought to happen commonly in abruptio placentae. Pritchard and Brekken[26] have firmly laid this concept to rest: hemorrhage in abruptio placentae is often massive and more often underestimated and undertreated.

Coagulopathy can contribute to aggravate hemorrhagic problems, but as discussed before this complication has quick resolution on delivery of the placenta and becomes significant only if operative treatment is necessary. Postpartum uterine atony and Couvelaire uterus certainly happen with abruptio placentae. Amniotic fluid embolization, which most likely increases with abruption,[24] is a catastrophic complication that cannot be anticipated. Also, it is important to remember that the Rh-negative mother with abruptio placentae may have had massive fetomaternal transfusion and require larger than usual RhoGAM dosage to avoid isoimmunization.

For the management of some maternal complications of abruption, the reader is referred to Chapter 13 and the discussion of the management of patients with severe bleeding earlier in this chapter. With respect to the fetus, the overwhelming majority of complications result from prematurity and hypoxia. Hypovolemic shock of the newborn is rare but may be associated with any maternal antepartum hemorrhage. A fetal and neonatal coagulopathy has been suggested in connection with abruption but is very infrequent.

Prognosis for future pregnancies

According to Pritchard et al,[27] 14% of future pregnancies in patients with abruptio placentae will finish in spontaneous abortion and 9.3% of the patients will have repeated abruption. It has also been suggested that the risk of repetition after two consecutive pregnancies with abruptio placentae is 25%. A great deal of discussion has been directed toward management of subsequent pregnancies. Delivery before term has been recommended because of the significant

risk of repeated abruption and because the repeat abruption may be more severe than the first. Again, no data can substantiate this recommendation. Most likely, corrections of premorbid factors such as poor nutrition, low weight gain, and smoking would have a far greater effect on reducing the incidence of recurrence than early delivery with its potential for fetal morbidity.

■ VASA PREVIA

Vasa previa is an anomaly in which the umbilical vessels have a velamentous insertion on a low-lying placenta and traverse the membranes in the lower uterine segment in front of the fetal presenting part. Under this condition the vessels may be lacerated at the time of artificial or spontaneous rupture of the membranes, causing fetal exsanguination and death. Because of the absence of the protective Wharton's gelatin, the vessels may also become lacerated and bleed before rupture of the membranes occurs. Fetal hypoxia and eventual fetal death may be caused when the cord vessels are compressed by the fetal presenting part, particularly during uterine contractions. With all these possibilities, it is not surprising that fetal mortality in vasa previa reaches 75% to 100%. There is little, if any, increase in maternal complications. Fortunately, vasa previa is a rare condition (1 out of 2000 to 3000 deliveries).

The diagnosis of vasa previa should be considered in all cases of third trimester bleeding and in all cases of fetal distress with monitoring characteristics of cord compression. If both conditions exist in the same patient, that is, vaginal bleeding and fetal distress, the possibility of vasa previa is greater. Vaginal blood should be examined immediately for fetal hemoglobin (see box on p. 281). Emergency delivery of the fetus should be effected if there is evidence of fetal bleeding.

■ ANTEPARTUM BLEEDING OF UNKNOWN ETIOLOGY

After exclusion of placenta previa and abruptio placentae in the bleeding patient, the tendency is to breathe a sigh of relief and send the patient home. Willocks[32] reported an incidence of premature delivery of 17% in his population of women with antepartum bleeding of unknown etiology, and an overall perinatal mortality of 14.2%, far higher than in the general population. Roberts[28] presented similar data with a perinatal mortality of 6%, 72% of which resulted from premature delivery. Although these risks are less than with other antepartum problems already discussed, caution and appropriate monitoring of these patients should be exercised.

Other etiologies for antepartum bleeding as proposed by Abdul-Karim and Chevli[1] are as follows:

Cervicitis
Cervical erosions
Endocervical polyps
Cancer of the cervix
Vaginal, vulvar, and cervical varicosities
Vaginal infections
Foreign bodies
Genital lacerations
Bloody show
Vasa previa
Degenerating uterine fibroids

This confirms that at one point in the management of third trimester bleeding there is a need for a direct cervical examination with a speculum. These entities most probably represent less than 1% of all bleeding cases but would certainly alter therapy. Except for vasa previa, only a few of these complications pose a risk to fetal life, unless there is massive hemorrhage.

■ REFERENCES

1. Abdul-Karim RW, Chevli RN: Antepartum hemorrhage and shock. Clin Obstet Gynecol 1976;19:533.
2. Beller FK, Uszynski M: Disseminated intravascular coagulation in pregnancy. Clin Obstet Gynecol 1974; 17:250.
3. Blair RG: Abruption of the placenta. A review of 189 cases occurring between 1965 and 1969. J Obstet Gynaecol Br Commonw 1973;80:242.
4. Breen JL, Neubecker R, Gregori CA, et al: Placenta accreta, increta, and percreta. Obstet Gynecol 1977; 49:43.
5. Brenner WE, Edelman DA, Hendricks CH: Characteristics of patients with placenta previa and results of expectant management. Am J Obstet Gynecol 1978; 132:180.
6. Crenshaw C, Jones DED, Parker RT: Placenta previa: a survey of twenty years experience with improved perinatal survival by expectant therapy and cesarean delivery. Obstet Gynecol Surv 1973;28:246.
7. Fish JS, Bartholomew RA, Colveir ED, et al: The role of marginal sinus rupture in antenatal hemorrhage. Am J Obstet Gynecol 1951;61:20.
8. Fox H: Placenta accreta, 1945-1965. Obstet Gynecol Surv 1972;27:475.
9. Grieve JFK: Prevention of gestational failure by high protein diet. J Reprod Med 1974;13:170.
10. Hibbard BM, Jeffcoate TN: Abruptio placentae. Obstet Gynecol 1966;27:155.
11. Hibbard LT: Placenta previa. Am J Obstet Gynecol 1969;104:172.
12. Howie RN, Liggins GC: Clinical trial of antepartum betamethasone therapy for prevention of respiratory distress in pre-term infants, in Anderson A, Beard R, Brundenell JM, et al (eds): *Pre-term labor*. London, The Royal College of Obstetricians and Gynecologists, 1977, p. 281.
12a. Johnson JW, Austin KL, Jones GS, et al: Efficacy of 17 alpha hydroxy progesterone caproate in the prevention of premature labor. N Engl J Med 1975;293:675.
13. Kalstone CE: Couvelaire uterus and placenta previa. Am J Obstet Gynecol 1969;105:638.
14. Kleiner GJ, Greston WM: Current concepts of defibrination in the pregnant woman. J Reprod Med 1976;17:309.
15. Knab DR: Abruptio placentae: an assessment of the time and method of delivery. Obstet Gynecol 1978;52:625.
16. Kurjak A, Barsic B: Changes of placental site diagnosed by repeated ultrasonic examination. Acta Obstet Gynecol Scand 1977;56:161.
17. Liggins GC, Howie RN: A controlled trial of antepartum glucocorticoid treatment for prevention of the respiratory distress syndrome in premature infants. Pediatrics 1972;50:515.
18. Lunan CB: The management of abruptio placentae. J Obstet Gynaecol Br Commonw 1973;80:120.
19. Naeye RC, Harkness WL, Utts J: Abruptio placentae and perinatal death: a prospective study. Am J Obstet Gynecol 1977;128:740.
20. Naeye RL: Placenta infarction leading to fetal or neonatal death: a prospective study. Obstet Gynecol 1977;50:583.
21. Nelson HB, Huston JE: Placenta previa: a possible solution to the associated high fetal mortality rate. J Reprod Med 1971;7:188.
22. Niswander KR, Gordon M, Drage J: The effect of intrauterine hypoxia on the child surviving to 4 years. Am J Obstet Gynecol 1975;121:892.
23. Ogita S, et al: A simplified method for measuring fetal hemoglobin. Obstet Gynecol 1976;48:237.
24. Peterson EP, Taylor HB: Amniotic fluid embolism: an analysis of 40 cases. Obstet Gynecol 1970;35:787.
25. Pritchard JA: Haematological problems associated with delivery, placental abruption, retained dead fetus, and amniotic fluid embolism. Clin Haematol 1973;2:563.
26. Pritchard JA, Brekken AL: Clinical and laboratory studies on severe abruptio placentae. Am J Obstet Gynecol 1967;97:681.
27. Pritchard JA, Ruble M, Corley M, et al: Genesis of severe placental abruption. Am J Obstet Gynecol 1970;108:22.
27a. Pritchard JA, McDonald PC: *Williams Obstetrics*, ed. 15. New York, Appleton-Century-Crofts, 1976, p. 407.

28. Roberts G: Unclassified antepartum hemorrhage incidence and perinatal mortality in a community. J Obstet Gynaecol Br Commonw 1970;77:492.

29. Semmens JP: A second look at expectant management of placenta previa. Postgrad Med 1968;44:207.

30. Sher G: Pathogenesis and management of uterine inertia complicating abruptio placentae with consumption coagulopathy. Am J Obstet Gynecol 1977;291:164.

31. Sher G: A rational basis for the management of abruptio placentae. J Reprod Med 1978;21:123.

32. Willocks J: Antepartum hemorrhage of uncertain origin. J Obstet Gynaecol Br Commonw 1971;78:987.

16

■ ■ ■

ABNORMALITIES OF LABOR

Fernando Arias

Labor is a complex physiologic process by which the products of conception (fetus, amniotic fluid, placenta, membranes) are expelled from the uterus into the outside world. This process is clinically characterized by increased frequency, intensity, and duration of uterine contractions, by progressive effacement and dilation of the cervix, and by descent of the fetus through the birth canal.

Most of the present understanding of labor and its abnormalities is the product of the work of Emanuel A. Friedman. Since 1954 this investigator has been publishing his clinical research about labor, and by doing so he has built up a scientific work that remains unchallenged in its dimensions and in the validity of its conclusions. Friedman gave scientific basis to the clinical evaluation of labor and made it possible for everybody to understand labor and its abnormalities. Most of this chapter is a reiteration of Friedman's findings (for additional information on the subject see his original work and especially his book *Labor: Clinical Evaluation and Management*,[1a] which is a milestone in the history of modern obstetrics).

■ A GRAPHIC REPRESENTATION OF LABOR: THE FRIEDMAN CURVE

When progression in cervical dilation and descent of the presenting part during normal human labor are plotted against time, a graphic

representation (partogram) of the labor process is construed (Fig. 16-1). By looking at this graph it is apparent that during normal labor cervical dilation follows a sigmoid-shaped curve (Fig. 16-1, line A) where it is possible to recognize three distinct parts: (1) the initial part of the sigmoid where there is little progression in cervical dilation is called *latent phase;* (2) the part of the curve where there is a fast progression in dilation is called *active phase;* and (3) the final part of the sigmoid where the rate of cervical dilation becomes slow again is called *deceleration phase.* Descent of the presenting part (Fig. 16-1, line B) follows a hyperbolic-shaped curve with little initial change, followed by fast progress that starts at the beginning of the deceleration phase and continues linearly until the perineal floor (station +5) is reached.

There are variations in the partogram between nulliparous and multiparous patients and among individual patients with the same parity. Normal variations, however, are amenable to statistical analysis that in turn makes it possible to recognize the occurrence of abnormalities.

■ TYPES OF LABOR ABNORMALITIES

We prefer to classify the abnormalities of labor according to the period of labor in which they occur: the latent phase (Friedman's preparatory division), the active phase (Friedman's dilational division), and the second stage of labor (Fried-

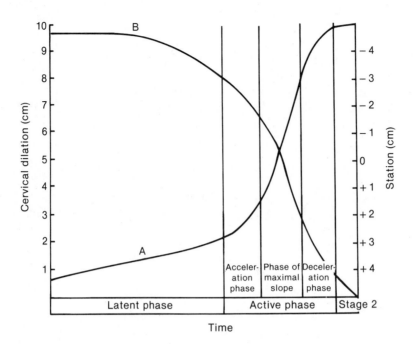

FIG. 16-1 ■ Graphic representation of labor (Friedman curve). Line *A*, progress in cervical dilation with time and line *B*, progressive descent of the presenting part with the progression of labor.

Labor abnormalities

PERIOD OF LABOR	ABNORMALITY
Latent phase	Prolonged latent phase
Active phase	Protracted active phase dilation Secondary arrest of dilation Prolonged deceleration phase
Second stage	Failure of descent Protracted descent Arrest of descent
All periods	Precipitate labor

---

man's pelvic division). The latent phase of labor, in which the cervix becomes prepared for the drastic anatomic changes that happen later, has only one abnormality, prolonged latent phase. The abnormalities of the active phase of labor, characterized by perturbations of the cervical dilation process are (1) protracted active phase dilation, (2) secondary arrest of dilation, and (3) prolonged deceleration phase. Abnormalities of the second stage of labor, characterized by defects in the descent of the presenting part, are (1) failure of descent, (2) protracted descent, and (3) arrest of descent. Finally, there is an abnormality characterized by a rapid labor, precipitate labor. A summary of the eight types of labor abnormalities is shown in the box on the left.

The abnormalities just mentioned are easily recognized if the obstetrician uses a graphic analysis of labor in which cervical dilation and descent of the presenting part are plotted in the ordinate and time in hours is plotted in the abscissa. The diagnosis of labor abnormalities in the absence of a graphic analysis of labor is imprecise and frequently in error.

Prolonged latent phase

Definition. The latent phase is the interval from the onset of labor to the beginning of the active phase (upswing of the cervical dilation tracing). The mean duration of the latent phase is 8.6 hours in the nullipara and 5.3 hours in the multipara; the 95th percentile limits are 20.6 hours for nulliparas and 13.6 hours for multip-

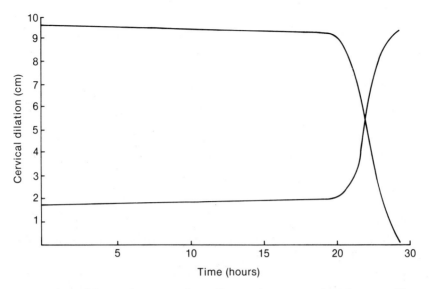

FIG. 16-2 ▪ Prolonged latent phase. A prolonged latent phase exists when the interval between the beginning of labor and the upswing of the cervical dilation curve exceeds 20 hours in the nullipara and 14 hours in the multipara.

aras. A prolonged latent phase exists when its duration exceeds the 95th percentile limits or from a practical viewpoint when it exceeds 20 hours in the nullipara and 14 hours in the multipara (Fig. 16-2).

Diagnosis. The most common problems associated with the diagnosis of a prolonged latent phase are the difficulties in defining the onset of labor and the beginning of the active phase. In many instances it is difficult to distinguish between false labor and a latent phase of labor. Also, sometimes it is difficult to decide if the labor is in a prolonged latent phase or an early secondary arrest of cervical dilation.

The problem of differentiating between a latent phase of labor and false labor is not critical as long as the obstetrician avoids any active intervention such as amniotomy or labor stimulation. In fact, both false labor and prolonged latent phase are benign conditions, and no harm occurs to either baby or mother from a wait-and-see policy. In contrast, intervention may lead to a series of complications and result in maternal and fetal morbidity.

The best criterion for recognizing false labor from a prolonged latent phase is retrospective: if a patient who has had regular uterine contractions without cervical changes ceases laboring after receiving 15 mg of morphine and 200

mg of secobarbital, she was in false labor. Unfortunately, a retrospective diagnosis is not useful in practice. The best way to avoid a mistake is by a clear definition of the beginning of labor. Friedman believes that the presence of regular uterine contractions, uncomfortable enough to make the patient come to the hospital, is the most reliable sign of the onset of labor. Other authors,[12] however, only accept as an adequate sign of the beginning of labor the observation of progressive effacement and dilation of the cervix.

A differential diagnosis of greater significance is between a prolonged latent phase and an early secondary arrest of cervical dilation. The first is a benign condition, whereas the latter implies a significant risk of cephalopelvic disproportion. This problem of diagnosis usually does not exist when the patient has been observed in the hospital for several hours and a definite upswing in the cervical dilation curve has been documented. The problem is common when patients are admitted to labor and delivery with 3 or 4 cm of dilation, advanced cervical effacement, regular uterine contractions, but no progress in cervical dilation is observed during the next few hours. These patients may be in secondary arrest of dilation or in a prolonged latent phase. Since under this set of circumstances there is no way of making a differential diagnosis, the best management is to assume that the worst (secondary arrest of cervical dilation) is happening and initiate the diagnostic and therapeutic measures necessary for patients affected with this condition.

Frequency. A prolonged latent phase is not a common event. According to Friedman, it affects 1.45% of nulliparas and 0.33% of multiparas. However, when cases of prolonged latent phase alone and cases of prolonged latent phase combined with other labor disorders are put together, the incidence increases to 2.31% in nulliparas and 0.44% in multiparas. Sokol et al[13] found a higher incidence for this disorder; it affected 3.6% of the nulliparas and 4.2% of the multiparas in their study, but they did not differentiate between a prolonged latent phase alone and a prolonged latent phase combined with other disorders.

Etiology. The most common (about 50% of the cases) etiologic agent of a prolonged latent phase in nulliparas is early and excessive use of sedative and analgesics during labor.[3] In these cases resumption of normal labor usually occurs after the medications wear off. The second most common cause in nulliparas is the presence of a thick, uneffaced, unripe cervix at the beginning of labor.

The most common cause of prolonged latent phase in multiparas is false labor. Although false labor only occurs in about 10% of nulliparas initially diagnosed as in a prolonged latent phase, it occurs in more than 50% of multiparas with the same diagnosis. This difference in the incidence of false labor between nulliparas and multiparas shows how difficult it is to diagnose the beginning of labor in multiparous patients.

Management. There are two modes of management for patients with a prolonged latent phase: (1) rest and (2) oxytocin stimulation. Both methods have approximately the same effectiveness and are capable of eliminating the labor abnormality in about 85% of the cases. The selection of management should be based on considerations such as the state of fatigue and anxiety of the patient, the basic etiology of the problem (excessive sedation, unripe cervix), and the convenience for the patient and obstetrician.

If rest is chosen as the mode of management, 15 mg of morphine IM should be given followed by oral administration of 200 mg of secobarbital.

This treatment is effective: the overwhelming majority of patients are sleeping within 1 hour after treatment and awake 4 to 5 hours later in active labor or in no labor. There are two eventual problems with this treatment. The first problem is the possibility of giving this relatively high dose of narcotics to a patient who in reality is in the active phase of labor and who may deliver a depressed baby within a short period after treatment. This problem can be avoided by careful evaluation of the patient before administration of the drugs. If the problem occurs, the pediatrician should be notified before delivery so that he or she can be ready to administer adequate treatment to the infant if necessary.

The second problem with the rest approach to the management of patients in a prolonged latent phase is that the obstetrician, reluctant to use the generous amounts of medication just recommended, may give instead smaller doses that are often ineffective and may contribute to making the problem worse. The dose just recommended is adequate for most patients and should be lower only in the case of small, thin women.

If oxytocin stimulation is chosen as the mode of treatment, an intravenous drip of the medication must be used, and labor must be monitored with electronic instruments. The patient is already in labor and may not need a large amount of medication to move into the active phase. Oxytocin must be started at 0.5 to 1.0 mU/minute and increased gradually at 20- to 30-minute intervals. The majority of patients in the latent phase respond to dosages no larger than 8 mU/minute.

A therapeutic error that should be avoided with patients in prolonged latent phase is amniotomy in an attempt to accelerate labor. Amniotomy for this purpose is of no value, according to Friedman. Also, since the prognosis for patients in a prolonged latent phase is benign and the treatment of the disorder is usually successful, there is no justification for cesarean section in these cases unless there is an indication different from the labor abnormality. To perform a cesarean section because of a prolonged latent phase reveals poor judgment.

Prognosis. A prolonged latent phase is a benign abnormality that entails little or no risk for mother and baby. The great majority (75%) of patients with this abnormality continue laboring normally once they come out of the latent phase and have normal vaginal deliveries. A minority come out of the prolonged latent phase only to develop another abnormality such as secondary arrest of cervical dilation (6.9% of the patients) or a protracted active phase (20.6%). The prognosis is not benign for patients who develop other labor abnormalities because frequently (about 50% of the cases) they require termination of pregnancy by cesarean section. Finally, about 10% of patients with a prolonged latent phase are in fact in false labor.

Protracted active phase

Definition. A protracted active phase is characterized by a rate of cervical dilation in the active phase of labor that is less than 1.2 cm/hour in the nullipara and less than 1.5 cm/hour in the multipara (Fig. 16-3, line A).

Diagnosis. The diagnosis of protracted active phase has the following three requirements:

1. The patient must be in the active phase of labor. Sometimes patients in the latent phase at 3 or 4 cm of dilation may be erroneously diagnosed as having protracted active phase when in fact the upward swing of the cervical dilation curve (characteristic of the beginning of the active phase of labor) has not yet occurred.

2. The patient must not have reached the deceleration phase. Sometimes confusion occurs between prolonged deceleration phase (an arrest disorder) and protracted active phase (a protraction disorder). This happens more often in patients with combined labor abnormalities (ie, protracted active phase plus prolonged deceleration phase), but such confusion should not occur if close attention is given to the characteristics of the labor curve. In the case of prolonged deceleration a lack of cervical dilation at the end of the first stage of labor is apparent, whereas in the case of the protraction disorder a characteristically slow progress in cervical dilation affecting the whole length of the active phase is seen.

3. The patient must have a minimum of two pelvic examinations 1 hour apart. The diagnosis is much more precise, however, if the slope of cervical dilation is measured from a labor curve constructed from the findings of three or four pelvic examinations carried out during a 3- to 4-hour period.

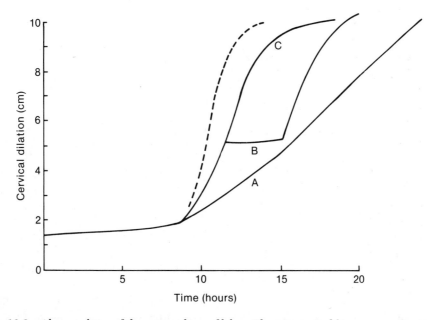

FIG. 16-3 ■ Abnormalities of the active phase of labor. The interrupted line, a normal pattern of cervical dilation during the active phase of labor. Line *A*, cervical dilation in a patient with protracted active phase dilation. Line *B*, cervical dilation in a patient with secondary arrest of cervical dilation; the postarrest slope of the dilation curve is normal. Line *C*, the cervical dilation pattern of a patient in a prolonged deceleration phase; in these cases dilation is normal until it reaches 8 or 9 cm, then it becomes abnormally slow.

Frequency. Protracted active phase is present in about 2% to 4% of all labors. In more than 70% of the cases this abnormality occurs in combination with arrest disorders or with a prolonged latent phase.

Etiology. Excessive sedation, conductive anesthesia, fetal malposition, and cephalopelvic disproportion are the most common etiologic agents. Disproportion is present in 28.1% of the cases. Occipitotransverse (OT) and occipitoposterior (OP) presentations are found in 70.6% of the cases.[4]

Management. As in the management of other labor aberrations, in the case of protracted active phase the treatment depends on the etiology of the disorder. Since the frequency of disproportion is high, it must be a prime suspect, and clinical evaluation of the fetus-pelvic relationship must precede any therapeutic procedure. If the Hillis-Müller maneuver (described later) shows a roomy pelvis, the possibility of excessive sedation or anesthesia or the presence of an abnormal fetal position are the next factors to consider.

If excessive sedation or regional anesthesia is the probable causal agent, waiting for spontaneous abatement of the labor-inhibiting factor is the adequate course of action. If fetal malposition (OP or OT) is present, the patient should be supported and reassured until she reaches a point in labor at which intervention may be possible (see Chapter 17). If disproportion is present (as documented by Ball pelvimetry), the pregnancy must be terminated by cesarean section.

Frequently it is impossible to identify a causal factor for patients in protracted active phase. The pelvis is roomy, there is a clear downward thrust with the Hillis-Müller maneuver, the fetal head position is normal, and the patient is not under the influence of labor-inhibiting factors. In these cases an intrauterine pressure catheter (IUP) should be inserted to obtain a precise evaluation of the uterine contractility. If the contractions are more than 3 minutes apart, last less than 40 seconds, and provoke a rise in IUP of less than 50 mm Hg, it is proper to assume that a deficiency in the expulsive power of the uterus is the cause of the problem, and gentle stimulation with oxytocin is in order. If the contractions are adequate, no benefit will be obtained from oxytocin augmentation, amniotomy, or rest

and sedation, and these patients will continue with their slow progression in cervical dilation until delivery.

If protracted active phase is part of a combined labor disorder, the patient must be managed according to the norms given for the treatment of the most serious of the combined problems. For example, if protracted active phase and arrest of cervical dilation are present in a given patient, the management must follow the norms given for secondary arrest of cervical dilation, the more serious of the two disorders.

Prognosis. Almost 70% of patients in protracted active phase subsequently develop an arrest disorder (arrest of cervical dilation or arrest of descent). The other 30% continue with their slow progress, and the prognosis, both maternal and fetal, is good as long as the delivery is atraumatic.

The prognosis for patients who develop arrest patterns after protracted active phase is poor: 42% require cesarean-section delivery, and 20% have midforceps deliveries. The delivery prognosis is influenced markedly by the presence of an adequate postarrest slope of cervical dilation. Also, combined disorders have a poor prognosis when they are diagnosed before the cervix reaches 6 cm of dilation. Another important factor in the prognosis is the parity of the patient: most multiparas (83.3%) with combined protraction and arrest disorders respond to therapy and dilate further; only about 24% of them require cesarean-section delivery.

Secondary arrest of cervical dilation

Definition. Secondary arrest of cervical dilation occurs when the dilation of the cervix stops for 2 or more hours during the period of maximal slope in the active phase of labor (Fig. 16-3, line B).

Diagnosis. The diagnosis of secondary arrest of dilation requires a minimum of two vaginal examinations 2 hours apart, documenting the lack of cervical dilation during this period. The arrest of dilation must occur during the phase of maximal slope of dilation to avoid confusion with prolonged latent phase (a disorder that occurs when the phase of maximal slope has not yet started) or prolonged deceleration (a disorder that occurs when the phase of maximal slope is over).

Frequency. The most common disorder occurring during the active phase of labor is secondary arrest of dilation. Sokol et al[13] found this problem in 6.8% of nulliparas and in 3.5% of multiparas. These figures are significantly lower than the frequency of 11.7% in nulliparas and 4.8% in multiparas found by Friedman and Kroll[2] using the data of the Collaborative Perinatal Study. In any case this labor abnormality occurs more in nulliparas and is a frequent component of situations in which several labor abnormalities are present simultaneously.

Etiology. The most important fact in secondary arrest of cervical dilation is that in about 50% of the cases the etiologic factor is cephalopelvic disproportion. As is discussed later, this high incidence of disproportion makes it imperative to evaluate rigorously the fetus-pelvic relationship in every patient exhibiting this abnormality of labor.

In the original work by Friedman and Sachtleben[5] 44.6% of all patients with secondary arrest of cervical dilation had documented cephalopelvic disproportion. Other prevalent etiologic agents are malposition of the fetal head, excessive narcosis, and regional anesthesia; quite often patients are affected by a combination of two or more of these factors, including disproportion.

Management. The first thing to do once the diagnosis of secondary arrest of cervical dilation has been established is to evaluate the fetus-pelvic relationship. The objective is to document the presence of disproportion to avoid unnecessary and potentially dangerous augmentation of labor. The problem lies in the lack of sensitivity of the presently available methods for assessing the fetus-pelvic relationship. In fact, clinical evaluation of this variable is at its best imprecise, and there are serious questions about the reliability of the assessment by means of x-ray examination.

The most important clinical maneuver for evaluating the fetus-pelvic relationship is the Hillis-Müller test. To carry it out the obstetrician does a pelvic examination immediately before or at the beginning of a uterine contraction. When the contraction is at its peak, an attempt is made to push the fetal presenting part into the pelvis by pressing on the uterine fundus with the free hand. The hand in the vagina is used to determine whether or not there is downward mobility of the presenting part into the maternal pelvis when pressure is applied to the fundus. If the presenting part does not move or moves very little, the possibility of fetus-pelvic disproportion becomes high. In contrast, if the presenting part moves easily into the pelvis, the chances of disproportion are low.

Patients with secondary arrest and limited mobility with the Hillis-Müller test should be subsequently evaluated by x-ray pelvimetry. What must be evaluated is the fetus-pelvic relationship and not the maternal pelvis alone. It makes little sense to measure the diameters of the bony pelvis and determine the absence or presence of disproportion by comparing these measurements against some arbitrary standards when they should be evaluated in relation to the dimensions of the fetal head. This is the basic reason the Ball method, as described and modified by Friedman and Taylor,[10] is the best radiologic technique for assessing a patient with arrest of cervical dilation. Two films (an anteroposterior and a lateral centered at the pelvis) are necessary, and both must be taken with the patient in a standing position. The distance from the x-ray source to the film must be constant (40 to 44 inches) and must be known by the obstetrician, since the nomograms available for calculation are based on one of these two values. The values for the anteroposterior and transverse diameters of the inlet, the interspinous diameter, and the circumference of the fetal head are obtained and corrected using the object-film distance. Finally, the corrected pelvic diameters are converted to capacities and the head circumference to volume, and these values are compared to evaluate the cephalopelvic relationship. If the head volume exceeds the inlet capacity by more than 50 ml or the interspinous capacity by more than 200 ml, absolute disproportion is present. If the head volume exceeds the capacity of the inlet by less than 50 ml or the capacity of the middle of the pelvis by 150 to 200 ml, the case is one of relative disproportion. If the inlet capacity is equal to or greater than the head volume or if the interspinous capacity is up to 150 ml smaller than the head volume, no disproportion exists.

Ball pelvimetry makes it possible to diagnose absolute cephalopelvic disproportion and avoid further attempts for a vaginal delivery in about one third of the patients with secondary arrest of cervical dilation. Another one third of these patients have borderline disproportion, and another third have no disproportion. Those patients with confirmed diagnosis of disproportion must have cesarean-section delivery without further delays.

Patients with a positive Hillis-Müller test (adequate downward movement of the fetal head with fundal pressure) and those with adequate or borderline Ball pelvimetry require augmentation of labor under invasive monitoring (IUP catheter and fetal scalp electrode). A majority of these patients have poor uterine activity manifested by contractions that are infrequent (more than 3 minutes apart), short (total duration of 40 seconds or less), and mild (less than 50 mm Hg at the peak). In the majority of these cases improvement of the uterine activity with judicious administration of intravenous oxytocin is effective in overcoming the arrest disorder and achieving a normal vaginal delivery.

A few patients with secondary arrest of cervical dilation and normal or borderline pelvimetry (by both Hillis-Múller and Ball x-ray examinations) show adequate uterine contractility (contractions every 2 to 2½ minutes, lasting 60 seconds, with more than 50 mm Hg pressure at the peak) when the IUP catheter is applied. These cases are controversial: for some obstetricians the uterus is working adequately, and further stimulation is inadvisable and may be dangerous; for others the uterine activity is not adequate, since it has not dilated the cervix, and in the absence of clinical and radiologic evidence of disproportion further stimulation is indicated. We share the second opinion and believe that many of these cases can be successfully managed with *gentle* oxytocin augmentation. The word *gentle* is stressed because oxytocin augmentation in patients who already have good uterine activity may be dangerous and should be carried out with the utmost care. The medication must be started at a rate of 0.5 mU/minute, and if a careful evaluation fails to reveal hyperstimulation or fetal distress, periodic increases of 0.5 mU should be carried out at least 20 minutes apart. In these cases a maximal dosage of 5 mU/minute of oxytocin should not be exceeded.

The question is how long and how much is necessary to augment labor in patients in whom oxytocin stimulation has been chosen as the op-

timal course of action. According to Friedman and Sachtleben,[6] almost all patients respond within 6 hours to stimulation, although 85% of those who do respond do so within 3 hours. A positive response is characterized by an upswing of the cervical dilation curve. Therefore 3 hours of adequate postarrest uterine activity constitutes an adequate trial of labor for patients with secondary arrest of cervical dilation being managed with oxytocin augmentation. If no change in cervical dilation is observed after 3 hours of augmented labor, further attempts to achieve a vaginal delivery are unwarranted, and the patient should have cesarean section-delivery.

When the patient responds to oxytocin augmentation, the slope of the postarrest curve of dilation may be equal to or larger than that observed before the arrest. In these cases the prognosis is good, and the chances for vaginal delivery are excellent. When the patient does not respond to oxytocin stimulation or the postarrest slope of cervical dilation is less than it was before the arrest, the situation has to be carefully reevaluated because in many of these cases disproportion was missed in the initial evaluation. The Hillis-Müller maneuver must be repeated, and the Ball pelvimetry films must be carefully reviewed in search of sources of error. As a general rule, the working diagnosis in these patients should be disproportion, and the treatment should be operative delivery. The burden of the proof lies with the person who has a different diagnosis or wants to opt for a different form of therapy.

There are some differences in the nature and outcome of secondary arrest of cervical dilation depending on how early or late the arrest occurs in the course of labor. In fact, early arrests are often caused by disproportion and require operative delivery more frequently than arrests occurring late in the active phase of labor. Also, when an early arrest responds to oxytocin stimulation, the postarrest slope of dilation is usually greater than the prearrest slope, and the chances for vaginal delivery are excellent. In other words, few early arrests are correctable, but those that respond to oxytocin do so with a high efficiency.

The recurrence of a secondary arrest of cervical dilation must be treated by cesarean section, unless it is possible to demonstrate the existence of an etiologic factor different from dis-

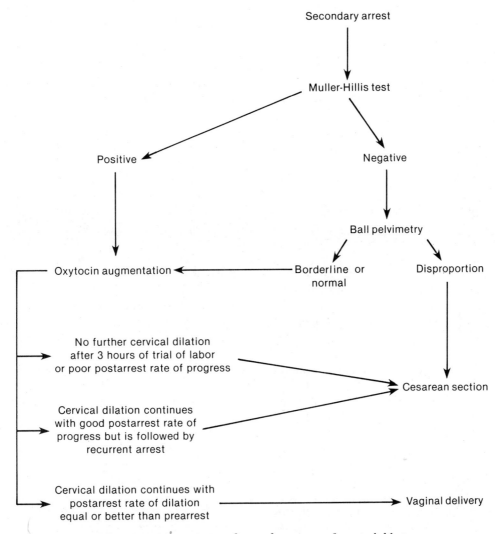

FIG. 16-4 ■ Management of secondary arrest of cervical dilation.

proportion (epidural anesthesia, excessive sedation) and responsible for the recurrence of the arrest. As was true in the case of patients who do not respond after 3 hours of oxytocin stimulation, in cases of recurrent arrest of dilation the burden of proof is with the individual who believes in an etiology different from disproportion and opts for a plan of management other than abdominal delivery. A summary of the management plan for secondary arrest is found in Fig. 16-4.

Prognosis. The high incidence of disproportion among patients with secondary arrest of cervical dilation makes the prognosis of the situation guarded. With the use of Ball pelvimetry it is possible to determine the existence of absolute disproportion in 25% to 30% of all patients affected by this labor disorder. After an adequate trial of labor, another 10% to 15% of patients—most of them with borderline fetus-pelvic disproportion—are therapeutic failures and require abdominal delivery. The rest of the patients, about 55%, deliver vaginally.

Prolonged deceleration phase

Definition. Prolonged deceleration phase (Fig. 16-3, line C) is characterized by a prolongation of the deceleration phase for more than 3 hours in the nullipara or more than 1 hour in the multipara. Under normal circumstances the mean duration of the deceleration phase is 54 minutes in the nullipara and 14 minutes in the multipara.

Diagnosis. The diagnosis of a prolonged deceleration phase requires a minimum of two pelvic examinations 3 hours apart in the nullipara and 1 hour apart in the multipara. In reality more than two pelvic examinations are usually carried out during the time required to establish the diagnosis.

In the course of normal labor the deceleration phase is difficult to detect unless frequent pelvic examinations are carried out at the end of the active phase. However, when an abnormality of the deceleration phase occurs, it is readily detectable unless its occurrence is shadowed by the presence of concomitant labor abnormalities. This association occurs frequently, and in about 70% of the cases prolonged deceleration is associated with protracted active phase dilation or with arrest of descent. In these cases the diagnosis is not always made because more emphasis is given to the definition and management of the associated disorder.

Frequency. Sokol et al[13] observed a prolonged deceleration phase in 0.8% of nulliparas and in 1.7% of multiparas. Friedman[1a] found that up to 5% of all labors may be complicated by this disorder. In any case it is the least frequent of all labor abnormalities.

Etiology. The most common cause of this labor abnormality is fetal malposition. In fact, 40.7% of multiparous with a prolonged deceleration phase have infants in OP, and 25.4% have infants in OT positions. In nulliparas with this labor disorder 60% have infants in OT and 26.3% in OP positions. Fetus-pelvic disproportion is the etiologic factor in about 15% of both nulliparas and multiparas exhibiting this labor abnormality. There is evidence suggesting that prolonged deceleration is a frequent abnormality in labors complicated by shoulder dystocia.

Management. The management of a prolonged deceleration phase depends primarily on the characteristics of the descent of the presenting part. In fact, if the prolonged deceleration occurs in the presence of adequate descent, and especially if the presenting part is below the level of the spine, the possibility of disproportion is small, and the prognosis for vaginal delivery is good. In contrast, if a prolonged deceleration phase occurs when the presenting part is at a high station, and especially if it is accompanied by arrest of descent, the condition is serious, and the possibility of cephalopelvic disproportion is large. In the first case (arrest at +1 or a lower station) fetal malpositions (OP or OT), heavy sedation, or epidural anesthesia are the most frequent causes of the labor abnormality, and gentle stimulation with oxytocin or waiting for sedation or anesthetic block to abate are usually adequate modes of management. In the second group of patients (those with the presenting part above 0 station) Ball pelvimetry should be immediately obtained and further labor allowed only if disproportion is ruled out.

The patient's parity should not influence the management of a prolonged deceleration phase. In fact, the incidence of cephalopelvic disproportion is similar for nulliparas (15.8%) and multiparas (15.3%) exhibiting this labor disorder.

Prognosis. More than 50% of nulliparas and about 30% of multiparas with a prolonged deceleration phase require instrumental delivery, according to Friedman.[1a] Midforceps (usually forceps rotations) were necessary in 40% of nulliparas and in 16.9% of multiparas, and cesarean section was performed in 16.7% of nulliparas and in 8.5% of multiparas.[1a] This difference in outcome between nulliparas and multiparas probably reflects the more frequent and aggressive use of uterotonic stimulation in multiparas. Whatever the reason, the prognosis of this labor abnormality is worse for the nullipara than for patients who already have experienced childbirth.

Failure of descent

Definition. The progressive caudal advancement of the presenting part in the maternal pelvis (descent) is an important characteristic of normal labor.[7] Descent usually starts during the phase of maximal cervical dilation and is easily observable during the deceleration phase and especially during the second stage of labor. In some patients descent does not occur at all, failure of descent (Fig. 16-5, line A).

Diagnosis. The diagnosis of this abnormality requires documentation that descent has not occurred during the second stage of labor. In the majority of cases failure to descend is associated with other labor abnormalities: 94.1% of the patients have secondary arrest of cervical dilation, and 78.4% have associated protraction disorders. In the majority of cases the diagnosis can be made with two vaginal examinations 1 hour apart during the second stage of labor.

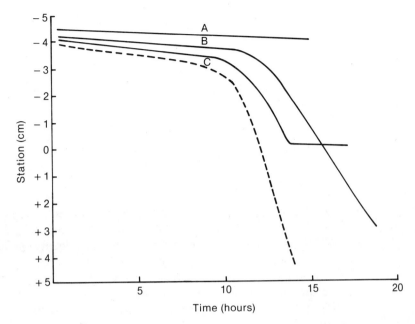

FIG. 16-5 ■ Abnormalities of the second stage of labor. The interrupted line, the descent of the presenting part during normal labor. Line *A*, failure of descent, a situation in which descent does not occur. Line *B*, protracted descent, a situation in which descent is abnormally slow. Line *C*, arrest of descent, a situation in which there is no progress in the movement of the fetus through the birth canal for at least 1 hour.

Frequency. According to Friedman,[1a] failure of descent affects 3.6% of all labors.

Etiology. The overwhelming majority of patients with failure of descent have cephalopelvic disproportion. In Friedman's experience disproportion can be documented radiologically in 54% of these patients, although it is present by clinical criteria in almost all cases.

Management. The patient with failure of descent must have immediate cesarean-section delivery. The incidence of disproportion as the etiologic agent of this disorder is so high that it is better to err by performing an unnecessary cesarean section on the occasional patient who might have had a vaginal delivery if allowed to labor than risk the increased frequency of complications that would occur with labor in the large majority of patients who have disproportion.

Prognosis. Since cesarean section is required for the management of failure of descent, the prognosis is guarded.

Protracted descent

Definition. Protracted descent is an abnormally slow rate of descent of the presenting part.

Its definition changes according to the patient's parity: in nulliparas it exists when the maximal slope of descent is 1.0 cm/hour or less; in multiparas protracted descent exists when the maximal slope of descent is 2.0 cm/hour or less (Fig. 16-5, line *B*).

Diagnosis. As in the case of protracted active phase dilation, it is necessary to measure the slope of descent to make the diagnosis of protracted descent. That slope can be calculated from data collected in two pelvic examinations 1 hour apart, but the precision of the diagnosis increases considerably if the observation period is for 2 hours and includes a minimum of three pelvic examinations.

The normal slope of descent for a nullipara is 3.3 cm/hour; the 5th percentile value is 0.96 cm/hour. In multiparas the normal slope of descent is 6.6 cm/hour, and the 5th percentile value is 2.1 cm/hour. Values under 1 cm/hour for the nullipara and under 2 cm/hour for the multipara are abnormal.

Frequency. According to Friedman and Sachtleben,[8] protracted descent occurs in 4.7% of all labors.

Etiology. Cephalopelvic disproportion, excessive sedation, regional block anesthesia, and fetal malposition are factors associated so frequently with protracted descent that they should have etiologic significance. Disproportion is present in 26.1% of nulliparas with this disorder of labor and in 9.9% of multiparas. This fact implies that the problem is more serious when it occurs in the nullipara.

Similar to arrest of descent, protraction in the caudal movement of the presenting part often occurs when the infant is macrosomic (weight greater than 4000 grams). In Friedman's and Sachtleben's study[8] 9% of the infants born to mothers with protracted descent weighed more than 4000 grams as compared with an incidence of 4.2% in patients without labor abnormalities. Minor fetal malpositions (OP, OT, asynclitism), which in most cases are of little importance when they occur in normal-size infants, become major causal factors for abnormal labor when they occur in macrosomic babies. A fetal malposition in an oversize infant represents on many occasions the difference between a normal vaginal delivery and a cesarean-section delivery.

The popularization of epidural anesthesia in recent years has become a major etiologic factor for descent disorders during labor. In fact, epidural blocks frequently impair the ability of the patient to push during the second stage of labor. This inability has its origin in the interruption of the pushing reflex or in partial paralysis of the abdominal muscles of the parturient or in a combination of these two factors. Patients receiving epidural anesthesia during labor exhibit more descent disorders than patients without epidural blocks, and they have a higher incidence of operative and forceps deliveries.

A frequent etiology of protracted descent in the multipara is a failure of the expulsive forces of the uterus during the second stage of labor. In fact, multiparas who have been contracting adequately during the active phase sometimes have diminished uterine activity when they become fully dilated and the presenting part is at a relatively high station (-1 to $+1$). This can be documented clinically (the contractions become significantly infrequent and of shorter duration) by means of an IUP catheter. The solution for this minor problem is gentle oxytocin stimulation.

Management. The first order of business in the patient with protracted descent is to rule out

obvious reasons for the problem such as epidural anesthesia, excessive sedation, fetal malpresentation, and fetal macrosomia. If these factors are not present, disproportion should be suspected, especially in the primipara for whom its incidence is about 30%, and clinical pelvimetry (Hillis-Müller maneuver) should be carried out. If clinical pelvimetry is inadequate, it should be followed by Ball pelvimetry. Radiologic evaluation is also necessary when the protraction pattern becomes an arrest pattern, a fact that happens in a high percentage of patients with protracted descent and macrosomic infants.

Treatment must be directed to the suspected or confirmed etiologic agent: epidural block or excessive sedation must be managed with an abatement policy; disproportion requires cesarean-section delivery; poor uterine contractility demands oxytocin stimulation. Cesarean-section delivery is also the management choice in cases of macrosomia combined with fetal malposition.

Prognosis. The delivery prognosis in patients with protracted descent depends to a large extent on the further development of an arrest pattern. Patients in whom descent is continuous, even if the slope of descent is abnormal, have a good prognosis for uncomplicated vaginal delivery (about 65% of the cases). Another 25% of these patients require midforceps intervention. If an arrest pattern superimposes on protracted descent, the prognosis becomes bleak: 43% incidence of cesarean section; 18% incidence of midforceps interventions. Furthermore, a perinatal mortality of 69 per 1000 and a 32% incidence of low Apgar scores occur in patients with protracted descent if labor has been stimulated with oxytocin and delivery includes intervention with midforceps.

Arrest of descent

Definition. As explained before, most of the descent of the presenting part takes place at the end of the first stage and especially during the second stage of labor. Thus failure of descent, arrest of descent, and protracted descent are typically disorders of the second stage of labor. Arrest of descent occurs when there is no progress in the movement of the fetus through the birth canal for 1 hour as documented by appropriately spaced vaginal examinations (Fig. 16-5, line C).

Diagnosis. The diagnosis of arrest of descent

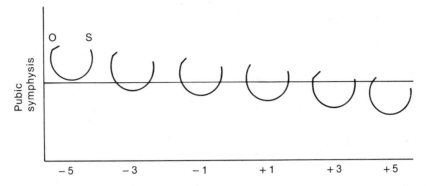

FIG. 16-6 ■ Assessing the station of the presenting part by abdominal examination. The graph shows the progressive descent of a fetal head (*O*, occiput; *S*, sinciput) through the pelvis. The head eventually crosses a line that represents the *pubic symphysis*. The station is evaluated using a range of −5 when the head is floating to +5 when the head is deep inside the true pelvis. (From Crichton D: S Afr Med J 1974;48:784.)

requires a minimum of two pelvic examinations 1 hour apart. The evaluation of alterations in the fetal descent through the maternal pelvis is complicated by the existence of changes in the fetal head at the end of labor (molding, caput formation), which increases the possibility of physician error. In many cases a pelvic examination seems to reveal that progress is being made when in reality what has been felt as a positive change is just scalp edema and molding of the fetal scalp bones. This source of error is so common that Friedman recommends assessing the station of the presenting part by both abdominal and pelvic examinations in all cases of suspected abnormalities of descent.

To evaluate the descent of the presenting part by abdominal examination,[1] the first and second Leopold maneuvers should be carried out and the station assessed from −5 to 0 (Fig. 16-6). This method is not as precise as station assessment by pelvic examination, but with the use of both methods it is possible to minimize mistakes originating in the molding of the fetal head during labor.

Frequency. Arrest of descent occurs in about 5% to 6% of all labors.

Etiology. There are three main causes for arrest of descent: cephalopelvic disproportion, fetal malposition, and regional anesthetic blocks. In the nullipara, disproportion is the cause in more than 50% of the cases, and this incidence is even greater when the arrest occurs at a high station or when the patient is receiving uterotonic stimulation with oxytocin. Epidural anes-

thesia was present in 80.6% of the nulliparas with arrest of descent studied by Friedman and Sachtleben.[9] This does not mean that the regional block was the cause of the problem in all these patients, but indicates that in a high number of cases epidural anesthesia is a contributory factor. Similarly, fetal malpositions (OT or OP) were present in 75.9% of all patients with arrest of descent. However, almost all nulliparas with fetal malposition exhibited other factors operating simultaneously, and this situation makes it difficult to isolate the role of malposition as an etiologic agent of arrest of descent.

In multiparas with arrest of descent the incidence of disproportion is only 29.7%. The proportion of patients with fetal malpositions or under epidural anesthesia is similar to that found in nulliparas.

Management. The first step after making a diagnosis of arrest of descent is to search for etiologic factors. The presence of an obvious reason for the abnormality such as epidural anesthesia or fetal malposition must not, however, distract the observer from ruling out the presence of disproportion. A Hillis-Müller maneuver must be performed, and only if easy downward movement of the fetal presenting part occurs, should the assessment be oriented toward factors other than disproportion. If the Hillis-Müller test gives a negative result, Ball pelvimetry must be carried out immediately and the pregnancy terminated by cesarean section if disproportion is present.

When disproportion has been ruled out by

clinical and x-ray pelvimetry, abatement of sedation and regional blocks if present or uterotonic stimulation are indicated. In both instances careful fetal and maternal monitoring is required. It has been shown that the fetus becomes progressively acidotic during labor with the lower pH values occurring during the second stage.[11] Therefore if a policy of abatement of labor inhibitors or one of augmentation of uterine contractions is chosen as treatment, invasive monitoring using a fetal scalp electrode and IUP catheter is mandatory. Furthermore, if the second stage becomes abnormally prolonged (more than 2½ hours in the nullipara, more than 50 minutes in the multipara), fetal scalp samples should be obtained every 30 minutes to assess the acid-base status of the fetus, even if the electronic monitoring trace does not reveal significant abnormalities.

In cases in which disproportion has been effectively ruled out by clinical and Ball pelvimetry and excessive sedation or segmental anesthesia are not present, oxytocin augmentation is indicated even if the uterine contractions seem to be normal as evaluated with the IUP catheter. However, oxytocin must be administered carefully, starting at low dosages (0.5 to 1.0 mU/minute) with increases separated by at least 20 minutes.

Most of the patients who are going to respond to the abatement of inhibitory anesthesia or sedation or to oxytocin augmentation do so in 1 to 1½ hours (0.96 ± 0.23 hour for oxytocin; 1.36 ± 0.19 hours for abatement). If no response is noticed 2 hours after the beginning of therapy, the situation should be carefully reevaluated in search of undetected disproportion. At this moment the burden of proof rests on the physician who believes that disproportion is not present. In fact, unless a meticulous analysis shows that disproportion does not exist, the pregnancy should be terminated by cesarean section without further attempts to obtain a vaginal delivery.

Prognosis. Patients with arrest of descent have a guarded prognosis. The main reason for this is the high frequency of disproportion as the etiologic agent of this abnormality of labor. In Friedman's and Sachtleben's study[9] 30.4% of patients with arrest of descent required cesarean section, 37.6% were delivered with midforceps, 12.7% had forceps rotations, and 5.1% had failed forceps.

The following are the most important prognostic indexes in patients with arrest of descent:

1. Fetal station at the time of arrest (the higher the station the greater the possibility of disproportion)
2. Duration of the arrest (the longer the duration the greater the possibility of disproportion)
3. Characteristics of the postarrest progression (if the postarrest descent rate is equal to or larger than the prearrest slope, the prognosis for atraumatic vaginal delivery is good)

Arrest of descent is associated with significant maternal and fetal morbidity independently of the need for operative intervention. Postpartum bleeding is the most common maternal complication (12.5% of the cases). Fetal distress, as evidenced by a low Apgar score, is a common problem (21.9% of the cases). Shoulder dystocia with its associated morbidity (Erb's palsy, clavicular fractures, fetal trauma, etc) occurs in 14.1% of the cases.

Precipitate labor

Definition. According to Friedman,[1a] the 95th percentile for the rate of dilation of the cervix during labor is 6.8 cm/hour in nulliparas and 14.7cm/hour in multiparas. For the descent of the presenting part these limits are 6.4 cm and 14.0 cm respectively. Therefore for practical purposes precipitate labor (not to be confused with precipitate delivery) is characterized by rates of dilation and descent greater than 5 cm/hour in nulliparas and 10 cm/hour in multiparas. In most cases precipitate dilation and precipitate descent occur simultaneously.

Diagnosis. Usually the diagnosis of precipitate labor is made in retrospect when the labor curve of a patient who delivered after a fast labor is analyzed.

Etiology. Etiologic factors are unclear. Oxytocin stimulation may be a trigger for this disorder, although in the series of Friedman[1a] only 11.1% of all patients with precipitate labor received oxytocin.

Management. If precipitate labor is diagnosed before delivery and especially if there are electronic monitoring signs of fetal distress, labor should be inhibited with beta mimetic agents. Terbutaline (250 to 500 μg intravenous push) or ritodrine (300 μg/minute IV) are effective drugs for decreasing the frequency, duration, and intensity of the uterine contractions. These drugs paralyze the uterus momentarily, and when labor restarts, it usually has lost its tumultuous character.

Prognosis. The prognosis for vaginal delivery is good. Occasionally labor is so fast that the patient has a precipitate delivery in bed. Following delivery the obstetrician must directly inspect the cervix for lacerations, since they occur frequently in patients with precipitate labor.

The fetal and neonatal prognosis is guarded. Frequently the fetus does not tolerate the hypoxic insult generated by frequent and intense uterine contractions, and the result is intrapartum distress, neonatal depression, and hyaline membrane disease.

■ **REFERENCES**

1. Crichton D: A reliable method of establishing the level of the fetal head in obstetrics. S Afr Med J 1974;48:784.
1a. Friedman EA: *Labor: Clinical Evaluation and Management*, ed 2. New York, Appleton-Century-Crofts, 1978.
2. Friedman EA, Kroll BH: Computer analysis of labor progression. IV. Diagnosis of secondary arrest of dilatation. J Reprod Med 1971;7:176.
3. Friedman EA, Sachtleben MR: Dysfunctional labor I. Prolonged latent phase in the nullipara. Obstet Gynecol 1961;17:135.
4. Friedman EA, Sachtleben MR: Dysfunctional labor. II. Protracted active phase dilatation in the nullipara. Obstet Gynecol 1961;17:566.
5. Friedman EA, Sachtleben MR: Dysfunctional labor. III. Secondary arrest of dilatation in the nullipara. Obstet Gynecol 1962;19:576.
6. Friedman EA, Sachtleben MR: Dysfunctional labor. V. Therapeutic trial of oxytocin in secondary arrest. Obstet Gynecol 1963;21:13.
7. Friedman EA, Sachtleben MR: Station of the fetal presenting part. I. Pattern of descent. Am J Obstet Gynecol 1965;93:522.
8. Friedman EA, Sachtleben MR: Station of the fetal presenting part. V. Protracted descent patterns. Obstet Gynecol 1970;36:558.
9. Friedman EA, Sachtleben MR: Station of the presenting part. VI. Arrest of descent in nulliparas. Obstet Gynecol 1976;47:129.
10. Friedman EA, Taylor MB: A modified nomographic aid for x-ray cephalo-pelvimetry. Am J Obstet Gynecol 1969;15:111.
11. Modanlou H, Yeh SY, Hon EH, et al: Fetal and neonatal biochemistry and Apgar scores. Am J Obstet Gynecol 1973;117:942.
12. Pritchard JA, MacDonald PC: *Williams Obstetrics*, ed 16. New York, Appleton-Century-Crofts, 1980, p. 375.
13. Sokol RS, Stojkov J, Chik L, et al: Normal and abnormal labor progress. I. Quantitative assessment and survey of the literature. J Reprod Med 1977;18:47-53.

17

■ ■ ■

ABNORMAL FETAL
PRESENTATIONS AND POSITIONS
DURING LABOR

Fernando Arias and William L. Holcomb, Jr.

The usual fetal presentation at the time of parturition is a vertex (cephalic) presentation, and the usual mechanism of labor involves internal rotation of the presenting vertex to an occipitoanterior position with subsequent delivery. Situations that deviate from this are known as abnormal fetal presentations. They are a management problem for the obstetrician and the subject of this chapter. The term *abnormal* should not imply pathology. For example, with some pelvic shapes, delivery with the occipitoposterior presentation is easier than with the occiput in the more common anterior position.

■ BREECH PRESENTATION

Breech presentation occurs in 3% to 4% of all deliveries. It is a well-established fact that fetal and neonatal mortality and morbidity are considerably higher for the fetus in breech presentation than for the fetus in vertex position. For example, at McDonald House of the University Hospitals of Cleveland the overall fetal mortality for breech deliveries between 1962 and 1969 was 25.4% compared to 2.6% for nonbreech deliveries.[3] In the Royal Women's Hospital of Melbourne breech deliveries represented only 3.3%

of the total number of deliveries but accounted for 24.3% of the total perinatal mortality.[8] This poor fetal outcome persists even when some other factors such as prematurity and congenital abnormalities are excluded.[1,22]

Problems

A considerable part of the fetal and neonatal morbidity and mortality found in breech presentations may be accounted for by the presence of associated factors capable of independently generating significant mortality and morbidity. The most important of these factors are preterm delivery, congenital malformations, preterm rupture of membranes, placenta previa, and abruptio placentae.

Preterm delivery. The prevalence of preterm birth among infants delivered in breech presentation varies from 20.1%[30] to 41.6%.[19] Therefore a significant proportion of the morbidity and mortality associated with the breech presentation is a consequence of preterm birth rather than the presentation. In most studies a birth weight of less than 2500 grams is used as the definition of preterm. This has led many investigators to correct their studies on breech pre-

TABLE 17-1 ■ Relationship between perinatal mortality and fetal weight in breech babies

Birth weight (grams)	Number of infants	Perinatal loss (%)
1000 to 1499	61	67.2
1500 to 1999	44	20.5
2000 to 2499	72	13.9
2500 to 2999	145	3.4
3000 to 3499	192	0.5
3500 to 3999	122	0.8
4000 +	28	7.1

Modified from De Crespigny, LJC, Pepperell RJ: Obstet Gynecol 1979;53:141.

TABLE 17-2 ■ Relationship between severe congenital malformations and fetal weight in breech babies

Birth weight (grams)	Number of infants	Lethal anomalies (%)
1000 to 1499	61	16.4
1500 to 1999	44	4.5
2000 to 2499	72	4.1
2500 to 2999	145	2.0
3000 to 3499	192	0.5
3500 to 3999	122	0.8
4000 +	28	0

Modified from De Crespigny, LJC, Pepperell RC: Obstet Gynecol 1979;53:141.

sentation by excluding from consideration those infants with a birth weight under 2500 grams.

Most studies on the outcome of preterm breech infants have concluded that (1) the fetal hazards and perils of breech presentation are increased when preterm birth is an added factor, and (2) the perinatal outcome of the preterm infant delivered in a breech position is worse than could be expected on the basis of the prematurity alone.

The first point of the dangers of breech presentation being more when preterm birth is an added factor has been repeatedly shown in the literature. As can be seen in Table 17-1, breech infants weighing less than 2500 grams have a higher perinatal mortality than heavier infants. It is also clear from these data that perinatal mortality in breech infants is in a close inverse relationship with the birth weight.

The second point of the perinatal outcome of the preterm breech infant being worse than expected from the prematurity alone is a conclusion reached in several studies in which the outcome of preterm breech and preterm vertex infants has been compared. For example, in the study of breech delivery by Kauppila,[20] the perinatal mortality of preterm (601 to 2600 grams) breech infants was 50.3% in contrast with 23.4% for preterm infants in the vertex position.

Congenital malformations. Congenital malformations, another factor associated with breech presentation, are capable of generating significant independent mortality and morbidity. It is a sobering experience for any obstetrician to perform a cesarean section in a young primigravida in an attempt to improve the outcome of a fetus in breech presentation, only to find out that the infant has multiple congenital abnormalities incompatible with life. In fact, congenital malformations occur more often in breech than in vertex presentations, and their incidence has a strong inverse correlation with fetal age (Table 17-2).

In Goldenberg's and Nelson's study[15] the frequency of major congenital abnormalities for preterm breech and preterm vertex infants delivered vaginally was 6.2% and 2.3%, respectively. In Kauppila's series[20] the incidence of congenital malformations was 10.2% for breech infants under 2500 grams and 8.3% for those above 2500 grams. In another series[14] congenital abnormalities accounted for 23.6% of all perinatal deaths in a group of preterm single breech births. Thus the conclusion is that congenital abnormalities occur frequently in babies in breech presentation, and their occurrence has a strong inverse correlation with fetal weight at birth. From a practical point of view the obstetrician should consider that the chances of a major congenital malformation may be as high as 15% in breech infants of less than 1500 grams.

The predominant major congenital malformations in breech infants involve the central nervous system (hydrocephaly, anencephaly, and meningomyelocele). The most common abnormality is, however, dislocation of the hip, a process that affects more females than males (ratio 3:1). Anomalies of the gastrointestinal tract; the respiratory, cardiovascular, and urinary systems; and multiple abnormalities are also rela-

tively common. Many of these abnormalities can
be detected by careful ultrasound and x-ray evaluation; these tests are mandatory for the adequate management of patients with breech presentations.

Preterm rupture of membranes. There is no
clear evidence that preterm rupture of the
fetal membranes (PROM) occurs more often in
breech than in vertex presentations. Brenner et
al[3] found that rupture of the membranes was
significantly increased in breech presentations
only after 36 weeks of gestation (25.1% in breech
versus 15.8% in nonbreech). Jurado and Miller[19]
found a 1.5 greater incidence of rupture of the
membranes before labor in breech versus nonbreech presentations, but no analysis was made
of the statistical significance of this difference.
The same authors also point out that 8 out of 12
fetal deaths in patients with ruptured membranes and breech presentation were the result
of intrauterine infection.

Rupture of the membranes causes special
problems in breech presentation because of the
high proportion of preterm babies that exists
within a population of breech infants. These preterm infants become infected more often and
with greater severity than term infants because
of a decreased antibacterial effect of amniotic
fluid and immature immunological responses.
Therefore sepsis is an important cause of perinatal mortality in all breech studies.

PROM in breech babies leads to "occult" prolapse of the cord, a problem that is just beginning to be recognized in the literature. In these
cases electronic monitoring of the fetus shows
variable decelerations appearing spontaneously
or with contractions, and the vaginal examination fails to provide evidence of cord prolapse.
Delivery usually ends with the birth of a severely depressed infant, and no evidence is generally found of the nature of the accident causing
the variable decelerations and the fetal hypoxia.
The problem is usually attributed to an occult
cord prolapse.

Placenta previa and abruptio placentae. Jurado and Miller[19] found the incidence of placenta
previa in breech presentation (3.4%) sevenfold
higher than vertex presentation. Brenner et al[3]
found an incidence of placenta previa 1.6% and
abruptio placentae 6.0% in breech presentations
in contrast with incidences of 0.6% and 1.8%
for vertex presentations, respectively. In these

cases the complications associated with placenta
previa or abruptio placentae are the primary determinants of the fetal outcome rather than the
breech presentation itself.

Other causes of perinatal mortality and morbidity

Even if the factors just mentioned (prematurity, congenital abnormalities, PROM, and placental abnormalities) are taken out of consideration, "corrected" mortality and morbidity in
breech births are greater than in vertex presentations. This is most probably caused by a series
of problems, some of them occurring exclusively
and others happening frequently in breech presentations.

Prolapse of the umbilical cord. Prolapse of
the umbilical cord is a dangerous accident that
occurs in about 6% of all breech deliveries and
has a fetal mortality of 30% to 50%. In frank
breech deliveries (lower extremities flexed at the
hips and extended at the knees) prolapse of the
cord happens in about 1% of the cases, but in
complete breech presentations (one or both
knees flexed and one foot or both feet or knees
lying below the breech) it happens in 10% to
15% of the cases. Fortunately, frank breech is
the most common type of presentation found in
breech infants, as shown in the following material:

Type	Frequency
Frank breech	64%
Double footling	10%
Single footling	14%
Complete breech	12%

Nonfrank breech presentations occur more often in preterm than in term infants, as shown

TABLE 17-3 ■ Frequency of frank breech and nonfrank breech presentations in relation to fetal weight

Weight (grams)	Frank breech %	Nonfrank breech %
500 to 999	27	73
1000 to 1499	37	63
1500 to 1999	40	60
2000 to 2499	59	41
2500 to 2999	67	33

Modified from Goldenberg RL, Nelson KG: Am J Obstet
Gynecol 1977;127:240.

in Table 17-3. Therefore the clinician should expect a greater incidence of prolapse cord in preterm than in term breech infants. Kauppila[20] found that there was a 6.1% incidence of prolapsed cord in breech infants weighing more than 3500 grams as compared to an incidence of 2.9% ($p > 0.01$) in breech infants under 3500 grams. Other studies have also pointed to the frequent occurrence of prolapsed cord in multiparas with breech infants.

Entrapment of the fetal head. There is no adequate description in the literature of the incidence, methods of management, and outcome of infants when the fetal head is entrapped during a breech delivery. Several papers, however, mention this complication, and almost every obstetrician who has delivered breech infants, especially preterm breech infants, has had the experience of the entrapped head. This complication is an important cause of fetal asphyxia that is second to prematurity as the leading factor in perinatal mortality for breech infants.

The reason for the occurrence of this complication has to do with the relative size of the fetal head and buttocks of the preterm infant. The smaller diameter of the pelvic pole makes it possible to delivery the pelvis and the body of a breech infant through a partially dilated cervix that does not permit the delivery of the larger cephalic pole. The consequences are delayed head delivery, fetal asphyxia, brain damage, and death. The problem occurs more often in the preterm infant because the difference between head and body diameters is larger than in term infants.

There is no accepted method of identifying in advance the breech infant who is going to have an entrapped head at the time of delivery. The best policy is to assume that every preterm breech infant has an excellent chance of developing this complication and that the risk increases with smaller infant size, nulliparity of the mother, and footling presentations. The only preventive treatment is surgical intervention, discussed later.

The classic and most rapid and effective approach for treating entrapment of the fetal head is the use of Dührssen's incisions in the incompletely dilated cervix. However, this maneuver may become complicated by extension of the incisions into the lower uterine segment and may have a deleterious effect on the future re-

productive capacity of the mother by causing cervical incompetence. Therefore, the best approach is the use of an effective and rapid-acting uterine and cervical relaxant: intravenous terbutaline (300 μg intravenous push) or intravenous diazoxide (300 mg intravenous push) paralyzes the myometrium and permits the extraction of the trapped head with gentle pulling. Terbutaline is preferred to diazoxide because of less pronounced cardiovascular effects. Another powerful uterine relaxant is the general anesthetic halothane. However, its use requires adequate conditions for maternal general anesthesia with endotracheal intubation and usually cannot be administered as quickly as the intravenous injection of terbutaline. Only if the pharmacologic maneuver fails and there is still hope of delivering a healthy baby should the obstetrician use the surgical approach with Dührssen's incisions to the cervix.

Fetal trauma. The frequent occurrence of fetal trauma during vaginal breech delivery is well documented in the literature. For example, in Potter's and Adair's[26] study on perinatal mortality traumatic hemorrhage was the cause of death in 43.4% of infants dying during breech delivery. Thus fetal trauma is the third most frequent cause of perinatal death (after prematurity and asphyxia) in the breech infant.

A traumatic injury often found is to the central nervous system. This occurs frequently during vaginal deliveries of breech infants with hyperextended heads, a condition complicating about 5% of all term breeches. In a recent study[4] a perinatal mortality of 13.7% and an incidence of medullary and vertebral injuries of 20.6% were found in vaginal deliveries of breech infants with hyperextended heads. These figures are impressive and justify the need for an x-ray examination to rule out the presence of a hyperextended head before allowing labor to continue.

A large proportion of the traumatic injuries to the breech fetus is the result of manipulations by the obstetrician in the course of vaginal breech deliveries. Occipital osteodiastasis (separation of the squamous and lateral portions of the occipital bone) is, for example, one injury that occurs from pressure of the fetal head against the mother's pubis and is usually caused by suprapubic pressure on the fetal head at the time of delivery.[33] Separation of the bone causes tentorial tears and intraventricular and subdural hemorrhages.

The peripheral nervous system is also frequently injured (Erb's palsy, facial nerve paralysis) during vaginal breech delivery, and muscle trauma is common and severe. Ralis[28] found in an autopsy study that the hemorrhages in injured muscles of infants who died after breech delivery were equivalent to between 20% and 25% of the infants' total blood volume. The muscle damage was predominant in the lower limbs, genitalia, and the anal region. Also, the intraabdominal solid organs (liver, adrenal, spleen) may suffer traumatic damage during breech delivery; Potter and Adair[26] recorded 24 hepatic and four adrenal lethal injuries in their series.

The mechanism of trauma during breech delivery is directly related to the amount of obstetric manipulation during delivery,[31] which in turn is directly related to the difficulties encountered during that process. The manipulation most strongly associated with traumatic injury is the total breech extraction. This procedure is so traumatic that it is contraindicated except in certain cases of fetal distress or for the delivery of second twins.[25] Vaginal delivery of the breech infant carries a considerable risk of traumatic injury to the fetus under the circumstances described in the following paragraphs.

Unrecognized cephalopelvic disproportion (CPD). A condition often associated with fetal trauma during breech delivery is unrecognized CPD. The unmolded fetal head requires wide pelvic diameters to negotiate the bony pelvis without traumatic manipulation. Multiparity does not guarantee the existence of adequate pelvic diameters for a nontraumatic breech delivery unless the birthweight of a previous infant was larger than the size of the present breech infant. Difficult breech vaginal deliveries were as frequent in nulliparous as in multiparous patients in Kauppila's[20] large series. If CPD goes unrecognized, the delivery of shoulders and head will be delayed with the occurrence of fetal asphyxia, which may lead to fetal death or to serious neurologic sequelae. Therefore adequate evaluation of the maternal pelvic diameters, especially in relation to the fetal head size, is an important prerequisite for the vaginal delivery of a breech infant.

Trapping of the fetal head by an incompletely dilated cervix. Entrapment of the fetal head was described previously. It is a complication that affects primarily the delivery of preterm breech infants.

Delay in delivery of the head because of extension of the fetal arms. A complication usually related to obstetric manipulation during delivery and predominantly seen in cases of total or partial breech extraction is delay in delivery of the head because of extension of the fetal arms. Intervention by pulling the baby's body during breech extraction may cause extension and elevation of the fetal arms with placement of one or both of the infant's arms in apposition with its neck (nuchal arm).[16] The result is an increase in the diameter of the cephalic pole and the impossibility of delivering the baby's head unless the arms are displaced from their abnormal position before the delivery of the head. In some cases the arms can be displaced relatively easily; in other cases it is necessary to fracture the fetal humerus or clavicle before being able to displace the arms; and in other cases, in spite of all efforts, there is considerable delay in delivering the infant's head with resulting fetal asphyxia and intrapartum death. Extension of the arms complicated 5.2% of nulliparous and 9.7% of multiparous full-term partial breech extractions in Kauppila's series.[20]

Excessively rapid delivery of the fetal head. Another situation associated with considerable risk of traumatic injury to the breech fetus is excessively rapid delivery of the fetal head. This problem may be minimized by using Piper's forceps. This is an instrument designed for the purpose of avoiding dangerous delays in the delivery of the head. Milner[23] demonstrated that Piper's forceps delivery of the head is safer than delivery without the instrument for infants weighing between 1000 and 3000 grams. The Piper's forceps is also useful in preventing trauma to the fetal mouth and throat during the Mauriceau maneuver and the intracranial bleeding associated with the sudden "popping out" of the fetal head through the vaginal introitus.

During the Mauriceau maneuver the middle finger of the obstetrician is introduced into the mouth of the infant while the body rests on the palm of the hand and the forearm. The index and the annular fingers are placed at each side of the baby's nose and press on the upper maxillary bone. Two fingers of the other hand are hooked over the infant's neck and used to apply downward traction. Sometimes voluntary or involuntary traction is exerted with the finger placed in the infant's mouth for the purpose of obtaining maximal flexion of the fetal head, and a frequent result is traumatic injury to the baby's mouth and pharynx. Routine use of Piper's forceps eliminates this complication.

Management

Management of breech presentations is an important and complex obstetric problem for which, unfortunately, much of the information available for making decisions comes from retrospective and uncontrolled studies. The problem is simple for all those who think that the treatment of all breech presentations is cesarean-section delivery. In our opinion, however, a large proportion of breech infants can be delivered vaginally without increasing perinatal morbidity and mortality and without exposing the mother to the immediate and long-term risks associated with cesarean section.

The obstetrician faces the problem of what to do with a breech presentation under two different sets of circumstances. One is when a patient has a persistent breech presentation in the last 6 weeks of gestation. The second situation is when a breech presentation is found unexpectedly at the time of active labor.

Antepartum management. It is common for the obstetrician to find patients with infants in breech presentation in the course of routine prenatal evaluations during the last 4 to 6 weeks of gestation. Once the breech presentation has been detected, the next prenatal visit is anxiously awaited by parents and physician with the idea that spontaneous rotation has taken place. Although spontaneous rotation is the usual outcome of this situation, when the fetal malpresentation persists during several weeks, the chances of spontaneous rotation becomes small, and the obstetrician is left with two alternatives: (1) to do nothing and postpone the management decisions until labor begins or membranes rupture or (2) to proceed to an external cephalic version.

If the first alternative is chosen, the patient should be informed of the risks and dangers associated with breech presentations and with breech delivery. She also should be informed that a decision about the route of delivery (vaginal or abdominal) is made at the beginning of

labor. She should be instructed to report to the hospital as soon as labor begins or as soon as the membranes rupture. The advantage of this approach is that is provides a maximal time for a spontaneous rotation. The main disadvantage is the possibility of rupture of the membranes and prolapse of the umbilical cord, especially when the presenting part is not well applied against the cervix. It is a terrible experience to wait for spontaneous version of a breech infant at term and lose the baby because of a cord prolapse after spontaneous rupture of the membranes.

External cephalic version is another approach to the antepartum management of breech presentations that attempts to avoid the disadvantages of the expectant approach. For this purpose an ultrasound examination is performed at 36 weeks of gestation to find out by applying the following criteria if it is feasible to perform the external version.

1. A problem indicating cesarean-section delivery, such as:
   a. Placenta previa
   b. Contracted pelvis
2. A problem indicating vaginal delivery, such as:
   a. Fetal death
   b. Severe congenital abnormality (anencephaly, etc)
3. A condition generating difficulties for the performance of the procedure, such as:
   a. Rupture of the membranes
   b. Oligohydramnios
   c. Lack of uterine relaxation (patient in labor)
   d. Multiple pregnancy
   e. Anterior placenta
   f. Pregnancy close to term with engaged breech
4. A condition generating increased maternal or fetal risks with the procedure, such as:
   a. Rh negative mother*
   b. Severe pregnancy hypertension
   c. Severe intrauterine growth retardation
   d. Fetus with hyperextended head

If none of these conditions are present, external cephalic version may be performed following the next protocol.

1. The procedure should be carried out in the labor and delivery area at 36 weeks of gestation. An ultrasound examination for careful assessment

---

*If the mother is Rh negative, this contraindication may be bypassed with the use of RhoGAM if a Fetaldex test shows that fetoplacental bleeding did occur during the procedure.

of the fetal position and to rule out congenital abnormalities and electronic monitoring of the fetal heart rate (FHR) and uterine activity should precede the maneuver.

2. An intravenous infusion of terbutaline (5.0 to 8.0 µg/minute) with the patient lying on her left side with her feet slightly elevated should be started. The infusion needs to be continued for 15 minutes. Maternal pulse should be between 100 and 120 beats/minute.

3. When the uterus is completely relaxed, version by dislodging the breech from the pelvis using both hands should begin. Moving the fetus forward using manual pressure only on the breech needs to be continued. Once the baby has reached a transverse position, the rotation is completed by pushing up the breech with one hand and pushing down the fetal head with the other hand. Fetal heart activity must be constantly monitored during the maneuver with real-time ultrasound.

4. *The procedure should be interrupted if* (1) the version is not easy, (2) the mother is in pain, (3) there is a marked increase or decrease in FHR or an irregular rhythm of the fetal heart.

5. FHR monitoring should be continued for 1 hour after completing the procedure. The patient should be allowed to walk and eat, and FHR monitoring repeated for a short period before discharge.

6. If the mother is Rh negative, a sample of blood must be analyzed by Kleinhauer-Betke stain after the procedure. RhoGAM must be given if there is evidence of fetal-maternal transfusion.

The reason external cephalic version is not universally advocated for the management of breech presentations before labor is that obstetricians are afraid of the 1% to 4% chance of complications (including fetal losses as high as 1.7%) reported in the literature in association with the procedure. The literature is controversial with some investigators enthusiastically favoring external version[10,29] and others[2] finding no advantage to its use. A recent work[32] demonstrated that external version reduces the incidence of intrapartum breech presentations and suggests that the procedure is safer than reported in the old literature. In our opinion, external cephalic version is a reasonable management alternative for most persistent breech presentations.

External version is facilitated greatly by the use of uterine relaxants during the procedure and should be carried out under continuous real-time ultrasound monitoring of the fetus. The fetal manipulation should be gentle, and the procedure must be stopped if the mother is in pain or if there is a significant (more than 15%) increase or decrease in FHR frequency. The procedure should be carried out in the labor and delivery area where immediate intervention is possible in the case of severe fetal distress.

A special case in the antepartum management of breech presentations is the patient with a footling breech or any other unstable breech presentation, who has contraindications for external version or who has had a failed attempt to external version. If pregnancy is allowed to continue until the onset of spontaneous labor, there is a substantial risk of cord prolapse after rupture of the membranes. It is better to perform an amniocentesis and deliver by cesarean section as soon as lung maturation is adequate.

Intrapartum management. If a breech presentation is suspected or diagnosed in a patient who is in the latent or active phase of labor, the uterus should be paralyzed by administering a tocolytic agent (terbutaline 300 mg intravenous push) to have time for a systematic evaluation of the situation. The majority of the questions in that evaluation are answered with the help of a fetogram and an ultrasonic study of the fetus, procedures that should be carried out immediately after stopping labor with the tocolytic agent. The first question to be answered is the following:

> **Is there evidence of major congenital abnormalities in the fetus?**

The ultrasound and the fetogram are valuable in determining the presence or absence of anencephaly, microcephaly, hydrocephaly, and limb-reduction defects. The ultrasound examination is also useful to rule out other anomalies such as polycystic kidney disease, meningomyelocele, and fetal ascites.

The presence of a normal ultrasound and fetogram does not necessarily exclude all fetal congenital malformations, especially chromosomal defects. However, these tests are useful in ruling out some of the most frequent abnormalities, and they should be the first step in the evaluation of the breech infant.

If the answer to the question of whether or not the infant has a gross congenital abnormality is affirmative, the mother should be informed of the situation, and in most cases vaginal delivery may be offered as the best management alternative. If no abnormalities are detected in evaluation of the fetus, the next question is the following:

What is the fetal weight?

For management purposes, the weight of the infant in breech presentation should be categorized into one of the following groups: (1) less than 2000 grams, (2) between 2000 and 3500 grams, and (3) larger than 3500 grams.

Accurate evaluation of fetal weight is difficult, and the lack of precision is greater in breech than in vertex presentations. To evaluate the size of the infant, the obstetrician should use all the available information (history, examination, x-ray films, sonogram). We have found the ultrasound examination (biparietal diameter and abdominal circumference) particularly helpful in the evaluation of fetal size, especially in infants weighing less than 2500 grams.

If the estimated fetal weight is more than 3500 grams, pregnancy should be terminated by cesarean section. A large weight (greater than 3500 grams) is another indication for the surgical delivery of the infant in breech presentation. As shown in Table 17-1, a perinatal mortality of 0.5% for breech infants between 3000 and 3499 grams begins to increase when the birth weight exceeds the latter figure. This is mainly the result of fetal asphyxia caused by difficulties in the delivery of the head and fetal trauma secondary to difficult vaginal deliveries.

If the fetal weight is less than 2000 grams, the breech infant should be delivered by cesarean section. The controversy over vaginal versus abdominal delivery of the preterm breech infant has not yet been settled. An illustrative paper about the problems involved in this decision is that of Cruikshank and Pitkin.[7] The authors point out that a large proportion of the perinatal mortality associated with the vaginal delivery of preterm breech infants is a consequence of (1) prematurity, (2) congenital abnormalities, (3) maternal disease (diabetes, Rh incompatibility, etc), (4) placental complications, and (5) unknown etiology (macerated fetus); these causes of perinatal mortality are not preventable by cesarean-section delivery. However, other important causes of perinatal mortality and morbidity in the preterm breech infant such as prolapse of the cord, entrapment of the fetal head by an incompletely dilated cervix, and fetal trauma during vaginal delivery are preventable by surgical intervention. Since there is no way to predict which particular breech infant is going to suffer from one or more of these preventable complications, the best approach is—after congenital abnormalities have been ruled out—to deliver abdominally all preterm breech infants weighing less than 2000 grams.

When counseling the parents about the need for surgical intervention for the preterm breech birth, it is important to remember that the infant's chances for survival and for short- and long-term morbidity are closely related to birth weight. The closer the infant is to 1000 grams of estimated fetal weight, the smaller the chances for survival and the larger the possibilities of significant morbidity. The closer the infant is to 2000 grams, the better the chances for survival and for decreased morbidity.

There has been considerable improvement in the last decade in the survival and morbidity figures for the tiny baby. However, the prognosis for the infant under 800 grams remains poor, and only under exceptional circumstances should the mother be counseled to suffer the short- and long-term morbidity of a cesarean-section delivery for the sake of improving the survival chances of a marginal baby. Infants with a birth weight between 500 and 800 grams have only about a 40% chance for survival, and less than 50% of the survivors are neurologically intact. This gives a bleak prognosis for survival with unimpaired brain function. Many parents opt for abdominal delivery in spite of the overall poor prognosis for the fetus, but in our opinion this is a bad decision.

If the fetal weight is between 2000 and 3500 grams, the following should be the next question:

Is there hyperextension of the fetal head?

Hyperextension of the fetal head is another clear indication for operative delivery of the breech infant even in situations looking extremely favorable for vaginal delivery. If there is no hyperextension of the fetal head, and the fetal weight is between 2000 and 3500 grams, the next question is the following:

Is the infant a nonfrank breech or a frank breech?

Since nonfrank breech presentations are accompanied by prolapse of the umbilical cord in an excessively large number of cases, all nonfrank breech pregnancies should be terminated by cesarean section. If the infant is in a frank breech presentation, the head is flexed, and the weight is between 2000 and 3500 grams, the next question is the following:

Is the maternal pelvis size adequate for the delivery of a breech infant?

The criteria for judging the adequacy of a maternal pelvis for breech delivery are much more stringent than those used for vertex delivery. The reason is that during a vertex delivery the fetal head suffers a process of accommodation to the maternal pelvis (molding), which allows vaginal delivery in spite of pelvic diameters that sometimes are equal to or even smaller than the cephalic diameters of the fetus. During breech delivery the unmolded fetal head should rapidly pass through the pelvis without any previous accommodation. The minimal diameters adopted by Collea et al[6] in a randomized study of vaginal versus cesarean-section delivery for term

infants in frank breech presentations were the following:

Inlet	
Transverse	11.5 cm
Anteroposterior	10.5 cm
Midpelvis	
Transverse	10.0 cm
Anteroposterior	11.5 cm

The history of a vaginal delivery of an infant with a weight equal to or greater than the estimated fetal weight of the present pregnancy is even better than x-ray pelvimetry criteria in assessing the adequacy of the maternal pelvis. However, if the past obstetric history contains only deliveries of infants weighing less than that estimated for the present pregnancy, x-ray pelvimetry should be obtained to assess more critically the adequacy of the bony pelvis. In nulliparous patients we look first to the appearance of the ischial spines in the fetogram. If the spines are prominent and the bispinous diameter in the fetogram is less than 10 cm, the pelvis is considered narrow and the patient should have a cesarean-section delivery. If the spines are not prominent, pelvimetry is obtained.

Needless to say, the role of x-ray pelvimetry in the management of breech presentation is highly controversial, and several investigators believe that this method is inadequate for selecting those patients who will have difficulties during labor. However, we feel that until proven otherwise by controlled studies, the technique allows the detection of inadequate pelvic diameters in certain patients (50% in the study of Collea et al[6]) and makes it possible for them to avoid the perils of a trial of labor. *If the maternal pelvis is judged to be inadequate, the pregnancy*

FIG. 17-1 ■ Intrapartum management of breech presentations.

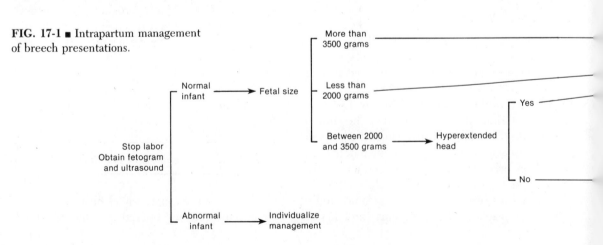

should be terminated by cesarean section. If the pelvic dimensions are adequate, labor should be allowed to continue and vaginal delivery expected.

Once the patient has been selected for vaginal delivery in accordance with the multiple criteria just described, the obstetrician should not be afraid to use oxytocin to augment labor if this is necessary for the treatment of prolonged latent phase or protracted active phase of labor. Other abnormal labor patterns such as secondary arrest of cervical dilation or abnormalities of descent are an indication for cesarean section.

Labor in breech presentation should be monitored electronically and the pregnancy terminated by surgical intervention if there is clear evidence of fetal distress. Mild variable decelerations happen frequently in the course of labor when the infant is in breech presentation. Variable decelerations are indicative of fetal distress if they become severe, coexist with a low fetal pH, or are concomitant with poor beat-to-beat variability of the fetal heart trace. Blood sampling from the buttock is feasible in breech infants to assess fetal pH.

A summary of the overall plan of management for breech presentation at the time of labor appears in Fig. 17-1. For technical details on delivering a breech infant see the corresponding chapter in *Williams Obstetrics*.[27]

■ PERSISTENT OCCIPITOPOSTERIOR (OP) POSITION

Persistent OP position is a rather common intrapartum problem that in the great majority of cases resolves spontaneously but in others is a cause of unnecessary instrumentation and fetal-maternal trauma. In about 5% of all term labors

the occiput fails to spontaneously rotate to an anterior position, a situation that is characterized clinically by protracted descent or arrest of descent of the presenting part. The persistent OP malposition is often solved with midforceps rotation and midforceps delivery, maneuvers that are potentially harmful for both fetus and mother.

Etiology

There is no clear explanation for the lack of spontaneous internal rotation in cases of persistent OP malpositions. The problem occurs more often in small women, in blacks, and when the fetus is large. It seems to be associated with the presence of relatively narrow transverse diameters of the midpelvis,[18] but the evidence in this respect is not solid. The pelvic shape is not the only factor in the etiology of the OP position, and there is no association between this malposition and CPD. OP positions occur up to three times more often in patients laboring under conduction anesthesia, a fact that suggests a possible etiologic role for a deficiency of the expulsive forces of labor.

Labor abnormalities

The most common labor abnormalities in patients with persistent OP malposition are protracted descent and arrest of descent of the presenting part. Prolonged latent phase, prolonged active phase, and prolonged deceleration phase may also occur, but descent problems are predominant. Malposition of the fetal head should be suspected when the fetal head remains at −1 or 0 station during the last few centimeters of cervical dilation, and the suspicion should be stronger if the presenting part remains high after

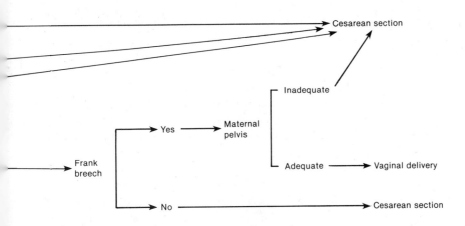

complete cervical dilation. Frequently the lack of descent is attributed to incomplete cervical dilation because there is a persistent anterior rim of the cervix that fails to disappear in spite of what seems to be adequate uterine contractions. The truth of the matter is that the disappearance of this anterior rim of the cervix does not influence the characteristics of the labor abnormality. Every time this clinical situation appears (anterior rim of cervix, high presenting part) the presence of an OP malposition should be strongly suspected and the diagnosis confirmed by pelvic examination or by real-time ultrasound.

Management

During the early part of this century several reports described dangers and perils in persistent OP positions. Today it is known that most of these complications are unrelated to the fetal position and that the main problem with the malposition is the inadequate intervention of the obstetrician and the use of instrumental maneuvers that may cause serious fetal and maternal morbidity. The first rule in the management of this situation is therefore not to intervene—especially with midforceps rotations—without carefully weighing other management alternatives that may be less hazardous for mother and infant.

Before anything else the obstetrician should make a decision about the possibility of CPD in the patient with persistent OP position and abnormal labor. If the infant is large, the mother is short, and the presenting part is above 0 station, CPD should be strongly suspected and x-ray pelvimetry obtained. Also, if the Hillis-Müller maneuver (pushing the head into the pelvis during a uterine contraction to ascertain its downward thrust by means of vaginal examination) fails to show a downward thrust of the fetal head, CPD should be suspected and x-ray pelvimetry obtained. The majority of patients with persistent OP malposition have no clinical evidence of a narrow pelvis, and to obtain x-ray pelvimetry in all of them is unnecessary. The clinician should select those patients at high risk of CPD and limit the x-ray examination to that specific group. Ideally, the x-ray assessment of the bony pelvis should include a simultaneous evaluation of the volume of the fetal head (Ball pelvimetry) and the relation of that volume to the capacity of the pelvis. If the cephalopelvi-

metry shows disproportion, cesarean section delivery is indicated immediately.

As just mentioned, the large majority of patients with persistent OP malposition do not require pelvimetry because clinical evaluation shows the presence of an adequate bony pelvis. In many of these cases it is clear that there is a deficiency in the expulsive forces of the uterus, which is important in perpetuating the malposition and prolonging the labor abnormality. Frequently the patient is under epidural anesthesia or heavily sedated, and her uterine contractions are mild to moderate and short in duration. Sometimes the patient is obese, the fetus is large, and the quality of contractions is difficult to determine, but they do not seem to last long enough. In any case if a deficiency in the expulsive forces of the uterus is suspected, the next thing to do is to insert a catheter and quantify the intrauterine pressure. Also, internal monitoring of the FHR should be carried out at this time in anticipation of a prolonged second stage of labor requiring careful fetal monitoring.

If the uterine work is deficient, labor augmentation with intravenous oxytocin is the treatment of choice; in many cases this is followed by spontaneous rotation of the head to an occiptoanterior (OA) position and vaginal delivery. In other cases there is no spontaneous rotation, but the improvement in the expulsive forces of the uterus makes the head descend to a point at which the infant may be delivered in OP position. In this latter case a generous episiotomy should precede vaginal delivery to avoid a perineal tear.

If there is no disproportion and the uterine work is adequate, the patient with persistent OP malposition should be allowed to labor unless signs of fetal distress appear. If left alone, the large majority (59%) of patients with OP malpositions and adequate uterine contractions deliver spontaneously with the fetus still in OP position.[17] Other patients rotate spontaneously and deliver, sometimes precipitously, with the fetus in OA position. The question in these cases is how long a patient should be allowed to remain in the second stage of labor before there is a significant risk of fetal or maternal complications. According to Friedman,[11] the upper limit of normalcy for the duration of the second stage of labor is 2½ hours for the nullipara and 50 minutes for the multipara. These figures correspond to the mean duration of the second stage plus two standard deviations from the mean and were obtained in a large population of nulliparous and multiparous patients. However, immediate intervention (forceps or cesarean-section delivery) is not necessarily justified when the upper limit of the normal duration for the second stage of labor has been reached and there are no signs of fetal distress. Studies[5] have shown that in the absence of signs of fetal distress the second stage of labor may be prolonged for several hours without unfavorable effects on the infant. Therefore it seems unwarranted to terminate a pregnancy simply because the length of the second stage of labor has reached an arbitrary limit. However, a decision favoring prolongation of the second stage of labor beyond the limits of normalcy should be balanced against evidence[24] showing that there is a progressive decrease in fetal blood pH values during the second stage. Also, it is possible that the slow but progressive acidosis of the second stage may not be reflected in dramatic fetal monitoring changes such as those seen during acute episodes of fetal hypoxia. If this is true, prolongation of the second stage may be dangerous unless the fetal status is monitored with periodic scalp blood pH determinations.

When a patient reaches the upper limit of normal duration for the second stage of labor, our policy is one of meticulous reevaluation of the overall situation. The possibility of CPD should be strongly considered, and cephalopelvimetry should be obtained even if clinical evaluation points to the existence of an adequate pelvis. If x-ray pelvimetry was obtained at the beginning of the problem, the films should be measured again, preferably by another observer, and the relation between pelvic and fetal head volumes recalculated. The fetal status should also be carefully reevaluated and a scalp pH sample obtained even if the direct electronic monitoring trace is normal. The intrauterine pressure catheter should be calibrated, and a judgment should be made about the quality of the uterine work. At the end of this reevaluation, cesarean section should be undertaken unless the obstetrician can be certain that there is nothing to impede further progress other than the fetal head malposition.

If there is no obstructed labor, it is permissible to allow patients with persistent OP malpositions to continue laboring, despite the fact that the upper limits of normal duration for the second stage of labor have been exceeded, as long as the following conditions are fulfilled:

1. Cephalopelvimetry of good quality shows that disproportion is not present.
2. The Hillis-Müller maneuver is positive, and it is reasonable to believe that prolongation of labor has a good chance of ending in vaginal delivery.
3. The direct FHR monitoring trace is completely normal.
4. Fetal scalp pH is measured every hour in the nullipara and every 30 minutes in the multipara once the upper limit of duration for the second stage of labor has been exceeded and the pH remains above 7.25 with no significant decrease (greater than 0.03 pH units) between successive samples.

If further descent occurs and the fetal head reaches the perineum, a digital rotation to the OA position[21] should be attempted to facilitate the spontaneous expulsion of the fetus. The following is the technique for digital rotation from OP to OA position:

1. The vertex should be at a low station, visible at the introitus.
2. Using the right hand for a left-sided position and the left hand for a right-sided position, the lambdoid suture should be identified and the tip of the middle finger placed exactly at the angle of the lambdoid suture with the tip of the index finger directly alongside the middle finger on the upper lambdoid suture.
3. The hand that is outside the vagina should be applied in the form of a fist against the anterior shoulder of the infant.
4. Simultaneously, the two fingers placed on the lambdoid suture should exert a steady rotary motion in a direction at right angles to the saggital suture (clockwise) with the fist pushing the fetal shoulder transversly (counterclockwise) in the direction of the occiput. The counterpressure to the rotary motion of the internal fingers brings about flexion of the head and correction of asynclitism. The two pressures must be exerted simultaneously.

If the digital rotation fails and the maternal expulsive efforts are not enough to achieve spontaneous delivery in the OP position, miniature spatulas or low forceps should be used and the infant delivered in OP without further attempts to rotate the fetal head with instruments. If the arrest of descent has not changed after a total of 4 hours of second stage in the primipara and 2

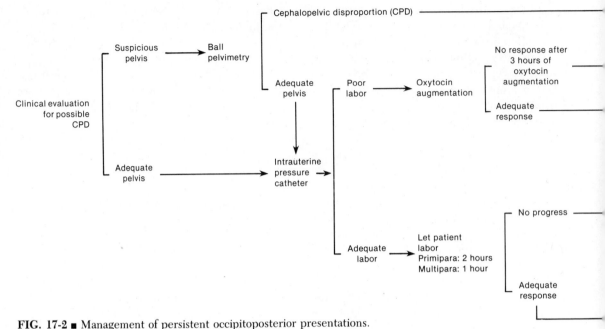

FIG. 17-2 ■ Management of persistent occipitoposterior presentations.

hours in the multipara, the pregnancy should be terminated by cesarean section.

A summary of the plan of management for persistent OP malposition is shown in Fig. 17-2. The emphasis of the protocol is to avoid midforceps rotations. Several authors, especially Friedman and Sachtleben[12,13] have demonstrated that the adverse short- and long-term effects of labor abnormalities occur predominantly in babies submitted to midforceps operations.

■ OTHER ABNORMAL PRESENTATIONS

Shoulder, face, and compound presentations are rare events in obstetrics. Their management is reviewed briefly here.

Shoulder presentation (transverse lie)

Shoulder presentation occurs in approximately 0.3% of singleton pregnancies and more frequently in the second twin of multiple births (about 10% of the cases). Shoulder presentation, often called *transverse lie,* implies that the long axis of the fetus is perpendicular to the long axis of the mother. In the majority of cases the shoulder is the presenting part. However, in many other cases the infant has his hand and arm prolapsed into the vagina, or occasionally there is no presenting part in the pelvis (fetal back over the pelvic inlet). In other unfortunate cases the

fetal back is up against the uterine fundus and the small parts are over the inlet, and the patient arrives with the umbilical cord prolapsed into the vagina and no presenting part in the pelvis. An ultrasound examination or a fetogram confirms the diagnosis. Transverse lies are usually associated with multiparity, and more than 80% of the cases occur in patients who are para III or more. They also frequently occur in preterm infants (up to 38%) and in women with placenta previa (up to 10%).

Cesarean section is the method of choice for the delivery of a fetus in transverse lie with two exceptions, grossly immature fetuses (less than 800 grams) and macerated fetuses up to 1250 grams, both of which can be delivered vaginally. In all other circumstances, even in neglected shoulder presentations with fetal death in uterus and chorioamnionitis, cesarean section is the recommended procedure. The alternative is a destructive procedure with vaginal removal of the dead fetus; this is more hazardous than a cesarean section and may cause more maternal morbidity.

A lower segment transverse uterine incision is safer for the mother than a low vertical cesarean section (less risk of uterine rupture in subsequent pregnancies), but it cannot be used in most cases of transverse lie. Often it is difficult to extract an infant in transverse lie through a

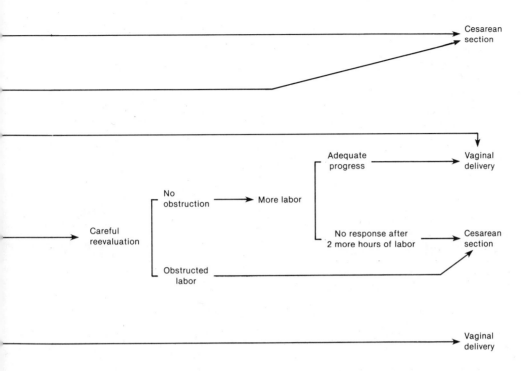

low transverse incision, especially when the fetal back is over the pelvic inlet. However, if the low uterine segment is developed, the position of the head and feet is remembered by the surgeon at the time of the operation, and the surgeon remains calm, a good number of transverse lies can be delivered with a low transverse uterine incision.

Face presentation

Face presentation is also rare with an incidence of 0.2%. It is characterized by an extreme extension of the fetal head so that the face rather than the skull becomes the presenting part. Any factor that favors the extension or prevents the flexion of the fetal head, such as congenital goiter or anencephaly, may be an etiologic factor in cases of face presentation. Like shoulder presentation, face presentation is associated with maternal multiparity. The lack of resistance of the anterior abdominal wall in multiparas allows the fetus to sag forward and extend the cervical spine. Occasionally, face presentations occur in association with CPD; a combination of an inlet contraction and a macrosomic infant may occur in up to 39.4% of all cases of face presentation.

The clinical diagnosis of a face presentation is made by vaginal examination and confirmed by fetogram or ultrasound. The presentation is often confused with a breech, a mistake that is easily avoided by remembering two rules.

1. The anus has sphincter tone. The mouth does not.
2. The anus is in line with the ischial tuberosities. The mouth and the malar prominences form a triangle.

In handling face presentations spontaneous vaginal delivery can be expected in 60% to 80% of the cases.[9] When the position is mentoposterior (fetal chin in the posterior part of the maternal pelvis), up to 50% of these patients rotate spontaneously to mentoanterior position allowing vaginal delivery. This usually happens during the second stage of labor. Thus there is no reason to intervene early in cases of mentoposterior positions if dilation of the cervix and descent of the head are proceeding normally.

Maneuvers to convert a face presentation to a vertex or to convert manually or instrumentally a mentoposterior to a mentoanterior position should be avoided. If a patient with a face presentation is making progress during labor, she should be left alone. If arrest of labor (dilation or descent) occurs, cesarean section is indicated.

Compound presentations

Compound presentations are rather uncommon situations in which one or two of the fetal extremities enter the pelvis simultaneously with the presenting part. The problem occurs in 0.1%

of all deliveries. The most common combinations are vertex-hand, breech-hand, and vertex-arm-foot; the most common complication is umbilical cord prolapse, which may occur in up to 20% of the cases. Compound presentations are usually associated with multiparity, prematurity, twin gestation (usually the second twin), and CPD (narrow inlet).

In the large majority of cases the prolapsed extremity does not interfere with the normal course of labor and vaginal delivery. In the case of vertex-hand presentation, the hand of the newborn may look swollen and bluish for 24 to 48 hours after birth, but recovery without sequelae is the rule. Breech-hand presentations (the second most common) should be managed with the same criteria used to manage any breech presentation without consideration for the presence of the hand in the pelvis. Vertex-foot and vertex-arm-foot presentations require a gentle attempt at repositioning the lower extremity if it does not slip out of the way spontaneously during labor. If this attempt fails and the foot or arm does not move inside the uterus, cesarean section is necessary unless the fetus is extremely small (less than 800 grams).

■ REFERENCES

1. Bilodeau R, Marier R: Breech presentation at term. Am J Obstet Gynecol 1978;130:555.
2. Bradley-Watson PJ: The demeaning value of external cephalic version in modern obstetric practice. Am J Obstet Gynecol 1975;123:237.
3. Brenner WE, Bruce RD, Hendricks CA: The characteristics and perils of breech presentation. Am J Obstet gynecol 1974;118:700.
4. Caterini H, Langer A, Sama JC, et al: Fetal risk in hyperextension of the fetal head in breech presentation. Am J Obstet Gynecol 1975;123:632.
5. Cohen WR: Influence of the duration of second stage labor on perinatal outcome and puerperal morbidity. Obstet Gynecol 1977;49:266.
6. Collea JV, Ratin SC, Weghorst GR, et al: The randomized management of term frank breech presentation: vaginal delivery vs. cesarean section. Am J Obstet Gynecol 1978;131:186.
7. Cruikshank OP, Pitkin RM: Delivery of the premature breech. Obstet Gynecol 1977;50:367.
8. De Crespigny LJC, Pepperell RJ: Perinatal mortality and morbidity in breech presentation. Obstet Gynecol 1979;53:141.
9. Duff P: Diagnosis and management of face presentation. Obstet Gynecol 1981;57:105.
10. Fall O, Nilsson BA: External cephalic version in breech presentation under tocolysis. Obstet Gynecol 1979;53:712.
11. Friedman EA: *Labor: Clinical Evaluation and Management*. New York, Appleton-Century-Crofts, 1967, pp. 36-37.
12. Friedman EA, Sachtleben MR: Station of the fetal presenting part. VI. Arrest of descent in nulliparas. Obstet Gynecol 1976;47:129.
13. Friedman EA, Sachtleben MR, Bresky PA: Dysfunctional labor. XII. Long-term effects on infant. Am J Obstet Gynecol 1977;127:779.
14. Galloway WH, Bartholomew RA, Coluin ED, et al: Premature breech delivery. Am J Obstet Gynecol 1967;99:975.
15. Goldenberg RL, Nelson KG: The premature breech. Am J Obstet Gynecol 1977;127:240.
16. Hall EJ, Kohl SA, O'Brien F, et al: Breech presentation and perinatal mortality. Am J Obstet Gynecol 1965;91:665.
17. Haynes DM: Occiput posterior position. JAMA 1954:156:494.
18. Holmberg NG, Liliequist B, Magnusson S, et al: The influence of the bony pelvis in persistent occiput posterior position. Acta Obstet Gynecol Scan (Suppl) 1977;66:49.
19. Jurado L, Miller GL: Breech presentation. Am J Obstet Gynecol 1968;101:183.
20. Kauppila O: The perinatal mortality in breech deliveries and observation on affecting factors: a retrospective study of 2227 cases. Acta Obstet Gynecol Scand (Suppl) 1975;39:1.
21. Lowenstein A, Zevin R: Digital rotation of the vertex. Obstet Gynecol 1971;37:790.
22. Lyons ER, Papin FR: Cesarean section in the management of breech presentation. Am J Obstet Gynecol 1978;130:558.
23. Milner RDG: Neonatal mortality of breech deliveries with and without forceps to the aftercoming head. Br J Obstet Gynaecol 1975;82:783.
24. Modanlou H, Yeh SY, Hon EH, et al: Fetal and neonatal biochemistry and Apgar scores. Am J Obstet Gynecol 1973;117:942.
25. Morley GW: Breech presentation: a 15-year review. Obstet Gynecol 1967;30:745.
26. Potter EL, Adair FL: Clinical pathological study of the infant and fetal mortality for a ten-year period at the Chicago Lying-In Hospital. Am J Obstet Gynecol 1943;45:1054.
27. Pritchard JA, MacDonald PC: *Williams Obstetrics*, ed 16. New York, Appleton-Century-Crofts, 1980, pp. 889-902.
28. Ralis ZA: Birth trauma to muscles in babies born by breech delivery and its possible fatal consequences. Arch Dis Child 1975;50:4.
29. Ranney B: The gentle art of external cephalic version. Am J Obstet Gynecol 1973;116:239.
30. Sinder A, Wenstler NE: Breech presentation with follow-up. Obstet Gynecol 1965;25:322.
31. Tank ES, Davis R, Holt JF, et al: Mechanisms of trauma during breech delivery. Obstet Gynecol 1971;38:761.
32. Van Dorstein JP, Schifrin BS, Wallace RL: Randomized control trial of external cephalic version with tocolysis in late pregnancy. Am J Obstet Gynecol 1981;141:417.
33. Wigglesworth JS, Husemeyer RP: Intracranial birth trauma in vaginal breech delivery: the continued importance of injury to the occipital bone. Br J Obstet Gynaecol 1977;84:684.

18

■ ■ ■

FETAL DISTRESS

Fernando Arias and Obi C. Okehi

Fetal distress is a state of jeopardy of the fetus that if undetected and untreated leads to fetal death or causes significant neonatal mortality and morbidity. Most of the common causes of fetal distress are extrinsic to the fetus and exert their deleterious effect by interfering with the fetal gas exchange. Variations in the nature, duration, and severity of the hypoxic insult lead to a wide range of fetal consequences. For example, hypoxia may be severe but transient and well tolerated; it may be severe and persist long enough to kill the fetus in utero; it may be chronic and sublethal and lead to permanent neurologic damage and mental disabilities during extrauterine life. The role of the obstetrician is to recognize those conditions causing fetal jeopardy, continuously evaluate their effect on the fetus, and determine the most adequate time for delivery of the compromised infant.

A large part of the obstetric research during the last two decades has been directed toward developing new and more accurate means for detecting and evaluating the severity of fetal distress. In the early 1970s electronic monitoring of the fetal heart became available, and its enthusiastic adoption by physicians and hospitals has resulted in drastic changes in the practice of obstetrics in the United States. However, it was soon found that electronic monitoring of the fetal heart did not provide unequivocal answers to the problem of intrapartum evaluation of the fetus. Unfortunately, during the process of learning about the limitations of this technique we have seen a dramatic increase in the incidence of cesarean sections being carried out because of erroneous diagnosis of fetal distress. Today it is clear that electronic monitoring of the fetus is valuable because of its ability to diagnose fetal normalcy and predict the occurrence of a normal outcome (few false negative results, high negative predictive value), but it is inaccurate for making a positive diagnosis of fetal distress or for predicting a poor fetal outcome (high number of false positive results, low positive predictive value). Fortunately, the development of fetal scalp pH measurements has made it possible to increase significantly the accuracy of the diagnosis of fetal distress.

■ FETAL GAS EXCHANGE AND pH REGULATION

The large majority of agents causing fetal distress act through a common mechanism of interference with the fetal gas exchange and pH regulation. To understand better the characteristics of the fetal situation under different stressful conditions a brief review of some basic concepts about these aspects of fetal physiology is in order.

CO_2 exchange and respiratory acidosis

In a significant number of cases interferences with the fetal gas exchange primarily affect the ability of the fetus to eliminate acid waste in the

331

Fetal side

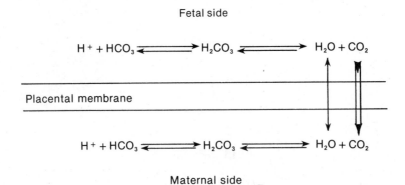

FIG. 18-1 ▪ Fetal bicarbonate buffer system. The H^+ ions produced in the intermediate metabolism of the fetus are transformed into CO_2. This CO_2 is transferred by a pressure gradient into the maternal circulation and eventually eliminated by the maternal lungs. The fetus cannot control the elimination of its CO_2 and is easily affected by conditions that impair fetal transfer of CO_2 to the placenta (cord compression) or interfere with maternal CO_2 elimination (asthma).

form of CO_2. In such cases the initial biochemical changes are similar to those seen in adult respiratory acidosis, and the dominant phenomena are an increase in fetal PCO_2 and a drop in pH. Later the increase in PCO_2 causes increased fetal concentration of H^+ ions and a decrease in base with further lowering of the pH so that the picture is that of a mixed respiratory and metabolic acidosis. Typical examples of this situation are found in cases of umbilical cord compression and maternal status asthmaticus.

It is apparent that, although at the beginning of fetal distress it may be possible to find biochemical evidence of a primary respiratory or metabolic drop in pH, in the majority of cases the clinician encounters a mixed respiratory *and* metabolic acidosis. This has its explanation in the mechanism for fetal CO_2 elimination and its relation to pH. As shown in Fig. 18-1, any excessive H^+ production by the fetus (metabolic acidosis) drives the equation toward the right and causes an increase in PCO_2. Any interference with CO_2 elimination (respiratory acidosis) causes in turn a drive of the equation toward the left with formation of H^+.

The fetal acid-base balance depends on a bicarbonate buffer system that is not as efficient as it is outside the uterus because the ability to quickly eliminate CO_2 into the atmosphere by the respiratory system, a factor that gives a unique buffering capacity to the bicarbonate system, does not exist during intrauterine life. Fetal

CO_2 is eliminated by diffusion throughout the placenta as molecular CO_2 and eventually disposed of by the maternal respiration, but since the fetus cannot influence the maternal respiratory rate, maintenance of the fetal acid-base balance is dependent on mechanisms over which the fetus has no control.

Fetal CO_2 diffusion through the placenta is possible because of the existence of a CO_2 gradient between the fetal and the maternal circulations. Fetal PCO_2, measured in scalp blood, is 38 to 44 mm Hg, whereas maternal PCO_2 is 18 to 24 mm Hg; this difference generates the driving force that makes possible the transfer of fetal CO_2 to the maternal circulation. Any significant decrease in this gradient because of increased maternal PCO_2, such as happens in cases of maternal respiratory failure, impairs fetal CO_2 elimination and may be potentially lethal. When the maternal PCO_2 reaches 35 to 40 mm Hg, measures to improve maternal CO_2 elimination (endotracheal intubation and mechanical ventilation) should be taken to avoid fetal acidosis and death. It is clear from Fig. 18-1 that little is achieved in attempting to treat fetal acidosis by maternal administration of bicarbonate, since the diffusion of H^+ and HCO_3^- through the placenta is slow and therapeutically ineffective. It makes more sense to treat fetal acidosis by asking the mother to hyperventilate, thus decreasing maternal PCO_2 and improving the placental gradient in favor of fetal CO_2 elimination.

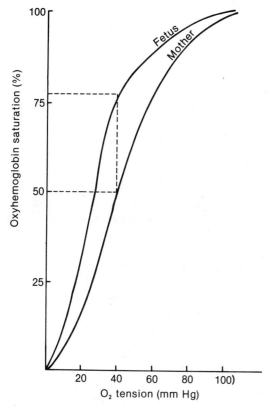

FIG. 18-2 ■ Fetal and maternal oxyhemoglobin dissociation curves. The high oxygen affinity of fetal hemoglobin allows the fetus to have an adequate oxygen saturation at O_2 tensions that are inadequate to maintain a normal oxygen concentration in the maternal blood.

O_2 exchange and metabolic acidosis

Decreased oxygen transfer to the fetus is another important cause of fetal distress. A normal fetus requires 5 to 10 ml O_2/kg/minute to sustain normal growth, development, and normal pH, and it seems that the limiting factor in O_2 transfer to the placenta is the maternal blood flow rather than the resistance to diffusion of the placental membrane. Decreased O_2 supply to the fetus may occur suddenly (abruptio placentae, hypertonic labor, spinal shock syndrome), but it may be also the consequence of a chronic, sublethal process (maternal hypertension) that progressively taxes the fetal economy. In both cases O_2 deficiency causes a metabolic switch to anaerobic metabolism with the generation of 2 moles of lactate and 2 moles of H^+ per each mole of glucose used for energy generation purposes. The H^+ generated reduces the concen-

tration of buffer base (bicarbonate and protein) producing initially a biochemical picture of metabolic acidosis. Later, however, the excessive H^+ being produced generates equimolar amounts of CO_2 and drives the equation in Fig. 18-1 toward the right, resulting in a biochemical profile of mixed metabolic and respiratory acidosis. If the insult is acute and severe (abruptio placentae), there is no time for adequate metabolic adaptation to the sudden decrease in P_{CO_2}, and signs and symptoms of fetal distress are readily apparent. If the insult is chronic and sublethal (maternal chronic hypertension), the fetus will temporarily adapt to the situation. However, the inefficient generation of adenosine triphosphate (ATP) caused by the chronic oxygen deprivation is apparent, since fetal growth and the capacity of the fetus to tolerate even minimally stressful situations are seriously compromised.

Fetal compensating mechanisms can deal more effectively with deficiencies in oxygen supply than excesses in H^+ production or defects in CO_2 elimination. The high oxygen affinity of fetal hemoglobin allows an adequate saturation of the fetal blood in spite of significant decreases in maternal P_{O_2} (Fig. 18-2). For example, at a maternal P_{O_2} of 40 mm Hg the fetus is still capable of keeping about 75% of its hemoglobin saturated with oxygen. Similarly, and this is the rationale for maternal oxygen therapy when there is impairment in the O_2 transfer to the fetus, increases in maternal P_{O_2} result in increases in the oxygen content of the fetus. In contrast, compensation for rises in fetal H^+ or fetal P_{CO_2} is limited to improving the delivery of CO_2 to the placenta by increasing the fetal heart rate (FHR). The rebound tachycardia seen after episodes of cord compression most probably represents such a mechanism of compensation.

In other cases fetal distress appears as a consequence of interference with both fetal oxygenation and fetal P_{CO_2} elimination. The effects on the fetus are marked, and the metabolic events leading to fetal death may occur rapidly. A typical example of this situation is hypertonic labor in which the availability of oxygen to the fetus and the ability to dispose of the fetal P_{CO_2} are compromised. The biochemical profile in this situation is that of a mixed respiratory and metabolic acidosis.

■ ANTEPARTUM FETAL DISTRESS

Fetal hypoxia and acidosis may occur during the antepartum period, but they are detected more often during labor because uterine contractions are a stress for the fetus, which challenges compensation mechanisms to a maximum. The fetus with marginal compensatory capacity tolerates poorly the stress of labor and shows signs of distress. It becomes important to identify before parturition those fetuses at high risk for intrapartum problems to avoid the dangers of labor for those unable to tolerate uterine contractions and the dangers of cesarean section for those with enough functional reserve to tolerate labor safely.

Antepartum fetal distress occurs mostly in high-risk pregnancies. The possibilities of a hypoxic insult to the fetus during a normal pregnancy are extremely rare, and the occurrence of fetal distress in a normal pregnancy is an indication for initiating an extensive search for the presence of an undiagnosed maternal disease or a fetal abnormality responsible for the unexpected event. Intrapartum fetal death at term and in the absence of risk factors occurred in less than 1 per 25,000 patients in the Collaborative Perinatal Study.[18]

Clinical indicators

Fetal movement and uterine growth are the only two valuable clinical indicators of the fetal status during the antepartum period. Other indicators (FHR, antepartum meconium) are of questionable value. Similar to laboratory methods used for the same purpose, clinical indicators of the fetal status are valuable in confirming the presence of a normal pregnancy but lack specificity in assessing the existence of distress. They are important because their alteration is a red flag for the obstetrician who must immediately move to assess the fetus with laboratory examinations.

Fetal movement. Maternal reports of fetal movement (FM) are perhaps the most valuable index of fetal well-being. If the mother feels the fetus moving and denies any decrease in the amount or intensity of the movement, the fetus is healthy and in no distress. In contrast, if the mother perceives a definite decrease in fetal motility, the fetus may be in trouble.[27,30,31] At each prenatal visit the obstetrician must ask the mother about fetal movement and be seriously concerned if she reports a decrease, especially if she is a high-risk patient and there is other clinical or laboratory evidence suggesting fetal distress. When maternal reporting of adequate movements coincides with laboratory tests suggesting fetal jeopardy, the obstetrician should doubt the accuracy of the laboratory tests and suspect false positive test results.

The main problem limiting the use of FM as a clinical tool is the difficulty in quantification and establishment of normal limits. Additional problems are variations in subjective perception from one mother to the next and the fact that FM normally tends to decrease at the end of pregnancy. Several efforts have been made to solve the problem of quantification. For example, Pearson and Weaver[27] studied the FM occurring daily between 9 AM and 9 PM from 32 weeks of gestation until delivery in 61 patients who delivered healthy infants. They found that the median FM value was 90/12 hours at 32 weeks, falling to 50/12 hours at 40 weeks. Their lower limit of normal was 10 FM/12 hours. Seven patients who had a precipitous drop in FM to levels below this lower limit had complete disappearance of movement for 12 to 48 hours and finally cessation of fetal heart activity. Sadovsky and Polishuk[30] reported a normal range for FM of 4 to 1440 and indicated that there is no significance to the absolute amount of FM unless it completely ceases during a period of 12 hours. This 12-hour period when there is cessation of movement with the fetal heart still audible has been called *movements alarm signal* and suggests the presence of serious fetal complications. Spellacy et al[34] studied FM in patients lying on their left side for 10 minutes three times each day (morning, noon, and evening). They found that there was a diurnal variation with the amount of FM being significantly more during the evening. Less than 10 movements in 10 minutes was considered abnormal. The results suggest that evening FM determination for 10 minutes may help in the detection of developing fetal problems.

Any pregnant patient who complains of decrease or cessation of fetal movement must be taken seriously and given a nonstress test (NST). The finding of a "reactive" NST is extremely reassuring; the absence of reactivity must be followed with a contraction stress test (CST) (discussed later in this chapter).

Uterine growth. A considerable amount of information about the fetal well-being may be obtained by measuring the height of the uterine fundus at each prenatal visit. The uterine height must be measured in centimeters from the symphysis pubis to the fundus, always using the same technique. Measurements in centimeters have the advantage of usually equaling the gestational age, especially between 20 and 36 weeks. The patient must be in the supine position, and the legs must be kept straight to avoid the upward displacement of the symphysis that occurs when the knees are bent. The measurements must be performed along the longitudinal axis of the uterus except in the third trimester when they must be taken along the longitudinal axis of the fetus. If a pregnant patient is going to be seen by several physicians, they should agree to take the measurements the same way.

If the uterus is not growing at the expected rate or if there is an arrest in uterine growth, the clinician must be concerned about the possibility of retarded fetal growth,[4,39] a condition in which antepartum fetal distress often occurs (see Chapter 8). Unfortunately, there are many variables interfering with the assessment of fetal growth by measuring the uterine height. We have already mentioned variations in the technique used to measure the uterus. In addition, maternal obesity, excessive or decreased amounts of amniotic fluid, multiple pregnancies, and abnormal fetal presentations are other factors that contribute to determining the height of the uterus and introduce error in the clinical evaluation of fetal growth. However, despite its variability, measurement of the uterine height is the best clinical index of normal, excessive, or decreased fetal growth.[4,39] A normal increase in uterine height is reassuring, and a subnormal growth is an alarm signal demanding further investigation of fetal well-being.

Meconium staining of the amniotic fluid. The presence of meconium in the amniotic fluid has been traditionally accepted as a sign of fetal distress. Meconium may be found in amniotic fluid obtained from patients *before term and not in labor, intrapartum* after spontaneous or artificial rupture of the bag of waters, or in the fluid of patients who are *postterm and not in labor*.

Sometimes meconium is found in the amniotic fluid of normal or high-risk patients who require amniocentesis for evaluation of fetal lung mat-

uration. More rarely meconium may be seen in amniotic fluid obtained from patients during second trimester amniocentesis, usually for the purpose of antenatal diagnosis of chromosomal abnormalities. The finding of meconium in these situations is perturbing because of the natural tendency to consider its presence indicative of fetal distress. However, the significance of this finding is unknown. There is no evidence showing that the presence of meconium in the fluid before term and when the patient is not in labor is a reliable sign of fetal distress. Most studies on meconium staining have been carried out in patients with intrapartum meconium or prolonged pregnancies, and therefore the tendency to consider antepartum meconium as a bad sign is nothing but an extrapolation of studies done under different circumstances. We are aware of only one study about meconium staining of fluids obtained during second trimester amniocentesis,[13] and it shows that this finding has no significance and may only reveal that a transient hypoxic episode occurred before the amniocentesis.

The fact that perinatal mortality is increased in babies showing meconium staining at birth when compared with infants who are not meconium stained cannot be ignored. In one retrospective study[11] the meconium stained group had a neonatal mortality of 3.3% as opposed to 1.7% in the nonstained group. In the stained group cardiovascular malformations (13.9%), Rh isoimmunization (22.4%), chorioamnionitis (37.7%), and preeclampsia (11.1%) were significantly higher. However, this study did not differentiate between antepartum and intrapartum meconium and did not indicate in how many instances meconium staining was associated with the stigmata of postmaturity.

In general, the absence of meconium in amniotic fluid obtained before the initiation of labor in normal and high-risk patients is a reassuring sign pointing to the lack of acute or chronic fetal distress. The presence of meconium suggests the existence of a state of chronic fetal hypoxia or the prior occurrence of acute repetitive hypoxic episodes on the fetus. The significance of the finding is greater when it occurs in high-risk patients and when the meconium is heavy (darkly stained, dark green or black, thick, and tenacious). The presence of light meconium (lightly stained, yellow or greenish) in the amniotic fluid before term and when the patient is not in labor does not constitute absolute evidence of fetal distress and it is not an indication for pregnancy termination. However, further testing of fetal well-being is necessary; if other tests also point to the existence of fetal distress, delivery may be indicated; if other tests fail in confirming the presence of fetal distress, there is no need for pregnancy termination.

Auscultation of the fetal heart. Auscultatory determination of the FHR has little value in the assessment of fetal well-being or in the diagnosis of fetal distress. If the mother says that FM is normal, there is no point in listening to the fetal heart except as a reassuring gesture and because fetal arrhythmia or fetal bradycardia may occasionally be detected. When fetal arrhythmia is detected, it is a source of preoccupation for mother, father, and obstetrician; it produces additional expenses in mostly unnecessary testing and consultation; and it generates the possibility of iatrogenic premature delivery. The outcome of pregnancy in cases of fetal arrhythmias, however, is almost invariably good. More than 90% of the fetuses with arrhythmias or bradycardias discovered in antenatal visits in otherwise normal pregnancies are healthy, and the problem usually disappears at birth.[35]

Auscultation of the fetal heart during prenatal visits has more value as an index of fetal well-being if it is used as a fetal reactivity test.[25] For this purpose the clinician must listen to the fetal heart before and after moving the baby. If the fetus responds to movement with an increase in the frequency of heart beats, this is an excellent sign of fetal well-being. If there is a negative or dubious response of the FHR movement, the fetus may be in distress and an NST should be obtained. Quite often the fetus that has been found to be nonreactive to movement when listened to with the stethoscope is found to be reactive and healthy when examined with the electronic monitor. Therefore office fetal reactivity testing with the stethoscope has a limited value, and only positive responses may be accepted. We use this testing mostly in healthy, normal patients as a complement to the traditional auscultation of the fetal heart.

Laboratory indicators

Several different laboratory tests have been proposed as indicators of fetal distress or fetal

well-being during the antepartum period. In this section only those tests that have tolerated the passage of time and are commonly available in hospitals taking care of pregnant women (ultrasound, estriol, human placental lactogen, and antepartum electronic monitoring) are reviewed.

Ultrasound. Observation of the fetus and the placenta by real-time ultrasound is becoming an increasingly used method for the diagnosis of antepartum fetal distress. Analysis of the biophysical profile of the fetus, based on observation of the fetal body movements, fetal breathing movements, fetal tone, amount of amniotic fluid and fetal reactivity, allows an accurate identification of the distressed fetus.[20] Also, ultrasound is useful for the follow-up of fetal growth. The presence of an ultrasonic growth pattern suggestive of intrauterine growth retardation must be taken seriously because of the high incidence of antepartum and intrapartum fetal distress occurring in these babies (see Chapter 8).

Estriol. Determinations of urinary and plasma estriol for the purpose of evaluating the fetal status have been extremely popular among obstetricians during the last 10 years, and innumerable papers have been written about the subject. Today it is clear that estriol measurements do not provide current and precise information about the fetal status, they have little value in the management of high-risk situations, and their use as the only method of fetal evaluation may lead to unnecessary surgery and iatrogenic preterm delivery.[9]

There are several reasons for estriol measurements being unreliable when in theory they should be an excellent index of the function of the fetoplacental unit. Urinary estriol determinations are handicapped by the inadequacy of 24-hour urine collections, changes in glomerular filtration rate, and the existence in the urine of substances (glucose, methenamine) that interfere with some of the methods of measuring. Serum levels are affected by maternal liver function, status of the maternal enterohepatic circulation, maternal glomerular filtration rate, and minute-to-minute variations in concentration that may be the result of a pulsatile release of the steroid by the placental tissue. Serum and urine are affected by maternal ingestion of ampicillin and glucocorticoids. It is necessary to add to all these factors the existence of different laboratory techniques for determining estriol, the large intraassay and interassay variations of estriol assays, and the wide dispersion of values found in normal pregnant patients. Finally, the frequency of sampling is important because the predictive value of the test is diminished, at least in pregnant patients with diabetes, if the intervals between samples is longer than 24 hours.

In our opinion estriol measurements have a limited role in the diagnosis of antepartum fetal distress. Normal, rising estriol values are reassuring when they occur in a high-risk pregnancy in which clinical evaluation and serial sonography show normal fetal growth and the mother perceives an adequate amount of FM. Under similar circumstances low or dropping estriol values are not adequate evidence of fetal distress. Low or dropping estriol values should be taken as additional evidence of fetal distress only in high-risk patients with sudden or severe deterioration of the maternal disease, in patients with serial ultrasound suggesting fetal growth retardation, or in patients with abnormal antenatal electronic fetal monitoring. In cases in which the clinical and biophysical evaluations point toward the presence of fetal distress, normal estriol values should be interpreted as false negative, and more invasive evaluation of the fetal status should be carried out. From these examples it is clear that the information obtained through the use of estriol determination is helpful only when it agrees with other clinical and biophysical indicators. Therefore the use of estriol measurements as a single routine test for the screening of fetuses at risk of antepartum distress or for the diagnosis of fetal distress is unjustified.

Human placental lactogen. Human placental lactogen (HPL) determinations may have some value in the assessment of the fetal status in patients who have small, fibrotic, infarcted placentae associated with pregnancy hypertension,[32] intrauterine growth retardation,[33] and postterm pregnancies.[12] As is discussed in detail in the chapters of this book dealing with these pregnancy problems, the finding of serial HPL values in the fetal danger zone (FDZ)—that is, less than 4 µg/ml after 30 weeks of gestation—suggests the existence of fetal deterioration. Unfortunately, the opposite is not true. The presence of normal HPL values in pregnancies complicated by hypertension, growth retardation, or

postmaturity does not rule out the possibility of antepartum fetal distress.

HPL measurements should not be used as a single criterion to determine the need for pregnancy termination. When HPL values fall into the FDZ in the course of any of the three pregnancy complications just mentioned (hypertension, growth retardation, suspected postmaturity), the fetal status must be evaluated further by electronic monitoring and biophysical profile. Only if these tests show signs of fetal distress will delivery be indicated.

HPL determinations are useless for fetal evaluation when the placenta is functioning well and fetal distress is not placental in origin. Using HPL measurements in attempts to detect fetal distress in patients with problems such as Rh isoimmunization, drug addiction, diabetes, and fetal congenital anomalies is not only an unnecessary expense but may be a dangerous mistake. In pregnancy problems different from hypertension, growth retardation, and postmaturity normal or elevated HPL values may coexist with fetal distress, and the latter may be undetected because of a false sense of security generated by the normality of the test.

Electronic monitoring. There are two methods for antepartum evaluation of the fetus using electronic monitoring: (1) fetal reactivity determination or NST and (2) CST (mostly oxytocin stress testing).

FHR reactivity determination (NST). NST has been the favorite monitoring technique for fetal evaluation in European countries, but only relatively recently has it been introduced in the United States. The rationale behind the method is that reactive fetal tachycardia in response to spontaneous or induced FM is an important sign of fetal well-being and an indicator of a normal intrapartum course. In contrast, absence of fetal heart reactivity is a sign suggestive of the possibility of fetal distress.

To carry out the test (see box on p. 338) the patient is placed in the semi-Fowler's position, and the tocodynamometer and ultrasound transducer of an electronic monitor are placed on the patient's abdomen. The patient is instructed to push the 50 mm Hg calibration button of the monitor whenever she notices fetal activity. In most patients the tocodynamometer also picks up some of the FM. The occurrence of five or more FHR accelerations within a 20-

How to do an NST

1. Place patient in the semi-Fowler's position. Use pillows under one of her hips to displace the weight of the uterus away from the inferior vena cava. Take the patient's blood pressure every 10 minutes during the procedure.
2. Apply the tococardiographic equipment to the maternal abdomen, and observe the uterine activity and FHR for 20 minutes. Instruct the patient to push the calibration button of the uterine contraction tracing every time she feels FM.
3. A reactive test is present when five or more FHR accelerations are clearly recorded during a 20-minute period, each of 15 or more beats per minute and lasting 15 or more seconds, usually occurring simultaneously with episodes of fetal activity.
4. If no spontaneous FM occurs during the initial 20 minutes of observation, the test is continued for another 20 minutes, and during this period FM is provoked by external manipulation. If there is no acceleration with spontaneous or repeated external stimuli during a 40-minute period, the test is considered nonreactive.
5. The test is unsatisfactory if the quality of the monitor trace is inadequate for interpretation.

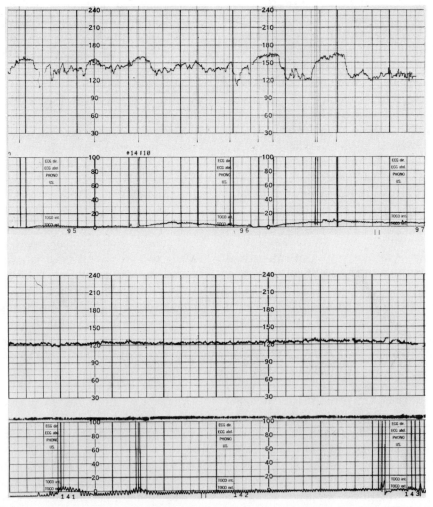

FIG. 18-3 ■ Reactive and nonreactive nonstress test (NST). Upper panel, reactive NST. There are several accelerations of the fetal heart of 15 or more beats per minute, lasting 15 or more seconds associated with fetal movements. Lower panel, nonreactive NST. There is absent long-term variability and decreased short-term variability; no accelerations are present in association with fetal movements.

minute period, each 15 or more beats per minute and lasting at least 15 seconds, is called a *reactive* test. If no FM is noticed during 20 minutes, the fetus must be stimulated by external manipulation and the observation time extended to 40 minutes. If movement and FHR accelerations, as just defined, occur after external manipulation, the test is also called *reactive* (Fig. 18-3, upper panel). If no movement is noticed spontaneously or after repeated external manipulation or if there is no FHR acceleration with movement, the test is abnormal and called *nonreactive* (Fig. 18-3, lower panel). Occasionally there are technical problems making it difficult or impossible to interpret the test. In this case the result is called *inadequate*.

Most of the literature on NST[14,24,29,38] indicates that a reactive NST correlates favorably with a normal intrapartum course and a good perinatal outcome. In other words, a reactive NST has the same prognostic value as a negative oxytocin stress test. In the extensive experience of the investigators at the University of Southern California[26] four fetal deaths occurred in a group of 1547 patients with reactive NST, and six occurred in 851 patients with negative oxytocin challenge tests (OCTs). There were no significant differences in fetal outcome between the negative NST and the negative OCT groups.

A reactive NST and a negative OCT are valid for 1 week. This means that the chances of fetal demise in the week following a reactive NST are extremely small. The finding of a nonreactive NST is not by itself a sign of fetal distress or an indication for pregnancy termination. When patients are further tested with the CST, a high proportion of them (74.3% to 88%) have a false positive NST. Therefore if an abnormal (nonreactive) NST is found in a patient, a CST must be performed, and further management depends on the results of the latter test.

The reactivity of the FHR to stimuli different from movement has also been used as an index of fetal well-being. The fetus may react to amniocentesis and to sound with FHR acceleration, and this response may be as valuable as a reactive NST. However, none of the tests using a stimulus different from movement have been generally accepted as a substitute for NST.

CST (OCT). The CST is useful for detecting fetal distress in the antepartum period. This test is based on experimental evidence showing that the uteroplacental blood flow decreases or ceases during uterine contractions. Therefore contractions originating spontaneously or by means of oxytocin subject the fetus to a repetitive hypoxic stress. The ability or lack of ability of the fetus to tolerate this stress is a measure of the fetal status. A normal, healthy fetus tolerates uterine contractions without difficulty, and this is shown by the absence of periodic changes in FHR. In contrast, a fetus in distress often is not able to tolerate the decrease in oxygen supply that occurs during contractions and shows late decelerations.

To carry out an OCT (see box on p. 340) the patient is instructed to come to the laboratory with an empty stomach (the fetus is less active after meals). She is placed in the semi-Fowler's position, and the monitoring equipment is applied to her abdomen as described for the NST test. The maternal blood pressure is taken every 10 to 15 minutes during the test to detect drops of blood pressure that may account for false positive results. The patient is observed for 15 to 20 minutes, and a reassessment of acceleration with movements is made as if doing an NST test. Also, during this period of observation it is possible to detect some patients who have spontaneous uterine contractions at the time of the test and do not require oxytocin stimulation. If there is no spontaneous uterine activity during the observation period and the fetus remains nonreactive, oxytocin is administered IV via piggy back using a Harvard pump and beginning at a rate of 0.5 mU/minute. The rate is doubled every 15 to 20 minutes until three contractions lasting 40 to 60 seconds are produced within a 10-minute period.[28] Usually the test does not require more than 8 to 12 mU of oxytocin per minute to obtain an adequate uterine response.

In many patients it is unnecessary to use oxytocin, and contractions may be elicited by gentle massage of the patient's nipples with a warm towel. Once an adequate number of contractions are obtained (three in 10 minutes), the administration of oxytocin is interrupted, but monitoring is continued until the contractions are more than 10 minutes apart. If hypertonic labor results as a consequence of oxytocin administration or breast stimulation or if the patient continues with contractions every 2 or 3 minutes after stopping the oxytocin, it is advisable to administer a single subcutaneous injection of 250

How to do a CST or an OCT

1. Place patient in semi-Fowler's position. Use pillows under the patient's hip or side to displace the weight of the uterus away from the inferior vena cava. Take the patient's blood pressure every 10 minutes through the test.
2. Apply the tococardiographic equipment to the maternal abdomen, and observe the uterine activity and the FHR for approximately 15 to 20 minutes. Many patients who are receiving the test because of a nonreactive NST show adequate fetal reactivity during this observation period and do not require oxytocin stimulation. Other patients show spontaneous uterine activity of sufficient frequency and duration and do not require oxytocin administration.
3. Start intravenous oxytocin administration using a Harvard pump at 0.5 mU/minute. Double the rate every 15 to 20 minutes until three contractions lasting 40 to 60 seconds occur within a 10-minute period. If late decelerations appear before this duration and frequency of contractions have been achieved, the administration of oxytocin must be interrupted. Massage of the nipples with a warm towel by the patient may be all that is necessary to provoke uterine contractions and avoid the use of oxytocin.
4. Usually the test requires between 1½ and 2 hours. The amount of oxytocin required to obtain adequate uterine contractility is generally below 16 mU/minute.
5. After completing the test, monitoring of FHR and uterine contractions should continue until they return to baseline. If uterine activity persists, the subcutaneous administration of 250 mg of terbutaline is usually sufficient to paralyze the uterus.

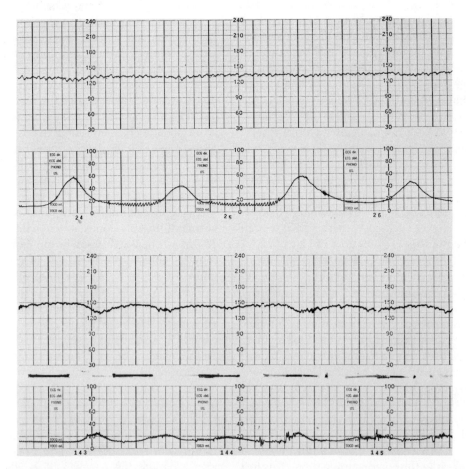

FIG. 18-4 ■ Negative and positive contraction stress test (CST). Upper panel, negative CST. Long-term variability is absent, short-term variability is decreased, but there are no decelerations associated with the uterine contractions. Lower panel, positive CST. Long- and short-term variability are decreased, and every uterine contraction is followed by a deceleration of the fetal heart rate.

μg of terbutaline to paralyze the uterus. The test is interpreted as negative (Fig. 18-4, upper panel), positive (Fig. 18-4, lower panel), suspicious, or unsatisfactory.

negative Three contractions in 10 minutes with no late decelerations.

positive Persistent late decelerations.

suspicious Nonpersistent late decelerations or late decelerations associated with uterine hyperstimulation.

unsatisfactory Unreadable FHR tracing or insufficient uterine activity.

The OCT is an invasive test that may cause complications such as induction of preterm labor, uterine rupture in patients with a scar in the uterus, vaginal bleeding in patients with placenta previa, and severe fetal distress. To avoid these complications the clinician should know the following list of contraindications to the OCT.

Placenta previa
Previous classic cesarean section
Rupture of the fetal membranes
Polyhydramnios
Preterm labor
Multiple pregnancy

The evidence mentioned before[26] indicating that a reactive NST is as good as a negative OCT has led to the use of NST as the primary screening test for fetal distress in complicated pregnancies. The proponents of this approach argue that the OCT is an invasive procedure with a large number of potential iatrogenic complications and requires a minimum of 2 hours for its performance. They also argue that there is no reason to use the OCT as a screening test, since the NST is noninvasive, noniatrogenic, carried out in a relatively short period of time, and if reactive, is usually as good as the OCT. According to these authors, the use of the OCT must be limited to further evaluation of the fetus with a nonreactive NST. A large proportion (more than 80%) of these patients with nonreactive NST have negative OCT and may continue being followed with a weekly NST. A suspicious, a hyperstimulated, or an unsatisfactory OCT requires repetition within 24 hours.

The combination of a nonreactive NST and a positive OCT is usually indicative of the existence of fetal distress, especially if other clinical indexes (decreased or absent FM, rapid deterioration of maternal condition, inadequate growth of the uterus) or laboratory indexes (HPL values in the FDZ, ultrasonic suggestion of growth retardation) further point to that diagnosis. In these cases pregnancy must be terminated. Attempts to prolong pregnancy are futile, and the infant is better off within a neonatal intensive care unit than in the hostile intrauterine environment. If the patient has a favorable cervix for induction (Bishop score greater than 6) and there are no obstetric contraindications for vaginal delivery, a trial of labor with invasive fetal monitoring is justified. In this case, after completing the preparations for a cesarean-section delivery, the mother is turned to the lateral position, oxygen is given by mask, the membranes are ruptured, and a fetal scalp electrode and intrauterine pressure catheter are put in place. Then oxytocin induction of labor is started. If monitoring signs of fetal distress appear, the induction of labor is discontinued, the uterus is paralyzed with subcutaneous terbutaline, and the infant is delivered by cesarean section. In a few instances the fetus does not show late deceleration during labor and may be delivered vaginally.

In our opinion the CST is a better test than the NST for primary fetal surveillance in all those situations in which oxytocin administration is not contraindicated or the uterus contractions are not potentially dangerous. The rationale behind that opinion is that the process of fetal hypoxia follows a rather defined sequence in its manifestations. Increased severity of fetal hypoxia goes from tracings in which the variability is normal or decreased and late decelerations are present to traces in which variability is decreased or absent and late decelerations are present. In other words, late decelerations are an earlier sign of fetal distress than lack of variability. The sign that appears first rather than late should be used for screening purposes. However, the problem with using the CST as a primary tool for fetal surveillance are the time required and the need for physician availability.

Some investigators have introduced modifications to the NST with the aim of increasing its specificity, thus making it a better tool for primary fetal surveillance. A popular modification is the use of a scoring system in which several variables, different from accelerations with movements, are evaluated.[15,19] Nonstressed monitoring is useful in evaluating FHR variability, which is a valuable index of fetal well-being. Short- and long-term FHR variability can be measured accurately only with the use of fetal scalp electrode, fetal phonocardiogram, or abdominal fetal electrocardiogram. However, some of the new external monitoring equipment allow an excellent estimation of FHR variability. Other variables that may be observed in the NST tracing are the basal FHR frequency, the number of FMs, and the presence of absence of spontaneous decelerations. If initial results are confirmed by more extensive investigation, it is possible that scored NST testing will become the most adequate means for primary antepartum evaluation.

Another approach to increasing the specificity of the NST is by making it a part of a biophysical profile of the fetus.[20] This seems to be a highly reliable technique of antepartum evaluation, but similarly to the OCT, it is time-consuming and requires expertise of the operator.

■ INTRAPARTUM FETAL DISTRESS

Intrapartum fetal distress is a term used to indicate the presence of fetal hypoxia and acidosis during labor. In the majority of cases intrapartum fetal distress is the consequence of a severe derangement of the normal metabolic exchange process between mother and fetus. Patients with intrapartum fetal distress usually fall within two large categories.

In one category the fetal-maternal exchange has been chronically affected during intrauterine life, and the stress of labor becomes the ultimate insult causing the profound derangement that manifests itself as intrapartum fetal distress. This is the case in patients with chronic or acute hypertensive disease, diabetes mellitus, hemolytic disease, etc, whose chronic fetal distress has usually been manifested in the antepartum period by the presence of abnormal fetal growth or amniotic fluid changes. With superimposition of the stress of labor some of these patients exhibit monitoring signs of intrapartum fetal distress. How much uterine activity is necessary to produce fetal distress in these patients depends to a large extent on the severity of the fetal compromise.

In the second category monitoring signs of fetal distress appear during labor, complicating otherwise normal pregnancies for which there is no reason to suspect a chronic impairment of the fetal-maternal exchange. In these cases fetal distress often is iatrogenic (oxytocin stimulation, regional anesthesia) or is caused by a sudden insult to the umbilical cord or the placenta (abruptio placentae, occult or apparent cord prolapse) or corresponds to unrecognized chronic fetal-maternal exchange impairment. In these patients the stress caused by the uterine contractions is an important factor in increasing the severity of the fetal compromise. The following is a summary of various common causes of fetal distress in the two categories just discussed.

A. Occurring in pregnancies with chronic impairment of the fetal-maternal exchange
1. Maternal causes
a. Toxemia of pregnancy
b. Diabetes and pregnancy
c. Chronic hypertension and pregnancy
d. Cardiac disease (Class II or more) and pregnancy
e. Hemoglobinopathy
2. Fetal causes
a. Hemolytic disease (erythroblastosis)
b. Multiple pregnancy (twin transfusion)
c. Prematurity
3. Placental causes
a. Anatomic abnormalities of the placenta (previa, circumvallata, battledore, velamentosa)
b. Postmaturity
c. Primary placental insufficiency
B. Occurring in pregnancies without evidence of chronic impairment of the fetal-maternal exchange
1. Iatrogenic causes
a. Oxytocin stimulation of labor
b. Regional anesthesia
c. Paracervical block anesthesia
d. Systemic hypotensive agents
2. Acute cases
a. Abruptio placentae (usually occurring in patients with chronic fetal-maternal exchange impairment because of maternal or placental causes)
b. Cord accident (occult or apparent prolapse, true knot)
C. Unrecognized chronic impairment of the fetal-maternal exchange

The diagnosis of intrapartum fetal distress is *suggested* by the following:
1. The presence of heavy meconium
2. The presence of one or several of the following electronic monitoring patterns:

a. Persistent late decelerations of any magnitude
b. Persistent *severe* variable decelerations
c. Prolonged bradycardia
d. Decreased or absent beat-to-beat variability

The diagnosis of intrapartum fetal distress is *almost certain* under the following circumstances:

1. There is an abnormal fetal pH in fetal scalp samples.
2. There is no improvement or there is a recurrence of the abnormal monitoring pattern after tocolytic therapy.

The electronic monitoring criteria *suggesting* intrapartum fetal distress are unreliable and fraught with individual biases. *Only one out of every five fetuses with monitoring signs suggesting fetal distress has a low pH.* Therefore intervention is necessary for only 20% of those patients showing monitoring signs of distress. Electronic monitoring during labor has its best use in determining the fetus that is normal; the reliability of the formerly considered classic or pathognomonic signs of intrapartum distress is extremely questionable. Each one of the variables suggesting or indicating fetal distress during labor is discussed in the following paragraphs.

Intrapartum meconium

Most of the recent literature tends to disregard the importance of intrapartum meconium as a sign of fetal distress unless there are monitoring signs pointing toward this diagnosis.[1,22] A recent study presented a classification of meconium during labor and its correlation with the fetal outcome.[21] Meconium staining was classified as *early* (noted before or during the active phase of labor) or *late* (passed in the second stage of labor after clear fluid had been previously noted). Early meconium was subdivided into *light* (lightly stained yellow or greenish) or *heavy* (darkly stained dark green or black, usually thick and tenacious). Meconium was observed in 646 (22%) pregnancies with cephalic presentation, and it had the following distribution:

Early (78.8%) ⟨ Light (53.6%)
　　　　　　　　Heavy (25.2%)
Late (21.2%)

The incidences of 1- and 5-minute Apgar scores below 7 and intrapartum and neonatal deaths were significantly greater in patients with *early heavy* meconium than in similar controls matched by age, parity, and birth weight. *Early heavy* and *late* meconium were also associated with a significantly greater incidence of meconium aspiration syndrome.

From this study it may be concluded that in about 50% of all cases (the early light group) intrapartum meconium staining may be disregarded as a nonsignificant finding. In contrast, *early heavy* or *late* meconium staining should be considered suggestive of fetal distress, and detection must be followed with invasive fetal monitoring and the adoption of precautions to prevent meconium aspiration at the time of delivery. For more on meconium aspiration see Chapters 8, 9, and 19.

Late decelerations

The presence of recurrent FHR drops immediately following the peak of uterine contractions, the so-called *late decelerations* (Fig. 18-5), has been traditionally considered a good indicator of fetal distress. This has been demonstrated in human and animal studies showing significantly greater hypoxic morbidity and mortality in fetuses exhibiting late decelerations during labor when compared with those not exhibiting the same monitoring pattern.[3,7,23] Unfortunately, the strength of the correlation *late decelerations to fetal distress* has generated an unwritten policy of *late decelerations equal emergency delivery by cesarean section* in a large number of obstetric units in the United States. This policy has been the source of multiple unnecessary surgical deliveries. Late decelerations and fetal distress are often transient, and also frequently the consequence of preventable or treatable iatrogenic intervention. For example, late decelerations may occur in up to 25.8% of all patients receiving epidural anesthesia during labor[7] and may be corrected by repositioning the patient and giving intravenous fluids to compensate for the effect of peripheral blood pooling.[37] Late decelerations are also present in the majority of patients who develop hypertonic labor spontaneously or as a consequence of oxytocin administration during labor.[16] In the latter case the decelerations disappear with measures that decrease uterine

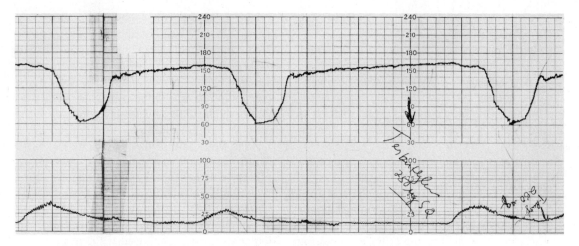

FIG. 18-5 ■ Late decelerations. Absent long- and short-term variability and severe late decelerations after each uterine contraction. This is an ominous trace.

contractility. Also, late decelerations often follow maternal administration of hypotensive agents such as diazoxide and hydralazine, but they disappear after elevation of the maternal blood pressure to levels compatible with adequate uteroplacental perfusion.

In summary, late decelerations are an important sign of fetal distress, but their existence is *not* synonymous with the need for emergency surgical intervention. They must be interpreted within the context of the overall situation of the individual patient in labor, and they should be followed by fetal scalp pH determinations to avoid unnecessary surgical interventions.

Severe variable decelerations

Variable decelerations (Fig. 18-6) are so named because of the inconsistency of their relation to the uterine contractions and the variability of their configuration. There is evidence from animal and human studies that variable decelerations occur as the result of compression of the umbilical cord causing baroreceptor and chemoreceptor stimulation that provokes transient vagal bradycardia. Variable decelerations are the most common periodic change seen during labor, and in more than 50% of the cases it is impossible to correlate the variable decelerations with entanglement of the cord around the fetal neck or the fetal parts.[36] Most probably stimuli different to cord compression may also cause the vagal response that is recognized in the monitor trace as a variable deceleration.

When severe variable decelerations occur, the patient must be immediately examined to rule out a cord prolapse or a funic presentation (umbilical cord present in the pelvis before the body of the infant), either of which is an indication for cesarean section. If the pelvic examination is negative, positional changes, tocolytic therapy, and fetal scalp pH measurements must be carried out. If the severe variable deceleration pattern is recurrent or uncorrectable or the scalp pH shows fetal acidosis, the infant must be delivered by cesarean section. Severe variable decelerations during the second stage of labor may be benign provided the mother has no high-risk factors, they do not continue for more than 10 minutes, and there are no other indicators of fetal distress such as decreased variability, poor recovery of the FHR after the deceleration, or thick meconium staining.

Fetal bradycardia

Not all cases of fetal bradycardia have the same significance with respect to fetal well-being, and it is necessary to recognize at least the following four different situations.

1. *Baseline bradycardia* corresponds to an FHR of less than 120 beats/minute present since the beginning of labor without coexistent periodic changes and with adequate beat-to-beat variability. Baseline bradycardia is a benign pattern[17] that does not demand further intervention unless there are superimposed severe decelerations or lack of beat-to-beat variability.

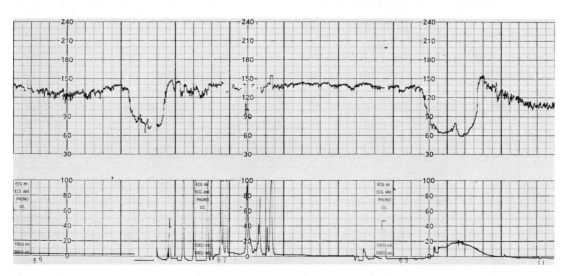

FIG. 18-6 ■ Two variable decelerations, both moderate, with the long- and short-term variability normal. Variable decelerations are characterized by the shape of the deceleration and may occur before, during, or after a contraction. They are mild if they last less than 30 seconds regardless of the level or if the fetal heart tone drop is above 80 beats/minute regardless of duration. They are moderate if the drop in fetal heart rate is to less than 80 beats/minute regardless of duration. They are severe if the drop in fetal heart tone is to less than 70 beats/minute for more than 60 seconds.

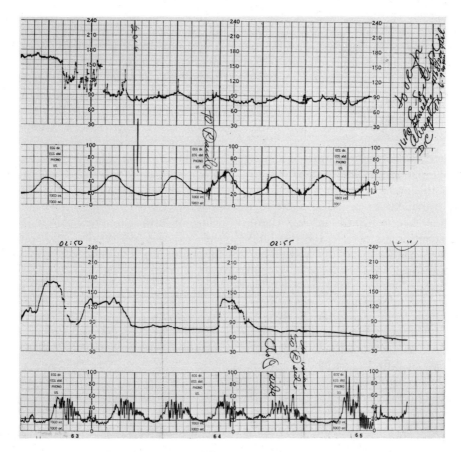

FIG. 18-7 ■ Prolonged fetal heart rate bradycardia following variable decelerations. The main difference between these two traces is the lack of variability of the fetal heart rate trace in the lower panel, whereas in the upper panel variability (although decreased) is still present. In both traces labor is hypertonic. Both patients had quick cesarean-section delivery. A partial abruption was found in the upper case, and the baby had Apgar scores of 6 and 7. An occult cord prolapse was the diagnosis in the lower case, and the baby had Apgar scores of 1 and 5.

2. *Prolonged end-stage deceleration* is a sudden, prolonged drop in FHR that happens in some patients who are close to the time of delivery.[5] The FHR during the episode is anywhere between 40 and 90/minute. This bradycardia does not have pathologic significance if the patient is low-risk and the trace before the deceleration did not show decelerations and had normal variability. However, it is alarming and often influences the obstetrician to terminate the pregnancy with a midforceps operation.

3. *Sudden, prolonged FHR bradycardia in the postterm infant* concomitant with lack of beat-to-beat variability is an ominous pattern.[8] This pattern may or may not be preceded by mild late decelerations and usually does not respond to tocolytic therapy.

4. *Prolonged FHR bradycardia following late or variable decelerations* is an ominous pattern that should be interpreted as a manifestation of exhaustion of the fetal reserve (Fig. 18-7). Immediate administration of tocolytic therapy followed by cesarean section if there is no response to the beta mimetic agent is the treatment of choice.

Decreased or absent beat-to-beat variability

FHR variability is one of the most important pieces of information that the obstetrician can obtain from the examination of a monitoring trace. FHR variability is an index of the fetal reserve or tolerance to hypoxic insults. Therefore the presence or absence of FHR variability confers special significance to any of the other signs of fetal distress reviewed before. Meconium staining of the amniotic fluid, late decelerations, variable decelerations, and fetal bradycardia become ominous signs if they occur concomitantly with decreased or absent beat-to-beat variability. As mentioned before, the best way to evaluate beat-to-beat variability is when the FHR trace is obtained with a fetal scalp electrode. Thus in all intrapartum high-risk situations fetal monitoring should be direct to adequately observe this important dimension of fetal well-being.

In some instances decreased FHR variability is not equivalent to fetal distress. FHR variability is a phenomenon resulting from the constant physiologic balance between sympathetic and parasympathetic impulses on the fetal myocardial frequency. Thus, variability decreases under the effect of medications such as atropine, propranolol, diazepam, meperidine, scopolamine, phenobarbital, and morphine, drugs often used for high-risk patients in labor. FHR variability is also dependent on the degree of maturation of the fetal neurovegetative system and is decreased in preterm infants. Fetal tachycardia also decreases the beat-to-beat intervals, but in this case poor variability does not necessarily mean fetal hypoxia. Finally, normal, term fetuses have transient episodes of decreased or absent variability that correspond to periods of fetal sleep. All these causes of decreased FHR variability must be taken into consideration at the time of evaluating a trace with decreased variability.

Fetal pH determination

The normal values for blood gases and pH in the umbilical vein, umbilical artery, and fetal scalp samples are shown in Table 18-1. Most investigators agree that a fetal scalp pH value below 7.20 is indicative of fetal acidosis and that values between 7.20 and 7.25 are suspicious or "preacidotic" and require further evaluation (see box on p. 347). Fetal scalp pH, however, is not an absolute index of fetal distress: 6% to 20% of patients with fetal scalp pH measurements within normal range have infants with low Apgar scores; also, 8% to 10% of all infants delivered because of low pH values have normal Apgar scores at birth.[6] In spite of these false positive and false negative results, fetal scalp pH measurements are the most accurate method for de-

TABLE 18-1 ■ Normal values for fetal blood gases

	Fetal scalp		Umbilical cord	
	First stage of labor	Second stage of labor	Artery	Vein
pH	≥7.30	≥7.28	≥7.26	≥7.32
Po_2	21.10	19.10	17.60	27.80
Pco_2	45.10	47.80	48.70	38.90
Base deficit	5.40	6.10	8.80	6.60

termining the existence of fetal distress. A comparison between scalp measurements and electronic monitoring has shown that 32 out of 37 fetuses found to be acidotic by fetal scalp pH measurements had abnormalities of the FHR tracing, but only 32 out of 138 fetuses with abnormal FHR tracings were found to be acidotic by pH measurements.[17] The following are common causes for false positive and false negative fetal scalp measurements:

1. Mother in the dorsal position (falsely low pH)
2. Maternal alkalosis (falsely normal or elevated fetal pH)
3. Slow rate of collection of scalp blood into the collection tube (falsely low pH)

The possibility of error is always present, especially when the biochemical information does not agree with the clinical and monitoring data.

The diagnostic value of fetal scalp pH determinations increases if several sequential measurements are performed to determine the trend of the acid-base status of the fetus. For example, an isolated pH value of 7.22 does not necessarily mean that the fetus is acidotic. The same pH value has greater significance if in two previous observations the pH was 7.28 and 7.25. In this case the trend is toward progressively lower pH values, and intervention is justified at a pH of 7.22, even though by definition this value still is not in the acidotic range.

To obtain a fetal scalp blood sample for pH measurement the patient is placed in the left lateral knee-chest position with the right leg elevated by the patient with the help of a nurse. This position is preferred to avoid the hemodynamic changes caused by the supine position and the eventual effects on the uteroplacental circulation. An amnioscope (metal or plastic) is introduced into the posterior fornix of the vagina, and its anterior border is guided with the clinician's finger until it is placed inside the cervix. There are amnioscopes with different diameters to be used according to the degree of cervical dilation. Scalp sampling is rarely successful, however, before the cervix has reached 3 to 4 cm of dilation. Once the amnioscope is in contact with the fetal head, a light source is attached to the instrument, and the fetal scalp is cleaned of amniotic fluid and blood using cotton swabs. Next the fetal scalp is sprayed with ethyl chloride to cause hyperemia. This is an important step, since the objective of the procedure is to obtain a sample of "arteriolized" venous blood that implies the production of vasodilation and hyperemia in the tissue to be sampled. The excess of ethyl chloride is removed with cotton swabs, and an incision of about 3 to 5 mm is made in the scalp using a specially designed guarded blade that is only 2 mm long and is not supposed to penetrate the scalp aponeurosis. The incision must be made in the upper part of the circumferential area of the scalp seen through the amnioscope to facilitate the collection of blood in a preheparinized capillary tube. The new instruments for bedside determination of fetal scalp pH require only 15 μL of blood for an accurate pH measurement. There are disposable kits containing all the necessary elements for fetal scalp sampling.

The number of reported complications with fetal scalp sampling is small. The most common are bleeding and infection in the incision site. Bleeding at the time of the procedure usually subsides after a few minutes of pressure with a cotton swab. If the incision is bleeding at the

How to act in answer to fetal scalp pH values

If the pH is greater than 7.25 ⟶	Continue to observe
If the pH is between 7.25 and 7.20 ⟶	Repeat in 30 minutes
If the pH is less than 7.20 ⟶	Repeat immediately in the cesarean-section room and proceed with the surgery if the repeated value remains under 7.20
If the pH is less than 7.16 ⟶	Deliver immediately by cesarean section

FIG. 18-8 ■ Management of the patient showing electronic monitoring signs of fetal distress during labor.

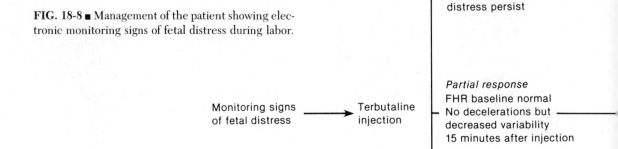

No response
Signs of fetal
distress persist

Partial response
FHR baseline normal
No decelerations but
decreased variability
15 minutes after injection

Complete response
No fetal distress signs
including adequate beat-
to-beat variability

Monitoring signs → Terbutaline
of fetal distress   injection

time of delivery, pressure will stop the bleeding in most cases, but if necessary, a small metal clip may be used for suturing. It is probably wise not to use vacuum extraction after scalp sampling to avoid further bleeding and eventual formation of cephalohematoma.

Response to tocolytic therapy

As was mentioned in the introduction to this chapter, fetal distress is often transient, iatrogenic, and correctable without need for emergency cesarean section. In our opinion,[2] inhibition of uterine activity with beta adrenergic receptor stimulators is useful to distinguish between patients with persistent deficits of the fetal-maternal exchange and patients with transient impairment who have no need for emergency cesarean section.

If the electronic monitoring indicators of intrapartum fetal distress persist after discontinuation of oxytocin, positional changes, oxygen administration, and intravascular volume expansion with crystalloid solutions, labor must be interrupted with the administration of 250 μg (0.25 ml of a solution containing 1 mg/ml) of terbutaline via intravenous push or if an intravenous line is not available, via subcutaneous injection. An intravenous infusion of ritodrine at 300 μg/minute accomplishes the same purpose if terbutaline is not available. If the fetal distress pattern continues after uterine paralysis (usually obtained in less than 5 minutes after the

injection of terbutaline), the pregnancy must be terminated immediately by cesarean section, and the birth of a seriously depressed infant must be anticipated. If the fetal distress pattern is not completely abolished (FHR baseline back to normal range, absence of decelerations, *but persistent decreased or absent variability*) 15 minutes after terbutaline injection, the fetal scalp pH must be measured. Variability is the indicator of fetal distress that lasts longer after terbutaline injection, and it is necessary to wait at least 15 minutes before determining that decreased or absent variability persists. Further management of the situation is dependent on the results of scalp blood pH. If the pH is below 7.20, pregnancy must be terminated by cesarean section and the birth of a depressed infant should be anticipated. If the pH is between 7.20 and 7.25, a new sample of scalp blood must be obtained in 10 to 15 minutes. No change in pH or a lower pH value in the second sample is an indication for cesarean section. Improved pH values in the second sample are indicative of fetal recovery, and there is no need for surgical intervention. When the pH is greater than 7.25 or there is complete recovery of the monitoring signs of fetal distress including adequate beat-to-beat variability, the patient should be allowed to resume labor. In most of these cases with complete recovery there is a readily identifiable cause of fetal distress such as uterine hypercontractility, epidural block, paracervical block, etc,

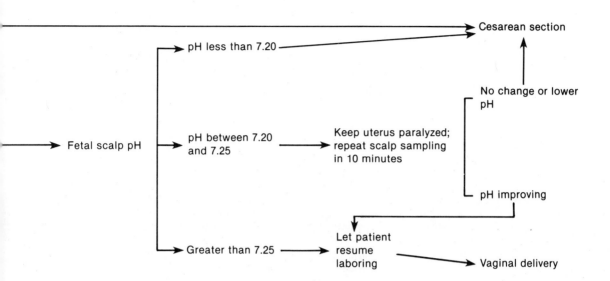

and if that cause is not recurrent, vaginal delivery of a healthy infant should be anticipated. Fig. 18-8 summarizes the management of intrapartum fetal distress using tocolytic therapy.

The use of tocolytics in the management of the fetus showing electronic monitoring signs of distress gives excellent results according to Esteban-Altirriba, et al.[10] The response was successful (increase in fetal pH after therapy) in 84.8% of cases of fetal distress secondary to excessive uterine activity, in 72% of cases of umbilical cord compression, and in 69.6% of fetal distress because of other causes. When fetal distress was secondary to placental insufficiency, a successful response was observed in only 31.4% of the cases. A favorable response happened more often (76.9%) if the fetal pH was between 7.20 and 7.24, but it still occurred in close to 50% of deeply acidotic (pH less than 7.20) fetuses. *Cesarean section can be avoided in about 50% of patients with monitoring signs of fetal distress with the use of fetal scalp sampling and tocolytic therapy.*

■ REFERENCES

1. Abramovici H, Brandes JM, Fuchs K, et al: Meconium during delivery: a sign of compensated fetal distress. Am J Obstet Gynecol 1974;118:251.
2. Arias F: Intrauterine resuscitation with terbutaline: a method for the management of acute intrapartum fetal distress. Am J Obstet Gynecol 1978;131:39.
3. Beard RW, Filshie GM, Knight CA, et al: The significance of the changes in the continuous fetal heart rate in the first stage of labor. Br J Obstet Gynecol 1971;78:865.
4. Belizan JM, Villar J, Nardin JC, et al: Diagnosis of intrauterine growth retardation by a simple clinical method: measurement of uterine height. Am J Obstet Gynecol 1978;131:643.
5. Bohem FH: Prolonged end stage fetal heart rate decelerations. Obstet Gynecol 1975;45:579.
6. Bowe ET, Beard RW, Finster M, et al: Reliability of fetal blood sampling. Am J Obstet Gynecol 1970; 107:279.
7. Cibils LA: Clinical significance of fetal heart rate patterns during labor. II. Late decelerations. Am J Obstet Gynecol 1975;123:473.
8. Cibils LA: Clinical significance of fetal heart rate patterns during labor. IV. Agonal patterns. Am J Obstet Gynecol 1977;129:833.
9. Duenhoelter JH, Whalley PJ, McDonald PC: An analysis of the utility of plasma immunoreactive estrogen measurements in determining delivery time of gravids with a fetus considered at high risk. Am J Obstet Gynecol 1976;125:889.
10. Esteban-Altirriba J, Cabero L, Calaf F: Correction of fetal homeostatic disturbances, in Aladjem S, Brown AK, Sureau C, (eds): *Clinical Perinatology*. St. Louis, The CV Mosby Co, 1980, pp. 100-115.
11. Fujikura T, Klionsky B: The significance of meconium staining. Am J Obstet Gynecol 1975;121:45.
12. Granat M, Sharf M, Diengott D, et al: Further investigation on the predictive value of human placental lactogen in high-risk pregnancies. Am J Obstet Gynecol 1977;129:647.
13. Karp LE, Schiller HS: Meconium staining of amniotic fluid at midtrimester amniocentesis. Obstet Gynecol 1977;50:475.
14. Koller WS, Curet LB: Fetal activity determination and oxytocin challenge tests for assessment of fetal well-being. Obstet Gynecol 1978;52:176.
15. Krebs HB, Petres RE: Clinical application of a scoring system for evaluation of antepartum fetal heart rate monitoring. Am J Obstet Gynecol 1978;130:765.

16. Kubli FW, Auttgers H: Iatrogenic fetal hypoxia, in Gevenes RH, Ruys JH (eds): *Proceedings of Symposium on Physiology and Pathology in the Neonatal Period*. Netherlands, Leiden University Press, 1971, p. 57.

17. Kubli FW, Hon HE, Khazin HF, et al: Observations on heart rate and pH in the human fetus during labor. Am J Obstet Gynecol 1969;104:1190.

18. Lilien AA: Term intrapartum fetal death. Am J Obstet Gynecol 1970;107:595.

19. Lyons ER, Eylsma-Howell M, Sharisi S, et al: A scoring system for nonstressed antepartum fetal heart rate monitoring. Am J Obstet Gynecol 1979;133:242.

20. Manning FA, Platt LD, Sipos L: Antepartum fetal evaluation: development of a fetal biophysical profile. Am J Obstet Gynecol 1980;136:787.

21. Meiss PJ, Hall M, Marshall JR, et al: Meconium passage: a new classification for risk assessment during labor. Am J Obstet Gynecol 1978;131:509.

22. Miller FC, Sacks DA, Yeh SY, et al: Significance of meconium during labor. Am J Obstet Gynecol 1975;122:573.

23. Myers RE, Mueller-Heubach E, Adamsons K: Predictability of the state of fetal oxygenation from a quantitative analysis of the components of late deceleration. Am J Obstet Gynecol 1973;115:1083.

24. Nochison DJ, Turbeville JS, Terry JE, et al: The nonstress test. Obstet Gynecol 1978;51:419.

25. O'Leary JA, Mendenhall HW, Andrinopoulos GC: Comparison of auditory versus electronic assessment of antenatal fetal welfare. Obstet Gynecol 1980;56:244.

26. Paul RH, Miller FC: Antepartum fetal heart rate monitoring. Clin Obstet Gynecol 1978;21:375.

27. Pearson JF, Weaver JB: Fetal activity and fetal wellbeing: an evaluation. Br Med J 1976;1:1305.

28. Ray M, Freeman R, Pine S, et al: Clinical experience with the oxytocin challenge test. Am J Obstet Gynecol 1972;114:1.

29. Rayburn WF, Duhring JL, Donaldson M: A study of fetal acceleration tests. Am J Obstet Gynecol 1978; 132:33.

30. Sadovsky E, Polishuk WZ: Fetal movements in utero: nature, assessment, prognostic value, timing of delivery. Obstet Gynecol 1977;50:49.

31. Sadovsky E, Yaffe H: Daily fetal movement recording and fetal prognosis. Obstet Gynecol 1973;41:845.

32. Spellacy WN, Buhi WC, Birk SA: The effectiveness of human placental lactogen measurements as an adjunct in decreasing perinatal deaths. Am J Obstet Gynecol 1975;121:835.

33. Spellacy WN, Buhi WC, Birk SA: Human placental lactogen and intrauterine growth retardation. Obstet Gynecol 1976;47:446.

34. Spellacy WN, Cruz AC, Gelman SR, et al: Fetal movements and placental lactogen levels for fetal-placental evaluation. Obstet Gynecol 1977;49:113.

35. Sugarman RG, Rawlison KF, Schiffrin BS: Fetal arrhythmias. Obstet Gynecol 1978;52:301.

36. Tejani JA, Mann LI, Sanghavi M, et al: Association of umbilical cord complications and variable decelerations with acid-base findings. Obstet Gynecol 1977;49:159.

37. Thomas G: Etiology, characteristics and diagnostic relevance of late deceleration patterns in routine obstetrical practice. Br J Obstet Gynaecol 1975;82:121.

38. Tushuisen PBTH, Stoot JEGM, Ubach JMH: Clinical experience in non-stressed antepartum cardiotocography. Am J Obstet Gynecol 1977;128:507.

39. Westin B: Gravidogram and fetal growth. Acta Obstet Gynecol Scand 1977;56:273.

19

■ ■ ■

OBSTETRIC EMERGENCIES

Mark M. Jacobs

This chapter covers several obstetric emergencies not discussed elsewhere in this book. The key to successful management of any medical or obstetric emergency lies first, in identifying the patient at risk beforehand; second, in taking necessary precautions to prevent the emergency, and last, in early recognition and treatment. Treatment for common obstetric emergencies should be logically thought out in advance by each practitioner. Creative and original thinking is impossible under conditions of great stress; it is far better to have a logical plan that can be rapidly implemented. Additionally, it is the responsibility of the obstetrician or practitioner to ensure that the necessary drugs, equipment, and support personnel are available to provide effective treatment for common obstetric emergencies.

■ PULMONARY EDEMA
Incidence

In a population of obstetric patients the incidence of pulmonary edema from all causes is between 0.5 and 2.0 per 1000 deliveries.

Pathophysiology

Cardiogenic pulmonary edema results from left ventricular failure caused by primary myocardial disease, or it may be secondary to exaggeration of the physiologic high cardiac output state of pregnancy. This exaggeration may be caused by volume overload, beta-adrenergic tocolytic agents, thyrotoxicosis, or profound anemia. With heart failure, pulmonary capillary hydrostatic pressure becomes elevated, and intravascular fluid moves into the pulmonary interstitial spaces and then the alveoli. Noncardiogenic pulmonary edema results from injury to the endothelium of pulmonary capillaries, and it is the result of many causes, such as the following[9]:

Aspiration
  Gastric contents
  Hydrocarbons
  Smoke
  Salt and/or fresh water
Embolization
  Thrombi of leukocytes and/or platelets (disseminated intravascular coagulation)
  Amniotic fluid
  Fat (long bone fracture)
Drugs
  Beta mimetics
  Opiates
  Lidocaine
  Thiazide

The result is leakage of fluid and protein into the pulmonary interstitium and then into the alveolar space. Sources of endothelial injury common in obstetric patients include gastric aspiration, drug toxicity, amniotic fluid embolism, sepsis, disseminated intravascular coagulopathy from any cause and possibly beta-adrenergic to-colytic agents.[1,6]

Patients at risk and possible preventive measures

Cardiogenic pulmonary edema. Identification of patients with intrinsic myocardial disease early in pregnancy is crucial. However, patients with cardiac disease who remain completely asymptomatic during gestation rarely have massive decompensation intrapartum or postpartum. Most patients who develop cardiogenic pulmonary edema do so because of the administration of beta-adrenergic tocolytic agents. Analysis of most cases of pulmonary edema associated with tocolytic therapy suggests that fluid and electrolyte retention as a result of the administration of intravenous beta agonist tocolytic agents and crystalloid solutions leads to high output left ventricular failure. Patients with medical or obstetric factors that predispose them to high output cardiac failure have relative or absolute contraindications to beta-adrenergic tocolytic agents. Risk factors for cardiopulmonary complications of beta mimetic tocolytic therapy are the following:

Symptomatic cardiac disease, especially ventricular outflow obstruction
Cardiac rhythm or conduction disturbance
Thyrotoxicosis
Severe pregnancy-induced hypertension
Anemia
Hypervolemia
Multiple gestation
Diabetes

Patients with right or left ventricular outflow obstruction are at risk for sudden death if they receive beta agonists. There is no evidence that any of the selective beta₂ agonists are more or less likely to produce pulmonary edema in the obstetric patient. Also, there is conflicting evidence regarding a possible synergistic effect of glucocorticoids and beta agonists in the production of pulmonary edema. All obstetric patients receiving these agents should be considered at risk for the development of pulmonary edema.

It is our belief that pulmonary edema is an almost entirely preventable complication of preterm labor therapy. The cornerstone of prevention is the rational use of these powerful drugs (see box below). Patient selection is of primary importance; those with contraindications must not receive these drugs. Any investigations necessary to rule out heart disease should be rapidly performed, including an electrocardiogram (ECG), a chest x-ray film, or an echocardiogram. Patients with cardiac conduction defects revealed by ECG but with no other evidence of cardiac disease should not receive tocolytic agents because they may develop unexpected episodes of life-threatening tachyarrhythmias, including ventricular tachycardia. Also, liberal use of amniocentesis should be practiced to establish fetal pulmonary maturity, especially if the response to tocolytic agents is not satisfactory.

Patients must be carefully monitored for the development of fluid retention: daily weights, hematocrit determinations, and strict input and output records are mandatory. Total intravenous

---

Rational use of beta mimetics

Proper patient selection
    Exclusion of high-risk patients
    Usage only if there is a high probability of significant neonatal morbidity with preterm
        delivery
    Liberal use of amniocentesis to assess lung maturation
Dose and duration
    Not more than 24 to 48 hours of total intravenous treatment
    Maternal pulse less than 120 beats/minute
Monitoring of patient
    Daily weight, hematocrit value, input and output measurements
    Attention to minor symptoms, especially chest pain and shortness of breath
Discontinuance of drugs
    Sooner rather than later

crystalloids should not exceed 1200 ml/24 hours in the first several days of therapy. The intravenous phase of tocolytic therapy should not, except in rare cases, last longer than 24 to 48 hours. Most cases of pulmonary edema occur after prolonged intravenous tocolytic administration. Situations in which the benefits of prolonged intravenous therapy outweigh the risks are few. In addition to maternal risks, there are theoretic and clinical grounds for suspecting that long-term beta agonist therapy may impair neonatal pulmonary function.

Maternal pulse must not exceed 120 beats/minute for prolonged periods. Many patients become "hyperdynamic" and display signs of tremor, diaphoresis, and tachycardia in response to beta$_2$ agonists. Patients who clinically manifest nonspecific beta-adrenergic stimulation in response to selective beta$_2$ tocolytic agents should be carefully watched as they may be at high risk for cardiopulmonary complications. In humans most uterine beta$_2$ receptors are probably occupied, and maximal effective tocolysis is achieved as maternal heart rate reaches 120 beats/minute. Even if a small increment in tocolytic effect can be achieved with doses of beta mimetics producing a maternal pulse greater than 120, these doses cannot safely be maintained and signal a poor response to therapy. Additionally, with the exception of preterm labor complicated by placenta previa and vaginal bleeding, total abolition of uterine contractions is usually not necessary. Patients may in most cases be safely weaned from intravenous to oral tocolytic agents if uterine contractions do not produce cervical change over 6 to 12 hours.

Noncardiogenic pulmonary edema. All obstetric patients should be considered at risk for noncardiogenic pulmonary edema, especially secondary to pulmonary endothelial injury caused by aspiration of gastric contents, amniotic fluid embolization, anesthetic drugs, sepsis, and disseminated intravascular coagulopathy.

Prevention of noncardiogenic pulmonary edema largely rests on the prevention of aspiration of gastric contents and the removal of the cause of disseminated intravascular coagulation or sepsis. Obstetric patients should be regarded as having a full stomach, no matter how distant their last meal. There is virtual uninhibited reflux of gastrointestinal contents between the small bowel and the stomach. Studies have clearly demonstrated that pulmonary injury is pH dependent: little injury is seen above pH 2.5, and severe chemical pneumonitis occurs below that level. It is important therefore to increase gastric pH by oral administration of antacid when the risk of aspiration is high, such as before general or conduction anesthesia or in preeclampsia. Some obstetricians advocate the routine administration of oral antacids every 3 hours to all patients in labor.

Careful management of the maternal airway is required during general anesthesia, including endotracheal intubation for even the lightest planes of general anesthesia. Patients with seizures are at high risk for aspiration, and patients who have seizures should be treated as if aspiration has occurred and require careful observation. Simply turning a patient with a seizure face down and protecting her head is effective prevention for aspiration and head injury. Seizures in the obstetric population are generally self-limited and rarely last more than 2 to 3 minutes; immediate medical treatment to terminate seizures is needed in only 5% of the cases. The prevention of seizures in obstetric patients involves mainly the early recognition and proper treatment of preeclampsia and the liberal use of magnesium sulfate for hypertensive patients in labor.

Recognition

Fulminant pulmonary edema from any cause is not difficult to detect; respiratory distress is extreme and physical examination unambiguous. Auscultation of the chest discloses diffuse wet rales, and frothy pink pulmonary edema fluid is seen when endotracheal intubation is performed. The clinical challenge is to detect pulmonary edema in its early stages when treatment may be maximally effective. This task is difficult as the early signs of pulmonary edema in obstetric patients are subtle and generally masked. Many normal obstetric patients have basilar rales, a third or fourth heart sound, jugular venous distention, dependent edema, increased heart and respiratory rales, subjective shortness of breath, and orthopnea. Early clinical signs of pulmonary edema are therefore easily overlooked. It is extremely important to give careful attention to any new signs or symptoms suggestive of pulmonary edema or to a change in those that are already present.

Several authors have divided clinical manifestations of respiratory insufficiency associated with pulmonary edema into stages that relate to the progression of the disorder and to its severity and prognosis. The early detection of pulmonary edema rests on a high index of suspicion, and in patients at risk detection depends on the liberal use of arterial blood gas determinations and chest radiographs. Patients in the earliest stage of pulmonary edema have few symptoms and a normal pulmonary examination; the only useful signs are that the respiratory rate and pulse are elevated. Persistent tachycardia or tachypnea must be explained in any patient and requires arterial blood gases to rule out early respiratory insufficiency. Arterial blood gases show a normal PaO_2 of 85 to 95 mm Hg and a decreased $PaCO_2$, usually below 30 mm Hg. The abnormality demonstrated is moderate hypoxemia and hypocapnia as a result of hyperventilation. Arterial blood gas determinations should be performed with the patient sitting upright as positioning has been shown to affect PaO_2 in pregnancy. During these early stages the chest x-ray film is normal.

In the next stage clinically apparent pulmonary edema occurs. Patients may manifest restlessness or agitation, and a few are able to identify shortness of breath as a primary complaint. The pulmonary examination may disclose scattered rales. The pulse and respiratory rate are definitely elevated, and the chest x-ray film may have faint infiltrates, difficult to identify in the typical supine portable film. Arterial blood gases are diagnostic in this stage but may initially appear normal with PaO_2 75 to 85 mm Hg and PaO_2 35 to 45 mm Hg. In the face of the increased ventilatory effort measured by the elevated respiratory rate, significant hypoxemia and hypercapnia exist, and respiratory insufficiency is well-established. A useful measure of defective O_2 exchange by the lung is the alveolar arterial oxygen gradient, normally no more than 10 mm Hg. Under normal circumstances, if PaO_2 is 90 mm Hg, alveolar PO_2 is 100 mm Hg. If inspired O_2 concentration is greater than 30%, the PaO_2 should be roughly six times the inspired O_2 concentration; that is, if 40% of O_2 is delivered, PaO_2 should be about 240 mm Hg. An alveolar-arterial oxygen difference greater than 20 mm Hg in a sitting pregnant patient is markedly abnormal.

Severe or late stage pulmonary edema is characterized by easily recognizable signs and symptoms to both patient and physician. Pulmonary examination and chest x-ray films are typical,

and arterial blood gases show PaO_2 less than 80 mm Hg and $PaCO_2$ greater than 45 mm Hg. It cannot be overemphasized that patients with previously normal cardiopulmonary function who progress to moderate or severe stages have a life-threatening disorder that demands immediate attention.

Treatment

Once pulmonary edema is recognized, treatment and further diagnostic maneuvers must proceed concurrently. Most important in immediate management are adequate ventilation and oxygenation, proper fluid therapy, treatment of hypotension, and ensuring fetal well-being. However, even with early treatment, it is typical for pulmonary edema to worsen before improvement is seen.

Ventilation and oxygenation. Patients with mild or moderate pulmonary edema can be managed with supplemental O_2 by mask or nasal prongs. Frequent assessment of arterial blood gases is performed to ensure that undetected worsening of respiratory insufficiency does not occur. Patients with profound respiratory distress or with room air arterial blood gases reflecting PaO_2 less than 65 mm Hg or $PaCO_2$ greater than 45 mm Hg should be intubated. The patient should not be allowed to tire and suffer cardiorespiratory arrest. Adequate ventilation may not occur unless effective positive end expiratory pressure (PEEP), usually 6 to 10 cm of H_2O is applied. Anesthesia machines and bagging devices do not supply effective PEEP unless equipment with special valves is available, and most intubated patients who need PEEP receive ventilation more effectively with mechanical ventilators. Also, it is best to move a mechanical ventilator to the patient if at all possible, rather than move an unstable patient to an intensive care unit.

Volume status. Unless there is evidence that hypervolemia exists, it is dangerous to empirically administer diuretics to obstetric patients with pulmonary edema. In patients with pulmonary edema blood volume may be low, normal, or high depending on whether cardiogenic or noncardiogenic pulmonary edema exists.[11] If diuretics are administered to a patient with noncardiogenic pulmonary edema and low blood volume, cardiac output and tissue oxygen delivery may fall, resulting in profound hypotension, worsening hypoxia, and possibly death. Assessment of central venous or left heart filling pressure by central venous or Swan-Ganz catheter should be performed first.[2] If evidence of hypervolemia is present—central venous pressure (CVP) greater than 12 cm H_2O or left ventricular end diastolic pressure greater than 18 to 20 cm H_2O—10 to 20 mg of intravenous furosemide may be administered, which reduces preload by diuresis and by increasing venous capacitance. As long as blood pressure is adequate, there is no immediate need to treat low central venous or left ventricular end diastolic pressure.

Hypotension. As previously mentioned, hypotension and reduced cardiac output in the face of hypoxemia may be rapidly fatal. Swan-Ganz catheterization in such instances is mandatory, but a CVP line may provide useful information. If systolic blood pressure falls below 90 mm Hg and central venous or left ventricular end diastolic pressure is less than 5 to 7 cm, crystalloids, albuminated saline solution, or blood should be administered. If blood volume is normal or high, hypotension should be treated with inotropic agents, drugs that raise blood pressure by increasing cardiac output through increased force of myocardial contraction. Dopamine or dobutamine singly or in combination are the drugs of choice.

Fetal considerations. The diagnosis of respiratory insufficiency or pulmonary edema does not necessarily mandate immediate delivery of the fetus. The fetus is well-adapted to hypoxia, and maternal PaO_2 greater than 65 mm Hg and $PaCO_2$ less than 45 mm Hg should be well-tolerated. However, viable fetuses must be monitored carefully. If fetal distress is diagnosed and thought to result from maternal respiratory insufficiency that can be quickly treated, it is better to do so before delivery. Surgical stress before maternal stabilization may be unnecessarily morbid for mother and fetus.

■ DISTRESSED NEWBORN
Incidence

The incidence of distressed newborns requiring immediate assistance in an unselected population of obstetric patients, as measured by 1-minute Apgar scores of less than 6, is 3% to 5%. This incidence climbs to 20% to 40% in a population of high-risk gravidas. The importance of skilled and immediate intervention for the distressed newborn is well-established. The longer the Apgar score remains low and asphyxia persists, the greater the incidence of subsequent seizures, cerebral palsy, mental retardation, and death.

Pathophysiology

Distress in the newborn period is the result of an inability of the fetus to establish extrauterine homeostasis and may or may not be preceded by fetal distress in utero. This failure to establish homeostasis is usually related to a lack of an essential substrate or an inability to deliver an essential substrate or metabolite. The necessary substrates include oxygen and glucose provided in a 37-degree neutral thermal environment. The essential delivery systems include the circulatory and gas exchange systems that not only deliver substrate but eliminate carbon dioxide produced by aerobic cellular metabolism. The following are common causes of neonatal distress:

Insufficient substrate
   Glucose—maternal diabetes, beta mimetic drugs
   Oxygen—sepsis, incorrect ventilation
   Oxygen and glucose—hypothermia, fetal asphyxia
   Calcium—prematurity, fetal asphyxia
Poor substrate delivery
   Structural disease of heart and great vessels
   Fetal distress in utero
   Persistent fetal circulation
   Sepsis
   Anemia
Drugs
   Magnesium sulfate
   Diazepam
   Halothane
   Morphine and/or meperidine

Insufficient substrate is present with fetal hypoglycemia. Hypoglycemia is associated with fetal hyperinsulinemia and maternal hyperglycemia from any cause, notably maternal diabetes or treatment with beta-adrenergic tocolytic agents. Also, hypoglycemia may be present subsequent to a long and difficult labor with or without in utero fetal asphyxia. The other important substrate, oxygen, may be present in inadequate amounts when demands are especially high, as in sepsis or hypothermia or with incorrect application of ventilatory assist devices, notably face masks and endotracheal tubes. A lack of calcium is rarely the primary cause of newborn distress but may accompany asphyxia, shock from any cause, and extreme prematurity. Hypocalcemia may result in continued neonatal depression until corrected.

Poor substrate delivery may be caused by structural or functional derangements of the cardiovascular and circulatory systems. Structural problems include airway or pulmonary hypoplasia, diaphragmatic hernia, choanal atresia, tracheoesophageal fistula, and congenital or iatrogenic pneumothorax. Functional pulmonary problems include hyaline membrane disease, pneumonia, or pulmonary edema. Although structural cardiovascular derangements usually appear some time after birth, some may show up immediately with neonatal depression; this includes anomalies producing shunting around the lung, such as uncompensated transposition of the great vessels or pulmonary atresia. Functional cardiovascular problems appearing in the delivery room include myocardial depression caused by lactic acidosis from in utero asphyxia, sepsis, persistent fetal circulation from significant meconium aspiration, hypocalcemia, and profound anemia.

Patients at risk and possible preventive measures

Since a large proportion of distressed newborns have problems that are preventable, it is crucial to identify fetuses at risk for neonatal distress. Goodlin[2a] has made the observation that antenatal and neonatal distress are exceedingly rare in a healthy fetus who progresses through a normal labor. The task confronting the obstetrician is to identify the unhealthy fetus before labor and provide protection from the stress of an abnormal labor.

The most accurate tools for assessing fetal well-being are ultrasonic fetal evaluation and antepartum electronic fetal heart rate monitoring. Selecting patients to evaluate with these tools is based on the prejudices and practices of individual obstetricians. At a minimum obstetricians should monitor pregnancies at high risk for uteroplacental vascular disease, acutely complicated by maternal cardiopulmonary problems for which delayed fetal growth can be documented or the risk of congenital anomalies is high. At the other end of the spectrum some

physicians advocate routine ultrasonic screening and electronic fetal monitoring in labor. What should be fundamental is that if a fetus is identified as possibly being compromised before labor, if there is an abnormality of labor, if significant pharmacologic intervention (ie, stimulation of labor or conduction anesthesia) is contemplated, close fetal monitoring is mandatory. This monitoring may be by continuous electronic means or by trained nurses providing constant one-to-one patient care and adhering to a rigid protocol for auscultation of the fetal heart rate. Fetal blood obtained from scalp puncture may be analyzed for pH, P_{CO_2}, and P_{O_2}. When fetal distress is diagnosed, appropriate steps should be taken to treat an underlying correctable problem (see Chapter 18).

It is crucial that whenever the fetus is thought to be unhealthy because of structural defect, acquired disease, or acute fetal distress, early neonatal consultation should be obtained. It has been demonstrated that an obstetric-neonatal approach to the delivery and postnatal management of fetuses at high risk for neonatal distress yields the best results. This approach includes the presence of attending neonatal and obstetric staff at all high-risk deliveries, a policy linked to improved intact survival of these infants. Extensive facilitites for neonatal resuscitation must be available in labor and delivery areas. Some centers have a room in labor and delivery with a neonatal intensive care table, a respirator, a polygraph, facilities for umbilical arterial catheterization, drugs, intravenous fluids, and a blood gas machine. In such a setting with attending neonatal staff present, resuscitation is rapid, atraumatic, and optimally performed.

Recognition

Obstetricians increasingly find themselves not only under consumer pressure to allow labor to proceed with fewer medical interventions, but under medical and/or legal pressure to assure a perfect outcome for each pregnancy. These conflicting influences are most evident in the delivery room; many patients desire dim lights, delayed cord clamping, birth in bed, and immediate reception of their newborn. Most obstetricians and pediatricians prefer to examine the newborn quickly under good lighting, suction the nasopharynx, return the infant briefly to its parents, and then observe it in the nursery for

4 to 6 hours. If an infant is thought to be at risk for neonatal distress, it should be routine to have a "traditional" delivery in a delivery room with expeditious transfer of the newborn to a well-lighted neutral thermal environment for evaluation and resuscitation if needed. However, in a low-risk situation a thorough evaluation of the newborn can be accomplished under conditions compatible with a "nontraditional" birth.

At the moment of birth normal newborns have a heart rate over 100. If the cord is not divided and the neonate is not stimulated, spontaneous respirations are established in 30 to 60 seconds, and spontaneous movements or crying may not occur. Color is usually impossible to determine if the lights are low and is in the first 10 to 15 minutes the least important dimension of fetal well-being. Subtle but important clues exist to assure that the newborn is healthy. Muscle tone should be present in a healthy newborn and can gently and unobtrusively be tested by pulling on a limb or by observation of a grimace with gentle bulb suctioning. Continued observation of the newborn in its mother's arms with an examining hand on the newborn's thorax enables an estimation of heart rate, respiratory rate, limb movements, and skin temperature. By 2 minutes of age the newborn should be breathing quietly with a rate of 50 to 70/minute, have a heart rate of 130 to 170 beats/minute, and have good muscle tone. Forcing an infant to cry or searching for cyanosis is unnecessary if all is well. Failure to establish regular respirations, poor muscle tone, bradycardia, the presence of meconium staining, or signs of decreased lung compliance such as tachypnea, nasal flaring, or retractions mandates immediate resuscitative efforts.[3]

Treatment

In the immediate postnatal period the goal of resuscitation is to provide ventilatory, circulatory, metabolic, and thermal support. Although these are all administered concurrently, each is considered separately. It cannot be overemphasized that newborn resuscitation requires at a minimum two or three persons who have extensive practical experience plus the proper equipment and support personnel.

Ventilatory support. If ventilation cannot be established rapidly and atraumatically, neurologic damage and death may occur in minutes.

Most neonates can receive ventilation effectively with a bag and mask. Unfortunately, most clinicians who attend neonates in the delivery room are unfamiliar with the proper technique for doing so and rapidly abandon unsuccessful attempts at mask ventilation for hurried attempts at endotracheal intubation.

Endotracheal intubation of the newborn, except in rare instances, should be performed in an unhurried fashion for a neonate receiving a good supply of oxygen.[12] The airway of the newborn is easily occluded by extensive flexion of the head and undue pressure of the mask over the face. It is crucial to apply the mask without pressure, elevate the chin with the fingers, and maintain the head in a neutral position. It is necessary to perform 30 to 50 ventilations per minute and to not exceed 30 cm H_2O positive airway pressure. The best way to learn this technique is to arrange for instruction by a qualified anesthesiologist, pediatrician, or obstetrician. The results of self-instruction in this essential skill are observable daily in delivery rooms. During mask ventilation a clinician should evaluate breath sounds and heart rate continuously to assume adequacy of ventilation. If ventilation cannot be established rapidly by bag and mask, the flow of O_2 should not be increased because inspired pressure of greater than 30 cm H_2O can easily result in iatrogenic pneumothorax, greatly complicating resuscitative efforts. Under these circumstances major considerations are choanal atresia and in premature infants severe respiratory distress syndrome with poor lung compliance. Immediately after passing an endotracheal tube, its placement should be assured by continuous auscultation of lung fields and heart rate, the O_2 flow needs to be properly adjusted, and ventilation should begin. If the tube is passed too far, it commonly lodges in the right bronchus, blocking ventilation of the left lung. If left lung sounds are diminished, the endotracheal tube should be pulled back 1 to 2 cm.

Common errors in endotracheal intubation are hyperextension of the fetal head that obscures the larynx, persistence in failed attempts by one clinician for more than 30 to 45 seconds, and the use of stiff wires as guides. The fetal head should be in a neutral position with the blade of the laryngoscope pushing the tongue downward toward the patient's feet, and looking straight *down* the clinician views the cords. Using this technique the clinician discovers that a semirigid curved tube falls in place. One clinician who fails after 30 to 45 seconds of attempting intubation should yield to another. Stiff wire guides are unnecessary if proper technique and semirigid tubes are used.

If ventilation cannot be performed with a properly placed endotracheal tube, diagnostic possibilities include diaphragmatic hernia, pneumothorax, and pulmonary hypoplasia. If diaphragmatic hernia exists, the bagging attempts may have inflated the bowel present in the thorax, and decompression is necessary to allow adequate ventilation. For this purpose a nasogastric tube should be immediately passed and suction applied. The next step, if ventilation is still unsuccessful, is to assume that pneumothorax has occurred and to pass chest tubes bilaterally. This may be accomplished with special devices designed for this purpose or with a 16-gauge plastic catheter. It should be entered at the level of the nipple in the midaxillary line to avoid liver and spleen, and a 50 cc syringe used to aspirate any air present. A chest x-ray film should be obtained as rapidly as possible. Adequacy of ventilation and oxygenation can be assessed clinically by heart rate, breath sounds, and color of lips and tongue, but blood gas determinations should be performed as soon as possible.

Some infants require a few lung expansions to begin spontaneous respirations and movements and cry soon thereafter, making it possible to discontinue positive pressure ventilation almost immediately. However, if ventilation is adequate but neonatal depression is not immediately reversed, mechanical ventilation needs to be continued until a full neonatal evaluation can be made. If particulate or thick meconium staining is noted before delivery, the hypopharynx should be gently suctioned before the thorax is delivered and the infant intubated before ventilation. The endotracheal tube is used to suck the airway and should be removed while sucking. If meconium staining is present, the lungs should be reintubated, sucked, and then gently inflated with 100% O_2 by bag and mask. Infants with significant meconium aspiration may need continued intubation to establish adequate ventilation.[4]

Circulatory support. Indications for immediate circulatory support include bradycardia in the face of adequate ventilation, shock from any cause, and anemia. Methods to support neonatal circulation include closed chest cardiac massage, intravenous fluid therapy, and drugs. After ventilation is established, if the heart rate is less than 80, closed chest massage with thumb and forefingers should be performed at a rate of 120/minute.[13] Usually, as oxygen debt is repaid by rapid mechanical ventilation, acidosis resolves and heart rate improves. Bradycardia and asystole, which do not respond to compression and ventilation, should be treated with 0.1 to 0.2 ml of 1 per 10,000 epinephrine by cardiac puncture.[8] The treatment of neonatal arrhythmia is beyond the scope of this discussion.

Shock can be diagnosed with certainty only with measurement of systolic blood pressure by occlusion of the brachial or femoral artery with a pneumatic cuff and auscultation with a Doppler device or by a pressure transducer attached to an umbilical arterial catheter. All neonates requiring resuscitation should have a systolic blood pressure greater than 30 mm Hg. Clinically, shock should be suspected with pallor, cyanosis, poor apical impulse, distant heart sounds, poor capillary filling, and hypotonia. If shock is diagnosed, rapid and judicious volume expansion (10 ml/kg, repeated if needed) with crystalloids, albuminated saline solution, or blood through an umbilical venous catheter should be performed. Umbilical vein catheterization can be performed rapidly and safely in the delivery room. For this purpose an umbilical tape is loosely tied around the base of the cord, the skin is prepared with Betadine, the cord is cut evenly with a scalpel 3 to 4 cm from the abdominal wall, and a 3 to 5 French neonatal feeding tube is inserted into the vein. The catheter is pushed in only far enough to aspirate blood, which signifies success. To prevent blood loss the umbilical tie should be secured with a 3-0 silk suture and tightened. Those clinicians unfamiliar with this simple technique can gain proficiency by practicing with discarded umbilical cords.

Caution should be exercised with volume replacement in preterm infants, especially those less than 34 weeks of gestation, since too vigorous or unnecessary volume expansion can cause rebound hypertension that is associated with intraventricular hemorrhage. In the presence of shock continuous arterial blood pressure recording via pressure transducer attached to an umbilical artery catheter should be performed.

Infants who are distressed should have an immediate determination of central or peripheral hematocrit level. Asphyxiated and normal infants have values of 55% or greater. Although a normal hematocrit value does not rule out hypovolemia, one that is less than 40% suggests partially compensated hypovolemia or normovolemic anemia, both indications for transfusion in the setting of neonatal distress.

Thermal support. Hypothermia and hyperthermia may result in increased oxygen and glucose requirements, overwhelming neonatal reserves. The newborn gains or loses heat in three ways: *conduction* describes heat gain or loss by being in contact with an object (blanket, maternal abdomen); *convection* is heat gain or loss by movement of air (prevented by isolette chamber, fold down walls of intensive care nursery table); and *radiation* that is heat gain or loss from an object not in direct contact with the neonate, (cold glass walls of isolette, warm radiant heater). There will be heat loss under a radiant heater if a newborn is wrapped or draped for a procedure. In a convection heater, such as an iso-

lette, a newborn loses heat if naked through radiation to the cold isolette walls. It is important to determine fetal temperature and provide a neutral thermal environment. Because the net result, substrate deficiency, is the same, hypothermic neonates manifest signs indistinguishable from a hypoxic neonate—cyanosis, retractions, hypotension, and hypotonia.

Metabolic support. In previous years it was advocated by some that depressed neonates receive a "cocktail" of bicarbonate, calcium, glucose, and crystalloids, since most were deficient in many of these components. However, the connection of hypervolemia with intraventricular hemorrhage, bicarbonate with possible liver damage and parodoxical central nervous system acidosis, and glucose with prolonged and severe lactic acidosis has tempered the initial enthusiasm. Indications for metabolic support are limited now to instances of documented substrate deficiency.

All depressed newborns should have an immediate blood-glucose sampling and administration of 1 g/kg intravenous dextrose in 50%

TABLE 19-1 ■ Newborn support

VENTILATORY	
Bag and mask	Adequate in almost all situations; do not exceed 30 cm H_2O of inspired pressure; can effectively suffocate neonate if poor technique is used; contraindicated if there is known diaphragmatic hernia
Endotracheal tube	Must be used with meconium, diaphragmatic hernia, choanal atresia, severe respiratory distress syndrome, pneumothorax; should be performed if possible in a fetus receiving a good supply of oxygen; placement must be confirmed by radiographs
Ancillary techniques if ventilation cannot be established	
Gastric decompression	To rule out inflated bowel in chest
Chest tube placement	To rule out pneumothorax
CIRCULATORY	
Cardiac compression	If heart rate is below 80 with adequate ventilation
Epinephrine intracardiac	1-2 ml 1/10,000 solution
Volume expansion	10 ml/kg crystalloid, albuminated saline solution, or blood for shock (blood pressure <30) or anemia (hematocrit value <40%)
THERMAL	Provide neutral thermal environment; determine fetal temperature
METABOLIC	
Glucose	Administer for proven hypoglycemia; avoid hyperglycemia; use 1 g/kg of 50% dextrose
$NaHCO_3^-$	Correct respiratory acidosis; then give 2-4 mg/kg if needed

solution if two successive determinations are less than 45 mg/dl. A determination should be made again in 5 minutes to confirm delivery of dextrose and repeated every 30 minutes until stable blood glucose is achieved.

In severely asphyxiated or depressed newborns serial blood gas determinations guide administration of bicarbonate. As a rule, the respiratory component of any acidosis should be corrected by rapid mechanical ventilation. When $PaCO_2$ falls to 40 to 50 mm Hg, respiratory acidosis is corrected, and any remaining base deficit greater than -4 to -5 can be corrected with $NaHCO_3^-$, 1 to 2 mg/kg. Sodium bicarbonate solutions are hypertonic and must be administered slowly by the intravenous route.

If neonatal depression has been preceded by narcotic administration, it is best to administer naloxone, 0.1 mg/kg IM or by umbilical venous catheter. True asphyxia may also be accompanied by narcotic depression that may complicate resuscitation. Table 19-1 summarizes the treatment for the distressed newborn.

■ POSTPARTUM HEMORRHAGE
Incidence

Postpartum hemorrhage complicates approximately 10% of all deliveries and accounts for the liberal use of blood and blood products in obstetric units. Uncontrolled postpartum hemorrhage may account for as many as 50% of all maternal deaths.

Pathophysiology

Postpartum blood loss is a normal consequence of childbirth. It is now well-known that obstetric attendants routinely underestimate blood loss at vaginal and cesarean-section deliveries. Best estimations are that total blood loss after vaginal delivery is 700 ml, with 500 ml occurring during the first 24 hours and the rest over the following 5 to 7 days.[10] With cesarean-section delivery the average blood loss in several studies has been 1000 ml. With the physiologic expansion of blood volume seen in pregnancy, postpartum hemoglobin and hematocrit levels are equivalent to preterm values unless greater than average blood loss has occurred. Probably the best definition of postpartum hemorrhage would include postdelivery blood loss resulting in symptoms, blood replacement, or drop in hematocrit value greater than 20%.

Hemostasis after normal labor and delivery

occurs by two basic mechanisms. The first involves constriction of uterine blood vessels in the placental bed by myometrial fibers and does not require an intact coagulation apparatus. The point is well-illustrated in patients with disseminated intravascular coagulopathy who do not experience unusual uterine bleeding if adequate uterine contractions are maintained. Normally, endogenously released oxytocin, which can be augmented by maternal nipple stimulation, nursing, and perhaps even handling of the newborn, causes elevated uterine tone with superimposed rhythmic contractions sufficient to result in uterine hemostasis.

There are many reasons the uterus may fail to adequately contract in the immediate postpartum period; the following general areas are recognized:

Mechanical factors
  Retained intrauterine material
    Placental fragments
    Abnormal placentation (accreta, increta)
    Clot
    Polyp/myoma
  Extreme uterine dilation
    Multiple gestation
    Polyhydramnios
  Rapid uterine evacuation
    Precipitous delivery
    Forceps delivery
    Noncontractile placental bed
    Placenta previa
  Uterine wall defect
    Uterine inversion
Metabolic factors
  Uterine hypoxia, acidosis, decreased glycogen
    Diabetes, uncontrolled
    Sepsis
    Respiratory insufficiency
    Obstructed labor
  Uterine hypoperfusion
    Hemorrhage
    Severe preeclampsia
  Hypocalcemia
    Massive blood transfusion
Pharmacologic factors
  Oxytocic drugs in labor
  Magnesium sulfate
  Beta-adrenergic agents
  Diazoxide
  Halothane
  Calcium channel blockers

Mechanical factors include inability of the uterus to contract because of an unrecognized intrauterine object, commonly including placental fragments, blood clots, and myometrial polyps. Also, abnormal placentation such as placenta accreta or increta results in uterine atony. Often it has been observed that extreme uterine distention before labor, as in multiple gestation or polyhydramnios, may be accompanied by poor uterine tone postpartum. The etiology of this phenomenon is unclear. Although smooth muscle seems not to be as injured by overstretching as striated muscle, overstretching may disrupt the bundles of actin-myosin in individual smooth muscle cells and decrease the efficiency of uterine contractions. Another observed relation with uterine atony is rapid uterine evacuation as sometimes seen in precipitous forceps delivery. Presumably an orderly evacuation of the uterine contents with adequate opportunity for the myometrium to contract is important. If the placental implantation side is located in a noncontractile area of the uterus, as can occur with placenta previa or retroplacental myoma, hemostasis may not be achieved. Uterine rupture, and for that matter any uterine wall defect including hysterotomy, may prevent uterine contractions until the defect in the uterine wall is closed. Uterine inversion occurring with an incidence of 1 per 2000 deliveries prevents uterine contraction and may result in copious bleeding although, in many cases shock may be more profound and immediate than can be accounted for by blood loss. There is thought to be a neurogenic component to shock in inverted uterus. Uterine inversion is caused by improper management of the third stage of labor or in rare cases may occur spontaneously.

Metabolic factors may contribute to uterine atony. There must be an adequate supply of O_2 and fuel to support aerobic metabolism of myometrial cells for effective contraction to be maintained. Hypoxia or acidosis from any cause, including acute respiratory insufficiency, diabetic ketoacidosis, and sepsis, may disturb myometrial metabolism. Patients who deliver after difficult or obstructed labor may suffer from uterine atony. Although etiology is complex in these cases, muscle exhaustion, lactate buildup, and glycogen depletion may be implicated. Uterine hypoperfusion causes myometrial dysfunction. Patients who have hemorrhaged for other reasons may have uterine atony refractory to treatment because of uterine hypoperfusion. Because calcium is an important regulator of smooth muscle tone, hypocalcemia, which may

occur after many units of banked blood have been transfused, can be implicated in some cases of uterine atony.

Commonly used drugs may have important effects on postpartum uterine tone. The use of large dosages of oxytocin to stimulate desultory or obstructed labor may result in relative oxytocin insensitivity postpartum. It is not clear if this tachyphylactic effect to exogenously administered oxytocin results from down-regulation of oxytocin receptors or simply from individual variability to oxytocin effects. Magnesium sulfate, administered to prevent or treat seizures in preeclampsia or as a tocolytic agent, may result in uterine atony by impairing the calcium-mediated activation of actin-myosin interaction. Beta-adrenergic tocolytic agents inhibit uterine contractility by increasing intracellular cyclic adenosine monophosphate. These drugs are given to inhibit preterm labor and treat fetal distress, and they may decrease effective uterine contractions for several hours.

Diazoxide, a potent antihypertensive agent, is also a powerful tocolytic drug inhibiting uterine contractions for up to 12 hours after an intravenous infusion. Halothane, a volatile anesthetic agent, also causes (at concentrations greater than 1% of inspired gas mixtures) uterine relaxation, and it is especially useful in situations in which rapid, reversible uterine relaxation is desirable. However, patients who are obese may accumulate this drug, which is fat soluble, and not display the rapid reversibility expected. Calcium channel blockers, such as verapamil and nifedipine, used in the United States for treating cardiac arrhythmias, are powerful tocolytic agents and may inhibit effective postpartum uterine contraction.

The second major mechanism of postpartum hemostasis involves the blood coagulation system. Coagulation is important in controlling bleeding from any and all disruptions of the birth canal, either spontaneous or surgical, from the lower uterine segment to the perineum. Small lacerations of the cervix, vagina, or perineum, which are confined to the mucosa and do not involve large blood vessels, seldom cause significant postpartum blood loss if blood coagulation is normal. However, if coagulopathy is present, even small lacerations may result in exsanguination. Lacerations of the birth canal are caused by the fetal presenting part—especially if it is unusually large or malformed—the use of forceps, or the use of vacuum extractors.

Defects in the coagulation system are not uncommon, and it is important to detect them before delivery. They consist of the following:

Disseminated intravascular coagulopathy
    Molar pregnancy
    Sepsis
    Amniotic fluid embolism
    Abruption
    Dead fetus in utero
    Severe preeclampsia
    Saline abortion
Defect in liver-dependent coagulation factors
    Lack of vitamin K (nutritional)
    Liver disease
    Warfarin
Defects in other coagulation factors
    von Willebrand's disease
Defects in platelets
    Immune thrombocytopenic purpura
    Aspirin use
    Preeclampsia

Disseminated intravascular coagulation (DIC) is the most common bleeding disorder seen in obstetric patients. Release of material with thromboplastin-like activity into the maternal circulation with subsequent activation of the coagulation and fibrinolytic systems occurs in molar pregnancy, amniotic fluid embolism, endotoxic shock, and fetal death in utero. Consumption of coagulation factors probably initiates DIC in abruptio placentae and hemorrhagic shock. The etiology of DIC in severe preeclampsia is unclear but may involve, as a first step, activation of platelet aggregation at the site of endothelial damage. Deficiency of clotting factors that are synthesized in the liver (factors II, VII, IX, and X) may occur with severe chronic or acute liver dysfunction, vitamin K deficiency, and the use of vitamin K antagonists such as warfarin.

The most common clotting-factor deficiency in young women is von Willebrand's disease, an acquired autosomal recessive disorder resulting in a relative, though not absolute, deficiency of factor VIII. Most patients have a family or personal history strongly suggesting coagulopathy, but a few patients who have never experienced serious injury or surgery may be undiagnosed. Fortunately, most patients with von Willebrand's disease have increased factor VIII activity during pregnancy.

Deficiency in platelet number or function may occur in pregnancy. Preeclampsia often results in relative thrombocytopenia, but seldom is the platelet count less than 50,000/mm^3, the level at which thrombocytopenia results in poor hemostasis. Immune thrombocytopenic purpura, an autoimmune disease often diagnosed in young women, is caused by circulating IgG antibodies to platelet antigens. These patients may have profound thrombocytopenia and are at risk of delivering infants with thrombocytopenia. Defects in platelet function occur with aspirin ingestion. Aspirin inhibits the enzyme cyclooxygenase and prevents the formation of thromboxane and other procoagulants that are potent stimulators of platelet aggregation.

Patients at risk and possible preventive measures

All parturients should be considered at risk for postpartum hemorrhage. Certain patients are at high risk because of medical and obstetric factors and need to have special precautionary measures taken. The risk factors for postpartum hemorrhage are as follows:

Medical factors
    Known or suspected preexisting bleeding disorder
    Liver disorder
    Nutritional deficiency
    Drugs with anticoagulant effect
    Anemia (hematocrit value less than 30%)
Obstetric factors
    Dysfunctional and/or obstructed labor
    Augmentation of labor
    Polyhydramnios
    Multiple gestation
    Rapid delivery
    Surgical delivery, vaginal or abdominal
    Preeclampsia
    Recent tocolytic therapy
    Magnesium therapy
    Dead fetus
    Grand multiparity
    Molar pregnancy
    Amnionitis
    Abruptio placentae or placenta previa
    History of postpartum hemorrhage

All patients must be assigned to low- or high-risk categories based on history, examination, and obstetric diagnosis. Low-risk patients should have blood type and antibody titer determined as early as possible in labor so that

TABLE 19-2 ■ Assessment of coagulation

Test	Normal value (pregnancy)	Significance of abnormal value
Fibrinogen concentration	>250 mg/100 ml	Consumption coagulopathy; rarely liver disease
Platelet count	>150,000/mm³	Consumption coagulopathy
		Idiopathic thrombocytopenic purpura
Bleeding time	<10 minutes	If PT and PTT are normal and platelet count is >70,000, there is a defect in platelet function; <70,000, inadequate platelet number
Prothrombin time (PT)	>75% of control	Consumption coagulopathy, warfarin, vitamin K deficiency, liver disease
Partial thromboplastin time (PTT)	<40 seconds	Consumption coagulopathy, liver disease, von Willebrand's disease, lupus anticoagulant
Fibrin split products	<12 mg	Consumption coagulopathy

potential problems with blood compatibility can be identified and efficiently solved. Hemoglobin and hematocrit values should be determined. During labor the risk assessment should be continually updated and the patient moved to a high-risk category if necessary.

The management of the third stage of labor is controversial, and many different approaches are used to accomplish placental delivery and minimize blood loss. We can provide no firm data that one mode is more efficacious than another. Fundamental in any approach is care to avoid undue traction on the umbilical cord to prevent uterine inversion, manual delivery of the placenta for excessive bleeding or prolonged third stage, immediate abdominal and/or vaginal uterine compression to assure adequacy of contraction, and careful manual and visual inspection of the birth canal if instrumental delivery was performed. Large episiotomies may result in blood loss approaching that found in cesarean section, about 1000 ml, and their repair should a⌐ᵗ be unduly delayed. Intramuscular or intravenous oxytocin should be used if the uterus is not firmly contracted.

Patients considered to be at high risk for postpartum hemorrhage must have several important precautionary measures taken. Blood products, including red blood cells, platelets, fresh frozen plasma, and cryoprecipitate, may be necessary and must be located and immediately available for use. Assessment of a coagulation profile including fibrinogen concentration, platelet count, prothrombin, partial thromboplastin, bleeding time, and fibrin split products

should be obtained as needed (Table 19-2). Next, it is crucial that adequate intravenous access is obtained before the patient becomes hypotensive. This may vary from one large bore 14- to 16-gauge free-flowing intravenous line to two such lines, a central venous catheter, or an arterial line. It cannot be overemphasized that all patients at high risk for postpartum bleeding—especially those who have complicating factors such as obesity, unstable cardiovascular status, preeclampsia, and coagulopathy—should have a minimum of two intravenous lines and preferably a central venous line.

Recognition and treatment

Whenever immediate blood loss exceeds 500 ml at vaginal delivery or whenever uterine atony or significant laceration of the birth canal is diagnosed, measures to treat postpartum bleeding should be initiated as follows:

1. Apply abdominal and/or vaginal uterine compression.
2. Insert one or two large bore intravenous lines, and begin oxytocin infusion (30 μg/1000 ml).

If not effective

1. Quickly manually explore the uterus for retained products or rupture.
2. Palpate and visualize vagina and cervix. Perform repairs as needed.
3. Reinstitute abdominal and/or vaginal compression of uterus.
4. Crossmatch blood.

If not effective

1. When stable, move to delivery room.

2. Administer methylergonovine maleate 0.2 mg to 0.4 mg IM or intrauterine, *or*
3. Administer prostaglandin F2α 2 mg intrauterine or the 15 methyl derivative of prostaglandin $F_{2\alpha}$ 250 μg IM. May repeat in 15 to 30 minutes.
5. Insert second intravenous line if not already done.

If not effective

1. Send coagulation panel to the laboratory.
2. Reexplore uterus and birth canal one more time; use blunt curette to assure that there are no retained products.
3. Begin transfusion of blood products.
4. Continue abdominal and/or vaginal massage.
5. Insert CVP and arterial line.

If not effective

1. Perform laparotomy.
2. Repair lacerations if present.
3. Tie hypogastric artery.
4. Massage uterus.

If not effective

1. Perform supracervical hysterectomy.

The most important treatment of postpartum hemorrhage is vigorous bimanual vaginal and/or abdominal uterine compression. This maneuver is effective in many cases and allows a precise diagnosis of uterine atony. Additionally, even if not successful as the sole treatment, it will reduce the rate of blood loss for almost any cause of uterine bleeding. Next, one or two intravenous lines should be inserted and an oxytocin infusion begun (30 μg/1000 ml of 5% dextrose in lactated Ringer's solution).

If uterine compression and intravenous oxytocin are not successful, the patient should have a rapid but thorough manual intrauterine exploration to rule out retained products and uterine rupture. Careful revisualization of the cervix and vagina for an undetected laceration is performed next. Blood is crossmatched and bimanual abdominal and/or vaginal uterine massage is continued. If blood loss continues, the patient should be moved to a delivery or operating room and given methylergonovine maleate 0.2 to 0.4 mg IM. If the patient is hypotensive, 0.4 mg of methylergonovine maleate IM should be administered; if normotensive, the smaller dose should be used first to avoid occasional rebound hypertension and should be repeated in 10 minutes. Prostaglandin $F_{2\alpha}$ (2 mg) may be admin-

istered by the transabdominal intramyometrial route.[5] This drug is relatively contraindicated in patients with asthma and seizure disorders. The injection may be repeated in 10 minutes if needed. Another useful prostaglandin for the treatment of postpartum uterine atony is the 15 methyl derivative of prostaglandin $F_{2\alpha}$. The dose is 250 μg IM, and it can be repeated every 30 minutes.

If bleeding still persists, a second intravenous line should be inserted and abdominal and/or vaginal uterine compression continued. Transfusion with type specific or O negative blood needs to be started. CVP and arterial lines should be inserted. Coagulation studies are sent to the laboratory and coagulation factors administered if needed, based on the laboratory and clinical situation. If the patient is bleeding from episiotomy, intravenous sites, or wounds, a clinical diagnosis of DIC should be made and fresh frozen plasma, cryoprecipitate, or fresh whole blood administered. In the delivery or operating room, and preferably under general anesthesia, the uterus and birth canal should be reexplored. A blunt curette is used to explore the endometrial cavity for retained products, rupture, or abnormal placentation.

If bleeding persists, laparotomy should be performed through a vertical midline incision and the uterine rupture repaired if discovered. If the uterus is intact, bilateral hypogastric artery ligation is performed. This procedure is accomplished by identification of the hypogastric artery and ureter, incision of the posterior peritoneum over the vessel, and passage of a silk or chromic tie around the artery 1 to 2 cm from its origin of the iliac artery. The pelvic arterial bed is rich in anastomosis, and the uterus still is perfused. However, the pressure head is much lower and without pulsatile properties, and hemostasis can be more reliably achieved with pressure alone. If bleeding still continues, a supracervical hysterectomy should be done and the surgical procedure terminated as rapidly as possible.

In the special case of postpartum hemorrhage caused by uterine inversion, treatment consists of uterine replacement and uterotonic agents. If the placenta is still adherent, it is best not to remove it until uterine replacement can be performed, or increased bleeding may ensue. The fundamental points in management include rapid recognition of the inversion, adequate anesthesia to aid replacement, and prophylactic antibiotics afterward. It is recommended that the portion of the uterus that inverted last should be replaced first so that double thickness of the myometrium is not created.[7] Halothane anesthesia in most cases causes sufficient uterine relaxation to allow replacement. Rarely, laparotomy may be required.

■ PELVIC HEMATOMA
Pathophysiology

Most pelvic hematomas are caused by injury to and rupture of a blood vessel without disruption of the overlying tissues.[10] Because of the greatly increased tissue elasticity and large potential communicating spaces within the pelvis, the likelihood of the development of hematoma after vessel injury is increased. Patients with coagulopathy are at increased risk of hematoma formation. Sources of injury to pelvic vessels include pressure exerted by the presenting part, forceps, vacuum extractors, and lacerations caused by paracervical or pudendal injection of anesthesia. In addition, hematomas may form at the apex of the episiotomies or lacerations. After cesarean section and more rarely after vaginal delivery, injury to the uterine vessels may result in retroperitoneal hematoma, which can cause serious diagnostic difficulties.

Patients at risk and possible preventive measures

Patients at risk include those with difficult or obstructed labor, instrumental delivery, coagulopathy, or lacerations of the birth canal. Any patients with unusual pelvic or perineal pain postpartum should be examined to rule out pelvic hematoma. Prevention entails careful use of forceps and vacuum extractors. As a rule, no instrument, forceps, vacuum extractor, or catheter should be placed in the vagina above the furthest level of the clinician's fingers; to do so invites vaginal injury and hematoma.

Recognition and treatment

Most hematomas are accompanied with pain, although a few result in such large blood loss that hypotension is the first sign. Careful abdominal, rectal, and vaginal examination is mandatory for proper diagnosis. Opinion varies as to whether all hematomas should be evacuated.

However, hematomas in the episiotomy site, those obviously enlarging, those causing disabling symptoms, and those infected should definitely be evacuated. In many cases bleeding vessels cannot be found, and deep mattress sutures and pressure dressings are used. Catheterization of the urinary bladder is needed for several days if repairs are extensive or vaginal packing is used.

Retroperitoneal hematoma is usually a diagnostic consideration when hypotension without external blood loss is present. Such patients, most of whom have had cesarean section, should have blood replacement and preparation for surgery. There is a role for conservative management of retroperitoneal hematoma under very narrow circumstances; (1) when intraperitoneal blood loss can be quickly ruled out in the delivery suite by paracentesis and sonography and (2) when the patient stabilizes after an initial transfusion of several units of blood. These patients must be carefully followed for further bleeding. However, most patients need laparotomy to identify and ligate bleeding vessels. In many cases it is necessary to perform bilateral hypogastric artery ligation with special care to avoid ureteral injury. If retroperitoneal bleeding ceases after hypogastric artery ligation, no further surgery or clot evacuation is needed; otherwise, an extensive, difficult, and sometimes unsuccessful retroperitoneal dissection may be necessary.

■ UMBILICAL CORD PROLAPSE
Pathophysiology

Whenever membrane rupture occurs, there is risk of umbilical cord prolapse. Conditions that increase this likelihood are an unengaged presenting part, presentations other than vertex, and greater than normal amounts of amniotic fluid. Compromised fetoplacental circulation can occur either because of cord compression or spasm. It should not be assumed that failure to palpate a pulsatile umbilical cord indicates fetal death because spasm may mask pulsations. Other methods should be used to assure fetal life.

Patients at risk and possible preventive measures

As just mentioned, patients with polyhydramnios, transverse or breech presentation, and an unengaged presenting part are at especially high risk for cord prolapse. A clinical association that has been noted is between umbilical cord prolapse and patients being managed conservatively for spontaneous preterm rupture of the membranes who have breech presentation. Such patients may experience "silent" dilation of the cervix and cord prolapse with only minimal uterine activity. It is important to monitor such patients carefully and perform speculum examination of the cervix for irregularity of the fetal heart rate.

Prevention rests on immediate vaginal examination of any patient who reports rupture of membranes. This examination is manual at term or by speculum in the case of preterm gestation. Fetal heart tones should be assessed and recorded. Additionally, any irregularity of the fetal heart rate, including bradycardia, variable decelerations, and tachycardia, should prompt an immediate search for a prolapsed cord. When it becomes necessary to artificially rupture membranes with an unengaged presenting part, the patient should be moved to a delivery room and placed in stirrups. With fundal pressure and bearing-down efforts the presenting part should be applied to the cervix, and with a speculum in place a needle should be used to puncture the membranes to prevent a sudden gush of fluid.

Treatment

The basic treatment of umbilical cord prolapse is relief of cord compression, confirmation of fetal life, and rapid cesarean section. Beta mimetic tocolytic agents such as terbutaline 125 to 250 μg delivered subcutaneously or in an intravenous bolus effectively stop contractions in 60 to 90 seconds for at least 15 minutes and may be a useful adjunct in the relief of cord compression. Manual elevation of the presenting part, however, should be performed until delivery whether or not tocolytic drugs are used.

Under certain conditions vaginal delivery may be considered in the presence of umbilical cord prolapse. During the final stage of breech delivery cord prolapse may occur, especially during the extraction of a breech second twin. Extraction can usually continue with general anesthesia using halothane for uterine relaxation if needed. Sometimes it is possible to use vacuum extraction or forceps in multiparous patients who experience cord prolapse in vertex presentation, who are late in labor, and who can deliver with assistance in 5 to 10 minutes. Although we cannot recommend this as a routine measure, it may be applicable in rare instances.

■ MATERNAL CEREBROVASCULAR ACCIDENTS
Pathophysiology

The incidence of all cerebrovascular diseases in pregnancy is between 1 per 5000 and 1 per 10,000 deliveries. Occlusive disease, commonly called *cerebral stroke*, may be caused by arteriosclerosis, embolism, vasculitis, or vasospasm. In one study 70% of pregnant patients with stroke had primarily arterial rather than venous occlusion, and in only one third of the patients could predisposing factors be identified. Intracranial hemorrhage may be caused by arterial or venous malformations, head trauma, or hypertension. It appears that saccular or berry aneurisms account for about half of the malformations that bleed during pregnancy, and arteriovenous malformations and angiomas account for the other half.[14]

Patients at risk and possible preventive measures

Since cerebrovascular accidents (CVAs) may account for 5% to 15% of all maternal mortality, increased awareness of this possibility is desirable among obstetricians. Patients at risk include many with the following obstetric problems:

Cerebral stroke
    Diabetes with vascular disease
    Collagen vascular disease
    Hyperlipidemia
    Sepsis
    Hypertension
    Hemoconcentration
    Preexisting risk factors with acute
        Hypotension
        Dehydration
        Hypoxemia
    Molar pregnancy
Cerebral hemorrhage
    Toxemia
    Hypertension
    Head trauma

Diabetic patients may have extensive arteriosclerosis at a relatively young age. Collagen vascular disease, most commonly systemic lupus erythematous, may cause cerebral vasculitis. Hyperlipidemia when uncontrolled may result in atheroma formation and hyperviscosity. Patients with a septic focus may suffer septic cerebral emboli. Chronic hypertension results in atherosclerotic changes in vessel walls and acutely in cerebral arterial spasm or rupture. Hemoconcentration, seen in diabetic ketoacidosis, hyperemesis, and preeclampsia, may cause hyperviscosity and thrombosis. Molar pregnancy can result rarely in trophoblastic embolization or cerebral metastatic disease and hemorrhage. Patients with predisposing risk factors who suffer acute cerebral hypoperfusion secondary to hypotension, dehydration, or hypoxemia are at increased risk.

Recognition and treatment

There are many different syndromes resulting from cerebrovascular accidents, but in pregnancy most cases involve sudden onset with major symptoms. Prominent are convulsion, alterations in consciousness, hemiparesis and hemiplegia, headache, and disturbances of vision and speech. Differential diagnosis may at times be difficult from migraine headache and preeclampsia, but usually persistence of neurologic symptoms for more than 1 hour seriously raises the possibility of a CVA. Computerized tomography of the head and arteriography confirm the diagnosis. Since 5% to 7% of all persons may have small asymptomatic arteriovenous malformations, it is crucial to prevent hypertensive crisis in pregnant patients. Diastolic blood pressure greater than 110 mm Hg must be treated promptly with antihypertensive drugs, preferably intravenous or intramuscular hydralazine.

Treatment of CVAs involves maintenance of mean arterial blood pressure at 90 mm Hg, ensuring adequate ventilation with intubation as needed, termination of prolonged seizures, and lowering of intracranial pressure with glucocorticoids and mannitol. Management of blood pressure may be extremely difficult, requiring drugs to lower and elevate it. Hypotension can be a sudden signal of imminent brain stem herniation from increased intracranial pressure,

which is lethal for mother and fetus. Thus if the fetus is viable and the maternal condition is grave, it is probably best to effect timely delivery, especially if the blood pressure has already been labile. Indicated neurosurgical diagnostic and therapeutic procedures should be performed regardless of the pregnancy. It is unclear if CVAs contraindicate vaginal delivery; on theoretic grounds it should, but no study has shown an advantage of cesarean section. Likewise, opinion is divided as to whether a prior CVA contraindicates subsequent pregnancy.

■ REFERENCES

1. Conners AF, McCaffee DR, Rogers RM: Adult respiratory distress syndrome. Disease a Month 1981;27(4):1.
2. Cotton D, Benedetti T: Use of the Swan-Ganz catheter in obstetrics and gynecology. Obstet Gynecol 1980; 56:641.
2a. Goodlin RC, Haesslein HC: When is it fetal distress? Am J Obstet Gynecol 1977: 128:440.
3. Gregory G: Resuscitation of the newborn, Anesthesiology 1975;43:225.
4. Gregory G, Gooding C, Phibbs R, et al: Meconium aspiration in infants: a prospective study. J Pediatr 1974;85:848.
5. Jacobs M, Arias F: Intramyometrial prostaglandin $F_{2\alpha}$ in the treatment of severe postpartum hemorrhage, Obstet Gynecol 1980;55:655.
6. Jacobs M, Arias F: Maternal cardiopulmonary complications of beta-adrenergic tocolytic therapy; in Berkowitz R (ed): *Intensive Care in Obstetrics*, New York, Churchill Livingstone, Inc, 1983, pp. 505-525.
7. Kitchen J, Thiagarajah S, May H, et al: Puerperal inversion of the uterus. Am J Obstet Gynecol 1975;123:51.
8. Levin D, Morrisi F, Moore G: *A Practical Guide to Newborn Intensive Care*, St. Louis, The CV Mosby Co, 1976.
9. Matthay M, Hopewell P: The adult respiratory distress syndrome: pathogenesis and treatment, in Simmons DH (ed): *Current Pulmonology*, New York, John Wiley & Sons, Inc, 1981, vol. 3, pp. 1-23.
10. Pritchard JA, MacDonald PC: *Williams Obstetrics*, ed 16. New York, Appleton-Century-Crofts, 1980, pp. 877-91.
11. Staub NC: Pulmonary edema, Physiol Rev 1976;54:678.
12. Ting P, Brady JP: Tracheal suction in meconium aspiration. Am J Obstet Gynecol 1975;122:767.
13. Todres D, Rogers M: Methods of external cardiac massage in the newborn infant, J Pediatrics 1975;86:781.
14. Tuttelman RM, Gleicher N: Central nervous system hemorrhage complicating pregnancy. Obstet Gynecol 1981;58:651.

INDEX

A

Abdominal circumference, fetal, 16
Abnormal antibodies, tests for identification of, 7
Abnormal fetal presentations; *see* Fetal presentations, abnormal
ABO incompatibility, 77
Abortion
  with Eisenmenger's syndrome, 191
  with fetoscopy, 30
  with genetic amniocentesis, 21-22
  with heart disease, 189
  for Marfan's syndrome, 193
  preterm labor associated with, 45
  spontaneous, 31-32, 237
  for toxoplasmosis, 214
  with twin gestation, 264-265
Abruptio placentae
  with anemia, 230-231
  asymmetric intrauterine growth retardation from, 155
  with breech presentation, 318
  classification of, 291-292
  clinical presentation of, 290
  complications with, 298
  definition and incidence of, 289-290
  diagnosis of, 290-291
  etiology of, 290
  fetal and neonatal outcome in, 291
  management of
    with fetal demise
      coagulopathy, 293-295
      delivery, 295-296
      evaluation and replacement of blood loss, 292
      fetal presentation and size, 295
      intravenous fluids and central venous pressure, 292-293
    with live fetus, 296-297
    in patients with hypertonic uterus, 296-297
    in patients with soft uterus, 297
  with placenta previa, 289
  preeclampsia complicated by, 112
  associated with preterm labor, 48
  prognosis for future pregnancies with, 298
AC; *see* Abdominal circumference
Acetest, 143
Acetylcholinesterase in amniotic fluid, 28
Acidosis, 134; *see also* Metabolic acidosis; Respiratory acidosis
Acquired heart disease, 194-198
Acquired immune hemolytic anemia, 236-237
Active phase of labor, 301, 302
  protracted dilation in, 305-306
  secondary arrest of dilation in, 306-309
Activity, control of, for cardiac disease during pregnancy, 184
Acute glomerulonephritis, 255-256
  and nephrotic syndrome, differential diagnosis between, 253
Acute nephrolithiasis, 256-257
Acute pyelonephritis, 222-223
Acute renal failure
  diagnosis of, 248-249

Acute renal failure—cont'd
  etiology of, 246-247
  pathophysiology of, 247-248
Acute tubular necrosis, 248, 251-252
  and prerenal azotemia, differential diagnosis between, 248-249
Acyclovir, 220
Adequate for gestational age infant, 38, 39
AFP; *see* Alpha fetoprotein
AGA; *see* Adequate for gestational age
Age
  advanced, pregnancy with, 23-24
  gestational; *see* Gestational age
  as risk factor
    for diabetes, 123
    for Down's syndrome, 24
    for preterm labor, 44
Albumin for management of nephrotic syndrome, 255
Alcohol; *see also* Fetal alcohol syndrome
  potential teratogenicity of, 34
  use during pregnancy, 10
Aldomet; *see* Methyldopa
Alpha fetoprotein
  in amniotic fluid, 21, 26-28
  for fetal surveillance, 14
  at different gestational ages, 26-27
  in maternal serum, 28
  with neural tube defects, 26-27
Alpha glycoproteins for fetal surveillance, 14
17 Alpha hydroxyprogestrone caproate; *see* Progesterone
American College of Obstetricians and Gynecologists, 33
  Committee on Terminology, 91, 92
  recommendation for employment during pregnancy, 9
  recommendation of phenobarbital for anticonvulsant therapy during pregnancy, 33
American Heart Association, 189
Amino acids in pregnancy, 121, 122
Aminoglycosides for urinary tract infections, 223
Aminophylline, 186
Aminopterin, 154
Amniocentesis; *see also* Amniotic fluid analysis
  genetic; *see* Genetic amniocentesis
  infection as complication of, 84
  for measurement of fetal lung maturity, 60
  for multiple gestation, 272
  patient preparation for, 83
  ultrasound for, 83, 85
Amniography
  for conjoined twins, 268
  for neural tube defects, 28
Amnionitis; *see also* Chorioamnionitis
  with multiple gestation, 266-267
  with premature rupture of membranes, 64
  unrecognized, 46
Amnioscopy, 66, 347
Amniotic cavity, fluorescein injection into, for diagnosis of premature rupture of membranes, 66
Amniotic fluid
  acetylcholinesterase in, 28
  alpha fetoprotein concentrations in, 21, 26-28
  antibacterial activity of, 64

Asymptomatic bacteriuria, 221, 222
ATN; *see* Acute tubular necrosis
Atrial fibrillation, 185-186
Atrial flutter, 186
Atrial septal defects, 192
Autosomal trisomy, 31
Azathioprine, 68, 236-237, 261

B

Background retinopathy, 134
Bacterial endocarditis, antibiotics for prevention of, 188
Bacteriuria, asymptomatic, 221, 222
Bacteroides fragilis, 67
Ball pelvimetry, 307
Battledore placenta, 48
BCN; *see* Bilateral cortical necrosis
Bed rest
  with multiple gestation, 270
  for prevention of preterm labor, 51
Bendectin, 33
Benzathine penicillin, 185
Benzoin, 211
Beta mimetics
  alternatives to, 54-55
  anemia with, 59
  blood or plasma sugar concentrations with, 59
  contraindications to, 54
  for expectant management of premature rupture of membranes, 70-71
  hemoglobin/hematocrit values with, 59
  measuring blood levels of, 57
  for multiple gestation, 270-271
  for premature labor, 83
  for preterm labor, 51-52
    in diabetic patients, 144
  risk factors for cardiopulmonary complications with, 352-353
  serum potassium levels with, 57-59
  side effects of, 57, 188
Beta thalassemia, DNA analysis for diagnosis of, 30
Beta thalassemia minor, 237
Betadine; *see* Povidone iodine
Betamethasone
  for expectant management of premature rupture of membranes, 71, 72
  for fetal lung maturity, 42-43 60
  for multiple gestation, 272
  in Rh sensitized pregnancies, 89
Betke-Kleihauer test, 80
Bicarbonate for neonatal depression, 360
Bicarbonate buffer system, 332
Bicornuate uterus, preterm labor from, 46
Bilateral cortical necrosis, 248, 251-252
Bilirubin content of normal amniotic fluid, 83
Biochemical tests for fetal surveillance, 13-14
Biophysical tests for fetal surveillance, 14-16
Biparietal diameter
  in diagnosis of intrauterine growth retardation, 157-158, 162-163
  gestational age, crown-rump length, femur length, correlation between, 6

Biparietal diameter—cont'd
  growth curve, 5
  as measurement of gestational age in genetic amniocentesis, 21
  in patients at risk of intrauterine growth retardation, 160-161, 162-163
  in twin gestations, 271
  ultrasound for determining, 4
Birth defects in preterm labor, 47-48
Birth order correlated with birth weight, 45
Birth weight
  correlated with birth order, 45
  and gestational age, correlation between, 38, 39
  low; *see* Low birth weight
  associated with maternal weight gain during pregnancy, 45
  associated with nutritional status, 153
  correlated with previous birth weights, 45
  sibling, concordance of, 149
Birth weight standards, 148-149
Bleeding; *see also* Hemorrhage
  antepartum, of unknown etiology, 298-299
  as contraindication to beta mimetics, 54
  diathesis, 239
  intracranial, in preeclampsia, 112
  postpartum, with multiple gestation, 266
  third-trimester, 278-300
    evaluation of, 283
    mild, 283, 286
    moderate, 283, 285-286
    severe, 283-285
Blighted ovum, 31, 32
Blindness with diabetic retinopathy, 135
Blood chemistry for acute renal failure, 249
Blood flow, cerebral, 92, 93
Blood gases
  fetal, normal values for, 346
  in pulmonary edema, 353
Blood group
  antigens, inheritance of, 75-76
  of father, 78
Blood loss
  evaluation and replacement of, with abruptio placentae, 292
  poor tolerance to, in patients with pregnancy-induced hypertension, 94
Blood pressure
  in abruptio placentae, 290
  diastolic, error in measurement of, 97
  elevation in pregnancy-induced hypertension, 97
  for hypertension with renal disease, 260
  as indication for delivery in preeclampsia, 107
  in nephrotic syndrome, 252
  sustained, 91
  systolic, associated with recurrence of eclampsia, 113
Blood samples in severe bleeding, 284
Blood smears for iron-deficiency anemia, 232
Blood sugar; *see* Glucose
Blood transfusions for sickle cell disease, 238
Blood types, 7
Blood volume in pregnancy, 182

Diabetic patient—cont'd
  management of—cont'd
    of puerperium, 140
    stable insulin-dependent, 127, 129-132
    unstable insulin-dependent, 127, 132-134
  metabolism in, 121-122
  prognostic signs in, 134
  risk factors for, 123
Diabetic retinopathy, 134-135
Diagnostic methods, weaknesses of, 156
Diagnostic radiation and pregnancy, risks of, 32-33
Dialysis for acute tubular necrosis and bilateral cortical necrosis, 251-252
Diamine oxidase test, 67
Diaphragmatic hernia, 358
Diastolic blood pressure, error in measurement of, 97
Diastolic murmurs, 183
Diathesis, bleeding, 239
Diazepam, 34, 101, 166
Diazoxide
  as cause of late decelerations, 344
  for control of blood pressure, 112
  for inhibition of uterine contractions, 361
  for preterm labor, 54-55
  side effects of, 104, 105
DIC: *see* Disseminated intravascular coagulation
Diet
  carbohydrate, for oral glucose tolerance test, 124
  compliance with, in unstable insulin-dependent diabetes during pregnancy, 133
  in management of nephrotic syndrome, 253
  in stable insulin-dependent diabetes, 130
Diethylstilbestrol, 287
  and abnormalities of uterus, 46
Differential count with premature rupture of membranes, 71, 72
Diffusion, facilitated, 121
Digital rotation from occipitoposterior to occipitoanterior position, 327
Digitalis, 185, 186
Digitalis toxicity, 185
Digoxin, 185, 186, 196
Dehydroepiandrosterone sulfate, 94
Dilantin; *see* Phenytoin
Dipalmitoyl lecithin, 40-41
Dipalmitoyl phosphatidylcholine, 40-41
Diphenylhydantoin; *see* Phenytoin
Disease(s)
  cardiac; *see* Cardiac disease; Heart disease
  causing hypertension, 92
  causing preterm labor, 47
  congenital heart, 190-191
    intrauterine growth retardation with, 154
  coronary artery, 197-198
  Ebstein's, 194
  heart; *see* Cardiac disease; Heart disease
  hyaline membrane; *see* Hyaline membrane disease
  hypoxic, symmetric intrauterine growth retardation from, 154-155
  minimal change, 253
  renal, and pregnancy, 246-262

Disease(s)—cont'd
  sickle cell, 237-238
    DNA analysis for diagnosis of, 30
  thromboembolic, 240-244
  TORCH, 200
  vascular; *see* Vascular disease
  von Willebrand's, 240, 362
Disseminated intravascular coagulation, 284, 293-295, 362
Disseminated intravascular coagulation profile, 284
  for abruptio placentae, 294, 296
Distressed newborns
  incidence of, 355
  pathophysiology of, 355-356
  patients at risk and possible preventive measures, 356
  recognition of, 356-357
  treatment of
    circulatory support, 358-359
    metabolic support, 359-360
    thermal support, 359
    ventilatory support, 357-358, 359
Diuretics
  contraindications to, 94, 116
  for hypertension with renal disease, 259, 260
  interference of, with insulin action, 134
  for nephrotic syndrome, 255
  for prerenal failure, 251
DNA analysis, 30
Dobutamine, 355
Dopamine, 355
Down's syndrome; *see also* Mental retardation
  causes of, 23-24
  paternal age as factor in, 23
  recurrence risk of, 24-26
DPL; *see* Dipalmitoyl lecithin
Drugs; *see also* Medications; specific drugs
  causing fetal heart rate variability, 346
  causing neonatal distress, 355
  interfering with insulin action, 134
  interrupting uterine contractions, 360, 361
  for penicillin-sensitive patients with syphilis during pregnancy, 219
  symmetric intrauterine growth retardation from, 154
  used during pregnancy, 9-10
    potential teratogenicity of, 33-34
Drying agents for herpes lesions, 211
Du antigen, 76
Dührssen's incisions, 319
DVT; *see* Deep vein thrombosis
Dysmaturity, 173
Dyspnea, 183

E
Ebstein's disease, 194
Echocardiograms, changes in, during pregnancy, 183-184
Eclampsia, 92; *see also* Preeclampsia-eclampsia
Eclamptic seizures, management of, 101-103
EDC; *see* Estimated date of confinement
Edema, 183; *see also* Pulmonary edema
Eisenmenger's syndrome, 191-192
Electrocardiograms, changes in, during pregnancy, 183-184
Electrolyte imbalance, preeclampsia complicated by, 108-109